Digital Forensics for the Health Sciences:

Applications in Practice and Research

Andriani Daskalaki
Max Planck Institute for Molecular Genetics, Germany

A volume in the Advances in Digital
Crime, Forensics, and Cyber Terrorism
(ADCFCT) Book Series

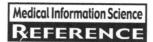

Medical Information Science
REFERENCE

Senior Editorial Director:	Kristin Klinger
Director of Book Publications:	Julia Mosemann
Editorial Director:	Lindsay Johnston
Acquisitions Editor:	Erika Carter
Development Editor:	Joel Gamon
Production Coordinator:	Jamie Snavely
Typesetters:	Keith Glazewski & Natalie Pronio
Cover Design:	Nick Newcomer

Published in the United States of America by
Medical Information Science Reference (an imprint of IGI Global)
701 E. Chocolate Avenue
Hershey PA 17033
Tel: 717-533-8845
Fax: 717-533-8661
E-mail: cust@igi-global.com
Web site: http://www.igi-global.com

Library of Congress Cataloging-in-Publication Data

Digital forensics for the health sciences : applications in practice and research / Andriani Daskalaki, editor.
    p. cm.
  Summary: "This book discusses current applications of digital forensics in health sciences as well as the latest research in this area, with coverage in basic concepts, best practices, common techniques, investigative challenges and, most important-ly, the major limitations of current tools and approaches"-- Provided by publisher.
  Includes bibliographical references and index.
  ISBN 978-1-60960-483-7 (hardcover) -- ISBN 978-1-60960-484-4 (ebook) 1. Radiography, Medical--Digital techniques. 2. Medical jurisprudence--Data processing. I. Daskalaki, Andriani, 1966-
  RC78.7.D35D52 2011
  616.07'572--dc22
                                    2010054472

This book is published in the IGI Global book series Advances in Digital Crime, Forensics, and Cyber Terrorism (ADCF-CT) Book Series (ISSN: 2327-0381; eISSN: 2327-0373)

British Cataloguing in Publication Data
A Cataloguing in Publication record for this book is available from the British Library.

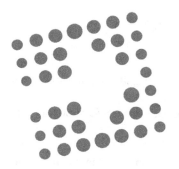

Advances in Digital Crime, Forensics, and Cyber Terrorism (ADCFCT) Book Series

ISSN: 2327-0381
EISSN: 2327-0373

MISSION

The digital revolution has allowed for greater global connectivity and has improved the way we share and present information. With this new ease of communication and access also come many new challenges and threats as cyber crime and digital perpetrators are constantly developing new ways to attack systems and gain access to private information.

The **Advances in Digital Crime, Forensics, and Cyber Terrorism (ADCFCT) Book Series** seeks to publish the latest research in diverse fields pertaining to crime, warfare, terrorism and forensics in the digital sphere. By advancing research available in these fields, the **ADCFCT** aims to present researchers, academicians, and students with the most current available knowledge and assist security and law enforcement professionals with a better understanding of the current tools, applications, and methodologies being implemented and discussed in the field.

COVERAGE

- Computer Virology
- Cryptography
- Cyber Warfare
- Database Forensics
- Digital Crime
- Encryption
- Identity Theft
- Malware
- Telecommunications Fraud
- Watermarking

IGI Global is currently accepting manuscripts for publication within this series. To submit a proposal for a volume in this series, please contact our Acquisition Editors at Acquisitions@igi-global.com or visit: http://www.igi-global.com/publish/.

Titles in this Series

For a list of additional titles in this series, please visit: www.igi-global.com

The Psychology of Cyber Crime Concepts and Principles
Gráinne Kirwan (Dun Laoghaire Institute of Art, Design and Technology, Ireland) and Andrew Power (Dun Laoghaire Institute of Art, Design and Technology, Ireland)
Information Science Reference • copyright 2012 • 372pp • H/C (ISBN: 9781613503508) • US $195.00 (our price)

Cyber Crime and the Victimization of Women Laws, Rights and Regulations
Debarati Halder (Centre for Cyber Victim Counselling (CCVC), India) and K. Jaishankar (Manonmaniam Sundaranar University, India)
Information Science Reference • copyright 2012 • 264pp • H/C (ISBN: 9781609608309) • US $195.00 (our price)

Digital Forensics for the Health Sciences Applications in Practice and Research
Andriani Daskalaki (Max Planck Institute for Molecular Genetics, Germany)
Medical Information Science Reference • copyright 2011 • 418pp • H/C (ISBN: 9781609604837) • US $245.00 (our price)

Cyber Security, Cyber Crime and Cyber Forensics Applications and Perspectives
Raghu Santanam (Arizona State University, USA) M. Sethumadhavan (Amrita University, India) and Mohit Virendra (Brocade Communications Systems, USA)
Information Science Reference • copyright 2011 • 296pp • H/C (ISBN: 9781609601232) • US $180.00 (our price)

Handbook of Research on Computational Forensics, Digital Crime, and Investigation Methods and Solutions
Chang-Tsun Li (University of Warwick, UK)
Information Science Reference • copyright 2010 • 620pp • H/C (ISBN: 9781605668369) • US $295.00 (our price)

Homeland Security Preparedness and Information Systems Strategies for Managing Public Policy
Christopher G. Reddick (University of Texas at San Antonio, USA)
Information Science Reference • copyright 2010 • 274pp • H/C (ISBN: 9781605668345) • US $180.00 (our price)

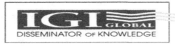
DISSEMINATOR OF KNOWLEDGE

www.igi-global.com

701 E. Chocolate Ave., Hershey, PA 17033
Order online at www.igi-global.com or call 717-533-8845 x100
To place a standing order for titles released in this series, contact: cust@igi-global.com
Mon-Fri 8:00 am - 5:00 pm (est) or fax 24 hours a day 717-533-8661

Editorial Advisory Board

Table of Contents

Foreword xvi

Preface xviii

Acknowledgment xx

Section 1
Digital Forensics Best Practices in Medicine

Chapter 1

Forensic Anthropology: Current Tools, Future Concepts 1

    Douglas H. Ubelaker, Smithsonian Institution, USA

    Julia A. Grossman, Smithsonian Institution, USA

Chapter 2

Laser Scanning Confocal Imaging of Forensic Samples and Their 3D Visualization 13

    Anya Salih, University Western Sydney, Australia

Chapter 3

Data Hiding in Digitized Medical Images: From Concepts to Applications 29

    Mehul S. Raval, Dhirubhai Ambani Institute of Information and Communication

      Technology, India

Chapter 4

Vertebral Morphometry in Forensics 48

    Giuseppe Guglielmi, University of Foggia, Italy & Scientific Institute Hospital, Italy

    Stefano D'Errico, University of Foggia, Italy

    Cristoforo Pomara, University of Foggia, Italy

    Vittorio Fineschi, University of Foggia, Italy

Chapter 5
Facial Reconstruction as a Regression Problem 68
   Maxime Berar, Université de Rouen, France
   Françoise Tilotta, Université Paris Descartes, France
   Joan A. Glaunès, Université Paris Descartes, France
   Yves Rozenholc, Université Paris Descartes, France
   Michel Desvignes, GIPSA-LAB, France
   Marek Bucki, Laboratoire TIMC-IMAG, France
   Yohan Payan, Laboratoire TIMC-IMAG, France

Section 2
Basic Research: A Bridge to Digital Forensics

Chapter 6
Montoring the Transcriptome 89
   Stilianos Arhondakis, Biomedical Research Foundation of the Academy of Athens, Greece
   Georgia Tsiliki, Biomedical Research Foundation of the Academy of Athens, Greece
   Sophia Kossida, Biomedical Research Foundation of the Academy of Athens, Greece

Chapter 7
Resolving Sample Traces in Complex Mixtures with Microarray Analyses 108
   George I. Lambrou, University of Athens, Greece
   Eleftheria Koultouki, University of Athens, Greece
   Maria Adamaki, University of Athens, Greece
   Maria Moschovi, University of Athens, Greece

Chapter 8
Predictive Dynamical Modelling MicroRNAs Role in Complex Networks 156
   Elena V. Nikolova, Bulgarian Academy of Sciences, Bulgaria
   Ralf Herwig, Max Planck Institute for Molecular Genetics, Germany
   Svetoslav G. Nikolov, Bulgarian Academy of Sciences, Bulgaria
   Valko G. Petrov, Bulgarian Academy of Sciences, Bulgaria

Chapter 9
Machine Learning for Clinical Data Processing 193
   Guo-Zheng Li, Tongji University, China

Section 3
Digital Forensics Applications in Dentistry

Chapter 10
Digital Applications in Forensic Odontology 217
 Robert E. Barsley, American Board of Forensic Odontology, Inc.
 David R. Senn, American Board of Forensic Odontology, Inc.
 Thomas J. David, American Board of Forensic Odontology, Inc.
 Franklin D. Wright, American Board of Forensic Odontology, Inc.
 Gregory S. Golden, American Board of Forensic Odontology, Inc.

Chapter 11
Dental Age Assessment (DAA) of Children and Emerging Adults: A Practical Guide 226
 Graham J. Roberts, King's College London Dental Institute, UK
 Aviva Petrie, UCL Eastman Dental Institute, UK

Chapter 12
Automating Human Identification Using Dental X-Ray Radiographs 280
 Omaima Nomir, Univeristy of Mansoura, Egypt
 Mohamed Abdel Mottaleb, University of Miami, USA

Chapter 13
Left-Right Asymmetries and Other Common Anatomical Variants of Temporomandibular
Articular Surfaces 315
 Aldo Scafoglieri, Vrije Universiteit Brussel, Belgium
 Peter Van Roy, Vrije Universiteit Brussel, Belgium
 Steven Provyn, Vrije Universiteit Brussel, Belgium & Haute École Paul Henri Spaak, Belgium
 Jonathan Tresignie, Vrije Universiteit Brussel, Belgium
 Jan Pieter Clarys, Vrije Universiteit Brussel, Belgium

Chapter 14
Forensic Statistics in Health Sciences... 326
 Amit Chattopadhyay, National Institutes of Health, USA

Compilation of References 345

About the Contributors 383

Index.. 393

Detailed Table of Contents

Foreword xvi

Preface xviii

Acknowledgment xx

Section 1
Digital Forensics Best Practices in Medicine

Chapter 1

Forensic Anthropology: Current Tools, Future Concepts 1
Douglas H. Ubelaker, Smithsonian Institution, USA
Julia A. Grossman, Smithsonian Institution, USA

Traditionally, methodology within forensic anthropology has involved very basic techniques of measurement, observation and interpretation. Rooted in the academic fields of anatomy and physical anthropology, forensic anthropology has grown to address problems of recovery, determination of species, estimation of age at death, sex, ancestry, stature, postmortem interval, and the evaluation of evidence relating to foul play and identification. Growth and expansion of the field into new areas of application have revealed new problems needing new methodological solutions. Striving to resolve these problems, anthropologists have turned to new technology, or approaches utilized in related academic areas that would be new to anthropology. This chapter explores aspects of those technological developments and how they have found a home in the practice of forensic anthropology.

Chapter 2

Laser Scanning Confocal Imaging of Forensic Samples and Their 3D Visualization 13
Anya Salih, University Western Sydney, Australia

In the last three decades, confocal microscopy has become a widely used technique in the fields of biological and medical sciences. Gradually, its use is becoming more widespread in forensic sciences as it offers numerous advantages over conventional wide-field microscopy. This chapter describes the application of confocal imaging in fluorescence and reflection modes and the analysis of the three-dimensional (3D) data sets of samples relevant to forensic medical investigations and cover practical applications of a powerful 3D visualization and analyses software. Furthermore, this chapter discusses several examples of confocal imaging for medical forensic applications, including the 3D analysis of finger prints, hair, skin abrasions and grass pollen exine morphology to provide new diagnostic and prognostic information.

Chapter 3
Data Hiding in Digitized Medical Images: From Concepts to Applications 29
    *Mehul S. Raval, Dhirubhai Ambani Institute of Information and Communication
        Technology, India*

This chapter envelopd data hiding techniques applied to medical images for improving their security and culminates with study of algorithms for reversible watermarking techniques and discussion on future of watermarking in medical domain. The chapter covers types of medical images, their security requirements and type of threats to them providing a sufficient background and reasoning for applying data hiding techniques to the medical images. Furthermore, the purpose of this chapter is to study requirements of data hiding techniques with respect to medical imaging and cover state of art methods in this domain. These techniques are developed from different application perspectives and will help to understand their limitations and strengths.

Chapter 4
Vertebral Morphometry in Forensics 48
    Giuseppe Guglielmi, University of Foggia, Italy & Scientific Institute Hospital, Italy
    Stefano D'Errico, University of Foggia, Italy
    Cristoforo Pomara, University of Foggia, Italy
    Vittorio Fineschi, University of Foggia, Italy

Imaging techniques (plain radiographs, multi slice computed tomography (MSCT), and magnetic resonance (MRI)) are being increasingly implemented in forensic pathology. These methods may serve as an adjuvant to classic forensic medical diagnosis and as support to forensic autopsies. It is well noted that various post processing techniques can provide strong forensic evidence for use in legal proceedings. This chapter reviews vertebral morphometry application in forensics, expressly used in the case of semi-automatic digital recognition of vertebral heights in fractures, by means of vertebral shape analysis which relies on six or more points positioned over the margins of each vertebrae T5 to L4 used to calculate anterior, medial, and posterior heights and statistical shape models. This approach is quantitative, more reproducible, and more feasible for large-scale data analysis as in drug trials, where assessment may be performed by a variety of clinicians with different levels of experience. Furthermore, the authors aim to verify by an experimental model if the technique could contribute, in present or in future, to investigate the modality of traumatic vertebral injuries which may explain the manner of death.

Chapter 5

Facial Reconstruction as a Regression Problem 68

    Maxime Berar, Université de Rouen, France
    Françoise Tilotta, Université Paris Descartes, France
    Joan A. Glaunès, Université Paris Descartes, France
    Yves Rozenholc, Université Paris Descartes, France
    Michel Desvignes, GIPSA-LAB, France
    Marek Bucki, Laboratoire TIMC-IMAG, France
    Yohan Payan, Laboratoire TIMC-IMAG, France

The authors in this chapter present a computer-assisted method for facial reconstruction: this method provides an estimation of the facial outlook associated with unidentified skeletal remains. Current computer-assisted methods using a statistical framework rely on a common set of points extracted from the bone and soft-tissue surfaces. Facial reconstruction then attempts to predict the position of the soft-tissue surface points knowing the positions of the bone surface points. The authors propose to use linear latent variable regression methods for the prediction (such as Principal Component Regression or Latent Root Root Regression) and to compare the results obtained to those given by the use of statistical shape models. In conjunction, the authors have evaluated the influence of the number of skull landmarks used. The proposed method is validated in terms of accuracy, based on a leave-one-out cross-validation test applied on a homogeneous database. Accuracy measures are obtained by computing the distance between the reconstruction and the ground truth. Finally, these results are discussed in regard to current computer-assisted facial reconstruction techniques, including deformation based techniques.

Section 2
Basic Research: A Bridge to Digital Forensics

Chapter 6

Montoring the Transcriptome 89

    Stilianos Arhondakis, Biomedical Research Foundation of the Academy of Athens, Greece
    Georgia Tsiliki, Biomedical Research Foundation of the Academy of Athens, Greece
    Sophia Kossida, Biomedical Research Foundation of the Academy of Athens, Greece

The technologies monitoring the transcriptome are under a continuous status of development and implementation, producing high amounts of expression data which require reliable and well structured databases. This chapter provides a general overview and a reliable guide of these technologies, as developed from early 90s' to today, and of the most important available expression databases. The first part aims at introducing the reader to the fundamental functional aspects of these technologies, which are under a continuous development in order to obtain a more accurate description of the transcriptome. The second part offers the necessary information to those who are interested into further exploiting expression data in their research.

Chapter 7
Resolving Sample Traces in Complex Mixtures with Microarray Analyses 108
George I. Lambrou, University of Athens, Greece
Eleftheria Koultouki, University of Athens, Greece
Maria Adamaki, University of Athens, Greece
Maria Moschovi, University of Athens, Greece

High throughput technologies have facilitated the study of thousands of factors simultaneously. A well-known method that has been utilized throughout recent years is microarray technology. Since their advent, microarrays have been used to discover differences between samples, for example, on the level of gene expression or polymorphism detection. This technique has found applications in many areas of life sciences, including forensics. Forensic samples may consist of tissue mixtures that need to be distinguished. In the present work the authors review the microarray technology and deal with the majority of aspects regarding microarrays. The authors focus on today's knowledge of separation techniques and methodologies of complex signal, i.e. samples. Overall, the authors review the current knowledge on the topic of microarrays and present the analyses and techniques used, which facilitate such approaches. The authors provide the theoretical framework on microarray technology and a review of statistical methods used for microarray analyses and of methods used for discriminating traces of nucleic acids within a complex mixture of samples.

Chapter 8
Predictive Dynamical Modelling MicroRNAs Role in Complex Networks 156
Elena V. Nikolova, Bulgarian Academy of Sciences, Bulgaria
Ralf Herwig, Max Planck Institute for Molecular Genetics, Germany
Svetoslav G. Nikolov, Bulgarian Academy of Sciences, Bulgaria
Valko G. Petrov, Bulgarian Academy of Sciences, Bulgaria

The aim of this chapter is to give an extended analytical consideration of a mathematical modelling of the microRNA role in complex networks. For this purpose, the authors widely use ordinary and partial differential equations for synthezing and analyzing the models of gene, microRNAs, and mRNAs concentration alterations as time-dependent variables related by functional and differential relations between them. The architecture of the models and the definitions of its components are inspired by the qualitative theory of differential equations. This chapter shows that it is possible to ensure the authenticity and validity of the following qualitative conclusions: (a) the rates of protein production decrease with the increasing constant production rate of microRNA at microRNA-mediated target regulation on mRNAs; (b) time delay has stabilization role in the interaction between the miRNA-17-92 cluster and the transcription factors E2F and Myc.

Chapter 9
Machine Learning for Clinical Data Processing.. 193
Guo-Zheng Li, Tongji University, China

This chapter introduces great challenges and the novel machine learning techniques employed in clinical data processing. It argues that the novel machine learning techniques including support vector machines, ensemble learning, feature selection, feature reuse by using multi-task learning and multi-label learning provide potentially more substantive solutions for decision support and clinical data analysis. The authors demonstrate the generalization performance of the novel machine learning techniques on real world data sets including one data set of brain glioma, one data set of coronary heart disease in Chinese medicine and some tumor data sets of microarray. More and more machine learning techniques will be developed to improve analysis precision of clinical data sets.

Section 3
Digital Forensics Applications in Dentistry

Chapter 10
Digital Applications in Forensic Odontology 217
    Robert E. Barsley, American Board of Forensic Odontology, Inc.
    David R. Senn, American Board of Forensic Odontology, Inc.
    Thomas J. David, American Board of Forensic Odontology, Inc.
    Franklin D. Wright, American Board of Forensic Odontology, Inc.
    Gregory S. Golden, American Board of Forensic Odontology, Inc.

Forensic Odontology or forensic dentistry is the use of dental expertise, dental findings, and dental facts in legal proceedings. The principal efforts of dentists, in this regard, are geared toward establishing the identity of unknown human remains or verifying the identity of visually unrecognizable human remains. The digital revolution has impacted all aspects of forensic odontology. This chapter discusses the impact on person identification through dental means, dental identification in mass or disaster victim incidents, establishing the age of an unknown individual or human remains through dental examination, digital photography in dentistry and forensic odontology, and the use of digital methods in the analysis and comparison of bite mark evidence.

Chapter 11
Dental Age Assessment (DAA) of Children and Emerging Adults: A Practical Guide 226
    Graham J. Roberts, King's College London Dental Institute, UK
    Aviva Petrie, UCL Eastman Dental Institute, UK

A variety of methods has been used to estimate dental age. Tooth development as a means of estimating age has been used for several centuries. The purpose of the chapter is to describe the method used at the Dental Paediatric Unit of King's College London Dental Institute and the UCL Eastman Dental Institute to carry out Dental Age Assessment (DAA). An important principle is the biological variability of growth of teeth, a factor inappropriately considered in many studies of Dental Age Assessment (DAA). This chapter serves to inform colleagues, lawyers, immigration workers, social workers, and subjects of unknown date of birth of the way in which DAA is conducted.

Chapter 12

Automating Human Identification Using Dental X-Ray Radiographs 280

    Omaima Nomir, Univeristy of Mansoura, Egypt

    Mohamed Abdel Mottaleb, University of Miami, USA

The goal of forensic dentistry is to identify individuals based on their dental characteristics. In this chapter, the authors present a system for automating that process by identifying people from dental X-ray images. Given a dental image of a postmortem (PM), the proposed system retrieves the best matches from an antemortem (AM) database. The system automatically segments dental X-ray images into individual teeth and extracts representative feature vectors for each tooth, which are later used for retrieval. The authors developed a new method for teeth segmentation, and three different methods for representing and matching teeth. Each method has a different technique for representing the tooth shape and has its advantages and disadvantages compared with the other methods. The first method represents each tooth contour by signature vectors obtained at salient points on the contour of the tooth. The second method uses Hierarchical Chamfer distance for matching AM and PM teeth. In the third method, each tooth is described using a feature vector extracted using the force field energy function and Fourier descriptors. During retrieval, according to a matching distance between the AM and PM teeth, AM radiographs that are most similar to a given PM image are found and presented to the user. To increase the accuracy of the identification process, the three matching techniques are fused together. The fusion of information is an integral part of any identification system to improve the overall performance. The authors introduce some scenarios for fusing the three matchers at the score level as well as at the fusion level.

Chapter 13

Left-Right Asymmetries and Other Common Anatomical Variants of Temporomandibular
Articular Surfaces 315

    Aldo Scafoglieri, Vrije Universiteit Brussel, Belgium

    Peter Van Roy, Vrije Universiteit Brussel, Belgium

    Steven Provyn, Vrije Universiteit Brussel, Belgium & Haute École Paul Henri Spaak, Belgium

    Jonathan Tresignie, Vrije Universiteit Brussel, Belgium

    Jan Pieter Clarys, Vrije Universiteit Brussel, Belgium

In this chapter, the authors describe systematically left-right asymmetries and other common anatomical variants of the temporomandibular articular surfaces as they can appear in daily clinical practice. Digital photography and macroscopic observation were used to evaluate morphologic features of TMJ surfaces of elderly subjects at 100 glenoid fossae and articular eminences of dried skull bases, and at 100 dried mandibles. The antero-posterior and medio-lateral diameter of the temporomandibular articular surfaces were measured using a digital caliper. Morphologic left-right asymmetries of the temporomandibular articular surfaces were frequently present in mandibular condyles and in glenoid fossae. In general, mandibular condyles showed more often morphologic left-right asymmetries than glenoid fossae. Anatomical variants of the articular surfaces of the left and right mandibular condyles resulted from differences in shape. An important incidence of left-right asymmetries and other common anatomical variants of the temporomandibular articular joint surfaces must be considered at observation and therapy of the temporomandibular joint; arthrokinematic functional consequences may result.

Chapter 14

Forensic Statistics in Health Sciences.. 326
    Amit Chattopadhyay, National Institutes of Health, USA

This chapter reviews the application of forensic statistical methods related issues such as: methods of deciphering evidence; DNA profile matching; searching a database of DNA profiles; scientific reliability; discrimination in presentation of statistical evidence in legal settings; assumptions in underlying statistical analysis when evidence is presented; precision & accuracy; role of using extreme values in evidence; and decision analysis in forensic science. The emphasis of the chapter is on concepts from statistical application, nature, and use of evidences in every day clinical practice and in the court of law. Another goal of the chapter is to serve as a central reference to access of information about resources related to this topic.

Compilation of References 345

About the Contributors 383

Index.. 393

Foreword

The book, *Digital Forensics for the Health Sciences: Applications in Practice*, should be of great interest to forensic investigators throughout the world. The editor, Dr. Andriani Daskalaki, who works in the field of molecular medicine and bioinformatics at the Max Planck Institute for Molecular Genetics, has gathered experts from across the globe to contribute. From England, Italy, France, India, China, the United States of America, Australia, Greece, Egypt, Belgium, and of course Germany, the contributors write about forensic topics including anthropology, odontology, medical imaging, genetics and the genome, microarray analysis, facial reconstruction, machine learning, and forensic statistics.

The book consists of three sections, the first of which is *Digital Forensics Best Practices in Medicine*. From the Smithsonian Institution comes a discussion of new techniques, technologies, and approaches to anthropology and outlines how some of these have become part of the practice of forensic anthropology. Three-dimensional visualization of forensic samples such as fingerprints, hair, and skin abrasions among others utilizing fluorescent and reflective confocal laser imaging coupled with new software is the focus of Australian contributors. From India, authors discuss the security of medical images such as adding non-visible watermarks to assure authenticity. The digital use of morphometry in forensics is discussed in an Italian contribution. And from France comes a discussion on the use of computer-assisted method for facial reconstruction.

The second section, *Basic Research: A Bridge to Digital Forensics* begins with a discussion of the possible forensic value of the (RNA) transcriptome authored by the first group of contributors from Greece. Other Greek authors discuss the growing importance of microarray analysis in distinguishing forensic samples. From Germany comes a discussion of extended analytical consideration of mathematical modeling the microRNA role in complex networks. Part two concludes with an offering from China discussing the growing role, challenges, and novel machine learning techniques in clinical data sets.

Section three is focused on *Digital Forensics Applications in Dentistry*. The United States submits an article discussing the impact of digital advances on techniques in dental identification, disaster victim identification, and bitemark comparison. The English contribution discusses biologic variability of the growth of teeth in dental age assessment methods. Egyptian contributors present a method for identifying individuals using an automated system to compare postmortem and antemortem dental radiographic images. Right-left asymmetries in the articular surfaces of the temporomandibular joint are investigated by authors from Belgium. The final chapter, also contributed from the USA, reviews the application of statistical methods and the assumptions which underlie statistical analysis in the presentation of evidence at trial.

Too often forensic scientists fail to look beyond their borders in their discipline, their country, or their continent. This book crosses those borders and ties us all together.

Robert E. Barsley
LSUHSC School of Dentistry, USA
July 2010

Robert E. Barsley, *DDS, JD is a 1977 graduate of the LSU School of Dentistry and a 1987 graduate of the Loyola University School of Law in New Orleans. He was admitted to the bar in Louisiana in 1987. He joined the faculty of the LSU School of Dentistry in 1980, advancing to the rank of Professor. He currently serves as Director of Oral Health Resources, Community and Hospital Dentistry. Dr. Barsley became a diplomat of the ABFO in 1985 and is currently the Vice-president. A past-president of the ASFO, he serves as forensic dental consultant for several parishes (counties) in Louisiana. He is a Magistrate Judge for Ponchatoula, Louisiana. He is a fellow of the American College of Dentists, the International College of Dentists, and the Odontology Section of the American Academy of Forensic Sciences and currently serves as Secretary of the AAFS and Treasurer of the Forensic Science Foundation. He has also served as a Robert Wood Johnson Foundation Congressional Health Policy Fellow in the office of Senator John Breaux. The author of numerous articles and chapters on the subject of forensic dentistry, he has lectured to national and international audiences concerning forensic dentistry. One of the lead dentists in the identification process resulting from Hurricane Katrina in 2005, he has confirmed the identity of hundreds of other bodies, has analyzed numerous bite mark cases, and testifies in court on a regular basis.*

Preface

Digital forensics deals with the acquisition, preservation, analysis and presentation of electronic data. The detailed documentation and analysis of human data with 3D-imaging and processing techniques has led to qualitative improvements in forensic pathologic investigation and documentation.

In the human genome are a considerable number of genetic variations. Modern DNA techniques apply powerful tools that enable the precise identification. Bioinformatics methods are applied to the analysis of large-scale gene expression data from high-throughput technologies like microarrays. These technologies provide information for thousands of genes in parallel and produce huge amount of data. Data-analysis tools are developed for processing and data mining of this data, and provide insights into complex biological and medical forensic questions.

OBJECTIVE OF THE BOOK

This book provides current applications of digital forensics in health sciences as well as the latest research in this area. The book covers basic concepts, best practices, common techniques, investigative challenges in research. Most important, it also examines the major limitations of current tools and discusses approaches that may help investigators to deal with the ever-increasing size and complexity of forensics targets. These approaches cover a wide spectrum, from imaged-based authentication to high-throughput technologies for forensic analysis.

The target audience of this book will be composed of professionals and researchers working in the field of digital forensics as well as in health sciences.

ORGANIZATION OF THE BOOK

The book is divided into 3 sections:

Section 1, *Digital Forensics: Best Practices in Medicine* introduces the basic concepts in the use of computational tools in medical forensics. Chapter 1 is an introductory chapter presenting the current tools and future concepts in forensic anthropology. Chapter 2 is focused on the application of laser scanning confocal imaging in forensics. The emphasis of Chapter 3 is on strength and limitations of data hiding techniques applied in medical images. Chapter 4 describes the use of the vertebral morphometry approach in Forensics, and Chapter 5 presents a computed-assisted method in facial reconstruction.

Section 2, *Basic Research: A Bridge to Digital Forensics* serves as a comprehensive introduction to computational methods supporting basic research. Chapter 6 provides a general overview on technologies applied to analyse gene expression data. Chapter 7 describes methods used for discrimitation traces of nucleic acids within a complex mixture of samples. Chapter 8 gives an extended analytical consideration of mathematical modelling in complex networks and Chapter 9 introduces the novel machine learning techniques applied in clinical data processing.

Section 3, *Digital Forensics Applications in Dentistry* includes five chapters. Chapter 10 describes the use of digital photography in dentistry and forensic odontology, and the use of digital methods in the analysis and comparison of bite mark evidence. Chapter 11 presents a guide for dental age assessment in children and emerging adults. Chapter 12 presents a system for automating identification of people from dental X-ray images. Chapter 13 describes common anatomical variants of the temporomandibular articular surfaces in daily clinical practice. Chapter 14 reviews the application of statistical methods in forensics.

The book *Digital Forensics for the Health Sciences: Applications in Practice* contains text information, but also a glossary of terms and definitions, contributions from international experts, in-depth analysis of issues, concepts, new trends, and advanced technologies in digital forensics. This edition focuses more directly and extensively than ever on applications of digital forensics in medicine.
Because of the diverse and comprehensive coverage of multiple disciplines in the field of medical digital forensics in this book, this book will contribute to a better understanding for current applications, research, and discoveries in this evolving, significant field.

In shaping this book, I committed myself to making the textbook as useful as possible to forensics specialists, clinicians, as well as advanced researchers coping with the demands of modern medical research.

I hope this book will be a helpful tool, not only for the medical doctor who needs an expert source of basic knowledge in digital forensics, but also for the computer scientist and biologist who need clear, concise, and balanced information on which to conduct their research.

Thanks to a very hard-working advisory editorial board of scientists, excellent authors who fulfilled our invitations, and a very efficient publisher providing clear procedures and practices for a quality production, readers may now enjoy chapters on some of the major ideas that have concerned digital forensics and its applications in health sciences.

Andriani Daskalaki
Max Planck Institute for Molecular Genetics, Germany

REFERENCES

Pollitt, Mark & Shenoi, Sujeet (2006). *Advances in Digital Forensics*. 1. Auflage, Springer-Verlag.

Acknowledgment

The editor sincerely acknowledges the help of all persons involved in the collation and review process of this book, without whose support the project would not have been satisfactorily completed. Deep appreciation and gratitude is due to Prof. Dr. Hans Lehrach, Director of the Department of Vertebrate Genomics (Max Planck Institute for Molecular Genetics) for giving me the opportunity to work in his department.

I wish to express my appreciation to my colleague Dr. Christoph Wierling, who has helped me with constructive criticism and helpful suggestions.

Special thanks also go to the publishing team at IGI Global, whose contributions throughout the whole process from inception of the initial idea to final publication have been invaluable. In particular to Joel Gamon, who continuously prodded via e-mail for keeping the project on schedule.

I would also like to thank my father, Dimitirios Daskalakis, for his unfailing support and encouragement during the months it took to give birth to this book.

In closing, I wish to thank all of the authors for their insights and excellent contributions to this book.

Andriani Daskalaki, PhD
Max Planck Institute for Molecular Genetics, Germany
June 2010

Section 1
Digital Forensics Best Practices in Medicine

Chapter 1
Forensic Anthropology:
Current Tools, Future Concepts

Douglas H. Ubelaker
Smithsonian Institution, USA

Julia A. Grossman
Smithsonian Institution, USA

ABSTRACT

Traditionally, methodology within forensic anthropology has involved very basic techniques of measurement, observation and interpretation. Rooted in the academic fields of anatomy and physical anthropology, forensic anthropology has grown to address problems of recovery, determination of species, estimation of age at death, sex, ancestry, stature, postmortem interval, and the evaluation of evidence relating to foul play and identification. Growth and expansion of the field into new areas of application have revealed new problems needing new methodological solutions. Striving to resolve these problems, anthropologists have turned to new technology, or approaches utilized in related academic areas that would be new to anthropology. This chapter explores aspects of those technological developments and how they have found a home in the practice of forensic anthropology.

GROUND PENETRATING RADAR (GPR)

In some recovery situations involving suspected buried human remains, GPR has emerged as a useful approach (Conyers, 2004; Conyers & Goodman, 1997; Vaughan, 1986). Basically, this technology employs an electromagnetic pulse directed into the ground. Measurement reveals information about the density of subsurface features and more important, details about variation in density. The technique is most effective in locating buried remains and the pit originally dug for the burial of those remains. The effectiveness of this approach rests on the principle that once a pit is dug to bury remains and the soil is placed back

DOI: 10.4018/978-1-60960-483-7.ch001

within it, the compactness of the replacement soil will differ from that of the soil in surrounding undisturbed areas. Use of GPR may detect this variation in soil compaction and thus reveal the location of the burial.

The effectiveness and utility of GPR depends upon the local environmental context and circumstances of burial (Holland & Connell, 2009; Ubelaker, 1999). The approach is most effective in homogeneous soils with minimal evidence of disturbance other than the burial itself. Use of GPR involves systematic survey of the targeted area, usually employing a grid system. Survey results then are carefully examined to detect variants of the apparent normal pattern. These variants then can be tested using traditional archeological approaches to discover the likely source of the variation. Of course, any prior soil disturbance (e.g. animal activity, pipeline excavation, construction activity) will likely be detected and need to be distinguished from a possible burial. The technique is of limited use in an area with a history of abundant soil disturbance.

MAGNETOMETRY

Clues regarding the location of clandestine graves can potentially be gathered using techniques of magnetometry. Effective use of a magnetometer may detect variations in the magnetic orientation of subsurface features (Bevan, 1983; Clark, 1996). The metal detector is a commonly employed device, effective at detecting metal materials buried in soil environments. The extreme differences in magnetic properties between buried metal and the surrounding soil facilitate detection using these instruments.

More sophisticated approaches to magnetometry allow variations in soil patterns of electromagnetic properties to be differentiated. Basically, these approaches will detect not only metal inclusions, but also subsurface variations in the magnetic properties of soil particles. Disturbance of the soil due to grave digging will change the magnetic properties of the disturbed particles. The magnetometer will detect the difference between the disturbed soil and the surrounding undisturbed area. This approach is most useful to detect a clandestine grave within a homogeneous soil environment with minimal disturbance and minimal metal inclusions (Holland & Connell, 2009; Ubelaker, 1999).

Use of magnetometer survey is similar to that described above with GPR. Usually, the survey is conducted within a grid system. The electromagnetic data are then plotted to reveal normal patterns and to detect significant variation. As with GPR, the success of magnetometer survey is very dependent on the local environmental conditions as well as the nature of the burial. Ideal use would involve detection of a recent burial laden with metal artifacts in an environment with no metal inclusions and no history of other soil disturbance. In contrast, if the soil environment tested has a history of abundant soil disturbance with considerable metal at various locations, the burial would be more difficult to detect.

SOIL RESISTIVITY

Another approach to detecting clandestine burials utilizes the technology of the resistivity meter. This device will measure the flow of electricity through the soil and potentially detect variations leading to the discovery of the grave excavation (Bevan, 1996; Clark, 1996). Key to this approach is a thoughtful survey strategy that will quantify normal values of the area and allow variant measurement to be detected (Holland & Connell, 2009). As with GPR and magnetometry approaches, soil resistivity survey works best in areas with minimal soil disturbance.

MICROSCOPY

Various forms of microscopy have become key elements of forensic anthropology methodology. Use of a high-quality dissecting microscope facilitates examination of human remains, especially in the detection of trauma. Although some forms of traumatic alteration and other aspects of morphological variation can be detected with the naked eye, considerably more detail emerges with microscopic examination (Ubelaker & Smialek, 2009). The microscope is especially useful to detect the subtle differences between genuine perimortem trauma and antemortem and postmortem alterations. Microscopic examination will not only allow detection of alterations that would otherwise be overlooked, but also facilitate interpretation (Ubelaker, 1998).

Microscopic examination of sections of bones and teeth can facilitate estimations of age at death (Bouvier & Ubelaker, 1977; Cho et al., 2002; Dudar et al., 1993; Ericksen, 1991; Kerley & Ubelaker, 1978; Stout et al., 1994). Research in this methodology continues, but technological advances involving large monitors, digital photography, and associated software improve objectivity and applications (Crowder, 2009). While such technological improvements are useful, definition and quantification of complex histological structures remain interpretive and require considerable experience.

Use of the microscope also has provided valuable perspective in evaluating if small fragments are of human or non-human origin. In particular, the microscopic detection of patterns of plexiform bone or banding patterns can be diagnostic for non-human status (Mulhern, 2009; Mulhern & Ubelaker, 2001; Mulhern & Ubelaker, 2003). Patterns of microscopic histological structures also can be suggestive of human status, although it is difficult to rule out some non-human animals (Mulhern & Ubelaker, 2003; Mulhern & Ubelaker, 2009).

SCANNING ELECTRON MICROSCOPY/ENERGY DISPERSIVE SPECTROSCOPY (SEM/EDS)

Frequently, forensic anthropologists are presented with fragmentary evidence thought to represent possible human remains. Such evidence is submitted because investigators recognize the potential to utilize DNA analysis for identification, even with fragments. Usually, these fragments are recovered from contexts that produce taphonomic alterations, making identification from morphological evidence alone very difficult. Many materials from the recovery site environment can appear similar to bone or tooth, especially after they have been burned or otherwise altered by taphonomic factors.

A solution to this problem has been found in the technology of scanning electron microscopy/ energy dispersive X-ray spectroscopy (SEM/ EDS). SEM/EDS can be used to document the spectra of recovered samples, which can reveal the proportions of elements present. Then, utilizing a large databank of analyses of known materials, the spectra within the unknown sample can be compared and identified. This technique has proven effective in separating bones and teeth from other materials, even when only very small fragments have been recovered (Ubelaker et al., 2002). Proportions of calcium and phosphorus are particularly important in the definition of bone or tooth fragments. In a survey of many different materials, bone and tooth could be distinguished successfully, even from fragments with similar morphology. Of these other materials, ivory, mineral apatite and some types of corals were most similar, but even these presented significant differences (Ubelaker et al., 2002).

PROTEIN RADIOIMMUNOASSAY (PRIA)

Although SEM/EDS is very effective to distinguish bone and tooth from other materials, it

3

will not reveal if remains are of human or non-human origin. A useful technique in this regard is protein radioimmunoassay (pRIA). Using very small quantities of sample, this technique will distinguish human from non-human, and will also determine the non-human animal present if necessary (Lowenstein et al., 2006; Reuther et al., 2006; Ubelaker et al., 2004).

Although this technique is relatively new in forensic applications, it can be traced back to studies by Lowenstein (1980) indicating that proteins such as collagen and albumin are preserved in ancient material, even in fossils. In a recent modification of this general approach aimed specifically at forensic materials, protein is extracted from the unknown forensic material and subsequently exposed to species-specific antisera raised in rabbits. This resulted in binding to the wells of the testing plate; the greatest binding occurring with the antibody that had the closest specificity to the antigen.

In the second phase of this technique, the bindings of the previous phase were exposed to an antibody to rabbit raised in donkeys which was marked with radioactive iodine-125. The greatest binding of this phase of the procedure occurs in the plate wells with the greatest amount of rabbit gamma globulin already bound after phase one. The radioactivity of the wells after phase two of the procedure can then be measured to determine the greatest quantity of bound material and thus the species.

Applications of this procedure to forensic materials have demonstrated great success in distinguishing human from non-human, even with degraded and ancient materials (Ubelaker et al., 2004). Novel applications include detection of protein residues on artifacts (Reuther et al., 2006; Lowenstein et al., 2006).

DNA

Molecular approaches have revolutionized forensic science identification and have impacted forensic anthropology along the way. Analysis and sampling procedures are in place to acquire the necessary anthropological information prior to the destructive DNA analysis. Coupled with anthropological information about the individual, DNA analysis strengthens the probability of positive identification (Ubelaker et al., 2009). Molecular approaches are also available to determine the sex of an individual when necessary and offer an alternative to pRIA in determining species (Baker, 2009). Combined anthropological and molecular research has clarified factors involved in DNA preservation (Misner et al., 2009).

The impact of recent developments in DNA technology on the practice of forensic anthropology is complex. To be sure, with DNA approaches to identification now available and increasingly routine, the need for some anthropological approaches to identification has been diminished. A primary example is photographic superimposition. Just a few years ago, photographic superimposition was frequently called upon to assist identification efforts when human remains were found including the skull and an antemortem photograph was available of a missing person thought perhaps to be represented by the remains. Today, if antemortem photographs are available, it is very likely DNA samples are also available. Since DNA analysis would likely result in a greater probability of identification, it would be the preferred method.

Overall however, the impact of DNA technology has proved to be very positive for forensic anthropology. Prior to obtaining comparative DNA samples, techniques of forensic anthropology are vitally needed to narrow the search for missing persons and to elucidate the characteristics of the person represented by the recovered remains. In some cases, if positive identification can be made easily from radiographic comparisons, the need for DNA analysis can be diminished or eliminated. Even with DNA identification, anthropological analysis can be useful to corroborate the results and help refine the probabilities involved.

DNA analysis has proven to be useful in special circumstances requiring accurate sex determination. Of course, if a skeleton is complete and the pelvis is intact, standard anthropological analysis is the method of choice to estimate the sex of the individual (Braz, 2009). However, some cases may involve fragmentary remains, skeletons lacking information from the pelvis or immature individuals for which sex cannot be estimated with great reliability. In such cases, if it is very important to determine the sex of the individual, then DNA approaches may be called for. The favored molecular approach to sex estimation involves analysis of the amelogenin gene (Baker, 2009). Errors using this technique are still possible, especially when working with degraded specimens, but generally fall within the range of .02 percent and 1.85 percent (Baker, 2009; Chang et al., 2003; Kashyap et al., 2006; Michael & Brauner, 2004; Steinlechner et al., 2002; Thangaraj et al., 2002).

One reason that forensic anthropological techniques remain important regarding identification issues is that it is difficult to predict from conditions of bone or tooth the quality and quantity of DNA recovery (Boles et al., 1995; Gill, 2006; Gotherstrom et al., 2002; Hagelberg et al., 1991; Holland et al., 2003; Holland & Parsons, 1999; Just et al., 2004; Kaestle & Horsburgh, 2002; O'Rourke et al., 2000; Parsons & Weedn, 1997; Primorac et al., 1996). Misner et al. (2009) reports that of the variables worthy of consideration in selecting samples for DNA analysis, bone type is paramount. Selection by bone type yielded superior results regardless of the extent of weathering and deterioration.

RADIOCARBON ANALYSIS

Although radiocarbon analysis has been utilized for decades to generate dates of archeological samples, only recently have its applications in forensic contexts been realized. Beginning in the 1950's, atmospheric testing of thermonuclear devices generated into the atmosphere large quantities of artificial radiocarbon. Through the food chain, this radiocarbon became incorporated into the tissues of all living organisms. The amount of atmospheric radiocarbon increased steadily until the 1960's when international test ban treaties were put in place. Levels have decreased steadily since, but remain above those prior to the early 1950's.

If radiocarbon analysis of tissues from a forensic case reveals elevated levels, the analyst knows that the individual represented was alive during the modern bomb-curve period (Ubelaker, 2001). Analysis of specific tissues that form and remodel in different ways can reveal relevant information to the estimation of the birth date and the death date (Ubelaker & Buchholz, 2006; Ubelaker et al., 2006).

Dental enamel forms while teeth are developing prior to age 20. Unlike bone, dental enamel does not remodel. Thus, the enamel in the teeth of adults represents the same tissue formed early in life and retains the radiocarbon values at the time of formation. Since the timing of dental formation is well known, values of radiocarbon in dental enamel can be used to estimate the approximate year of birth if the radiocarbon values fall within the bomb-curve. For example, if radiocarbon analysis of enamel from a tooth produced radiocarbon values that suggest formation at the apex of the bomb-curve in about 1963, the age of formation of that enamel can be subtracted from 1963 to estimate the approximate year of birth.

Bone does remodel, but in varying ways. The dense cortical bone found in diaphyses of long bones exhibits relatively slow turnover. In contrast, trabecular bone associated with red marrow has a relatively faster rate of turnover. Thus, radiocarbon values from trabecular bone will be closer to atmospheric values at the death date than will those derived from cortical bone. Within a single skeleton, radiocarbon analysis of dental enamel, cortical bone and trabecular bone from selected anatomical areas will facilitate interpretation of both the birth dates and the death dates. Age at death represents a factor, since with increasing age, bone turnover appears to slow and some recycling of previously incorporated radiocarbon likely occurs (Ubelaker & Buchholz, 2006; Ubelaker et al., 2006).

DATABASES AND STATISTICAL ANALYSIS

During the computer era, major advances have been made in forensic anthropology through rigorous statistical analyses of new databases. Technological advancements have made it possible to assemble very large databases that provide a realistic sense of human variation, error and accuracy of methods derived from them. These approaches have impacted most areas of forensic anthropology, but especially those leading to the biological profile of the individual represented by recovered remains. Large databases enable sampling problems and issues to be overcome. They facilitate rigorous statistical analysis enabling powerful discriminant functions and other tools to be generated. By incorporating diverse samples, they provide a realistic view of human variation in the variables examined.

Specific studies that have benefited from these developments are too numerous to mention. Some highlights include the custom discriminant function program FORDISC (Ousley & Jantz, 1996) greatly facilitating estimates of sex, stature and ancestry. Techniques of 3D geometric morphometrics have emerged which have enabled more sophisticated approaches to morphological assessment, especially for sex and ancestry estimation (Rosas & Bastir, 2002; Ross et al., 1999; Ross & Ubelaker, 2009). Bayesian statistics have opened new doors to estimation of stature and age at death (Konigsberg et al., 1998; Konigsberg et al., 2006). Mathematical approaches and quantification have improved identification methods by elucidating their accuracy (Boldsen et al., 2002; Christensen, 2004; del Angel & Cisneros, 2004;

Hoppa & Vaupel, 2002). Tests of intraobserver and interobserver error have clarified the quality of applications (Baccino et al., 1999). Techniques of computerized tomography, 3D imagery and magnetic resonance imaging show great promise for anthropological applications and already have impacted key areas (Meyers et al., 1999; Ross & Kimmerle, 2009).

Future applications likely will involve virtual collections. Traditionally researchers have sought out documented collections of human remains such as the Terry collection at the Smithsonian Institution in Washington, D.C. and the Todd collection in Cleveland, Ohio. As documented collections continue to grow in a variety of worldwide locations, access remains challenging due to restrictions of travel, time and resources. This situation is ripe for projects to develop virtual electronic access through websites by using currently available technology including 3D, CT scan and MRI (Kullmer, 2008). Coupled with archived information on measurements, observations, and collection history, these possible approaches could represent tremendous assets to those conducting research in forensic anthropology.

Electronic databases are not new to the general field of anthropology. The Centre for Social Anthropology and Computing (http://lucy.kent.ac.uk) has been archiving results of ethnographic fieldwork and posting shared research sources on the web since the late 1980s (Elton & Cardini, 2008). Data sets regarding cultural variation amongst humans can be found in The Human Relations Area Files (http://www.yale.edu/hraf/index.html) (Elton & Cardini, 2008).

Within the field of skeletal biology, an excellent example of electronic web-based collection access is provided by FOROST (www.forost.org). FOROST represents a free-access visual metabase of images of skeletal alterations, especially those of traumatic origin. A virtual link is provided to images and collections of specimens relating to forensic anthropology. The availability of such electronic access to collections (Delson et al., 2007) could represent a tremendous boon to research worldwide and accelerate the pace of improvement in methodology of forensic anthropology.

CRANIOFACIAL IMAGING

In the forensic context, applications of craniofacial imaging are concentrated in two areas: facial approximation and photographic superimposition (Ubelaker, 2009). The former represents the attempt to estimate the facial appearance of an individual from features of a recovered skull (Ubelaker, 2007b). The latter technique is employed to compare a photograph taken during life of a missing person with the image of a recovered skull (Ubelaker, 2007a). Both of these areas of applications of craniofacial imaging have benefited substantially from technological advances in recent years.

Traditionally, facial approximation has focused on facial proportions and unusual landmarks rooted in bones and teeth. The placement of tissue depth markers on the skull serves to guide the approximation of the outer contours of soft tissue. The actual approximation technique varies and can include full scale three-dimensional sculpting, composite drawing, computerized approaches or various combinations of these. While traditional approaches remain popular today, new research has focused extensively on computerized methods, especially those incorporating large databases to objectively project facial features (Evison & Vorder Bruegge, 2009).

Superimposition techniques basically provide a method to compare two objects and evaluate the extent of their similarities and differences. While these techniques can be employed using any two objects, they primarily are utilized to compare a recovered skull with an antemortem photograph. While the use of this technique has declined in frequency in recent years due to increased reliance on molecular analysis, technology has improved its

quality. Current computerized techniques enable sophisticated superimposition with comparison of select areas. Potentially, large computerized databases of facial images could lead to greater quantification of this approach with enhanced understanding of the accuracy of application.

While both of these areas of application remain strongly interpretive, technological advances have improved applications. In particular, data from computerized tomography and ultrasound studies have enabled large, sophisticated database construction (Clement & Ranson, 1998; De Greef et al., 2006; Manhein et al., 2000; Stephan, 2009; Vandermeulen et al., 2006; Wilkinson, 2004).

SUMMARY

The above discussion focuses on ten areas of technological development within forensic anthropology that have significantly impacted applications. There are more. With today's increased scrutiny on accuracy within forensic science, interest is elevated in whatever new approaches can augment the science. Forensic anthropology has been at the forefront of many of these developments. Clearly the welcome mat is out for enhanced technological advancement within forensic anthropology; many areas of application stand poised to benefit from innovative, enhanced methodology.

REFERENCES

Baccino, E., Ubelaker, D. H., Hayek, L. C., & Zerilli, A. (1999). Evaluation of seven methods of estimating age at death from mature human skeletal remains. *Journal of Forensic Sciences, 44*(5), 931–936.

Baker, L. (2009). Biomolecular applications. In Blau, S., & Ubelaker, D. H. (Eds.), *Handbook of forensic anthropology and archaeology* (pp. 322–334). Walnut Creek, CA: Left Coast Press, Inc.

Bevan, B. (1996). Geophysical exploration of the U. S. national parks. *Northeast Historical Archaeology*, *25*, 69–84.

Bevan, B. W. (1983). Electromagnetics for mapping buried earth features. *Journal of Field Archaeology*, *10*(1), 47–54. doi:10.2307/529747

Boldsen, J. L., Milner, G. R., Konigsberg, L. W., & Wood, J. W. (2002). Transition analysis: A new method for estimating age from skeletons. In Hoppa, R. D., & Vaupel, J. W. (Eds.), *Paleodemography: Age distributions from skeletal samples* (pp. 73–106). Cambridge, UK: Cambridge University Press.

Boles, T. C., Snow, C. C., & Stover, E. (1995). Forensic DNA testing on skeletal remains from mass graves: A pilot project in Guatemala. *Journal of Forensic Sciences*, *40*(3), 349–355.

Bouvier, M., & Ubelaker, D. H. (1977). A comparison of two methods for the microscopic determination of age at death. *American Journal of Physical Anthropology*, *46*(3), 391–394. doi:10.1002/ajpa.1330460303

Braz, V. S. (2009). Anthropological estimation of sex. In Blau, S., & Ubelaker, D. H. (Eds.), *Handbook of forensic anthropology and archaeology* (pp. 201–207). Walnut Creek, CA: Left Coast Press, Inc.

Chang, Y. M., Burgoyne, L. A., & Both, K. (2003). Higher failures of amelogenin sex test in an Indian population group. *Journal of Forensic Sciences*, *48*(6), 1309–1313.

Cho, H., Stout, S. D., Madsen, R. W., & Streeter, M. A. (2002). Population specific histological age-estimating method: A model for known African-American and European-American skeletal remains. *Journal of Forensic Sciences*, *47*(1), 12–18.

Christensen, A. M. (2004). The impact of Daubert: Implications for testimony and research in forensic anthropology (and the use of frontal sinuses in personal identification). *Journal of Forensic Sciences*, *49*(3), 427–430. doi:10.1520/JFS2003185

Clark, A. (1996). *Seeing beneath the soil: Preparing methods in archaeology* (2nd ed.). London: B.T. Batsford.

Clement, J. G., & Ranson, D. L. (1998). *Craniofacial identification in forensic medicine*. London: Arnold.

Conyers, L. B. (2004). *Ground-penetrating radar for archaeology*. Walnut Creek, CA: AltaMira Press.

Conyers, L. B., & Goodman, D. (1997). *Ground-penetrating radar: An introduction for archaeologists*. London: AltaMira Press.

Crowder, C. M. (2009). Histological age estimation. In Blau, S., & Ubelaker, D. H. (Eds.), *Handbook of forensic anthropology and archeology* (pp. 222–235). Walnut Creek, CA: Left Coast Press, Inc.

De Greef, S., Claes, P., Vandermeulen, D., Mollemans, W., Suetens, P., & Willems, G. (2006). Large-scale in-vivo Caucasian facial soft tissue thickness database for craniofacial reconstruction. *Forensic Science International*, *159S*, S126–S146. doi:10.1016/j.forsciint.2006.02.034

del Angel, A., & Cisneros, H. B. (2004). Technical note: Modification of regression equations used to estimate stature in Mesoamerican skeletal remains. *American Journal of Physical Anthropology*, *125*(3), 264–265. doi:10.1002/ajpa.10385

Delson, E., Harcourt-Smith, W. E. H., Frost, S. R., & Norris, C. A. (2007). Databases, data access, and data sharing in paleoanthropology: First steps. *Evolutionary Anthropology: Issues. News Review (Melbourne)*, *16*(5), 161–163.

Dudar, J. C., Pfeiffer, S., & Saunders, S. R. (1993). Evaluation of morphological and histological adult skeletal age-at-death estimation techniques using ribs. *Journal of Forensic Sciences*, *38*(3), 677–685.

Elton, S., & Cardini, A. (2008). Anthropology from the desk? The challenges of the emerging era of data sharing. *Journal of Anthropological Sciences, 86*, 209–212.

Ericksen, M. F. (1991). Histologic estimation of age at death using the anterior cortex of the femur. *American Journal of Physical Anthropology, 84*(2), 171–179.

Evison, M. P., & Vorder Bruegge, R. W. (2009). *Computer-aided forensic facial comparison.* Boca Raton, FL: CRC Press.

Forensic Osteology. (2010). *Home page information.* Retrieved from http://www.forost.org

Gill, J. R. (2006). 9/11 and the New York City Office of Chief Medical Examiner. *Forensic Science, Medicine, and Pathology, 2*(1), 29–32. doi:10.1385/FSMP:2:1:29

Götherström, A., Collins, M.J., & Angerbjörn, A. & Lidén, K. (2002). Bone preservation and DNA amplification. *Archaeometry, 44*(3), 395–404. doi:10.1111/1475-4754.00072

Hagelberg, E., Gray, I. C., & Jeffreys, A. J. (1991). Identification of the skeletal remains of a murder victim by DNA analysis. *Nature, 352*, 427–429. doi:10.1038/352427a0

Holland, M. M., Cave, C. A., Holland, C. A., & Bille, T. W. (2003). Development of a quality, high throughput DNA analysis procedure for skeletal samples to assist with the identification of victims from the World Trade Center attacks. *Croatian Medical Journal, 44*(3), 264–272.

Holland, M. M., & Parsons, T. J. (1999). Mitochondrial DNA sequence analysis–validation and use for forensic casework. *Forensic Science Review, 11*, 21–50.

Holland, T. D., & Connell, S. V. (2009). The search for and detection of human remains. In Blau, S., & Ubelaker, D. H. (Eds.), *Handbook of anthropology and archaeology* (pp. 129–140). Walnut Creek, CA: Left Coast Press, Inc.

Hoppa, R. D., & Vaupel, J. W. (Eds.). (2002). *Paleodemography: Age distributions from skeletal samples.* Cambridge, UK: Cambridge University Press. doi:10.1017/CBO9780511542428

Just, R. S., Irwin, J. A., O'Callaghan, J. E., Saunier, J. L., Coble, M. D., & Vallone, P. M. (2004). Toward increased utility of mtDNA in forensic identifications. *Forensic Science International, 146*(Suppl.), S147–S149. doi:10.1016/j.forsciint.2004.09.045

Kaestle, F. A., & Horsburgh, K. A. (2002). Ancient DNA in anthropology: Methods, applications, and ethics. *American Journal of Physical Anthropology, 119*(S35), 92–130. doi:10.1002/ajpa.10179

Kashyap, V. K., Sahoo, S., Sitalaximi, T., & Trivedi, R. (2006). Deletions in the Y-derived amelogenin gene fragment in the Indian population. *BMC Medical Genetics, 7*, 37. doi:10.1186/1471-2350-7-37

Kerley, E. R., & Ubelaker, D. H. (1978). Revisions in the microscopic method of estimating age at death in human cortical bone. *American Journal of Physical Anthropology, 49*(4), 545–546. doi:10.1002/ajpa.1330490414

Konigsberg, L. W., Hens, S. M., Jantz, L. M., & Jungers, W. L. (1998). Stature estimation and calibration: Bayesian and maximum likelihood perspectives in physical anthropology. *Yearbook of Physical Anthropology, 41*, 65–92. doi:10.1002/(SICI)1096-8644(1998)107:27+<65::AID-AJPA4>3.0.CO;2-6

Konigsberg, L. W., Ross, A. H., & Jungers, W. L. (2006). Estimation and evidence in forensic anthropology: Determining stature. In Schmitt, A., Cunha, E., & Pinheiro, J. (Eds.), *Forensic anthropology and forensic medicine: Complimentary sciences from recovery to cause of death* (pp. 317–331). Totowa, NJ: Humana Press, Inc.

Kullmer, O. (2008). Benefits and risks in virtual anthropology. *Journal of Anthropological Sciences, 86,* 205–207.

Lowenstein, J. M. (1980). Species-specific proteins in fossils. *Naturwissenschaften, 67*(7), 343–346. doi:10.1007/BF01106588

Lowenstein, J. M., Reuther, J. D., Hood, D. G., Scheuenstuhl, G., Gerlach, S. C., & Ubelaker, D. H. (2006). Identification of animal species by protein radioimmunoassay of bone fragments and bloodstained stone tools. *Forensic Science International, 159*(2), 182–188. doi:10.1016/j.forsciint.2005.08.007

Manhein, M. H., Listi, G. A., Barsley, R. E., Musselman, R., Barrow, N. E., & Ubelaker, D. H. (2000). In vivo facial tissue depth measurements for children and adults. *Journal of Forensic Sciences, 45*(1), 48–60.

Meyers, J. C., Okoye, M. I., Kiple, D., Kimmerle, E. H., & Reinhard, K. J. (1999). Three-dimensional (3-D) imaging in post-mortem examinations: Elucidation and identification of cranial and facial fractures in victims of homicide utilizing 3-D computerized imaging reconstruction techniques. *International Journal of Legal Medicine, 113*(1), 33–37. doi:10.1007/s004140050275

Michael, A., & Brauner, P. (2004). Erroneous gender identification by the amelogenin sex test. *Journal of Forensic Sciences, 49*(2), 1–2. doi:10.1520/JFS2003223

Misner, L. M., Halvorson, A. C., Dreier, J. L., Ubelaker, D. H., & Foran, D. R. (2009). The correlation between skeletal weathering and DNA quality and quantity. *Journal of Forensic Sciences, 54*(4), 822–828. doi:10.1111/j.1556-4029.2009.01043.x

Mulhern, D. M. (2009). Differentiating human from nonhuman skeletal remains. In Blau, S., & Ubelaker, D. H. (Eds.), *Handbook of forensic anthropology and archaeology* (pp. 153–163). Walnut Creek, CA: Left Coast Press, Inc.

Mulhern, D. M., & Ubelaker, D. H. (2001). Differences in osteon banding between human and nonhuman bone. *Journal of Forensic Sciences, 46*(2), 220–222.

Mulhern, D. M., & Ubelaker, D. H. (2003). Histologic examination of bone development in juvenile chimpanzees. *American Journal of Physical Anthropology, 122*(2), 127–133. doi:10.1002/ajpa.10294

Mulhern, D. M., & Ubelaker, D. H. (2009). Bone microstructure in juvenile chimpanzees. *American Journal of Physical Anthropology, 140*(2), 368–375. doi:10.1002/ajpa.20959

O'Rourke, D. H., Hayes, M. G., & Carlyle, S. W. (2000). Ancient DNA studies in physical anthropology. *Annual Review of Anthropology, 29,* 217–242. doi:10.1146/annurev.anthro.29.1.217

Ousley, S. D., & Jantz, R. L. (1996). *FORDISC 2.0: Personal computer forensic discriminant functions.* Knoxville, TN: University of Tennessee Press.

Parsons, T. J., & Weedn, V. W. (1997). Preservation and recovery of DNA in postmortem specimens and trace samples. In Haglund, W. D., & Sorg, M. H. (Eds.), *Forensic taphonomy: The postmortem fate of human remains* (pp. 109–138). Boca Raton, FL: CRC Press.

Primorac, D., Andelinovic, S., Definis-Gojanovic, M., Drmic, I., Rezic, B., & Baden, M. M. (1996). Identification of war victims from mass graves in Croatia, Bosnia, and Herzegovina by the use of standard forensic methods and DNA typing. *Journal of Forensic Sciences, 41*(5), 891–894.

Reuther, J. D., Lowenstein, J. M., Gerlach, S. C., Hood, D., Scheuenstuhl, G., & Ubelaker, D. H. (2006). The use of an improved pRIA technique in the identification of protein residues. *Journal of Archaeological Science, 33*(4), 531–537. doi:10.1016/j.jas.2005.09.008

Rosas, A., & Bastir, M. (2002). Thin-plate spine analysis of allometry and sexual dimorphism in the human craniofacial complex. *American Journal of Physical Anthropology, 117*(3), 236–245. doi:10.1002/ajpa.10023

Ross, A. H., & Kimmerle, E. H. (2009). Contribution of quantitative methods in forensic anthropology: A new era. In Blau, S., & Ubelaker, D. H. (Eds.), *Handbook of forensic anthropology and archaeology* (pp. 479–489). Walnut Creek, CA: Left Coast Press, Inc.

Ross, A. H., McKeown, A. H., & Konigsburg, L. W. (1999). Allocation of crania to groups via the New Morphometry. *Journal of Forensic Sciences, 44*(3), 584–587.

Ross, A. H., & Ubelaker, D. H. (2009). Effect of intentional cranial modification of craniofacial landmarks: A three-dimensional perspective. *The Journal of Craniofacial Surgery, 20*(6), 2185–2187. doi:10.1097/SCS.0b013e3181bf038c

Steinlechner, M., Berger, B., Niederstätter, H., & Parson, W. (2002). Rare failures in the amelogenin sex test. *International Journal of Legal Medicine, 116*(2), 117–120. doi:10.1007/s00414-001-0264-9

Stephan, C. N. (2009). Craniofacial identification: Techniques of facial approximation and craniofacial superimposition. In Blau, S., & Ubelaker, D. H. (Eds.), *Handbook of forensic anthropology and archaeology* (pp. 304–321). Walnut Creek, CA: Left Coast Press, Inc.

Stout, S. D., Dietze, W. H., Işcan, M. Y., & Loth, S. R. (1994). Estimation of age at death using cortical histomorphometry of the sternal end of the fourth rib. *Journal of Forensic Sciences, 39*(3), 778–784.

Thangaraj, K., Reddy, A. G., & Singh, L. (2002). Is the amelogenin gene reliable for gender identification in forensic casework and prenatal diagnosis? *International Journal of Legal Medicine, 116*(2), 121–123. doi:10.1007/s00414-001-0262-y

Ubelaker, D. H. (1998). The evolving role of the microscope in forensic anthropology. In Reichs, K. J. (Ed.), *Forensic osteology: Advances in the identification of human remains* (2nd ed., pp. 514–532). Springfield, IL: Charles C. Thomas.

Ubelaker, D. H. (1999). *Human skeletal remains: Excavation, analysis, interpretation* (3rd ed.). Washington, DC: Taraxacum.

Ubelaker, D. H. (2001). Artificial radiocarbon as an indicator of recent origin of organic remains in forensic cases. *Journal of Forensic Sciences, 46*(6), 1285–1287.

Ubelaker, D. H. (2007a). Cranial photographic superimposition. In C.H. Wecht (Ed), *Forensic sciences, volume 2.* (pp. 27C-1-27C-41). New York: Matthew Bender and Company.

Ubelaker, D. H. (2007b). Facial reproduction. In C.H. Wecht (Ed.), *Forensic sciences, volume 3.* (pp. 28E-1-28E-70). New York: Matthew Bender and Company.

Ubelaker, D. H. (2009). Approaches to facial reproduction and photographic superimposition. In Steadman, D. W. (Ed.), *Hard rvidence: Case studies in forensic anthropology* (2nd ed., pp. 248–257). Upper Saddle River, NJ: Prentice Hall.

Ubelaker, D.H. & B.A. Buchholz. (2006). Complexities in the use of bomb-curve radiocarbon to determine time since death of human skeletal remains. *Forensic Science Communications, 8,* online journal.

Ubelaker, D. H., Buchholz, B. A., & Stewart, J. E. B. (2006). Analysis of artificial radiocarbon in different skeletal and dental tissue types to evaluate date of death. *Journal of Forensic Sciences, 51*(3), 484–488. doi:10.1111/j.1556-4029.2006.00125.x

Ubelaker, D. H., Jumbelic, M., Wilson, M., & Levinsohn, E. M. (2009). Multidisciplinary approach to human identification in homicide investigation: A case study from New York. In Steadman, D. W. (Ed.), *Hard evidence: Case studies in forensic anthropology* (2nd ed., pp. 29–33). Upper Saddle River, NJ: Prentice Hall.

Ubelaker, D. H., Lowenstein, J. M., & Hood, D. G. (2004). Species identification of small skeletal fragments using protein radioimmunoassay (pRIA). *Proceedings of the American Academy of Forensic Sciences*, *10*, 327–328.

Ubelaker, D. H., & Smialek, J. E. (2009). The interface of forensic anthropology and forensic pathology in trauma interpretation. In Steadman, D. W. (Ed.), *Hard evidence: Case studies in forensic anthropology* (2nd ed., pp. 221–224). Upper Saddle River, NJ: Prentice Hall.

Ubelaker, D. H., Ward, D. C., Braz, V. S., & Stewart, J. (2002). The use of SEM/EDS analysis to distinguish dental and osseus tissue from other materials. *Journal of Forensic Sciences*, *47*(5), 940–943.

Vandermeulen, D., Claes, P., Loeckx, D., De Greef, S., Willems, G., & Suetens, P. (2006). Computerized craniofacial reconstruction using CT-derived implicit surface representations. *Forensic Science International*, *159S*, S164–S174. doi:10.1016/j.forsciint.2006.02.036

Vaughn, C. J. (1986). Ground-penetrating radar survey used in archaeological investigations. *Geophysics*, *51*(3), 595–604. doi:10.1190/1.1442114

Wilkinson, C. (2004). *Forensic facial reconstruction*. Cambridge, UK: Cambridge University Press.

KEY TERMS AND DEFINITIONS

3D Geometric Morphometrics: A measurement technique used to study the form of objects in three dimensions.

Anthropological Analysis: The study of remains using techniques of forensic anthropology.

Bayesian Statistics: An approach for statistical analysis of data.

Craniofacial Imaging: Methodology focusing on the relationship of the facial outward appearance of an individual to the underlying skeletal structure.

CT Scan: A computed tomography (CT) scan is an imaging method using X-rays to produce cross-sectional images of the inside of objects.

DNA Identification: A method of identification of an individual resulting from the comparison of DNA received from human remains with DNA from known individuals.

Forensic Anthropology: The application of knowledge and techniques of anthropology to modern medico-legal problems.

Ground Penetrating Radar: A geophysical method of using radar pulses to provide images of the subsurface of the ground. Used to locate clandestine burials.

Interobserver Error: The human error involved when different individuals attempt to collect the same data from measurements or observations.

Magnetometry: A method employing the use of the magnetic field to provide images of the subsurface of the ground. Used to locate clandestine burials.

MRI: Magnetic Resonance Imaging (MRI) is an imaging method using the magnetic field and radio waves to produce images of the inside of objects.

Tissue Depth Markers: Cylindrical shaped objects equal in length to the estimated depth of soft tissue overlying skeletal structures.

Chapter 2
Laser Scanning Confocal Imaging of Forensic Samples and Their 3D Visualization

Anya Salih
University Western Sydney, Australia

ABSTRACT

This chapter describes the application of confocal imaging in fluorescence and reflection modes and the analysis of the three-dimensional (3D) data sets of samples relevant to forensic medical investigations. In the last three decades, confocal microscopy has become a widely used technique in the fields of biological and medical sciences. Gradually, its use is becoming more widespread in forensic sciences as it offers numerous advantages over conventional wide-field microscopy. One of the key advantages is the generation of sharply focused 3D data stacks of imaged material, without out-of-focus blur. The technique generates digital optical sections from sample surface down to a depth of 100-300 μm from which a multitude of structural, sculptural and optical parameters in 3D and 4D can be obtained and analysed. This chapter discusses several examples of confocal imaging for medical forensic applications, including the 3D analysis of finger prints, hair, skin abrasions and grass pollen exine morphology to provide new diagnostic and prognostic information. The chapter also covers practical applications of a powerful 3D visualization and analyses software.

INTRODUCTION TO CONFOCAL MICROSCOPY TECHNIQUE

Over the past three decades, confocal microscopy has revolutionized biological sciences and has become a common technique in many scientific disciplines as it rapidly overcame the popularity of conventional optical microscopes. Its development involved a timely convergence of a multitude of disciplines – biology, optical physics, computer sciences, chemistry, mathematics, engineering, etc. The result was a dramatic transformation of

DOI: 10.4018/978-1-60960-483-7.ch002

the study of cells and tissues in biological and bio-medical sciences. The pace of the development of confocal imaging in the forensic sciences is accel-erating, although its use is still relatively uncom-mon. It is beginning to be employed in instances when detailed inorganic sample, histological and cellular studies can provide forensic pathologists with the diagnostic techniques that add a wealth of 3D digital data and help in resolving difficult cases. The technique appears to be especially powerful when 3D microstructural information is required or when screening for molecular or pathological abnormalities occurring as a result of injuries or poisoning (Turillazzi et al., 2008).

The superiority of confocal imaging is largely due to the ease of obtaining high-resolution sub-surface images of specimens with minimal prepa-ration, without the need for chemical fixation or embedding. This is achieved by the elimination of image degrading out-of-focus light and by controllable the depth of field. Light detection is limited to a confocal volume within a sample by positioning a pinhole in front of the detector. The pinhole focuses the light emitted or scattered from the specimen before it reaches the detector. A confocal microscope, thus, provides an almost perfectly focused plane (the z-plane) without contribution of out-of-focus light from above or below it, although generally some out-of-focus light is usually detected. Acquiring the best ob-jectives for the system is still important because the degree of z-plane optical resolution depends almost entirely on the aperture of the objective used, called the Numeric Aperture (N.A.). The higher N.A., the less out-of-focus light and the greater the z plane resolution.

A sequence of optical sections (i.e., sequential images) collected at incremental steps perpendicu-lar to the optical axis of a specimen makes up a z-series (Figure 1). The series of steps are driven by a computer-controlled stepping motor that changes the focus by predetermined increments, set up

Figure 1. Confocal imaging of a live cell by opti-cal sectioning (A) and 3D reconstruction of the sections using image analysis software (Imaris, Bitplane). Image by Christopher Hammang

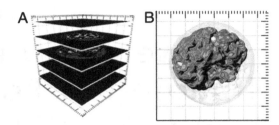

by the microscope operator, that be as low as 0.1 micrometer or 10s of micrometers. The specimen is thus imaged in 3D (xyz) by performing serial optical sections without the need to physically cut through it, providing a non-invasive capabil-ity. The optical sectioning capability of confocal microscopes enables imaging and analysis of cellular, tissue or sample architecture, as well as any pathological alteration, without having to physically cut the specimen and in an environ-ment with minimal alteration to biological reality. Even thick and relatively opaque specimen can be visualized by confocal imaging.

Specimen may also be viewed in a four-di-mensional mode (4D microscopy, xyzt) – a z-series data is collected at time intervals producing a 4-dimensional data set with three spatial dimen-sions (x, y, and z), the time being the fourth di-mension. The 3D and 4D data sets can be viewed as stereo pairs imaged at each time point, can be played back as a movie, or, imaged as xyz 3D reconstructions over a time series or as a 2D montage. Optical slice series through cells or tis-sues and 3D representation contains a great deal more information about the structure, morphol-ogy, sub-cellular location of fluorescence, local-ization of various cellular constituents and their relationship and special distribution (Figure 1 B).

IMAGING MODES

Confocal Fluorescence Imaging

The confocal technique incorporates several different image collection modes. The most widely used technique is the fluorescence mode, so that the specimen needs to be either autofluorescent or it must be stained with a fluorescent stain which can be specific to a particular cellular or tissue part, compartment, organelle or molecule. Hundreds of different stains are now available commercially – see for example, the Molecular Probes (Invitrogen Life Sciences) website (http://www.invitrogen. com/site/us/en/home/brands/Molecular-Probes. html) with 1000s of fluorophores for a variety of applications.

The most basic fluorescence imaging mode is to excite fluorescence by a single laser line and capture emissions by a single detector, generally a photomultiplier tube (PMT). PMTs are used because they are highly sensitive to finite numbers of photons. Fluorophore-specific optical filters, dichroic mirrors or spectral selection is subsequently used to direct the emitted light of a specific waveband into the PMT. In some cases, light is directed to an array of detectors, as is the case for Zeiss META confocal microscope. When several fluorophores are present, a more advanced imaging mode involves using a single laser line and detecting each emission band in different detectors or using excitation of multiple lasers, specific to each fluorophore, and imaging individual emissions in separate detectors.

Multi-Photon Fluorescence Imaging

A second solution involves the use of a laser that can be modified to strike fluorescent dyes with two photons (or more) at once instead of only one. The possibility of two photons striking simultaneously is rare, and it can only occur at the focal plane (as long as the projected laser light fills the back aperture of the objective). These are called two-photon, or multiphoton confocals.

Two-photon imaging does not require a pinhole to obtain optical sections and 3D resolution. Since there is no absorption in out-of-focus emissions from the specimen, more of the excitation light penetrates through the specimen to the plane of focus and this allows for greatly increased specimen penetration. The depth of imaging using multiphoton microscopy is therefore two to three times greater than using confocal microscopy and it is very useful for analyzing tissues and thick samples (Williams et al., 2001).

Transmitted Light Imaging

Another common imaging mode in confocal microscopy is transmission imaging, resulting in specimen image as obtained in conventional transmission light microscopy. This mode is useful when superimposed with images from fluorescence or reflectance modes. Any of the transmitted light imaging modes commonly employed in microscopy can be used in the LSCM, including phase contrast, differential interference contrast (DIC), dark field, or polarized light. A transmitted light detector is used to collect light passing through the specimen, and a fiber optic light guide transmits the signal to one of the photomultiplier tubes in the microscope system's scan head. The transmitted light images and confocal epifluorescence images can be acquired simultaneously using the same illumination beam, ensuring that all of the images are in registration. When the images are combined or merged using image processing software, the precise location of labeled cells within the tissues can be mapped. An informative approach in some studies is to combine a transmitted light, non-confocal image of a specimen with one or more confocal fluorescence images of labeled cells in the same specimen (Figure 2). Use of this approach would allow, for example, determining the spatial and temporal aspects of the migration of a subset of labeled cells within a population of unlabeled cells for a period of hours or even years.

A color transmitted light detector has now been introduced that collects the signal transmitted in the red, green, and blue (RGB) color channels to create a real color image in a way that is similar to some digital color cameras. Such a detector is especially useful to pathologists, who are accustomed to viewing true colors in tissues in transmitted light and overlaying these images with fluorescence data.

Reflectance Confocal Imaging (RCI)

Imaging can also be done in reflectance or backscattering mode creating excellent images of surface and subsurface structures. The advantage of RCI is that the specimen does not need to be autofluorescent or stained. Alternately, specimens can be stained with a reflective probe, such as by immunogold labeling or embedding silver grains. Another advantage of the reflective imaging method is that photobleaching is not a problem. The backscattered light image is often used to determine specimen's surface topography in the materials sciences but is also widely used with biological specimens to investigate the internal cellular structure. Surface and subsurface structures with different refractive indices can be visualized. To collect a backscattered light image the irradiating laser line needs to be scattered from the sample. Specific optical filters and dichroic mirrors are selection so that the irradiating laser

line is directed back up through the scan head to the PMT while the excitation laser light is blocked. Reflectance imaging has been used very successfully in forensic sciences to image specimen or their parts with light scattering properties.

Spectroscopic Confocal Techniques

The exciting development in confocal imaging is the addition of a suite of techniques that can be used to provide analytical information about the sample, in addition to the ready capability to produce excellent structural images. This mode of imaging analysis is only briefly covered in this chapter, as this is an extensive and a growing field that will need far too much space to cover properly

Spectral imaging in xyλ scan mode provides information about the emission spectra of the sample. It is important that an appropriate dichroic beam splitter is selected that will not introduce spectral artifacts by blocking part of the emissions or allowing laser light into the detector. Once λ series are collected, spectral properties of the specimen can be analyzed in define regions of interests (ROIs) in selected areas. Data can be imported into Excel spread-sheet as ASCII text file. Confocal microspectral imaging can reveal the presence of various fluorophores, drugs with unique spectral signatures, contaminants and biochemical alteration of samples. This mode of imaging can provide information regarding the distribution of

Figure 2. Visualization of mitochondrial structure and localisation in an L6 cell by labeling with a fusion construct of coral GFP-type fluorescent protein mt-mEosFP targeting mitochondrial sequence from subunit VIII of cytochrome c oxidase. A. Mitochondria imaged by green fluorescence of EosFP at 488 nm laser excitation. B. Grey-scale image of the whole cell obtained by transmission imaging. C. The two images A and B superimposed

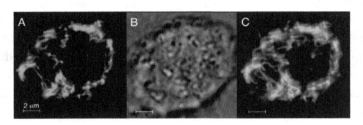

a substance in the entire volume of the sample. Other spectroscopic imaging modes include Raman confocal imaging (ref), fluorescence lifetime imaging (FLIM) (refs), fluorescence correlation spectroscopic (FCS) imaging (ref), etc. All these techniques can extend the diagnostic capability of confocal microscopes for a forensic pathologist.

Examples of Confocal Imaging Applications in Forensics

So far, confocal imaging within the field of forensic pathology has been used relatively rarely since the instruments are expense and require specialist training (Turillazzi et al., 2008). With the wider availability of confocal microscopes, their increasing ease of use and the enormous scope of applications, confocal imaging can be expected to be one of the common forensic techniques. Here, several examples of the application of confocal imaging in forensic medicine are demonstrated, showing how this technique can overcome particular diagnostic difficulties.

Some of the examples selected, such as pollen, hair and fingerprint analyses, require classification into databases and the digital format provided by confocal imaging greatly enhances the ability to store and analyze them. These examples fall into the category of forensic examinations that do not provide a direct statistical evaluation of their properties but depend on individual, qualitative characteristics. Such types of evidence material have been increasingly questioned as to their admissibility in court, particularly in United States, raising concerns of whether the examinations are strictly scientific or that they are subjective and unreliable. Even fingerprint analysis is beginning to be questioned so that in 2002 a US judge ruled that fingerprints did not meet the standards set for scientific testimony and that matching of fingerprints was subjective. It can therefore be expected that forensic pathologists will increasingly be required to provide diagnostic evidence that can be recognized as strictly scientific and not

subjective. The digitized mode of data collection, the wide availability of image data processing software and the interactive features of confocal instruments and their software will help to improve the utility of this method for forensic pathologists.

Confocal Imaging of Calcium Oxalate Crystals

Calcium oxalate crystals feature in several types of poisoning (e.g., Leth & Gregersen 2005) and their microscopic characterization and identification of localization in tissues aids in establishing a post-mortem diagnosis. Ingestion of calcium oxalate causes an intense sensation of burning in the mouth and throat, swelling, and choking. In greater doses, it causes a severe digestive upset, breathing difficulties and in severe cases, convulsions, coma, and death. Severe calcium oxalate poisoning can frequently lead to permanent liver and kidney damage. Calcium oxalate poisoning has even been reported responsible for a foodborne disease outbreak. On 24th February 2003, the manager of a cafeteria in Chicago contacted the city's Department of Health to report a spate of illnesses in people who had eaten at the facility. The analyses of the "Chinese braised vegetable" entrée that was eaten by the affected people by Food & Drug Administration's Forensic Chemistry Center, Cincinnati, found javelin-shaped crystals known as raphides, one of several crystal forms of calcium oxalate in plants, that caused the poisoning symptoms (Watson et al., 2005).

Seventy-five percent of flowering plants make one or more kinds of calcium oxalate crystals in specific tissues (Horner & Wagner, 1995; Lersten & Horner, 2000). Large quantities of calcium oxalate are found in their leaves, stems and roots: for example, in dumb cane (*Dieffenbachia*), leaves of rhubarb, various species of *Oxalis, Araceae* and agaves. If the stalk of *Dieffenbachia* is ingested, it causes very severe reactions due to the needle-like oxalate crystals that produce pain and swelling when they contact lips, tongue, oral mucosa, conjunctiva or skin. Ingesting *Arisaema* seed pod will also result in severe edema that takes twelve hours to subside.

Plant-derived calcium oxalate crystals have many shapes: 'crystal sand' has tetrahedral particle shape; some crystals have prismatic shapes; and druses form elaborate microstructures with rigid 'petals' that are sharp enough to lacerate the mouths of insects that ingest the plant. The biological function of these crystals has been proposed to be involved in defense, mechanical support, regulation of calcium balance, as well as sequestering of certain poisons, such as heavy metals (Horner and Wagner, 1995).

Calcium oxalate crystals are present in urine and are the most common constituents of human kidney stones (ref). Their formation is also one of the toxic effects of ethylene glycol (EG) poisoning (Leth & Gregersen, 2005). EG is a common ingredient in products such as antifreeze, hydraulic brake fluids, household cleaners and cosmetics. EG biotransforms into toxic metabolites, such as glycolic acid, which leads to a severe acidosis and precipitation of calcium oxalate in the kidneys and other tissues (Leth & Gregersen, 2005). Acute EG poisoning can cause central nervous system damage, severe metabolic acidosis, renal failure and death (Froberg et al., 2006). It is commonly found that internal examination of such patients is unremarkable except for edema of lungs and brain, and intense hyperemia (Froberg et al., 2006). The presence of calcium oxalate crystals in the urine leading to renal failure are characteristics of EG poisoning. Microscopic analysis of the urine typically reveals the presence of numerous calcium oxalate crystals and high numbers of erythrocytes (Eder et al., 1998). Histologic diagnosis in such cases relates to an acute tubular damage of kidneys, in association with calcium oxalate crystals deposition in tubular epithelial cells and their necrosis (Takahashi et al., 2008).

In a study by Pomara et al (2008) of tissues from a 33-year-old man who died from EG poisoning, confocal imaging and 3D reconstruction was performed on formalin fixed paraffin-embedded tissues sectioned at 4 μm and stained with hematoxylin-eosin. The specimens were analyzed by the confocal microscope (True Confocal Scanner, Leica TCS SP2) and showed precise localization of calcium oxalate crystals in renal tissue, associated with the renal tubular cell epithelium and localized inside the tubular cells. Confocal imaging showed precise localization of crystals within relatively thick renal sections and the analysis supported the hypothesis (McMartin & Wallace, 2005) that the crystals lead to mitochondrial damage that results in cell death, tubular necrosis that lead to renal failure.

The capability of 3D visualization of exact localization of oxalate crystals by confocal imaging technique can help overcome diagnostic difficulties of plant-derived or EG oxalate crystal poisoning, simplifying the histological preparation of samples. Here, an example of confocal imaging of oxalate crystals in plant tissues is presented, in which the fluorescence mode of imaging of cells was successfully combined with reflective imaging to visualize the crystals.

The genus *Lippia* (Verbenaceae) is a perennial herb that is extremely widespread, with approximately 240 species, occurring mainly in the tropics of America and Africa (Pascual et al., 2001). In Australia, *Lippia* has become an invasive species and causes serious environmental and pastoral problems in the Murray-Darling Basin. *Lippia* tissues have high concentrations of calcium oxalate, which makes it unpalatable to herbivores. In Africa, medicinal teas are made from *Lippia* leaves. The plant has a large number of subcutaneous glands, similar as those found in *Eucalyptus, Melaleuca* and *Citrus* spp. and that appear as cavities or ducts in the epidermis.

Confocal imaging to reveal the localization of calcium oxalate crystals was performed on live *Lippia* leaves that were unstained and roughly sectioned using a razor blade. Leaf sections mounted in water on glass slides were imaged at dual excitation by Leica TCS SP5 confocal microscope using excitation Diode 405 laser for reflection imaging (PMT1 set to capture laser emissions at 400-410nm) and Argon laser line of 488 nm to capture green autofluorescence at 495-520 nm and chlorophyll fluorescence at 670-700 nm. Leica TCS SP5 is equipped with an AOBS, the beam path is optimized automatically for the selected wavelength and no dichroic filters are required. Serial optical sections from the surface of the leaf were performed to 100 μm depth. *Lippia* epidermis was highly autofluorescent revealing numerous guard cells around stomatal pores and sharp setae overlaying the chloroplasts (Figure 3 B, C). Reflective imaging by 405 nm laser revealed that calcium oxalate crystals were more concentrated on the surface of leaves, within the surface ridges, glandular trichomes, guard cells and inside the spiky setae (Figure 3 A, D). The combination of reflective imaging of light scattering properties of calcium oxalate coupled with imaging of leaf autofluorescence proved to be a very effective technique to examine plant material for the presence and localization of calcium oxalate crystals.

Confocal Imaging of Pollen

Forensic pollen analysis, or forensic palynology, is the science of deriving evidence for court purposes from pollen and spores (Yoon, 1993; Horrocks et al., 1998). Pollen is extremely light and the slightest breeze makes it airborne; thus, vast pollen quantities become deposited on people's clothing, hair, skin and other surfaces. Since vegetation in any area consists of different pollen producing plants, the pollen found on a person in an area will be distinctive from other areas, not only at geographic scales, but often, at smaller spatial scales and presents a forensic evidence of person's or body's location and movement (Horrocks et al., 1998). Pollen has been important in medical forensic investigations and has been identified in nasal passages, in stomach contents, the digestive track during autopsy and in soil under the bones of human remains (Yoon, 1993; Quatrehomme et al., 1997; Horrocks & Walsh, 2001; Taylor & Skene, 2003; Gunn, 2009). It can provide information about whether a body has been moved since death and where it was located recently (Taylor

Figure 3. Confocal imaging of Lippia leave in reflective and fluorescence modes. (A) 405 nm laser light scattered by calcium oxalate reveals its localization in leaf epidermis, especially in long spiky setae. (B) Green autofluorescence at 488 nm excitation reveals cuticular ridging, guard cells, trichomes and (C) underlying chloroplasts in palisade layer. (D) Overlayed image

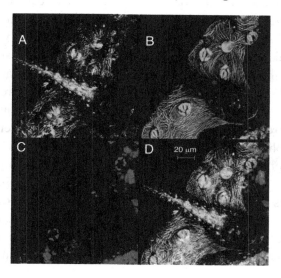

& Skene, 2003; Gunn, 2009). Pollen native to an area will still be in place months or even years later, taking seasons into account. It can, therefore, provide a time-frame for a person's death and estimated time elapsed since death (Taylor & Skene, 2003). Although still a rather under-utilized resource in forensic sciences (Bock & Norris, 1997), the use of pollen as associative or exclusionary evidence in courts is growing and as new technologies become available, its usage has vast potential.

The main obstacle of using pollen as evidence is the ability to identify pollen composition taxonomically and match it to its source. Moreover, even samples taken from the same locality can be quite varied – there may over 50 pollen species present in a sample and replicate samples from the same location may show pollen differences. Taxonomic identification of pollen is often complicated and even with complex and lengthy analysis, pollen of some plants cannot be resolved to the species level.

Examples of plants that are extremely difficult to taxonomically identify are grasses. Pollen of grasses (family Poaceae), whist being some of the most abundant, is morphologically very homogeneous, making taxonomic identification to the species or generic levels difficult. All grass species have pollen grains that are monoporate, with an operculum, an annulus, and a thin exine, with uniformly arranged supratectal processes or spinules (Wodehouse 1935). Finding the appropriate methodology to distinguish between species of wild grasses has become the subject of much research (Watson & Bell 1975; Peltre et al., 1987; Driessen et al., 1989). Whilst grass pollen grains usually exhibit exine surface reticulate patterning that are species specific (Grohne, 1957; Erdtman & Praglowski, 1959), it is not that easy to reveal the patterning. Pollen grains have to be treated by certain chemical methods that strip the outer waxy layer revealing the exine, but even then, the patterning characteristics have been often too subtle and difficult to quantify to provide reliable

taxonomic distinction using conventional light microscopy (Faegri & Iversen, 1989).

The use of confocal microscopy, in reflection mode, was shown to provide an excellent method to characterize grass pollen exine morphology at the surface and the sub-surface levels (Salih et al., 1997). Exine surface patterning for pollen from seven common grass species was imaged using the 488 nm line from a Krypton/Argon laser using x100 oil immersion objective (Zeiss Plan-Neofluor) and zoom setting of x6 (31 nm/pixel) by serial optical sections at incrementally increasing depths (i.e. approximately 0.2 μm increments). The serial images were then reconstructed using 3D software, VoxelView software package (VoxelView Ultra 2.1.2, Vital Images Pty. Ltd., Fairfield, Iowa, USA).

Confocal reflective imaging of chemically untreated grass pollen (*Paspalum dilatatum, Setaria gracilis, Bromus catharticus, Daclylis glomerata, Lolium perenne, Poa pratensis*) revealed clearly patterned exine of thickness 1.0 to 2.5 μm (Salih et al., 1997). The common characteristic found in all of the seven grass species examined was the presence of a distinct surface topography, made up of lumina of varying sizes and shapes, and surrounded by a network of reticulate elements of differing thicknesses (Salih et al., 1997). These provided criteria for taxonomic differentiation of the grass species examined. The reconstruction of the stacks of optical sections made through the exine permitted 3D visualization of not only the surface but also of sub-surface exine layer patterning. The reticulate elements formed distinct components that were thickened in places to form surface mounds having pentagonal, hexagonal or triangular arrangements, supporting either single or multiple surface knobs, which in turn were either blunt or sharply pointed, depending on the species examined (Figure 4).

Many of the above mentioned features revealed by confocal microscopy were found to correlate with findings from the more standard microscopic techniques currently used to identify the species of pollen grains, such as scanning electron microscopy (SEM). Confocal microscope imaged knobs on the surface of the mounds corresponded to spinules grouped on islands (or insulae) projecting from pollen surfaces, as identified by numerous SEM studies (e.g. Andersen & Bertelsen, 1972). The observed reticular patterns present in the species examined, may correspond to the intra-reticulate columellae, which are known to form a reticulate pattern below the exine surface (Praglowski & Punt, 1973; Faegri & Iversen, 1989). Further, the results of Salih et al. (1997) study indicated that the size and shape of the identified reticulate components may provide a means for taxonomic differentiation of grass pollens. A similar conclusion has been reached by the authors of various SEM studies of pollen, with suggestions that the shape and the size of the protruding island-like structures or insulae (Andersen & Bertelsen, 1972), the number of spinules per insula, and the width and sharpness of the incisions between the insulae are features having

Figure 4. Confocal reflective microscopy of grass pollen exine. (A) The uppermost surface of Bromus catharticus, with tips of large knobs protruding singly from mounds on exine surface and separated by polygonal or hexagonal deep lumina. (B) Oval, pentagonal or hexagonal lumina surrounded by reticulate elements supporting the surface knobs. Surface features of Lolium perenne exine with (C) crowded knobs and mounds and (D) circular lumina at 0.4 µm under surface

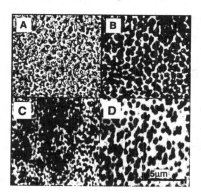

a certain amount of species specificity (Watson & Bell, 1975; Peltre et al., 1987; Rowley et al., 1988).

Confocal microscopy, however, has an advantage over SEM in terms of the methods of sample preparation, which permitted imaging of fresh grass pollen grains that were unacetolysed or otherwise chemically treated, in an aqueous environment. This is in contrast to the lengthy and chemically harsh preparation protocols which may significantly affect the specimen morphology required for SEM or TEM investigations (Hanks & Fairbrothers, 1970). As a further advantage of the confocal technique, all of the gathered images are in digital form, enabling both the 3D qualitative studies to be undertaken, as well as the quantitative comparison of exine patterns using image analysis and statistical software.

Confocal Imaging of Fingerprints

Fingerprints provide the most powerful forensic tool for identifying people because the ridge patterns of every print are unique. The ability to store and classify fingerprint data in searchable data-bases contributes to the powerful nature of fingerprint analysis (Egli et al., 2007). Fingerprints are either visible or latent; the former are made on contact with solid or semi-solid surfaces, have a 3D structure and do not require further enhancement to get visualized (Smith et al., 1993). On the other hand, latent fingerprints are invisible and require the application of dyes or powders to enable visualization and analysis by optical, physical and chemical methods (Smith et al., 1993).

The systematic classification of fingerprints is largely based on three categories of ridge patterns - loops, whorls and arches, as well as ridge bifurcations, islands and spurs and form the basis of automated fingerprint identification systems (AFIS) (Egli et al., 2007). However, the minimum number of fingerprint ridge characteristics needed to conclude a positive match is somewhat variable in different criminal laboratories and in courts of different countries. Moreover, there have been almost no studies to statistically evaluate the quantity of similar ridge characteristics occurring between different people. This fact, and the various cases of misidentification using AFIS, led to the need for other, more effective and advanced methods of fingerprint analysis.

Latent prints are the most common prints found at crime scenes, yet are the hardest to distinguish and consequently, there is a demand to improve their analysis in forensic science. Fingerprint detection using fluorescence analysis has been an extremely useful technique for latent fingerprint analysis, when conventional chemical enhancement methods fail. Application of fluorescence techniques and dusting powders, followed by photography, is the most common technique used (Sodhi & Kaur, 2001). The powdering technique relies on adherence of the powder to oily components of the print but has the major disadvantage in that contact between the brush and the print frequently causes degradation of the print (Sodhi & Kaur, 2001). Consequently, there has been an ongoing quest to develop a method of fingerprint analysis that avoids the use of fingerprint powders.

Effective storage of vast quantities of fingerprint data presents another problem. Fingerprints are traditionally stored as ink prints on paper, making automated matching difficult due to large file size of stored prints difficult, as well as time consuming, even though recent development of the computer and scanning techniques allowed fingerprints to be stored digitally.

The use of fluorescence-based techniques in fingerprint analysis continues to play a significant role in fingerprint detection when conventional chemical enhancement methods fail. When considering various modes of fingerprint analysis, clearly, these techniques continue to play a significant role in fingerprint detection when conventional chemical enhancement methods fail. As early as 1977, fingerprint auto-fluorescence by laser excitation was used to demonstrate the effectiveness of fluorescence imaging as a fingerprint detection method (Dalrymple et al., 1977). The majority of such earlier studies using fluorescence induced by

laser excitation were done using pre-processing procedures with various chemicals before detection to enhance sensitivity since autofluorescence fingerprints tends to be relatively weak (Menzel, 1977). Another study showed that confocal imaging in fluorescence mode of Rhodamine-treated fingerprints on clear plastic provided significant improvement over wide-field microscopy (Beesley et al., 1995). Interestingly, high contrast images at low magnification of latent fingerprints obtained in reflection mode of confocal imaging, showed that Rhodamine-treated fingerprints on the surface of a polished silicon wafer and glass could be effectively visualized by this method (Beesley et al., 1995). Reflective confocal imaging of fingerprints promises to offer a non-destructive technique that requires minimal sample preparation. It is possible to image fingerprints without powder pre-treatment (Salih & Hassick, unpublished), leading to cleaner images with reduced risk of contamination. The technique may be somewhat expensive for routine fingerprint analysis but in cases where a single fingerprint holds extra value, confocal reflective imaging can be a technique of choice. The additional data in the z plane and visualization and analysis in 3D digital mode enable further analysis including depth between and height of ridges. In cases, where only a partial print is recovered, the 3D digital data set can be analyzed by sophisticated image analysis software to provide additional information, increasing the probability of securing a conviction. The reflective confocal microscopy promises to be a powerful imaging technique for fingerprint analysis, providing superior information, data analysis, storage and retrieval over conventional methods.

Confocal Diagnostic Imaging of Hair

Hairs from humans or from animals are often recovered during forensic investigation and in fact, constitute one of the most common types of trace evidence (Nickell & Fischer 1999). Human hair morphology has been well characterized (Seta et al., 1988) since it is provides useful evidence and is very prevalent at crime scenes. Nuclear and mitochondrial DNA profiling of human hair in the 1980s and 1990s is considered a more efficient discriminating tool (Higuchi et al., 1988). However, DNA analysis of hair is complex and there is a problem in that nuclear DNA can only be accurately typed when the hair roots are in a specific growth cycle stage which is anagen or catagen, rather then the cycle most common for hair roots found at crime scenes which is telogen or resting phase (Linch et al., 1988). DNA profiling can be done by analyzing mitochondrial DNA from the hair shaft but this is a less reliable analysis than nuclear DNA and it is relatively complex (Graham, 2007).

For these reasons, forensic scientists continue to rely on morphological analysis of hair and the use of this technique has been accepted both scientifically and legally (Houck et al., 2002). However, in the last decade, hair microscopic profiling has become a controversial topic because hair morphology is very similar in appearance and often does not present sufficient discrimination. Its evaluation may be considered a subjective opinion as for example, criticism of forensic hair analysis for evidence was presented by the Royal Commission in Canada, followed by many cases in US and Europe, with suggestions that it should be altogether excluded from criminal trials (Taupin 2004). Forensic analysis of animal hairs collected from crime scenes also requires taxonomic identification of hairs to determine the species origin. It is often considered even more difficult than human hair profiling because of the variation that can exist within a species and even between hairs from the same animal (Moore, 1988; Petraco, 1987). Clearly, forensic hair analysis needs improving the various techniques of accurately characterizing, statistically analyzing and storing data.

The most common method for obtaining morphological analysis of the exterior of the hair shaft is by using conventional light microscopy technique (Seta et al., 1988; Robertson, 1999). Scale patterns are observed by embedding the hair

in a liquid medium, such as clear nail polish and allowing it to set. Once the polish has air-dried, the hair is removed, leaving a cast of the outer scales. Identification of human hair is done by comparing the scale patterns of the cuticle and the medullary index (i.e., the ratio of medulla to shaft size), which in humans is usually under 1/3 (Saferstein, 2004). Other features, particularly in animal hair studies, include hair length, maximum width along the hair shaft, cross sectional maximum diameter, cuticular thickness of a cross section, hair scale count (number of free edges of hair scale per unit length of 100 mm) are determined using a ruler and a microscope equipped with a micrometer. There are three basic scale structures of hair: coronal (crown-like), spinous (petal-like) and imbricate (flattened), with various combinations and variations of these types that can be used to determine the species. For instance, umbricate scales are found in humans (Saferstein, 2004).

More advanced analyses that revealed finer details of microstructure of hair scales became possible using scanning electron microscopy (SEM) techniques (Robbins, 1988; Van Neste & Houbion, 1989). This method, however, is somewhat lengthy, and a new option of using confocal imaging of untreated hair promises to be the technique of choice.

Advances in imaging techniques, combined with 3D image analysis, have lead to improvements in hair analysis. The first confocal imaging of hair in 1993 gave the 3D surface pattern similar, but somewhat inferior in quality, to images obtained by SEM (Corcuff et al., 1993). Confocal images of hair microstructure stained with Rhodamine B at excitation by 488 nm laser line, with subsequent image enhancement by software routines, served to improve image quality to resemble conventional SEM (Lagarde et al., 1994).

Even unstained hairs can be analyzed by confocal microscopy using reflection or back-scattering mode (Wessel et al., 2003). The procedure is to mount a hair sample on a glass slide and to use any of the available laser lines in reflection mode and

Figure 5. Confocal reflective imaging of hair scale microstructures. Spinous scales of (A) puma and (B) leopard hairs. (Image by Anya Salih, previously unpublished)

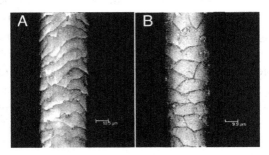

to take serial optical sections at incremental steps (0.3 micrometers) (Figure 5; Salih, unpublished). This technique reveals the detailed 3D architecture of hair scales and allows sub-surface imaging of the medulla. When hairs from several mammalian species were analyzed using this technique, clear qualitative differences were found in the scale morphology between cat, puma, leopard, cow, dog and human species (Figure 5).

The analysis to quantify the variations in hair scale morphology generated by confocal imaging of hair is still being developed. It can be envisaged that modern 3D analysis software solutions would be found that will involve shape characterization using complex Fourier analysis shape descriptors, such as first developed to measure the overall shape or form of structures - features such as angularity versus roundness, or focus on the still fine textural differences between shapes (Clark, 1981; Barrett, 1980). A useful image analysis technique was applied to analyze atomic force microscopy (AFM) generated hair images by characterizing the hair surface using multivariate approach to analyze an array of cuticular descriptors (Gurden et al., 2004). An algorithm capable of automatically scanning an AFM image and calculating descriptors at all possible locations was developed. Reflection confocal microscopy provides a quantitative, topographic imaging tool and an excellent alternative compared to SEM and AFM. The accuracy and sensitivity of this method promises a solution to quantitatively analyze of untreated hair samples.

To conclude this chapter, it can be foreshadowed that by incorporating novel imaging techniques, coupled with analytical instruments and powerful image data analysis, and by promoting cross-disciplinary interactions, confocal microscopy will increasingly find wider applications in forensic sciences and will emerge as an exciting, powerful and a widely used tool.

REFERENCES

Abelson, J. N., Simon, M. I., & Conn, M. P. (1999). Confocal microscopy. [Academic Press.]. *Methods in Enzymology*, 307.

Akiba, N., Saitoh, N., & Kuroki, K. (2007). Fluorescence spectra and images of latent fingerprints excited with a tunable laser in the ultraviolet region. *Journal of Forensic Sciences*, *52*(5), 1103–1107. doi:10.1111/j.1556-4029.2007.00532.x

Andersen, S. T., & Bertelsen, F. (1972). Scanning electron microscope studies of pollen of cereals and other grasses. *Grana*, *12*, 79–86. doi:10.1080/00173137209428830

Barrett, P. J. (1980). The shape of rock particles, a critical review. *Sedimentology*, *27*, 291–303. doi:10.1111/j.1365-3091.1980.tb01179.x

Beesley, K. M., Damaskinos, S., & Dixon, A. E. (1995). Fingerprint imaging with a confocal scanning laser macroscope. *Journal of Forensic Sciences, 40*(1), 10–17.

Bock, J. H., & Norris, D. O. (1997). Forensic botany: An under-utilized resource. *Journal of Forensic Sciences, 42*(3), 364–367.

Clark, M. W. (1981). Quantitative shape analysis: A review. *Mathematical Geology, 13*(4), 303–320. doi:10.1007/BF01031516

Combrinck, S., Duplooy, G. W., McCrindle, R. I., & Both, B. M. (2007). Morphology and histochemistry of the glandular trichomes of Lippia scaberrima (Verbenaceae). *Annals of Botany, 99*, 1111–1119. doi:10.1093/aob/mcm064

Corcuff, P., Gremillet, P., Jourlin, M., Duvault, Y., Leroy, F., & Leveque, J. L. (1993). 3D reconstruction of human hair by confocal microscopy. *Journal of the Society of Cosmetic Chemists, 44*, 1–12.

Dalrymple, B. E., Duff, J. M., & Menzel, E. R. (1977). Inherent fingerprint luminescence-detection by laser. *Journal of Forensic Sciences, 22*, 106–1510.

Driessen, M. N. B. M., Willemse, M. T. M., & van Luijn, J. A. G. (1989). Grass pollen grain determination by light- and UV-microscopy. *Grana, 28*, 115–122. doi:10.1080/00173138909429962

Eder, A. F., McGrath, C. M., Dowdy, Y. G., Tomaszewski, J. E., Rosenberg, F. M., & Wilson, R. B. (1998). Ethylene glycol poisoning: Toxicokinetic and analytical factors affecting laboratory diagnosis. *Clinical Chemistry, 44*, 168–177.

Egli, N. M., Champod, C., & Margot, P. (2007). Evidence evaluation in fingerprint comparison and automated fingerprint identification systems-modelling within finger variability. *Forensic Science International, 167*, 189–195. doi:10.1016/j.forsciint.2006.06.054

Erdtman, G., & Praglowski, J. R. (1959). Six notes on pollen morphology and pollen morphological techniques. *Botaniska Notiser, 112*, 175–184.

Fægri, K., & Iversen, J. (1989). *Textbook of pollen analysis* (4th ed.). Chichester, UK: J. Wiley & Sons.

Froberg, K., Dorion, R. P., & McMartin, K. E. (2006). The role of calcium oxalate crystal deposition in cerebral vessels during ethylene glycol poisoning. *Clinical Toxicology, 44*, 315–318. doi:10.1080/15563650600588460

Graham, E. A. M. (2007). DNA reviews: Hair. *Journal of Forensic Science, Medicine, and Pathology, 3*(2), 1556–2891.

Grohne, U. (1957). Die Bedeutung des Phasenkontrastverfahrens fur die Pollenanalyse, dargelegt am Beispiel der Gramineenpollen vom Getreideyp. *Photogr. Forsch, 7*, 237–248.

Gunn, A. (2009). *Essential forensic biology* (2nd ed., pp. 335–342). Ed Whiley Pty.

Gurden, S. P., Monteiro, V. F., Longo, E., & Ferreira, M. M. C. (2004). Quantitative analysis and classification of AFM images of human hair. *Journal of Microscopy, 215*(1), 13–23. doi:10.1111/j.0022-2720.2004.01350.x

Hadjur, C., Daty, G., Madry, G., & Corcuff, P. (2002). Cosmetic assessment of the human hair by confocal microscopy. *Scanning, 24*, 59–64. doi:10.1002/sca.4950240202

Hanks, S. S., & Fairbrothers, D. E. (1970). Effect of preparation technique on pollen prepared for SEM observation. *Taxon, 19*, 879–886. doi:10.2307/1218302

Higuchi, R., von Beroldingen, C. H., Sensabaugh, G. F., & Erlich, H. A. (1988). DNA typing from single hairs. *Nature, 332*, 543–546. doi:10.1038/332543a0

Horner, H. T., & Wagner, B. L. (1995). Calcium oxalate formation in higher plants. In Khan, S. (Ed.), *Calcium oxalate in biological systems* (pp. 53–72). CRC Book Press.

Horrocks, M., & Walsh, K. A. J. (2001). Forensic palynology: Assessing the value of the evidence. *Review of Palaeobotany and Palynology, 103*, 69–74. doi:10.1016/S0034-6667(98)00027-X

Houck, M. M., & Budowle, B. (2002). Comparison of microscopic and mitochondrial DNA hair comparisons. *Journal of Forensic Sciences, 47*(5), 1–4.

Kubinova, L., Janacek, J., Karen, P., Radochova, B., DiFato, F., & Krekule, I. (2004). Confocal stereology and image analysis: Methods for estimating geometrical characteristics of cells and tissues from three-dimensional confocal images. *Physiological Research, 53*(Suppl. 1), S47–S55.

Lagarde, J. M., Peyre, P., Redoules, D., Black, D., Briot, M., & Gall, Y. (1994). Confocal microscopy of hair. *Cell Biology and Toxicology, 10*, 301–304. doi:10.1007/BF00755774

Lee, H. C., & Gaensslen, R. E. (1991). *Advances in fingerprint technology*. Boca Raton, FL: CRC Press.

Lersten, N. R., & Horner, H. T. (2000). Types of calcium oxalate crystals in macro patterns in leaves of Prunus (Rosaceae: Prunoideae). *Plant Systematics and Evolution, 224*, 83–96. doi:10.1007/BF00985267

Leth, P. M., & Gregersen, M. (2005). Ethylene glycol poisoning. *Forensic Science International, 155*(2-3), 179–184. doi:10.1016/j.forsciint.2004.11.012

Linch, C., Smith, S., & Prahlow, J. (1998). Evaluation of the human hair root for DNA typing subsequent to microscopic comparison. *Journal of Forensic Sciences, 43*(2), 305–314.

McMartin, K. E., & Wallace, K. B. (2005). Calcium oxalate monohydrate, a metabolite of ethylene glycol, is toxic for rat renal mitochondrial function. *Toxicological Sciences, 84*, 195–200. doi:10.1093/toxsci/kfi062

Menzel, E. R. (1999). Fingerprint detection with lasers, 2nd ed. [New York: Marcel Dekker.]. *Journal of Forensic Sciences, 42*, 303–306.

Moore, J. E. (1988). A key for the identification of animal hairs. *Proceedings of the Forensic Science Society*, (pp. 335-339).

Neri, M. (2010). Beyond and together with autopsy techniques: Confocal scanning laser microscopy in forensic medicine. In Pomara, C., Karch, S. B., & Fineschi, V. (Eds.), *Forensic autopsy: A handbook and altas* (pp. 113–120). CRC press. doi:10.1201/EBK1439800645-c5

Nickell, J., & Fischer, J. F. (1999). *Crime science: Methods of forensic detection*. Lexington, KY: University of Kentucky Press.

Peltre, G., Cerceau-Larrival, M.-T., Hideux, M., Abadie, M., & David, B. (1987). Scanning and transmission electron microscopy related to immunochemical analysis of grass pollen. *Grana, 26*, 158–170. doi:10.1080/00173138709429945

Petraco, N. (1987). A microscopical method to aid in the identification of animal hair. *Microscope (Carshalton Beeches (Surrey)), 35*, 83–92.

Pomara, C., Fiore, C., D'Errico, S., Riezzo, I., & Fineschi, V. (2008). Calcium oxalate crystals in acute ethylene glycol poisoning: A confocal laser scanning microscope study in a fatal case. *Clinical Toxicology, 46*(4), 322–324. doi:10.1080/15563650701419011

Praglowski, J., & Punt, W. (1973). An elucidation of the microreticulate structure of the exine. *Grana, 13*, 45–50. doi:10.1080/00173137309428842

Quatrehomme, G., Lacoste, A., Bailet, P., Grevin, G., & Ollier, A. (1997). Contribution of microscopic plant anatomy to postmortem bone dating. *Journal of Forensic Sciences, 42*(1), 140–143.

Robbins, C. R. (1988). *Chemical and physical behavior of human hair* (2nd ed., pp. 1–36). New York: Springer-Verlag.

Robertson, J. (1999). Forensic and microscopic examination of human hair. In Robertson, J. (Ed.), *Forensic examination of hair* (pp. 79–154). London: Taylor & Francis.

Rowley, J. R., Skvarla, J. J., & Vezey, E. L. (1988). Evaluating the relative contributions of SEM, TEM and LM to the description of pollen grains. *Journal of Palynology, 23-24*, 27–28.

Saferstein, R. (2004). *Criminalistics: An introduction to forensic science* (8th ed.). Upper Saddle River, NJ: Pearson Education Inc.

Salih, A., Jones, A. S., Bass, D., & Cox, G. (1997). Confocal imaging of exine as a tool for grass pollen analysis. *Grana, 36*, 215–224. doi:10.1080/00173139709362610

Seah, L. K., Dinish, U. S., Phang, W. F., Chao, Z. X., & Murukeshan, V. M. (2005). Fluorescence optimisation and lifetime studies of fingerprints treated with magnetic powders. *Forensic Science International, 152*, 249–257. doi:10.1016/j.forsciint.2004.09.121

Seta, S., Sato, H., & Miyake, B. (1988). Forensic hair investigation. In Maehly, A., & Williams, R. L. (Eds.), *Forensic science progress*. Berlin, Heidelberg: Springer-Verlag.

Smith, W. C., Kinney, R. W., & De Partee, D. G. (1993). Latent fingerprints—a forensic approach. *Journal of Forensic Identification, 43*(6), 563–570.

Sodhi, G. S., & Kaur, J. (2001). Powder method for detecting latent fingerprints: A review. *Forensic Science International, 120*, 172–176. doi:10.1016/S0379-0738(00)00465-5

Takahashi, S., Kanetake, J., Kanawaku, Y., & Funayama, M. (2008). Brain death with calcium oxalate deposition in the kidney: Clue to the diagnosis of ethylene glycol poisoning. *Legal Medicine, 10*(1), 43–45. doi:10.1016/j.legalmed.2007.05.010

Taupin, J. M. (2004). Forensic hair morphology comparison-a dying art or junk science? *Science & Justice, 44*(2), 95–100. doi:10.1016/S1355-0306(04)71695-0

Taylor, B., & Skene, K. R. (2003). Forensic palynology: Spatial and temporal considerations of spora deposition in forensic investigations. *The Australian Journal of Forensic Sciences, 35*(2), 193–204. doi:10.1080/00450610309410582

Turillazzi, E., Karch, S. B., Neri, M., Pomara, C., Riezzo, I., & Fineschi, V. (2008). Confocal laser scanning microscopy: Using new technology to answer old questions in forensic investigations. *International Journal of Legal Medicine, 122*, 173–177. doi:10.1007/s00414-007-0208-0

Van Neste, D., & Houbion, Y. (1989). Office diagnosis of pathological changes in hair cuticular cell pattern. In Van Neste, D., Lachapelle, J. M., & Antoine, J. L. (Eds.), *Trends in human hair growth and alopecia research* (pp. 173–179). Dordrecht: Kluwer.

Watson, J. T., Jones, R. C., Siston, A. M., Diaz, P. S., Gerber, S. I., & Crowe, J. B. (2005). Outbreak of food-borne illness associated with plant material containing raphides. *Clinical Toxicology, 43*(1), 17–21.

Watson, L., & Bell, E. M. (1975). A surface-structural survey of some taxonomically diverse grass pollens. *Australian Journal of Botany, 23*, 981–990. doi:10.1071/BT9750981

Wessel, S., Pagel, M., Ritter, H., & Hohenberg, R. (2003). Topographic measurements of real structures in reflection confocal laser scanning microscope (CLSM). *Microscopy and Microanalysis, 3*, 162.

Williams, R. M., Zipfel, W. R., & Webb, W. W. (2001). Multiphoton microscopy in biological research. *Current Opinion in Chemical Biology*, *5*(5), 603–608. doi:10.1016/S1367-5931(00)00241-6

Wodehouse, R. P. (1935). *Pollen grains. Their structure, identification and significance in science and medicine*. New York, London: McGraw-Hill.

Yoon, C. K. (1993). Botanical witness for the prosecution. *Science*, *260*, 894–895. doi:10.1126/science.8493521

Zhuo, L., Hu, L. S., Zhou, L., Zheng, N., Liang, M., & Yang, F. (2009). Application of confocal laser scanning microscope in forensic pathology. *Fa Yi Xue Za Zhi*, *25*(6), 455–458.

KEY TERMS AND DEFINITIONS

Fluorescence: Emission of light that occurs almost instantly after light is absorbed by a specimen is called fluorescence. A wide range of specimens absorb light radiation, become "excited", and re-emit light. Emitted light is always longer wavelength than absorbed light. Fluorescent molecules have specific excitation and emission spectra.

Fluorescence Wide-Field Microscopy: Also known as epi-fluorescence microscopy, it is a technique in which the sample is irradiated with a specific band of wavelengths and the emitted fluorescence is separated from the excitation light and imaged. In samples greater than 2 micrometers, structural detail is lost because the emitted fluorescence occurs through the excitation volume and obscures resolution of features that lie in the objective focal plane.

Confocal Microscopy: Confocal microscopy differs from wide-field microscopy because out-of-focus light emitted by a specimen is blocked. It relies on fluorescence light emission by the specimen after irradiation by specific laser line.

It provides the ability to control depth of field, reduce background information outside of the focal plane and collect serial optical sections through the specimen. Confocal microscopy can be viewed as a 3D imaging technique which is coupled to a computer system to generate images of a specimen in 3D.

Reflectance Confocal Imaging (RCI): RCI is a non-invasive approach for *in-vivo* study of specimens. Laser light is scanned across a specimen and is reflected to varying degrees by structures with different refractive indexes. The light is captured by a detector and recomposed into a 2D gray scale image by computer software. Focusing the confocal microscope by adjusting the focal point on the z-axis, allows 3D visualization of the surface and sub-surface micro-structures, rendered at different contrast levels to a depth of over 200 μm.

Confocal Data Characteristics: Confocal data typically consists of a series of 2D grayscale images obtained as optical sections along the X, Y and Z-axes through a specimen, i.e., an image stack or series of data over the volume of a specimen. Image sizes are 256x256, 51x512 or 1024x1024 and up to 4096 x 4096; first number for pixels per line, second number for line per frame scanned. The use of red, green and blue (RGB) color is most informative for displaying the distribution of three fluorescent probes labeling a cell or from sample autofluorescence separated into different spectral bands.

Three Dimensional (3D) Reconstruction: A composite or projection view in the x, y, and z dimensions from a series of optical sections generated by confocal imaging can be reconstructed into a 3D view and enables multi-dimensional viewing. Composite views created from optical series enable structural and functional analysis of cells, tissues and whole specimens. The data can be displayed as 3D multicolor video sequences in real time.

Chapter 3
Data Hiding in Digitized Medical Images:
From Concepts to Applications

Mehul S. Raval
Dhirubhai Ambani Institute of Information and Communication Technology, India

ABSTRACT

This chapter envelops data hiding techniques applied to medical images for improving their security. It covers types of medical images, their security requirements and types of threats to them. This provides a sufficient background and reasoning for applying data hiding techniques to the medical images. The purpose of this chapter is to study requirements of data hiding techniques with respect to medical imaging and to cover state of art methods in this domain. These techniques are developed from different application perspectives helping to understand their limitations and strengths. The chapter culminates with study of algorithms for reversible watermarking techniques and discussion on future of watermarking in medical domain.

INTRODUCTION

Growth of digital technologies and communication networks has empowered the storage, transmission and retrieval of records from electronic database. This can have a wide spread applications in health sciences. ICT medical applications range from

DOI: 10.4018/978-1-60960-483-7.ch003

tele-medicine, tele-surgery, cooperative working, tele-diagnosis, to robotic surgery. Telemedicine or tele-diagnosis applications require transmission of medical images over a relatively insecure public domain computer networks. The demand will be similar to any public domain packet switched network like loss, retransmissions, compression and security issues. Transmission of data is also possible over more secure and private hospital networks. These kinds of networks may not have issues in terms of loss, retransmission, compression but malicious attempt to break into network for unauthorized access is a real threat. Thus there is a grave danger to shared Electronic Patient Record (EPR) in such situations and there is a need for security in both "online" and "offline" world. EPR is highly private in nature and its disclosure can cause severe personal, economic, social and political issues. EPR is converted into different types of file formats where it would be authorized and used by the medical practitioners. The involvement of physicians in authorization and format conversion process can be highly cumbersome for them. Thus one has to look for the techniques which are less demanding to physicians and at the same time provide adequate security to EPR. This chapter aims at providing the adequate security to the medical images through application of data hiding techniques.

Medical Imaging, Their Types and DICOM Format

Medical practitioners are dependent on images for diagnostics. Medical images cover a very wide spectrum within medical domain. Images capture morphology of internal parts and to an extent their functionality. Doctor concludes about proper functionality of the internal organs and lookout for pathological issues within them. Medical imaging uses conventional X ray techniques to images generated by computational techniques like Computer Tomography (CT). There are varieties of techniques belonging to computational category like Nuclear Magnetic Resonance (NMR), Positron Emission Tomography (PET) (Ryszard Tadeusiewicz, 2004). Many techniques use injection of reactive agent within body to obtain image. Ultra sonography (USG) is one such technique which uses absorption and reflection of ultra sound waves to generate images of internal body organs. Autoradiography visualization techniques utilize ionizing gamma radiation emitted by radioactive

organs. The radioactive material has to be inserted into patient body. Thermo vision images are also used to capture organization and functioning of internal parts of human body. All these medical imaging techniques provide immense knowledge to the medical practitioners and help them to conclusive diagnosis, and recovery plans from disease. Practitioner are increasingly refering to medical images when faced with a complicated problem. However medical images for individual are highly random and would further compound the problem for practiceners. A doctor looking at an medical images tries to understand the following issues:

1. How internal organs are appearing?
2. Why they are appearing in this specific manner?
3. What biological reasons can cause this shape, shade, brightening or change in texture?

One has to also concur with the fact that with increasing dependence on technology doctors have to quickly learn and unlearn new technology. This sometimes can be a cause for false diagnostics. Different modalities images have distinct requirements for storage and transmission. Thus there is a need for standard to ensure interoperability.

DICOM Formats

Digital Imaging and Communications in Medicine (DICOM) (DICOM Standard, 1993) is the standard created by American College of Radiology (ACR) and the National Electrical Manufacturers Association (NEMA) in 1993. The standard is created for transmission of medical images with metadata, storing, printing, and handling of medical image data. There are number of other bodies like ANSI, IEEE with whom liaison is done for development of this standard. DICOM standard defines the DICOM object format and communication protocol. Thus it solves the interoperability issues in the medical domain. DICOM object contains multiple attributes like personal details of the patient, pixel data, image properties, device properties. Pixel data can be compressed using standards like JPEG, JPEG 2000. DICOM have many services for transmission of data over the network. DICOM covers different types of modalities like endoscopy, microscopy, angiography, mammography, nuclear medicine, PET and many more. DICOM reserves standard port numbers for communication over the network. With DICOM standard medical imaging have gained acceptance in medical fraternity and there is a need for protection of infrastructure over which this image travel.

MEDICAL IMAGING AND INFORMATION ASSURANCE

Patient electronic record may contain details about diagnosis, images, doctors' notes, medicines, patient health, various clinical test records and patient medical history. There are strict legislations in various countries governing medical domain records. But merely complying with these legislations does not guarantee the security of medical data. There are much more complex requirements which can only be satisfied with planned and systematic approach of **Information Assurance** (C.D. Schou, 2004). Information assurance is required for protecting the critical information systems infrastructure. At the centre of information assurance is the five information security requirements which are:

1. **Confidentiality:** It allows only authorized users to have an access to the designated information.
2. **Integrity:** This control ensures that information has not been modified in any way during its transmission from source to destination.
3. **Authenticity:** This control ensures that information is issued from the right source and is about the intended entity only.
4. **Availability:** It is related to having an access to designated information systems and data under normal operative conditions.
5. **Non-repudiation:** It is an assurance whereby parties with mutual interest cannot back off from the claim of transaction that occurs in between them. It provides the confirmation of deliverance and identity proofs to each party involved in transaction.

There are various types of threats to each of these security services. For example keeping interest of medical information systems the following are common confidentiality and integrity threats which are as follows:

Confidentiality Threats

1. Illegal interception of the message on communication channel during its travel.
2. Illegal break-in the data base of the system.
3. Inserting a virus or a trojan into the system such that access is always open.
4. Compromise with the access control rights of the authorized personnel.
5. Rerouting the information along unauthorized paths.

Integrity Threats

1. Malicious manipulation of data by interception on the channel.
2. Destroying or modifying content of the database with unauthorized access.
3. Injecting worm, trojan, or virus into the data base for manipulations.

There are various types of mechanism to overcome these threats like confidentiality can be restored through controlled access and securing the protocol on the communication channel. The commonly used solutions are symmetric key or asymmetric key algorithms and digital signatures which are discussed next.

Symmetric Key Algorithms

These methods are based on algorithm for encryption and decryption with shared key in between two involved parties. The important issue with symmetric key algorithm is about key distribution and management. The issue becomes more serious when large number of people gets involved. It is also expected from the concerned parties to protect their keys and keep them secret. They also are advised to change their keys frequently to avoid any mishaps. As per classical Kerchoff's assumption key length would govern the security. Normally longer key lengths are desirable with minimum value of 128 bits. However longer key length means more algorithm processing time. Some typical symmetric key algorithms are DES and IDEA.

Asymmetric Key Algorithms

These methods are based on using two separate keys for embedding and extraction algorithms. One of the key is made public and other one kept secret. Sender will encrypt the message with the receiver public key. Encrypted message is transmitted and it is decrypted with the receiver own private / secret key. The asymmetric algorithms majorly involve mathematical operations of multiplication, division and exponentiation. The asymmetric key algorithms are basis for Deffi-Hellman, RSA algorithms.

Digital Signature

Medical image integrity control can be obtained by using Digital Signature (DS) which can be computed over whole of image or over some of its specific characteristics. If whole image content is used, then integrity check aims for "exact" authentication. Any difference in recomputed DS and embedded DS will indicate loss of integrity. Even a change in one bit will cause loss of integrity in case of exact authentication. However DS has an advantage that it is legally recognized in many countries.

The solution to restore integrity control is similar to restoring confidentiality measures. It must be kept in mind that designing for exact integrity control could be a very conservative approach. For example captured medical images have to undergo several non malicious and necessary steps during preprocessing. For example change in brightness level and in case of a very strict integrity control can flag off the loss of integrity which may not be the desired result. It is also very important to identify stage in processing which can be used to establish the integrity of the medical image and act as a reference stage / model for integrity control. However it can be very interesting to know about the short coming of these approaches.

Issues with Conventional Cryptographic Security Mechanism

Each of the conventional security mechanisms has their limitations. The cryptographic security mechanisms are no exceptions. During the storage and transmission cryptographic tools are extensively used. However "man in middle" can actually see the communication happening on to the channel, even though could be in encrypted form. These tools are also extremely sensitive to changes in the data formats and even a non malicious format change can trigger "alarm". These tools are also extremely susceptible to bit errors due to noisy communication channel. It will be more problematic when "exact" authentication is desirable and results may change due to error in one bit of information. Data is also available in "clear" at the receiver after its decryption and someone with unauthorized access can tap in. These tools require "communication with side information" meaning that there is always a need for a separate communication channel for transfer of side information like a key, or a signature. Looking into these issues watermarking is seen as a "complementary" technology to strengthen the security mechanism for medical images. Watermarking cannot replace the cryptographic mechanism but definitely can add a lot of advantage to its usage.

MEDICAL IMAGING AND WATERMARKING

Watermarking in general is looked upon as a technology for protection of copyright. Growing research interest in watermarking has led to development of several new ideas and proposals. Digitization of information in medical sciences has made watermarking an obvious choice to resolve several issues. Thus watermarking has emerged as an alternative mechanism to provide security to EPR. Watermarking involves insertion of some data known as watermark into the host content which could be image, video, text or audio clips. The broad objectives for watermarking in medical domain documents are as follows:

1. Data protection with integrity control.
2. Data protection with authenticity control.
3. Data protection with confidentiality control.
4. Data hiding for improving the usability of image with application like annotations.

Watermarking can be done in pixel / spatial domain or transform domain. Transform domain watermarking involves usage of frequency domain where in specific properties of transform can be exploited to strengthen the watermarking. Some of the important properties of watermark for medical domain are as follows (some of them are common with other application domain):

1. The inserted watermark should remain invisible.
2. It should be non-interfering with the host content.
3. It should have large embedding capacity.
4. It should improve security.

5. It should be robust.

The watermark has several advantages as compared to the other conventional security mechanisms like cryptography and they are summarized as below:

1. Watermarking allows security at the lowest level i.e. data level because watermark is embedded into the host.
2. It provides information protection even if the host presentation format is changed.
3. It provides security even if the data appears in "clear".
4. In case of cryptography, the encrypted text can be seen travelling on the communication channel but it may not be the case in invisible watermarking.

However there are several technical, legal, social challenges before the application of watermarking (G. Coatrieux, 2000; G. Coatrieux, 2006) and they are:

1. It is not recognized legally in many countries.
2. It introduces a completely new security layer and it is expected that it will provide protection during transmission, storage and processing without interfering with content.
3. The added watermark may change the data in irreversible fashion.
4. If the embedded watermark has high energy it may mask the lower energy details of the host.
5. The watermark insertion should preserve the "diagnosable" quality even if it alters the host document in an irreversible way.
6. Computational complexity for a real time performance is utmost important. Watermarking embedding and extraction algorithms should be designed in a manner to minimize the computational cost.

WATERMARKING TECHNIQUES IN MEDICAL DOMAIN FOR CONFIDENTIALITY, INTEGRITY AND AUTHENTICATION CONTROL

Three types of watermarking techniques have been identified for integrity and authentication control. These methods are as follows:

1. Reversible watermarking techniques.
2. Methods which embeds the watermark in Region of No Interest (RNI).
3. Methods which embeds the watermark in Region of Interest (ROI) with minimal distortion criteria in place.

Reversible Watermarking Techniques

In these techniques original contents are recovered after watermark is detected, decoded and removed from the medical image. However most of the reversible watermarking techniques suffer from very low embedding capacity and methods may sometimes generate unwarranted salt and pepper noise. These methods are can be used as a fragile domain watermarking methods thus it can provide solution for integrity and authentication control. Fragile domain watermarking can also be developed such that they provide integrity control only in case of severe intentional manipulations. For unintended non malicious manipulations data integrity should be preserved. For reversible watermarking security is similar to conventional cryptographic approach as after watermark is removed from the host, content is no longer secure. However if the watermark is recovered without any loss it is a parameter for image integrity. The advantages with reversible watermarking techniques are that image pre processing can be applied to whole of a medical image which may not be the case with RNI based methods. In RNI watermarking preprocessing has to be kept away from the RNI where watermark is embedded. Two types of reversible watermarking techniques exist:

1. Additive rule based
2. Substitution rule based

Additive Rule Based Reversible Watermarking Techniques

In case of an additive rule base, watermark w is added to the host medical image I with some watermark scaling factor α resulting in watermarked image I_w.

$$I_w = I + \alpha w \qquad (1)$$

These kinds of techniques are very popular in the spatial domain. Addition may lead to overshoot / undershoot in the pixel values and they may fall outside the prescribed range. The overshoot and undershoot can also occur in the transform domain. A strategy to overcome overshoot and undershoot issues includes utilizing modulo arithmetic. One of the approaches (C. W. Honsinger, 1999) is to use

$$I_w = (I + \alpha w) \bmod 2 \qquad (2)$$

where n is the number of bits required to represent grey scale. However due to sudden discontinuous jumps they tend to produce salt and pepper noise. An improvisation can be done if modulo rule is applied over smaller range of scale as compared to whole range at once (J. Fridrich, 2001). In another approach (G. Coatrieux, 2005) the host image pixels are identified which can undergo overshoot/undershoot if watermark is embedded in them. These pixels should be avoided for embedding the watermark. Watermark is inserted into the rest of the pixels. The pixel selection criteria can be shared with the decoder, which can be used to find the potentially watermark pixels while avoiding others. The method used by Xuan *et al.* (G.R. Xuan, 2006) utilize the shift in the range of histogram. This range can be found by looking for a gray scale with least and highest number of pixels. This range is shifted by adding or subtracting one gray level. Embedded data cannot be recovered unless the initial maxima are known to the receiver. Authors used wavelet domain which gives laplacian distribution to the coefficients and they are distributed around zero mean.

Substitution Based Reversible Watermarking Techniques

These methods replace the content of host image rather than modifying them. Fridrich *et al.* (J. Fridrich, 2001) tries to locate a bit plane in an image. If it is available then it can be losslessly compressed. The bit plane can also be replaced by the compressed version of the watermark. However the embedding capacity is extremely low. J. Tian (J. Tian, 2003) proposed an expansion embedding reversible watermarking technique. It shifts the binary representation of gray level value of pixel to the left. This creates a virtually new space for embedding. It applies this scheme to the difference of two pixel values. In similar manner Lee *et. al* (S. Lee, 2007) utilize expansion embedding to insert watermark into high frequency coefficients of 16 x 16 blocks. They have a very small location map which can very easily be shared. W. Pan *et. al* (W. Pan, 2009) tested the existing approaches in reversible watermarking on different modalities of images like MRI, PET and USG. They prepared a comparison matrix for these modalities images in terms of capacity and robustness. Their conclusion suggested that methods are dependent on watermarking algorithms and also the medical image modality. Zhicheng Ni *et. al* (Zhicheng Ni, 2008) developed a robust lossless data hiding technique, which is salt-and-pepper noise proof. They used a statistical quantity derived from patchwork theory, used a distribution for them and with error control coding like BCH codes obtained reversibility and robustness. It has been successfully applied to many images, thus demonstrating its generality. Their experiments indicated good perceptual quality and robustness

against compression. They showed authentication for losslessly compressed JPEG2000 images.

Watermarking in RNI

These methods embed the watermark in the area of medical images which are not critical from diagnostics perspective and hence will not significantly affect the final diagnostic outcome. The RNI normally corresponds to dark areas in medical images. Thus perceptual transparency criteria for watermark can be more lenient and there is no intrusion of watermark with area of interest. These watermarking methods can have a very high capacity due to reduced perceptual requirement and also they can provide good robustness. However the capacity of such methods is dependent on

1. Size of the RNI
2. Texture of RNI
3. Gray scale value within RNI

The embedding capacity is dependent on the modality of the medical image. The images drawn from different modalities will have different sizes of RNI. If the watermark amplitude is very high this methods can cause irritating salt and pepper pattern in the watermarked image. These methods can only be deployed if there is a presence of RNI in the medical image otherwise they are rendered unusable. Also there are some security issues involved with these methods like attacker can distort, already existing watermark by inserting new watermarks into RNI. Wakatani (Wakatani, A, 2002) suggested a medical image watermarking method that embeds watermark in the RNI. It preserves the image quality in RNI, but attackers can render this method useless by inserting multiple watermarks in RNI and also it is susceptible to copy attacks in RNI. Giakoumaki *et al.* (Giakoumaki, A., 2003) embeds watermark into wavelet domain. They used a multiple watermarking scheme and applied two watermarks to the medical images. They attained confidentiality and integrity control however image visual quality was mediocre with lower values of peak signal to noise ratio (PSNR).

Watermarking in ROI

These methods fall under the traditional watermarking paradigm. The aim of these methods is to reduce the distortion caused due to watermark embedding. The embedding of watermark can be into area of interest i.e. area which can be used for the diagnosis by the medical practitioner. Hence while designing these methods; one can consider Just Noticeable Difference (JND) of Human Visual System (HVS) or maximum power distortion criteria caused due to watermark embedding. Keeping the distortion level below computed threshold values will improve the quality of methods. The maximum power distortion can change even if medical image undergoes non malicious manipulation like intensity changes. A. Piva *et al.* (A. Piva, 2005) presented a data hiding schemes based on high capacity, perceptual transparency, and robustness. They evaluated scheme for embedding patient information into digital radiography medical images. Their algorithm was based on decision theory and they modeled this problem as a "communication problem with side information". The developed methods were tested for digital radiographies images. Jasni M Zain *et al.* (Jasni M Zain, 2006) made a case study to see whether medical diagnosis gets affected by the watermarking in different modalities of medical images. They embedded 256 bits watermark to RNI in different medical images and 48000 bits in both ROI and RNI. They presented watermarked medical images to various radiologists for blind evaluation. They claim that watermarking did not affect the clinical diagnosis of the experts. Radiologists also could not pinpoint difference in watermarked and original image and therefore conclusion was drawn that medical images are safe for digital watermarking embedding.

Watermarking Methods for Improving the Usability of Medical Images

The purpose of this type of approach is to make image more useful, instructive, and usable by insertion of information pertaining to it. Authors in (G. Coatrieux, 2009) embed the medical image with a summary of its associated data base. It improves the functionality of application like e-learning and tele-diagnosis. The summary of associated database was used as a watermark. Their aim of embedding such an information is to retrieve the images with similar / dissimilar diagnosis. Watermark provides the descriptors of images and the descriptors for the diagnosis. Watermark is embedded in the pixel domain. It also provides integrity and authenticity control. Authors also demonstrated an e-learning application for endoscopic application. Shan He *et al.* (Shan He, 2009) proposed a method which gives a high perceptual fidelity to the medical images. Their method utilizes watermarking for annotation and gives robustness to reasonable distortion. They used a perceptual model to quantify tolerable threshold of noise within the local regions. They used two watermarks: one indicating a presence of watermark and other with slightly high capacity (few dozen bits). Their objective is to embed 32 bits of metadata which remains robust to JPEG compression and cropping. Method used a database with large smooth regions. S. cheng *et al.* (S. Cheng, 2005) embedded indexing information in the host for identification. This can enable an efficient searching management of the given multimedia content. G. Coatrieux *et al.* (G. Coatrieux, 2005) extended the approach and suggested to embed the diagnostic information about the identified disease within the medical image. This can help in management of knowledge database. The medical image can contain an emblematic explanation of the attributes which makes searching in the database lot faster and meaningful. Thus it can improve the data mining and data base search applications. The security of the database can be improved and error controlling is possible.

PRACTICAL IMPLEMENTATION OF WATERMARKING SCHEME

Two schemes for watermarking are implemented to understand the concepts covered in the earlier parts of the chapter. Schemes implemented are:

1. Correlation based reversible watermarking technique
2. Reversible watermarking techniques using difference expansion (Tian, 2003).

Experimentation for reversible watermarking using difference expansion is based on the method proposed by J.Tian *et al* (2003).

Correlation Based Reversible Watermarking Technique

Medical images require "exact authentication" during transmission and any impairment to the image can have severe consequences. This work aims at providing an exact authentication to medical image through "reversible or erasable watermark". The features of this method are:

1. This method provides exact recovery of the original image at the recipient end after removal of watermark from the image.
2. The creator of the image computes a signature using information in an image and then embeds signature in an erasable manner within the image. This signature / hash / image-digest is unique for each image.
3. The recipient of the image extracts and records the embedded signature. The recipient removes the watermark and the resultant image is identical to original un-watermarked image.

4. Recipient computes a one way hash and compares it with a hash decoded from the signature. If the two hashes are identical, received image is authentic.
5. Watermark has same size as that of cover image. Predefined value of α is used in embedding and recipient knows this value (like a private key).

Watermark Embedding Algorithm

1. Compute forward DCT and extract DC coefficients.
2. Select ten highest DC coefficients to generate hash.
3. Use hash as a seed to generate a random pattern (W').
4. Generate the watermark (W) for the cover image (C) using the random pattern as follows:

W = W', if message-bit to be embedded is 1
W = -W', if message-bit to be embedded is 0

i.e. depending upon the bit to be embedded in C, select either W' or −W'. The watermarked image C_m is,

$$C_m = C + \alpha W \tag{3}$$

where α is a constant for scaling.

Watermark Extraction Algorithm

1. Any attack will introduce some distortion in C_m.
2. Generate watermark using seed (same value as in embedding).
3. Compute linear correlation between received image and watermark.
4. Bit detected is "1" if result of correlation exceeds threshold τ. Bit is "0" if correlation is below negative value of threshold (-τ).
5. Determine watermark W from detected bit,

Figure 1. Recovery in absence of any attack

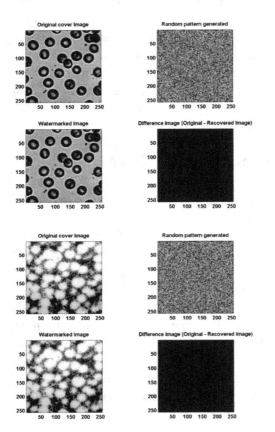

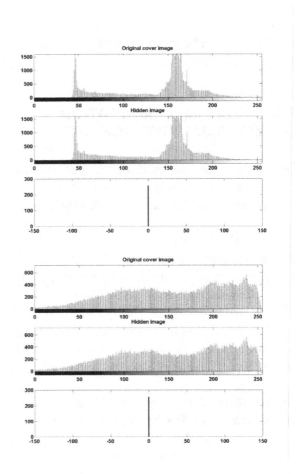

i.e. W = W', if bit is 1
  W = -W', if bit is 0

6. Subtract watermark W from received image

$$C' = C - \alpha W \tag{4}$$

7. Subtract received image from original (recovered) image to detect tampering. The difference image will be zero if C'=C. C'≠ C shows tampering at the locations.

The value of threshold τ is very critical. If it is too low, the false acceptance rate will be high. If it is too high, false rejection rate will be high. From the results of a number of experiments, a value was selected so as to minimize these error rates.

Experimentations

- After the removal of the watermark "original" image should be available to user. This is necessary in the medical field as "perfect diagnosis" is a must.
- Experimentation in this case is done on medical images of size 256 x 256, 178 x 178.
- The recovery of watermark is shown for
  - Absence of any attack.
  - JPEG compression with Q=100.
  - Low intensity noise addition (Gaussian and speckle).
  - Median filtering.

Figure 2. Image recovery with JPEG Compression with Q=100

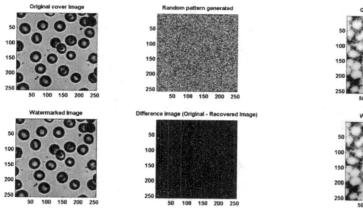

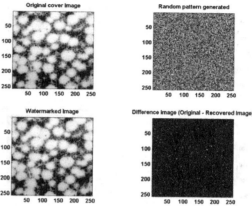

- Watermark used in this case is random noise pattern having same size as that of cover image.

The result of experimentation is shown in Figures 1-5. Table 2 reflects the performance parameter variation for different types of medical images under test. The results are displayed in the manner described in Table 1 for this method.

For histogram plots x axis shows gray scale value y axis shows number of occurrence for particular gray scale in image. Third histogram indicates plot for difference image.)

Observations

- This work deals with "exact authentication" and experimentation has succeeded in attaining the goal.
- After the removal of watermark from the image, in absence of any attack, original image is available.
- Histograms of original and watermarked image are identical.
- JPEG compression with Q=100 creates watermarked image identical to the original image. Difference image (between

Figure 3. Gaussian and Speckle Noise addition

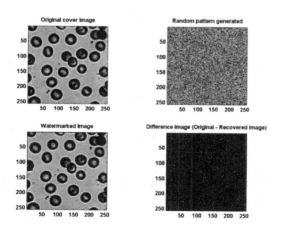

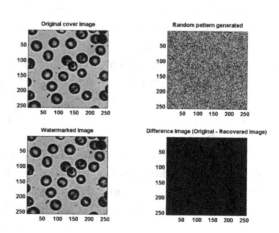

Figure 4. Localization of tampered area

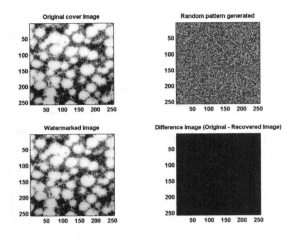

Figure 5. Median filtering to watermarked image

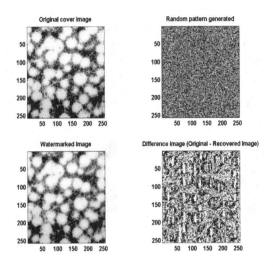

Table 1.

Original Image	Random Pattern as Water-mark
Watermarked Image	Difference Image

original and hidden image) generated by the algorithm reveals the changes. Thus, method developed is extremely sensitive to any trivial changes.

- Watermarked image is subjected to low intensity noise like Gaussian (zero mean and 0.000001 variance) and speckle. Such low intensity noise is deliberately added to generate perceptually identical water-marked image and cover image. The difference image discloses changes made to the original image.
- Localization of the tampered area is visible in the experimentation. This aids in detection of ruined part within image. The difference image indicates the region for distortion.
- Correlation based detector is used in this method. It indicates the presence or absence watermark depending on correlation value obtained. The threshold value at the

detector plays a very important role. Poor selection of threshold can result in false positive or negative errors.

REVERSIBLE WATERMARKING TECHNIQUES USING DIFFERENCE EXPANSION

Data Embedding and Extraction Algorithm

Difference Expansion basis: for a pair of pixel values *(x,y)* in a grayscale image, define their average *l* and difference *h* as,

$$l = \lfloor (x + y) / 2 \rfloor$$

$$h = x - y \tag{6}$$

The inverse transformation of (1) is

$$x = l + \lfloor (h + 1) / 2 \rfloor, y = l - \lfloor h / 2 \rfloor \tag{7}$$

The equation 6 and 7 are basis of difference expansion method.

Table 2. Performance parameter for erasable watermarking problem

SF	Seed for transmitter	Recovered Seed for receiver	Mean of original Cover Image	Mean of Hidden Image	Variance of Original Image	Variance of Hidden Image	MSE between Original and recovered Image
Spinegray.tif (without any attack)							
JPEG Compression Q=100							
1.0000	488.8224	488.8224	61.1028	61.1027	4258.7799	4258.9111	27.5417
Gaussian noise mean 0,variance 0.000001							
1.0000	488.8224	488.8989	61.1028	61.1124	4258.7799	4257.6130	19.8361
Salt and pepper Noise							
0.9700	488.8224	494.1494	61.1028	61.7687	4258.7799	4422.2634	121162.15
Localization							
1.0000	488.8224	488.8227	61.1028	61.1028	4258.7799	4258.7910	0.2028
Median Filtering							
1.0000	488.8224	488.7624	61.1028	61.0953	4258.7799	4253.3900	350.2500
Bacteriagray.tif (without any attack)							
1.0000	1006.4287	1006.4287	129.0000	129.0000	1417.2552	1417.2552	0.0000
JPEG Compression with Q=100							
1.0000	1006.4287	1006.4287	129.0000	129.0000	1417.2552	1418.0015	14.3920
Gaussian noise mean0,variance 0.000001							
1.0000	1006.4287	1006.4236	129.0000	129.0000	1417.2552	1417.3150	8.4432
Salt and pepper Noise							
0.9900	1006.4287	1006.1829	129.0000	129.0000	1417.2552	1574.7410	35116.5795
Localization							
1.0000	1006.4287	1006.4277	129.0000	129.0000	1417.2552	1417.2607	0.4318
Median Filtering							
1.0000	1006.4287	1006.5671	129.0000	129.0000	1417.2552	1393.6612	728.2159

Data Embedding

Split the original image into non-overlapping blocks with 8 x 8 pixels. Every block, is decomposed by 1-level IWT (Integer Wavelet Transform), and it produces a low frequency sub-band (4 x 4 matrix). Pair of diagonal pixels in a 4x4 block is checked for expandability. Grayscale-valued pair is expandable, if it satisfies the following condition,

$$0 \le \lfloor 2h + b \rfloor \le \min(2(255 - l), 2l + 1) \qquad (8)$$

for both $b=0$ and $b=1$.

If the pair of a diagonal pixels in 4x4 block are expandable, then we use '1' to stand for the attribute, else '0' is used to represent the attribute of that block. Data is embedded only in block with attribute '1'. Calculate the average and difference for the ith pair of pixels, by using equation (6).

$$h_i' = 2h_i + w_i$$

where w_i is the corresponding bit of data. Calculating new i^{th} pair of pixels (x_i', y_i') after embedding watermark by the following form.

Figure 6. Lena: Original image, watermarked image, histogram and binary data pattern

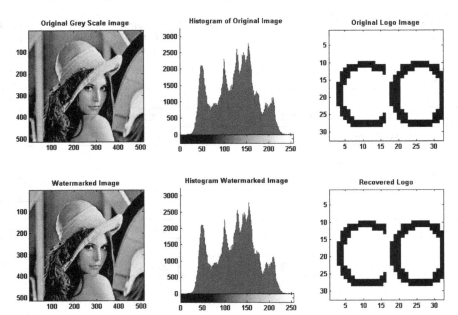

$$x_i^{'} = l_i + \left\lfloor (h_i^{'} + 1)/2 \right\rfloor, y_i^{'} = l_i - \left\lfloor h_i^{'}/2 \right\rfloor \qquad (9)$$

$$l^{'} = \left\lfloor (x^{'} + y^{'})/2 \right\rfloor, h^{'} = x^{'} - y^{'} \qquad (10)$$

Repeat the steps until all pixel pairs are processed. Perform the inversion to construct stego image by using new coordinates. The attribute signature will contain 4096 bits, one for each block. In this method this signature is shared with the receiver.

Data Extraction Algorithm

Split the original image into non-overlapping blocks with 8 x 8 pixels. The expansible blocks are decomposed by 1-level wavelet lifting scheme. The expansible blocks are found from attribute map which is shared with transmitter. For pair of pixels and of low frequency sub-band, the following procedures are adopted to extract data. Calculate the average and difference of the pair of pixels as

Extract data using $w = LSB(h^{'})$.   (11)

Experiments and Results

The proposed algorithm is tested on various images with size 512 x 512. The data to be embedded is a visible binary pattern of size 32 x 32. Various statistical parameters are derived like mean, variance, MSE in between the original and watermarked image to prove the statistical transparency of the algorithm. Test image, data to be embedded, recovered data, histograms of original and data embedded image is shown in Figures 6-9.

Table 3 indicates the various statistical parameters between the original image and stego image to prove the statistical and perceptual transparency. Perceptual transparency is quantified by computing a similarity Factor (SF) between the original and watermarked image.

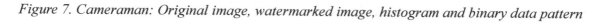

Figure 7. Cameraman: Original image, watermarked image, histogram and binary data pattern

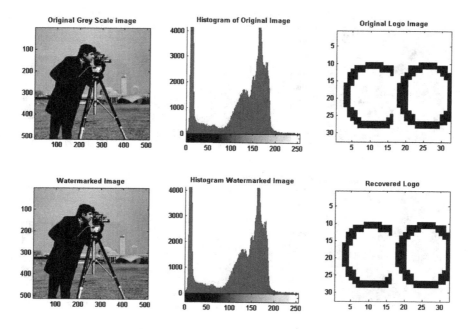

Figure 8. Mandrill: Original image, watermarked image, histogram and binary data pattern

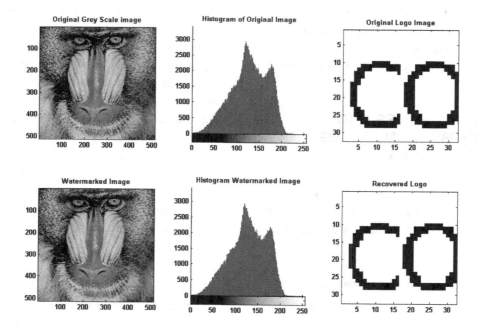

It is seen from the experimentation that stego image maintains an excellent perceptual and statistical transparency. The quantitative support to above reasoning is also visible from Table 3. The stego image exhibits an excellent perceptual quality indicated by Similarity Factor (SF) of 1

Figure 9. Pirate: Original image, watermarked image, histogram and binary data pattern

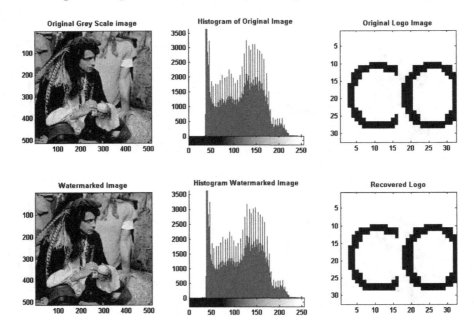

which is a normalized correlation. The method uses a wavelet lifting scheme thus its capacity can be improved. The low frequency band is used for embedding, thus the method can further be developed for high capacity robust applications.

ISSUES CHALLENGES AND FUTURE OF WATERMARKING IN MEDICAL DOMAIN

There is a tremendous scope for applying watermarking to medical field but it has not been fully explored. Many newer medical applications domains like in teaching, health care, research, administration, data base management, data archiving, data mining are opening and they are to be completely explored. Data hiding applications can provide a very good interface and security to the medical data base. However there are some important limitations of watermarking when applied to medical domain has to be considered:

- Capacity of the watermark without causing a significant damage to the diagnostic sensitivity is an utmost important issue.
- The computational cost of embedding and extraction watermarking also pays a signif-

Table 3. Indicating various parameters

Image	Mean Original	Mean Stego	Median Original	Median Stego	MSE	PSNR	SF
Lena	124.0500	124.0557	129	129	0.5881	50.4364	1
Cameraman	118.6496	118.6559	143	143	0.1980	55.1649	1
Mandrill	128.4792	128.4838	129	129	3.3244	42.9136	1
Pirate	111.6399	111.6452	117	117	1.0728	47.8254	1

icant role in deciding the responses from the physicians and popularity of watermarking approach. This cost can be more significant in case the 3D volume data processing like MRI or CT scan.

- There is no standardization as far as data hiding in medical domain is concerned. Due to methods tested under the limited set of conditions its universal appeal and applicability is always going to be questioned. Qualitative and quantitative evaluation of watermarking under different conditions and its uniform performance is highly desirable.

- The watermarking scheme should give uniform performance across different modalities of images like radiology, USG, MRI, PET.

It can be seen that for medical domain, data hiding schemes should be robust with minimal or no distortion at all. The developed methods should have universal nature and give similar performance across different modalities and applications. While designing the methods peculiarity about the medical image modality should be kept in perspective. This choice can be beneficial during selection of host coefficients used for embedding the watermark and indirectly it governs the robustness of method against lossy compression. The statistical parameter drawn for set of medical images are very different from the set of natural images and this fact should be considered while testing watermarking / data hiding methods for medical domain. The methods which are evolving seem to have fair amount of flexibility in terms of robustness, capacity and distortion criteria. The combination of different RNI, ROI and reversible watermarking techniques can have a large amount of flexibility in terms of above parameters. Watermarking along with the cryptographic solutions seems to be a proper approach till the watermarking or data hiding techniques gain technical and legal acceptability in the public at large. Even

the combination of data hiding techniques with biometrics can provide required flexibility for medical domain.

REFERENCES

Cheng, S., Wu, Q., & Castleman, K. R. (2005). Non-ubiquitous digital watermarking for record indexing and integrity protection of medical images. *Proceedings of ICIP*, *2*, 1062–1065.

Coatrieux, G., Lamard, M., Daccache, W., Puentes, J., & Roux, C. (2005). A low distortion and reversible watermark application to angiographic images of the retina. *Proceedings of the IEEE EMBC Conference, Shanghai, China, 2005*, (pp. 2224–2227).

Coatrieux, G., Lamard, M., Daccache, W., Puentes, J., & Roux, C. (2005). A low distortion and reversible watermark: Application to angiographic images of the retina. *Proceedings of the 27th IEEE EMBS Annual International Conference, 2005*, (pp. 2224-2227).

Coatrieux, G., le Guillou, C., Cauvin, J.-M., & Roux, C. (2009). Reversible watermarking for knowledge digest embedding and reliability control in medical images. *IEEE Transactions on Information Technology in Biomedicine*, *13*(2), 158–165. doi:10.1109/TITB.2008.2007199

Coatrieux, G., Lecornu, L., Roux, C., & Sankur, B. (2006). *A review of image watermarking applications in healthcare*. (pp. 4691–4694). 28th IEEE EMBS Annual International Conference, Aug 30-Sept. 3, 2006, New York.

Coatrieux, G., Maître, H., Sankur, B., Rolland, Y., & Collorec, R. (2000). Relevance of watermarking in medical imaging. (pp. 250–255). *Proceedings of the IEEE International Conference ITAB, USA*.

DICOM standard. (2010). *NEMA information*. Retrieved from http://medical.nema.org

Fridrich, J., Goljan, J., & Du, R. (2001). Invertible authentication. *Proceedings of International Conference SPIE, Security and Watermarking of Multimedia Content, San Jose, CA, Jan. 2001*, (pp. 197-208).

Giakoumaki, A., Pavlopulos, S., & Koutouris, D. (2003). A medical image watermarking scheme based on wavelet transform. *Proceedings of the 25th IEEE EMBS Annual International Conference, 17-21 Sept. 2003, Vol. 1*, (pp. 856-859).

He, S., Kirovski, D., & Wu, M. (2009). High-fidelity data embedding for image annotation. *IEEE Transactions on Image Processing, 18*(2), 429–435. doi:10.1109/TIP.2008.2008733

Honsinger, C. W., Jones, P., Rabbani, M., & Stoffel, J. C. (1999). *Lossless recovery of an original image containing embedded data*. US patent, docket no.:77102/E-D.

Lee, S., Yoo, C. D., & Kalker, T. (2007). Reversible image watermarking based on integer-to-integer wavelet transform information forensics and security. *IEEE Transactions Information Forensics and Security, 2*(3), 321–330. doi:10.1109/TIFS.2007.905146

Ni, Z., Shi, Y. Q., Ansari, N., Su, W., Sun, Q., & Lin, X. (2008). Robust lossless image data hiding designed for semi-fragile image authentication. *IEEE Transactions on Circuits and Systems for Video Technology, 18*(4), 497–508. doi:10.1109/TCSVT.2008.918761

Pan, W., Coatrieux, G., Montagner, J., Cuppens, N., Cuppens, F., & Roux, C. (2009). Comparison of some reversible watermarking methods in application to medical images. *Proceedings of the 31ˢᵗ IEEE EMBS Annual International Conference, September 2-6, 2009, Minneapolis, Minnesota, US*, (pp. 2172 – 2175).

Piva, A., Barni, M., Bartolini, F., & De Rosa, A. (2005). Data hiding technologies for digital radiography. *IEEE Proceedings of Visual Image Signal Processing, 152*(5), 604–610. doi:10.1049/ip-vis:20041240

Ryszard, T., & Marek, R. O. (2004). *Medical imaging understanding technology*. Springer Verlag.

Schou, C. D., Frost, J., & Maconachy, W. V. (2004). Information assurance in biomedical informatics systems. *IEEE Engineering in Medicine and Biology Magazine, 23*(1), 110–118. doi:10.1109/MEMB.2004.1297181

Tian, J. (2003). Reversible data embedding using a difference expansion. *IEEE Transactions on Circuits and Systems for Video Technology, 13*(8), 890–896. doi:10.1109/TCSVT.2003.815962

Wakatani, A. (2002). Digital watermarking for ROI medical images by using compressed signature image. *Proceedings of the the Annual Hawaii International Conference on System Sciences (HICSS) 2002, Jan.7-10*, (pp. 2043-2048).

Xuan, G. R., Yao, Q. M., Yang, C., & Gao, J. (2006). *Lossless data hiding using histogram shifting method based on integer wavelets*. (LNCS-4283). (pp. 323-332).

Zain, J. M., Fauzi, A. R. M., & Aziz, A. A. (2006). Clinical evaluation of watermarked medical images. *Proceedings of the 28th IEEE EMBS Annual International Conference, New York City, USA, Aug 30-Sept 3, 2006*, (pp. 5459-5462).

ADDITIONAL READING

Barni, M., & Bartolini, F. (2004). Data hiding for fighting piracy. *IEEE Signal Processing Magazine*, 28–39. doi:10.1109/MSP.2004.1276109

Chao, H.-M., Hsu, C.-M., & Miaou, S.-G. (2002). A Data-Hiding Technique with Authentication, Integration and Confidentiality for Electronic Patient Records. *IEEE Transactions on Information Technology in Biomedicine*, 6(1), 46–53. doi:10.1109/4233.992161

Cosman, P. C., Gray, R. M., & Olshen, R. A. (1994). Evaluating quality of compressed medical images: SNR, Subjective Rating, and Diagnostic Accuracy. *Proceedings of the IEEE*, 82(6), 919–932. doi:10.1109/5.286196

Cox, I., Miller, M., & Bloom, J. (2008). *Digital Watermarking and steganography 2/e Burlington M.A.* Morgan Kaufmann.

Eskicioglu, A. M., & Fisher, P. S. (1995). Image quality measures and their performance. *IEEE Transactions on Communications*, 43(12), 2959–2965. doi:10.1109/26.477498

Karunasekera, S. A., & Kingsbury, N. G. (1995). A Distortion Measure for Blocking Artifacts in Images Based on Human Visual Sensitivity. *IEEE Transactions on Image Processing*, 4(6), 713–724. doi:10.1109/83.388074

Luiz, O. M. K., Furuie, S. S., & Barreto, P. S. L. M. (2009). Providing Integrity and Authenticity in DICOM Images: A Novel Approach. *IEEE Transactions on Information Technology in Biomedicine*, 13(4), 582–589. doi:10.1109/TITB.2009.2014751

Zhou, X. Q., Huang, H. K., & Lou, S. L. (2001). Authenticity and Integrity of Digital Mammography Images. *IEEE Transactions on Medical Imaging*, 20(8), 784–791. doi:10.1109/42.938246

KEY TERMS AND DEFINITIONS

Content Authentication: This is one of the security controls ensuring legitimacy of the content being referred.

Copyright Protection: This protection enables the creator to establish rights over the generated digital content. Robustness is one of the important properties of copyright protection.

Data Hiding: This term encompasses the general domain for hiding the data within the digital content. It includes the domain of watermarking, steganography, fragile watermarking, and reversible watermarking.

Electronic Patient Record (EPR): This is the electronic version of patient medical record.

Information Assurance: This is a broad term indicating mechanisms and policies for protection of medical information infrastructure.

Medical Image: The two dimensional data indicating the information about the internals of human body.

Watermarking: This term is used for specifying the data hiding application meant to provide robust copyright protection to generated digital content.

Chapter 4
Vertebral Morphometry in Forensics

Giuseppe Guglielmi
University of Foggia, Italy & Scientific Institute Hospital, Italy

Stefano D'Errico
University of Foggia, Italy

Cristoforo Pomara
University of Foggia, Italy

Vittorio Fineschi
University of Foggia, Italy

ABSTRACT

Imaging techniques (plain radiographs, multi slice computed tomography (MSCT), and magnetic resonance (MRI)) are being increasingly implemented in forensic pathology. These methods may serve as an adjuvant to classic forensic medical diagnosis and as support to forensic autopsies. It is well noted that various post-processing techniques can provide strong forensic evidence for use in legal proceedings. This chapter reviews vertebral morphometry application in forensic, expressly used in the case of semi-automatic digital recognition of vertebral heights in fractures, by means of vertebral shape analysis which relies on six or more points positioned over the margins of each vertebrae T5 to L4 used to calculate anterior, medial, and posterior heights and statistical shape models. This approach is quantitative, more reproducible, and more feasible for large-scale data analysis, as in drug trials, where assessment may be performed by a variety of clinicians with different levels of experience. As a result, a number of morphometric methodologies for characterisation of osteoporosis have been developed. Current morphometric methodologies have the drawback of relying upon manual annotations. The manual placement of morphometric points on the vertebrae is time consuming, requiring more than 10 min per radiograph and can be quite subjective. Several semi-automated software have been produced to overcome this problem, but they are mainly applicable to dual X-ray absorptiometry (DXA) scans. Furthermore, this chapter aims to verify by an experimental model if the technique could contribute, in present or in future, to investigate the modality of traumatic vertebral injuries which may explain the manner of death.

DOI: 10.4018/978-1-60960-483-7.ch004

FORENSIC APPLICATION OF RADIOLOGY

The improvement and evolution of radiological sciences toward a broader definition of the technical parameters meant to study the details of the human body and its components, both in an anatomical–structural and physiological–physiopathological sense, brought radiology and forensic medicine closer together. In fact, the study and interpretation of anatomical reports is the principal aim in both.

The methodological and operational approach between the two disciplines has roots dating to the first uses of traditional radiology for the study and report of foreign bodies retained in the corpse. Back in the 1970s in the United States, the American College of Pathologists signaled the importance of the correct use of a preventive radiographic inquiry in some deaths and, concurrent with its introduction, studied the use of ecoguided techniques of anatomical sampling. In 1982 in Italy, Pierucci edited a handbook for the correct use of radiography in the study of deaths by firearms, which immediately gained credibility for the discipline. The prior identification of bullets held undamaged or in fragments was considered essential for a correct cross-sectional experiment. It was as essential as their consequential removal and report. In the 20 years and more since and especially in the last few years, the increasing availability—practically and economically—of eidologic exams has allowed the two disciplines to work in close collaboration, refining methods and gaining experience.

Postmortem radiography is an important part of a complete forensic examination. A radiology table or a portable x-ray machine should be always present in a modern autopsy service. The three-dimensional object is projected on a two dimensional plane and information about the position of an object that lies in the direction of the ray is lost unless a second projection, orthogonal to the first, is also obtained. Wide availability makes radiography a useful application in forensic pathology. A complete Rx examination (total body) is extremely useful for locating bullets or other metallic foreign objects, and its use is well known in forensic pathology for firearms-related fatalities or in cases of unknown or burned cadavers.

A routine anteroposterior and laterolateral radiograph is an acceptable approach to fetus autopsies also for the diagnosis of skeletal abnormalities. Lytic, inflammatory, degenerative, and developmental lesions of bones and joints are particularly best revealed by radiographs.

Computed tomography (CT) uses x-rays to obtain transverse (axial) images of body sections. The tube rotates around the longitudinal (z) axis of the cadaver lying on the CT table, transmitting radiation through the body from many angles. X-rays are absorbed according to the different radiographic density of tissues; those not absorbed reach the detector system beyond the cadaver, contributing to the absorption profile of one specific tube angle. The many profiles measured during one rotation are used by the computer to calculate a density map of the body section with discrete absolute density values of all image elements (voxels). Modern multidetector row scanners (multislice scanner, [MSCT]) are able to acquire information for several slices during one rotation, which can be used to improve z-axis, volume coverage, or speed.

Images of the slice thickness requested will then be calculated from those data at any selected z-axis position within the volume, according to the reconstruction interval chosen. This gives a resolution that is equivalent to isotropic imaging; voxels have similar dimensions in all three axes, for example, 1 mm. Isotropic voxels are ideal for image post-processing using multiplanar reformation to obtain images in sagittal, frontal, or oblique planes, or even three-dimensional presentation methods.

CT application on the postmortem examination allows forensic pathologists an excellent *in situ* reconstruction of injuries (i.e., traffic fatalities, mass disaster, falls) or a complete *in situ* study of a trajectory of bullets (firearm fatalities). It has also been stated that CT study of the cadaver in gunshot-related deaths can be useful in determining firearm distance by detecting gunshot residues deep in the entrance wound.

An unusual application of CT in forensic pathology is in the anthropologic study of body remains. In its original meaning, the word *virtopsy* (*virtual + autopsy*) was meant to refer to a futuristic approach to the cross-sectional experiment based on the use of MSCT equipment and magnetic resonance (1.5 Tesla GE scanner with spectroscopy software). Today, we could associate virtopsy with digital autopsy. Indeed, going through the contents of the scientific work produced until today, it is easy to understand how, in view of the outstanding work performed, digital autopsy hinges well on a basic notion of forensic medicine, that is, the investigation of scientific evidence as means of proof. The necroscopic technique aided by the digital investigation typical of a CT and MNR exam, appears to be really improved in terms of report investigation and inexpensiveness, first for the choice of the cross-sectional technique and, subsequently, for the explanatory capability of the iconography. It is easy to understand the reasons why some authors seek a CT study of the corpse with firearm deaths. A virtopsy can be configured as an observer-independent instrument, which does not alter the reality of the corpse and, since it is digitized and archived, is always repeatable and objectified, even if time has passed. Undoubtedly, the three-dimensional study of the human body (nowadays it is possible to provide up to 64 slices) allows for the finding metallic foreign bodies (e.g.,) and offers an excellent contribution to the exact recognition of intracorporeal internal trajectory (entrance wound) with a precision achieving levels that can be superimposed to the cross-sectional observation.

Actually, before stepping toward the future of the autopsy, it seems appropriate to wonder about its present: do we still need the autopsy? The most recent national and international literature clearly finds that the autopsy is not only necessary, but it must be considered indefeasible. Indeed, as noted earlier, the judicial autopsy is far from exhausting the investigations on the corpse. Autopsy, as an external exam of the corpse and a cross-sectional experiment, is just one (inescapable) approach to the corpse. Perhaps it is not the most important, but it is absolutely preliminary to the correct sampling, collection, and histological study of each organ or part of it.

Toxicological, genetic–forensic investigation, and so on to the most specialized exams of metabolomics or proteomics constitute today the right corollaries to a modern postmortem investigation. In the range of such auxiliary grafts to the main investigation (autopsy), the eidologic–forensic investigation raises to a new dimension, which can be counted with full rights among the means of research for scientific evidence (as such, legitimate and repeatable). Still more in a branch as forensic medicine, which feels the need of such a technique and of its employment as an instrument to reach scientific evidence, impossible to eliminate in the formal structuring of the methodology of penal action.

The awareness of the need for a great guarantee of validity (the best in a technical sense) and the capability to refer to more objective technical–scientific backups, improved the coroners' sensitivity in the last few years; anyway, the autopsy can be improved upon but not replaced. Description of macroscopic features like margins, edges, and auras are indispensable for a correct framing of the death (not just as the causative moment, but the information pertinent to the modus and time of the death).

Nevertheless, the ultimate impetus to the implementation of this methodology in forensic medicine came surely from the evolution of the imaging instruments typical of the CT means, that is, from the introduction of a new multilayer CT apparatus in which the procedure to capture the images is not restricted to single slices of predetermined thickness but to the evaluation of an entire "volume," which can even coincide with the whole human body.

Digital processing of images through last generation software reproduces the composite image in its tridimensionality and therefore are more usable to the unaccustomed eyes of those not specialized in radiology, such as coroners, judges, and lawyers.

Having such diagnostic support in the practice of forensic medicine on the occasion of a necroscopic examination is an extraordinary benefit, including the possibility to proceed to new evaluations, to verify at a later time, and to have multidisciplinary consults for complex investigations, even after the classic postmortem procedures are closed. The possibility also exists to use this instrument when religious or general cultural contexts do not allow traditional postmortem procedures.

Digital autopsy can provide surveys that could escape even the most careful and tried observation (a minuscule bony splinter, for instance, can easily avoid direct observation). Though accurate the digital autopsy is not an aseptic database that will return this piece of information for follow-up evaluation, allowing, for instance, further confirmation of the differential diagnosis between the entry and the exit wounds. However, the digital autopsy is, and will be, just a backup to the forensic medicine practice; it is not always available and it cannot be considered as an alternative to the usual postmortem procedures.

The questioning about the cost–benefit analysis is relevant, mostly because this is a work in progress and the case studies are still very limited. An undoubtedly unusual application of multilevel CT is the evaluation of skeletonized human remains, which pertains to archaeology and anthropology. This methodology could seem totally superfluous for the study of bones, since the visual ascertainment made by the coroner or by the anthropologist is, obviously, quite appropriate. And yet there could be some, even fundamental, elements unper-

ceivable to the ascertainment, being the destruction of reports inadmissible for inquiry purposes. The employment of this method has been on a large scale during the last few years because it is useful for various postmortem surveys (traumatic injuries in traffic accidents, drowning, hanging, infanticides, etc.) and even for studies on the living (abuse, assault with blunt instruments, etc.). However, in this particular phase of the debate, all the foresaid must lead to a correct interpretation and methodological–operational collocation of digital autopsy as an asset to two interdependent disciplines for the purposes of specific diagnostic conclusions. A radiographer cannot validate a postmortem result in a courtroom without necroscopic corroborations; similarly a coroner cannot validate a digital result without the assistance of a postmortem confirmation. This warning is certainly more binding for the medical examiner. The drive toward an objective and documentary direction of the forensic inquiry in the area of autopsy and histopathology aspires today to rise from a moment of convergence of standards to a guarantee of a correct survey of pathogenetic courses—starting with the immediate and direct injury, proceeding, through the possible intermediate pathologies, to the final event. Thus it is necessary, as scientific methodology obliges, to research and standardize the operativeness the two disciplines share, define spaces and borders for each of them, and pursue objectiveness empowered by investigation and study. By applying a logical postmortem intervention, we shall not forget that any modular control cannot, by itself, give an absolute guarantee. Form is not a substitute of essence. Operative protocols are no more than a collection of information, unable to ensure *ex nunc* that a physician using it will increase his or her skills, since these protocols are not an alternative to scientific knowledge, being procedures whose application can grant a complete exploitation of science's potential. Actually, beyond the apparent sternness of standards and protocols, the only real limit to the use of the cross-sectional experiment as an effective means to "discover the truth" is the lack of experience, training, and imagination of cross-sectional experts; in a single word: mastery.

Magnetic nuclear resonance (MNR) application in forensic pathology might represent the future. A more detailed imaging of the human body mixed with the possibility of histochemical study of cell by means of spectroscopy could help in a better definition of timing in postmortem modifications. MNR contributions to forensic pathology should be considered as a work in progress.

VERTEBRAL MORPHOMETRY: HISTORICAL PERSPECTIVE TO DIGITAL MORPHOMETRY

Vertebral morphometry is a quantitative method generally used to identify osteoporotic vertebral fractures that relies on the measurement of distinct vertebral dimensions, calculating relative changes. A vertebral fracture appears as an alteration in the shape and size of the vertebral body, with a reduction in vertebral body height, as a wedge, endplate (mono- or biconcave), or collapse vertebral deformity. In everyday clinical practice, vertebral fractures are usually diagnosed by visual inspection of the patient's spinal radiographs. However, this qualitative approach to identify vertebral fractures is regarded as subjective and therefore may lead to disagreement, especially when performed by inexperienced observers. Therefore, more than a decade ago the semiquantitative (SQ) and the quantitative (e.g., vertebral morphometry) methods of defining prevalence and incidence of vertebral fractures were proposed.

The visual semiquantitative (SQ) method described by Genant et al. is currently most widely used in multi-centre clinical trials[1]. Because both the number and the severity of prior vertebral fractures are important predictor variables, Genant et al. combined the information into one measure, the so-called spinal deformity index (SDI). For each vertebra, a visual semiquantitative grade of 0, 1, 2, or 3 is assigned for no fracture or mild, moderate, or severe fracture, respectively, and the SDI is calculated by summing the fracture grades of the 13 vertebrae from T4 to L4. An increase in SDI could occur either due to a new vertebral fracture or due to worsening of mild or moderate prevalent vertebral fractures.

Crans et al. demonstrated the prognostic utility of the SDI for assessing future vertebral fracture risk; patients with greater baseline SDI had the greater future risk for vertebral fractures. The SQ method represents a simple, but standardized approach that provides reasonable reproducibility, sensitivity, and specificity, allowing excellent agreement for the diagnosis of prevalent and incident vertebral fractures to be achieved among trained observers. However, this method has some limitations. In cases of subtle deformities, such as mild wedge-like deformities in the mid-thoracic region and bowed endplates in the lumbar region, the distinction between borderline deformity (grade 0.5) and definite mild (grade 1) fractures can be difficult and sometimes arbitrary. Accurate diagnosis of prevalent fractures, which requires assessment of normal variations and degenerative changes and distinguishing them from true fractures, still depends on the experience of the observer. Another limitation of visual SQ assessment is the relatively poor reproducibility in distinguishing the three different grades of vertebral fractures.

Vertebral morphometry was introduced as early as 1960 by Barnett and Nordin, who used a transparent ruler to measure vertebral heights on conventional lateral radiographs of the thoracolumbar spine. Vertebral morphometry may be performed on conventional spinal radiographs (MRX: morphometric X-ray radiography) or on images obtained from dual X-ray absorptiometry (DXA) scans (MXA: morphometric X-ray absorptiometry).

Morphometric X-Ray Radiography (MRX)

Quantitative vertebral morphometry involves making measurements of vertebral body heights. Before performing the vertebral heights measurement, the radiologist has to identify the vertebral levels; to make this easier, T12 and L1 should be visualized on both the lateral thoracic and lumbar radiographs. Identification of vertebral levels on radiographs of lumbar and thoracic spine may be difficult at times (e.g., anatomic variants of the lumbosacral transition or the thoracolumbar junction). The vertebral bodies should be marked so that they can be more easily identified in other reading sessions or when compared with follow-up radiographs. On lateral radiographs, with six-point placement- the most widely used technique-the four corner points of each vertebral body from T4 to L4 and an additional point in the middle of the upper and lower endplates are manually marked.

The manual point placement is done according to Hurxthal, who proposed excluding the uncinate process at the posterosuperior border of the thoracic vertebrae and the Schmorl's nodes and osteophytes from vertebral height measurement. When the outer contours of the endplate are not superimposed (incorrect patient positioning or severe scoliosis), the middle points are placed in the centre between the upper and the lower contour.

Digital Morphometry

More than a decade ago, some investigators developed a system for vertebral morphometry that is based on digital images displayed on a high-resolution workstation. Post-processing of the digital images can highlight the endplate and the four corners of vertebral bodies allowing points to be placed more precisely. The software automatically determines the midpoints between anterior and posterior corner points of the upper and lower endplates. Then the operator selects the true midpoints moving the calipers along a vertical line joining the vertebral endplates. The x and y coordinates of each point are stored in the computer, which calculates the posterior, middle, and anterior heights (Hp, Hm, Ha) of each vertebra, from T4 to L5, and specific indices derived from height measurements for defining vertebral deformities. There are many advantages in performing digital morphometry: magnification of the images to a specific level; selection of the contrast and brightness levels for optimum visibility of the cortical bone, a capability that is especially valuable when the film is of less than optimal quality; the images may be stored on optical disks, CD or DVD and can be remeasured on multiple occasions. Finally, measurement data can be captured directly from the images into a database, eliminating the need for data entry. The manual placement of the six measuring points represents a source of error in the measurement of the vertebral body because the placement can vary widely among various operators. The need to reduce these operator-dependent errors led to the development of a computer-assisted system.

The procedure is based on an algorithm that automatically locates the vertebral body contour in the digitized X-ray image and then is checked by the operator for accuracy.

Correction is possible through operator intervention at any time. The system also performs additional geometric calculations, enhancing the diagnostic capability of quantitative vertebral morphometry. This algorithm was used in the European Vertebral Osteoporosis Study (EVOS), but the reproducibility was worse than that with the manual placement technique. Because the six-point placement technique might not completely describe vertebral shape, Smyth et al. developed a technique based on use of an active shape model (ASM). An ASM is a statistical model to locate and measure the shapes of variable objects in images. It was applied to the measurement of vertebral shape on lateral spine DXA scans. The ASM technique obtained entire shape information, with accuracy as good as that with manual methods, but it can be performed more easily and rapidly. Therefore, digital morphometry with computer assistance and hierarchical segmentation of vertebrae from X-ray images represent useful tools to evaluate a large number of cases, allowing centralization of images for a large-scale clinical trial.

Recently a new digital technique for vertebral morphometry has been introduced in clinical practice using an instrument called MorphoXpress[2]. MorphoXpress (Procter & Gamble Pharmaceuticals, Rusham Park, Egham, UK) is a statistical model-based vision system to digitise and analyse plain film vertebral X-rays for semi-automated morphometric assessment. This system is based on a new technology that represents the next generation of statistical model-based techniques. To our knowledge, MorphoXpress is the first automated six-point morphometric system to operate on digitized plain film X-ray images, as opposed to DXA. Furthermore, unlike DXA, X-rays of the spine are still the only approved modality for diagnosis of vertebral fracture by the US Food and Drug Administration (FDA). This system works as follows: having defined a patient record, original lateral spine X-rays are digitized using a flatbed scanner connect to the personal computer that hosts the MorphoXpress software application, and analysis is initialized by the manual indication of the centres of the upper and lower vertebrae to be analyzed. The software then automatically finds the positions of the contours of the vertebrae, including the double endplate contours and part of vertebral process (Figure 1). This annotation is then used to determine landmarks for a standard six-point morphometry measurement, providing an optional confidence measure of correct registration for each vertebra. The software allows these points to be moved by the operator, if necessary, before the points are confirmed as being in correctly positioned. The positions of the confirmed points are then used by the software to calculate anterior, medial, and posterior vertebral heights, and these heights may also be used for the determination

Figure 1. Schematic representation of the vertebra showing automatic placement of the points used to define vertebral height and contour

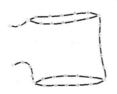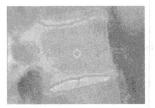

of a deformity metric. Finally, another advantage of this approach is given by the improvement of the workflow and in the overall positive results in terms of diagnostic accuracy (2.1% CV) and precision (1.68% CV).

The statistical modelling technique that has been applied to medical images is the Active Shape Model (ASM). The approach to model-based vision, including the one under investigation, uses the following frame work There are two distinct stages: a one-time 'model-building' stage and a 'runtime' stage. To build the model, a set of representative images of the anatomy to be modelled are annotated manually by an expert, i.e., training samples of the anatomy to be modelled are defined by a set of landmark points placed along the anatomical boundary. Each example is then described by a vector $x = [x_1, y_1, x_2, y_2, ..., x_n, y_n]$, where (x_i, y_i) is the position of the ith landmark on an example. In cases where certain boundaries are occluded or missing, the expert must use his/her anatomical knowledge to interpolate an estimated boundary. This set of annotated training images efficiently captures the expert's domain knowledge of how the anatomy of interest is presented in the chosen modality. The annotated objects are treated as a 'training set' and are aligned in scale and rotation, before a form of statistical decomposition is applied to describe the variation of the aligned shapes. This analysis results in the establishment of anatomical shape parameters, which can be understood as a set of independent weighted modes; adjusting the weights produces different shape examples. At runtime, the model is scaled, rotated, translated and further modified by adjusting the weights to create a statistically based best fit model describing the underlying patient image data. The shape captured by a statistical model may be described by a Point Distribution Model (PDM) that is generated by the statistical analysis of the variation in landmark point coordinates in a set of annotated images. The PDM represents shape in terms of a mean shape and a set of linearly independent modes of shape variation, requiring only the most significant variations of shape to be annotated. Any new shape, *x*, of the same type as those observed in the training set can then be generated by summing combinations of these modes of variation, contained within a matrix *P*, to the mean shape *xm*, with a vector of weight *b* controlling the influence of each mode: *x* = *xm* + *Pb*.

The accuracy and precision of semiquantitative and morphometric methods are heavily influenced by the quality of the spinal radiographs. Optimal radiographs can be achieved by training X-ray technologists and making sure that they are aware of the difference between radiographs for osteoporotic vertebral assessment and those for routine clinical practice, by using a standardized radiographic technique (Guglielmi et al., 2007), which includes both patient positioning and the choice of radiographic parameters. Currently, T4 to L4 are routinely used for vertebral morphometry, because of limitations in visualizing T1-T3 due to overlying of the shoulders and L5 due to overlying pelvis.

Morphometric X-Ray Absorptiometry (MXA)

To overcome some limitations of MRX, another method called morphometric X-ray absorptiometry (MXA) has been developed by the two major manufacturers of DXA equipment-Hologic, Inc. (Waltham, MA) and General Electric/Lunar (Madison, WI). In Hologic systems, two views

of the thoracic and lumbar spine are acquired: a posteroanterior (PA) scan and a lateral scan. The PA image is acquired in order to visualize spinal anatomy, such as scoliosis, to determine the centre line of the spine. This information is used in subsequent lateral scans to maintain a constant distance between the centre of the spine and the X-ray tube for all subjects at all visits, regardless of patient position or degree of scoliosis, thus eliminating the geometric distortion. Each lateral scan covers a distance of 46 cm, imaging the vertebrae from L4 to T4. The GE /Lunar scanner determines the starting position of the lateral morphometry scan by positioning a laser spot 1 cm above the iliac crest. The scan range for the GE-Lunar systems is determined by measuring the length between the iliac crest and the armpit. The lateral scan can be acquired using a single-energy X-ray beam with a very short scan time (12 s). However, the analysis may be affected by soft tissue artefacts in the image caused by prominent lung structures. These artefacts are absent in the dual-energy scans, which, however, take between 6 min (array mode) and 12 min (fast and high-definition modes). After the scan, the programme automatically identifies vertebral levels and indicates the centres of the vertebrae. The sixpoint placement for the determination of the vertebral heights is semiautomated. The operator uses a mouse pointing device to specify the 13 locations of the anterior inferior corner of the vertebrae from L4 to T4. Then the MXA software computes the positions of the remaining five vertebral points for each. To guide the operator during image analysis of follow-up scans, the vertebral endplate markers from the previous scan are superimposed on the current scan, improving long-term precision. After the analysis is finished, a final report is displayed. It gives information on the measured vertebral body heights and their ratios, and includes an assessment of the patient's fracture status based on normative data and different models for fracture assessment using quantitative morphometry (Figures 2-3).

Figure 2. The vertebral measurements are obtained automatically by the software and manually removed by the operator if necessary

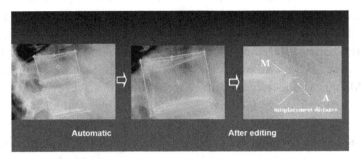

Comparison between MRX and MXA

Vertebral morphometry should be performed by trained observers resulting in good inter-observer measurement precision. Both MRX and MXA have a good precision, the intraoperator CV ranging from 1.2% for MXR to 3.4% for MXA, while the interoperator CV from 1.9% to 5.3 according to various authors. For MXA the precision obtained with two systems, Hologic and GE/Lunar, is similar. MXA overcomes some of the patient-positioning and exposure factor problems inherent in conventional radiography. Infact, the scanner arm of some models of densitometers can be rotated 90°, so that lateral scans can be obtained with the patient in the supine position without repositioning. A further advantage of MXA when using the scanning fan-beam geometry of DXA devices is the absence of distortions and magnification effects inherent in the standard X-ray technique. The main attraction of MXA is that the effective dose-equivalent to the patient is considerably lower than for conventional radiography. While MXA is able to assess the entire spine in a single image, in conventional radiography, radiographs of the lumbar and thoracic spine have to be performed separately, so the identification of the vertebral levels to perform MRX may be difficult at times. Furthermore, the improved image spatial resolution of the new DXA scan-

Figure 3. Schematic operation of the software. A 2-point initialisation is used to define the mid-points of the upper (L1) and lower (L4) vertebrae to be measured. A full annotation by model-fitting is then performed which is used to determine the positions of 6-point morphometry landmarks

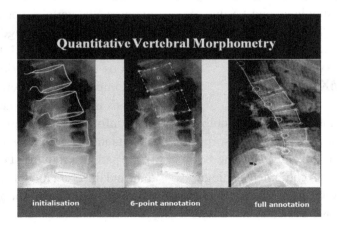

ners allows a better visualization of the upper thoracic vertebrae. So far, various comparative studies exist that have found excellent agreement between qualitative and quantitative radiographic assessment using fan-beam dual-energy DXA images. A large proportion of vertebrae are not visualized sufficiently for analysis on MXA scans, and this reduces the number of vertebral fractures identified, particularly in the upper thoracic spine (T4-T5). However, other authors have shown that high-speed fan-beam DXA imaging was feasible in a clinical population, allowing visualization of a substantial proportion of the vertebrae, using a rapid (10-s) single-energy imaging mode during suspended respiration.

FORENSIC APPLICATIONS OF VERTEBRAL MORPHOMETRY

Application in Fractures Detection

Because there is variation in vertebral size and shape at different levels of the spine (the anterior and posterior vertebral height increases from T3 to L2, but for L3-L5 the posterior height is lower than the anterior height) and vertebral size also varies between individuals (large people tend to have larger vertebrae), reference ranges should be established in the population under study, using the same technique, and derived from "normal" subjects or by "data trimming" of a population-based-sample. To determine the reference values of vertebral body heights, some authors have used a sample of premenopausal women, assuming that the prevalence of vertebral fractures is very low in this population. This approach may not be feasible for many studies because it involves radiation exposure for fertile women. Moreover, it has been demonstrated that vertebral heights change significantly with age, showing rates of loss of 1.2–1.3 mm/year. Age-related decrease of vertebral heights influences the definition of the normal range of vertebral shape, since a

deformity that may be in excess of 2 SD from the mean in younger subjects may be well within this limit 20 years later. Other authors have selected a subsample of postmenopausal women in which all vertebrae have been judged to be normal (un-fractured) on the radiographs by an expert reader. A third approach for defining normal vertebral dimensions uses the values of a population that includes postmenopausal women with and without vertebral fractures. Also, in a large study the authors have shown that reference ranges of vertebral heights derived from MRX studies may not be applicable to MXA, in view of the observed differences between their MXA mean values when compared with MRX values reported in the earlier studies. The differences observed led to a tendency for lower MXA critical values for detection of vertebral deformities, suggesting the use of technique-specific reference ranges. The preliminary report of an Italian multi-centre study showed that vertebral heights of 569 Italian normal women measured from T4-L4 using vertebral fracture assessment (VFA) on Lunar Prodigy (GE Healthcare) densitometers in all vertebrae were significantly smaller than the existing values collected from American normal women. Various morphometric algorithms to define vertebral fractures have therefore been developed[3].

Comparison of Semiquantitative (SQ) Visual and Quantitative Morphometric Assessment of Vertebral Fractures

A vertebral deformity is not always a vertebral fracture, but a vertebral fracture is always a vertebral deformity. Some comparative studies found a high concordance between different quantitative morphometric approaches and visual semiquantitative evaluation for prevalent vertebral fractures defined as moderate or severe. In these cases there was a strong association with clinical parameters (bone mineral density, height loss, back pain, incidence of subsequent deformities).

There are many causes of vertebral deformities, and the correct differential diagnoses for them can be achieved only by visual inspection and expert interpretation of a radiograph. In fact, there is a list of potential differential diagnoses for vertebral deformities, such as osteoporosis, trauma, degenerative disease, Scheuermann's disease, congenital anomaly, neoplastic disease, and haematopoietic disorders, infectious disease and Paget's disease, that should be taken into consideration, and the correct classification of vertebral deformities can be achieved only by expert interpretation of the radiograph. The quantitative morphometry is unable to distinguish osteoporotic vertebral fractures by vertebral deformities due to other factors, such as degenerative spine and disc disease. This limitation is a characteristic of any method of quantitative morphometry, but the limited spatial resolution of the DXA images in MXA may increase this problem. On the other hand, MRX, with its superior image quality, has the potential for qualitative reading of the radiographs to aid the differential diagnosis. In fact, although it is recognized that the visual interpretation of radiographs is subjective, it is also true that an expert eye can better distinguish between true fractures and vertebral anomalies than can quantitative morphometry. For example, the distinction between a fractured endplate and the deformity associated with Schmorl's nodes can only be made visually by an experienced observer, as is the case for the diagnosis of the wedge-shaped appearance caused by remodelling of the vertebral bodies in degenerative disc disease. Recently, a new algorithm-based approach for the qualitative (ABQ) assessment of vertebral fracture has been developed. The ABQ assumes that in every vertebral fracture, fracture of the endplate within the vertebral ring is always involved. Thus, by definition, wedge and crush fractures are also concave fractures, because they involve central depression of the endplate.

Comparing the ABQ approach, semiquantitative method (SQ) and quantitative morphometry (QM) for the identification of vertebral fracture in a population of elderly men showed that most of the men with vertebral fractures identified by SQ or QM, but not by ABQ were classified as having non-osteoporotic short vertebral height (SVH) by ABQ. These men did not have low BMD.

Assessment of Vertebral Fractures on DXA Images

Recently, the visual semiquantitative (SQ) method for identification of vertebral fractures has been applied to images of the spine acquired by fan-beam DXA devices. This method is called "instant vertebral assessment" (IVA) by Hologic or "vertebral fracture assessment" (VFA) by GE/Lunar. IVA has been compared with SQ evaluation of spinal radiographs demonstrating good agreement (96.3%, k=0.79) in classifying vertebrae as normal or deformed in the 1,978 of 2,093 vertebrae deemed analyzable on both the DXA scans and conventional radiographs. IVA showed good sensitivity (91.9%) in the identification of moderate/severe SQ deformities and an excellent negative predictive value (98%) to distinguish subjects with very low risk of vertebral fractures from those with possible fractures. The disagreement between the IVA and SQ methods resulted from the poor image quality, particularly in the upper thoracic vertebrae that were not visualized sufficiently for analysis. Although some vertebral fractures were missed by IVA, all patients with prevalent vertebral fractures were identified; therefore, for the identification of patients with fracture, visual assessment of DXA scans had 100% sensitivity and specificity. This means that if IVA had been used as a diagnostic pre-screening tool at the first assessment, all the patients with prevalent vertebral fracture would have been correctly referred for radiography to confirm the diagnosis. Also the "normal" subjects can then be excluded prior to performing conventional radiographs and further time-consuming and costly methods of vertebral deformity assessment such as SQ by an experienced radiologist and/or quantitative morphometry. Also, with its low radiation and good precision, IVA could be utilized to identify vertebral fractures in populations affected by conditions different from osteoporosis, but with high vertebral fracture risk, i.e., liver or kidney transplant patients.

Determination of Sex

The statistical examination of metrical data from human skeletal remains for determining sex has a long history in physical anthropology. Such analyses build on visually oriented studies—using directly observable anatomical markers to estimate sex—by providing methods that can be applied to a great variety of skeletal remains. Determination of sex is directly dependent upon the presence or absence of certain anatomical markers. However, the typical materials with which the physical anthropologist and archaeologist deal are seldom complete skeletal elements. In such contexts, it is prudent to devise analytical methods that are not compromised by specimen fragmentation. In addition, statistical analyses provide more replicable results and more reliable and quantifiable estimations than visual estimates. Because statistical analyses tend to follow visually oriented studies of an element, they commonly focus on the same bone. For example, visual tests that use anatomical attributes of the skull to estimate sex have been followed by statistical applications that use not only the same bone, but also use the same attributes. This analytic pattern seems to be changing. A few authors have taken into account some elements that do not possess directly observable anatomical indicators of sex, such as the humerus, the femur, the scapula, the metacarpals of hand, the talus or calcaneus, the first cervical vertebra, and the 12th thoracic and 1st lumbar vertebrae. The lower thoracic and lumbar vertebrae are often preserved well in archaeological skeletal assemblages and forensic contexts, because of their weight-bearing function and relative density.

Even when bone preservation is problematic for the axial skeleton, the 12th thoracic vertebra can be readily distinguished because of its unique morphology. The lower thoracic and lumbar vertebrae are highly sexually dimorphic according to work by Pastor on the Spitalfields and Terry samples. However, reliable metric methods on vertebrae are still in need of development, because it has been widely acknowledged that ancestral and regional variations in skeletal elements need to be considered when producing specific standards for accurate determination of sex.

Age determination of adult and fetal skeletons on the base of morphometry of vertebral column.

FUTURE PERSPECTIVE

To the best of our knowledge, more data are necessary to evaluate the time and effort involved in editing landmark using MorphoXpress. The data could be enhanced by recording the coordinates of the landmark as located from MorphoXpress and after any editing. That would provide statistics about the number of landmarks that needed editing and the differences in landmark locations. This would be a subject for future investigation of the efficacy of the new technology.

REFERENCES

Adams, J. E. (1997). Single and dual energy X-ray absorptiometry. In Guglielmi, G., Passariello, R., & Genant, H. K. (Eds.), *Bone densitometry: An update. European Radiology, 7(2), S20–S31.*

Aghayev, E., Yen, K., Sonnenschein, M., Jackowski, C., Thali, M., & Vock, P. (2005). Pneumomediastinum and soft tissue emphysema of the neck in post-mortem CT and MRI: A new vital sign in hanging? *Forensic Science International, 153,* 181–188. doi:10.1016/j.forsciint.2004.09.124

Andenmatten, M. A., Thali, M. J., Kneubuehl, B. P., Oesterhelweg, L., Ross, S., & Spendlove, D. (2008). Gunshot injuries detected by post-mortem multislice computed tomography (MSCT): A feasibility study. *Legal Medicine*, *10*, 287–292. doi:10.1016/j.legalmed.2008.03.005

Banks, L. M., van Juijk, C., & Genant, H. K. (1995). Radiographic technique for assessing osteoporotic vertebral fracture. In Genant, H. K., Jergas, M., & van Juijk, C. (Eds.), *Vertebral fracture in osteoporosis* (pp. 131–147). San Francisco: University of California Osteoporosis Research Group.

Barnett, E., & Nordin, B. E. C. (1960). Radiographic diagnosis of osteoporosis: New approach. *Clinical Radiology*, *11*, 166–174. doi:10.1016/S0009-9260(60)80012-8

Blake, G. M., Rea, J. A., & Fogelman, I. (1997). Vertebral morphometry studies using dual-energy X-ray absorptiometry. *Seminars in Nuclear Medicine*, *27*, 276–290. doi:10.1016/S0001-2998(97)80029-3

Blake, J. M., Jagathesan, T., Herd, R. J. M., & Fogelman, I. (1994). Dual X-ray absorptiometry of the lumbar spine: The precision of paired anteroposterior/lateral studies. *The British Journal of Radiology*, *67*, 624–630. doi:10.1259/0007-1285-67-799-624

Bruschweiler, W., Braun, M., Dirnhofer, R., & Thali, M. J. (2003). Analysis of patterned injuries and injury-causing instruments with forensic 3D/CAD supported photogrammetry (FPHG): An instruction manual for the documentation process. *Forensic Science International*, *132*, 130–138. doi:10.1016/S0379-0738(03)00006-9

Crabtree, N., Wrigh,t J., Walgrove, A., et al. (2000). Vertebral morphometry: Repeat scan precision using the Lunar Expert-XL and the Hologic 4500A. A study for the WISDOM RCT of hormone replacement therapy. *Osteoporosis International*, *11*, 537–543. doi:10.1007/s001980070098

Crans, G. G., Genant, H. K., & Krege, J. H. (2005). Measurement of vertebral heights. *Bone*, *37*, 175–179. doi:10.1016/j.bone.2005.04.003

de Bruijne, M., & Nielsen, M. (2004). Image segmentation by shape particle filtering. In *Proceedings of the 17th International Conference on Pattern Recognition 2004*, (pp. 722–725).

Di Maio, V. J. (1984). Basic principles in the investigation of homicides. *Pathology Annual*, *19*(2), 149–164.

Diacinti, D., Acca, M., & Tomei, E. (1995). Metodica di'radiologia digitale per la valutazione dell'osteoporosi vertebrale. *La Radiologia Medica*, *91*, 1–5.

Dirnhofer, R., Jackowski, C., Vock, P., Potter, K., & Thali, M. J. (2006). Virtopsy: Minimally invasive, imaging-guided virtual autopsy. *Radiographics*, *26*, 1305–1333. doi:10.1148/rg.265065001

Dolinak, D., Evan, M., & Lew, E. (2005). *Forensic pathology: Principles and practice*. Burlington, MA: Elsevier Academic Press.

Donchin, Y., Rivkind, A. I., Bar-Ziv, J., Hiss, J., Almog, J., & Drescher, M. (1994). Utility of postmortem computed tomography in trauma victims. *The Journal of Trauma*, *37*, 552–556. doi:10.1097/00005373-199410000-00006

Eastell, R., Cedel, S. L., & Wahner, H. (1991). Classification of vertebral fractures. *Journal of Bone and Mineral Research*, *6*, 207–215. doi:10.1002/jbmr.5650060302

Edmondston, S. J., Price, R. I., & Valente, B. (1999). Measurement of vertebral body height: Ex vivo comparison between morphometric X-ray absorptiometry, morphometric radiography and direct measurements. *Osteoporosis International*, *10*, 7–13. doi:10.1007/s001980050187

Ferrar, L., Jiang, G., & Eastell, R. (2003). Visual identification of vertebral fractures in osteoporosis using morphometric X-ray absorptiometry. *Journal of Bone and Mineral Research, 18*, 933–938. doi:10.1359/jbmr.2003.18.5.933

Finkbeiner, W. E., Ursell, P. C., & Davis, R. L. (2004). *Autopsy pathology: A manual and atlas.* Philadelphia: Churchill Livingstone.

Fogelman, I. (Ed.). (1998). *The evaluation of osteoporosis. Dual energy x-ray absorptiometry in clinical practice* (pp. 281–288). London: Martin Dunitz, Ltd.

Gallagher, J. C., Hedlund, L. R., & Stoner, S. (1988). Vertebral morphometry: Normative data. *Bone and Mineral, 4*, 189–196.

Gardner, J. C., von Ingersleben, G., & Heyano, S. L. (2001). An interactive tutorial-based training technique for vertebral morphometry. *Osteoporosis International, 12*, 63–70. doi:10.1007/s001980170159

Genant, H. K., Jergas, M., & Palermo, L. (1996). Comparison of semiquantitative visual and quantitative morphometric assessment of prevalent and incident vertebral fractures in osteoporosis. *Journal of Bone and Mineral Research, 11*, 984–996. doi:10.1002/jbmr.5650110716

Genant, H. K., Siris, E., & Crans, G. G. (2005). Reduction in vertebral fracture risk in teriaparatide-treated postmenopausal women as assessed by spinal deformity index. *Bone, 37*, 170–174. doi:10.1016/j.bone.2005.04.023

Genant, H. K., Wu, C. Y., & van Kuijk, C. (1993). Vertebral fracture assessment using a semiquantitative technique. *Journal of Bone and Mineral Research, 8*, 1137–1148. doi:10.1002/jbmr.5650080915

Guglielmi, G., Diacinti, D., van Kuijk, C., Aparisi, F., Krestan, C., & Adams, J. E. (2008). Vertebral morphometry: Current methods and recent advances. *European Journal of Radiology, 18*, 1484–1496. doi:10.1007/s00330-008-0899-8

Guglielmi, G., Palmieri, F., & Placentino, M. G. (2008). Assessment of osteoporotic vertebral fractures using specialized workflow software for six point morphometry. *European Journal of Radiology, 70*, 142–148. doi:10.1016/j.ejrad.2007.12.001

Guglielmi, G., Stoppino, L. P., & Placentino, M. G. (2007). Reproducibility of a semi-automatic method for 6-point vertebral morphometry in a multi-centre trial. *European Journal of Radiology, 69*, 173–178. doi:10.1016/j.ejrad.2007.09.040

Harke, H. T., Levy, A. D., Abbott, R. M., Mallak, C. T., Getz, M. J., & Champion, H. R. (2007). Autopsy radiography: Digital radiographs (DR) vs. multidetector computed tomography (MDCT) in high velocity gunshot wound victims. *The American Journal of Forensic Medicine and Pathology, 29*, 13–19.

Harvey, S. B., Hutchinson, K. M., & Rennie, E. C. (1998). Comparison of the precision of two vertebral morphometry programs for the Lunar Expert-XL imaging densitometer. *The British Journal of Radiology, 71*, 388–398.

Hayakawa, M., Yamamoto, S., Motani, H., Yajima, D., Sato, Y., & Iwase, H. (2006). Does imaging technology overcome problems of conventional postmortem examination? A trial of computed tomography imaging for post mortem examination. *International Journal of Legal Medicine, 120*(1), 24–26. doi:10.1007/s00414-005-0038-x

Hedlund, L. R., & Gallagher, J. C. (1988). Vertebral morphometry in diagnosis of spinal fractures. *Bone and Mineral, 5*, 59–67. doi:10.1016/0169-6009(88)90006-2

Howe, B., Gururajan, A., Sari-Sarraf, H., & Long, L. R. (2004). Hierarchical segmentation of cervical and lumbar vertebrae using a customized generalized Hough transform and extensions to active appearance models. In *Proceedings of IEEE 6*[th] (pp. 182–186). SSIAI.

Hurxthal, L. M. (1968). Measurement of vertebral heights. *AJR. American Journal of Roentgenology, 103*, 635–644.

Ith, M., Bigler, P., Scheurer, E., Kreis, R., Hoffman, L., & Dirnhofer, R. (2002). Observation and identification of metabolites emerging during postmortem decomposition of brain tissue by means of in situ 1H-magnetic resonance spectroscopy. *Magnetic Resonance in Medicine, 48*, 915–920. doi:10.1002/mrm.10294

Jackowski, C., Aghayev, E., Sonnenschein, M., Dirnhofer, R., & Thali, M. J. (2006). Maximum intensity projection of cranial computed tomography data for dental identification. *International Journal of Legal Medicine, 120*(3), 165–167. doi:10.1007/s00414-005-0050-1

Jackowski, C., Lussi, A., Classens, M., Kilchoer, T., Bolliger, S., & Aghayev, E. (2006). Extended CT scale overcomes restoration caused streak artifacts-3D color encoded automatic discrimination of dental restorations for identification. *Journal of Computer Assisted Tomography, 30*(3), 510–513. doi:10.1097/00004728-200605000-00027

Jackowski, C., Schweitzer, W., Thali, M., Yen, K., Aghayev, E., & Sonnenschein, M. (2005). Virtopsy: Postmortem imaging of the human heart in situ using MSCT and MRI. *Forensic Science International, 149*(1), 11–23. doi:10.1016/j.forsciint.2004.05.019

Jackowski, C., Sonnenschein, M., Thali, M. J., Aghayev, E., Allmen, G., & Yen, K. (2005). Virtopsy: Postmortem minimally invasive angiography using cross section techniques—implementation and preliminary results. *Journal of Forensic Sciences, 50*, 1175–1186. doi:10.1520/JFS2005023

Jauhiainen, T., Jarvinen, V. M., & Hekali, P. E. (2002). Evaluation of methods for MR imaging of human right ventricular heart volumes and mass. *Acta Radiologica, 43*(6), 587–592. doi:10.1034/j.1600-0455.2002.430609.x

Jergas, M., & San Valentin, R. (1995). Techniques for the assessment of vertebral dimensions in quantitative morphometry. In Genant, H. K., Jergas, M., & van Juijk, C. (Eds.), *Vertebral fracture in osteoporosis* (pp. 163–188). San Francisco: University of California Osteoporosis Research Group.

Kalender, W. A., & Eidloth, H. (1991). Determination of geometric parameters and osteoporosis indices for lumbar vertebrae from lateral QCT localizer radiographs. *Osteoporosis International, 1*, 197–200.

Kalidis, L., Felsenberg, D., & Kalender, W. A. (1992). Morphometric analysis of digitized radiographs: Description of automatic evaluation. In Ring, E. F. J. (Ed.), *Current research in osteoporosis and bone mineral measurement II* (pp. 14–16). London: British Institute of Radiology.

Kleerekoper, M., & Nelson, D. A. (1992). Vertebral fracture or vertebral deformity? *Calcified Tissue International, 50*, 5–6. doi:10.1007/BF00297288

Kosa, F., & Castellana, C. (2005). New forensic anthropological approachment for the age determination of human fetal skeletons on the base of morphometry of vertebral column. *Forensic Science International, 147*, 69–74. doi:10.1016/j.forsciint.2004.09.096

Lewis, M. K., & Blake, G. M. (1995). Patient dose in morphometric X-ray absorptiometry. *Osteoporosis International, 5*, 281–282. doi:10.1007/BF01774019

Ljung, P., Winskog, C., Persson, A., Lundstrom, C., & Ynnerman, A. (2006). Full-body virtual autopsies using a stateof-the-art volume rendering pipeline. *IEEE Transactions on Visualization and Computer Graphics, 12*(5), 869–876. doi:10.1109/TVCG.2006.146

Madea, B., Henssge, C., & Lockhoven, H. B. (1986). Priority of multiple gunshot injuries of the skull. *Zeitschrift fur Rechtsmedizin, 97,* 213–218.

Magid, D., Bryan, B. M., Drebin, R. A., Ney, D., & Fishman, E. K. (1989). Three-dimensional imaging of an Egyptian mummy. *Clinical Imaging, 13,* 239–240. doi:10.1016/0899-7071(89)90156-3

Mc Closkey, E. V., Spector, T. D., & Eyres, K. S. (1993). The assessment of vertebral deformity: A method for use in population studies and clinical trials. *Osteoporosis International, 3,* 138–147. doi:10.1007/BF01623275

Minne, H. W., Leidig, C., & Wuster, C. H. R. (1988). A newly developed spine deformity index (SDI) to quantitative vertebral crush fractures in patients with osteoporosis. *Bone and Mineral, 3,* 335–349.

Nelson, D., Peterson, E., & Tilley, B. (1990). Measurement of vertebral area on spine X-rays in osteoporosis: Reliability of digitizing techniques. *Journal of Bone and Mineral Research, 5,* 707–716. doi:10.1002/jbmr.5650050707

Nicholson, P. H. F., Haddaway, M. J., & Davie, M. W. J. (1993). A computerized technique for vertebral morphometry. *Physiological Measurement, 14,* 195–204. doi:10.1088/0967-3334/14/2/010

Njeh, C. F., Fuerst, T., & Hans, D. (1999). Radiation exposure in bone mineral density assessment. *Applied Radiation and Isotopes, 50,* 215–236. doi:10.1016/S0969-8043(98)00026-8

Notman, D. N., Tashjian, J., Aufderheide, A. C., Cass, O. W., Shane, O. C. III, & Berquist, T. H. (1986). Modern imaging and endoscopic biopsy techniques in Egyptian mummies. *AJR. American Journal of Roentgenology, 146,* 93–96.

O'Neill, T. W., Felsenberg, D., & Varlow, J. (1996). The prevalence of vertebral deformity in European men and women: The European vertebral osteoporosis study. *Journal of Bone and Mineral Research, 11,* 1010–1018. doi:10.1002/jbmr.5650110719

Oliver, W. R., Chancellor, A. S., Soitys, J., Symon, J., Cullip, T., & Rosenman, J. (1995). Three-dimensional reconstruction of a bullet path: Validation by computed radiography. *Journal of Forensic Sciences, 40*(2), 321–324.

Patriquin, L., Kassarjian, A., O'Brien, M., Andry, C., & Eustace, S. (2001). Postmortem whole-body magnetic resonance imaging as an adjunct to autopsy: Preliminary clinical experience. *Journal of Magnetic Resonance Imaging, 13,* 277–287. doi:10.1002/1522-2586(200102)13:2<277::AID-JMRI1040>3.0.CO;2-W

Pomara, C., & Fineschi, V. (2007). *Manuale atlante di tecniche autoptiche.* Padova: Piccin.

Pomara, C., Fineschi, V., Scalzo, G., & Guglielmi, G. (2009). Virtopsy versus digital autopsy: Virtuous autopsy. *La Radiologia Medica, 114*(8), 1367–1382. doi:10.1007/s11547-009-0435-1

Pomara, C., Karch, S. B., & Mallegni, F. (2008). A medieval murder. *The American Journal of Forensic Medicine and Pathology, 29,* 72–74. doi:10.1097/PAF.0b013e31816520bf

Poulsen, K., & Simonsen, J. (2007). Computed tomography as routine connection with medico-legal autopsies. *Forensic Science International, 171,* 190–197. doi:10.1016/j.forsciint.2006.05.041

Randall, B. B., Fierro, M. F., & Froede, R. C. (1998). Practice guideline for forensic pathology. *Archives of Pathology & Laboratory Medicine, 122,* 1056–1064.

Rea, J. A., Chen, M. B., & Li, J. (2000). Morphometry X-ray absorptiometry and morphometric radiography of the spine: A comparison of prevalent vertebral deformity identification. *Journal of Bone and Mineral Research, 15,* 564–574. doi:10.1359/jbmr.2000.15.3.564

Rea, J. A., Li, J., & Blake, G. M. (2000). Visual assessment of vertebral deformity by X-ray absorptiometry: A highly predictive method to exclude vertebral deformity. *Osteoporosis International, 11,* 660–668. doi:10.1007/s001980070063

Roberts, M., Cootes, T. F., & Adams, J. E. (2006). Vertebral morphometry: Semiautomatic determination of detailed shape from dual-energy X-ray absorptiometry images using active appearance models. *Investigative Radiology, 41*(12), 849–859. doi:10.1097/01.rli.0000244343.27431.26

Ros, P. R., Li, K. C., Vo, P., Baer, H., & Staab, E. V. (1990). Preautopsy magnetic resonance imaging: Initial experience. *Magnetic Resonance Imaging, 8,* 303–308. doi:10.1016/0730-725X(90)90103-9

Ross, S., Spendlove, D., Bolliger, S., Christe, A., Oesterhelweg, L., & Grabherr, S. (2008). Postmortem whole-body CT angiography: Evaluation of two contrast media solutions. *AJR. American Journal of Roentgenology, 190,* 1380–1389. doi:10.2214/AJR.07.3082

Sheng-Bo, Y., U-Young, L., Dai-Soon, K., Yong-Woo, A., Chang-Zhu, J., Jie, Z., et al. (2008). Determination of sex for the 12th thoracic vertebra by morphometry of three-dimensional reconstructed vertebral models. *Journal of Forensic Sciences, 53*(3), 620–625. doi:10.1111/j.1556-4029.2008.00701.x

Sidler, M., Jackowski, C., Dirnhofer, R., Vock, P., & Thali, M. J. (2007). Use of multislice computed tomography in disaster victim identification: Advantages and limitations. *Forensic Science International, 169,* 118–128. doi:10.1016/j.forsciint.2006.08.004

Smyth, P. P., Taylor, C. J., & Adams, J. E. (1999). Vertebral shape: Automatic measurement with active shape models. *Radiology, 211,* 571–578.

Steiger, P., Cummings, S. R., Genant, H. K., & Weiss, H. (1994). Morphometric X-ray absorptiometry of the spine: Correlation in vivo with morphometric radiography. *Osteoporosis International, 4,* 238–244. doi:10.1007/BF01623347

Steiger, P. & Wahner, H. (1994). Instruments using fan-beam geometry.

Thali, M. J., Braun, M., Markwalder, T. H., Brueschweiler, W., Zollinger, U., & Malik, N. J. (2003). Bite mark documentation and analysis: The forensic 3D/CAD supported photogrammetry approach. *Forensic Science International, 135,* 115–121. doi:10.1016/S0379-0738(03)00205-6

Thali, M. J., Braun, M., Wirth, J., Vock, P., & Dirnhofer, R. (2003). 3D surface and body documentation in forensic medicine: 3-D/CAD photogrammetry merged with 3D radiological scanning. *Journal of Forensic Sciences, 48,* 1356–1365.

Thali, M. J., Dirnhofer, R., Becker, R., Oliver, W., & Potter, K. (2004). Is virtual histology the next step after the virtual autopsy? Magnetic resonance microscopy in forensic medicine. *Magnetic Resonance Imaging, 22,* 1131–1138. doi:10.1016/j.mri.2004.08.019

Thali, M. J., Jackowski, C., Oesterhelweg, L., Ross, S. G., & Dirnhofer, R. (2007). Virtopsy: The Swiss virtual autopsy approach. *Legal Medicine, 9,* 100–104. doi:10.1016/j.legalmed.2006.11.011

Thali, M. J., Markwalder, T., Jackowski, C., Sonnenschein, M., & Dirnhofer, R. (2006). Dental CT imaging as a screening tool for dental profiling: Advantages and limitations. *Journal of Forensic Sciences, 51,* 113–119. doi:10.1111/j.1556-4029.2005.00019.x

Thali, M. J., Schweitzer, W., Yen, K., Vock, P., Ozdoba, C., & Spielvogel, E. (2003). New horizons in forensic radiology: The 60-second digital autopsy–full-body examination of a gunshot victim by multislice computed tomography. *The American Journal of Forensic Medicine and Pathology*, *24*, 22–27. doi:10.1097/00000433-200303000-00004

Thali, M. J., Taubenreuther, U., Karolczak, M., Braun, M., Brueschweiler, W., & Kalender, W. A. (2003). Forensic microradiology: Micro-computed tomography (micro-CT) and analysis of patterned injuries inside of bone. *Journal of Forensic Sciences*, *48*, 1336–1342.

Thali, M. J., & Vock, P. (2003). Role of and techniques in forensic imaging. In James, J. P., Busuttil, A., & Smock, W. (Eds.), *Forensic medicine: Clinical and pathological aspects* (pp. 731–745). San Francisco: GMM.

Thali, M. J., Yen, K., Plattner, T., Schweitzer, W., Vock, P., & Ozdoba, C. (2002). Charred body: Virtual autopsy with multi-slice computed tomography and magnetic resonance imaging. *Journal of Forensic Sciences*, *47*, 1326–1331.

Thali, M. J., Yen, K., Schweitzer, W., Vock, P., Boesch, C., & Ozdoba, C. (2003). Virtopsy, a new imaging horizon in forensic pathology: Virtual autopsy by postmortem multislice computed tomography (MSCT) and magnetic resonance imaging MRI)—a feasibility study. *Journal of Forensic Sciences*, *48*, 386–403.

Thali, M. J., Yen, K., Schweitzer, W., Vock, P., Ozdoba, C., & Dirnhofer, R. (2003). Into the decomposed body-forensic digital autopsy using multislice-computed tomography. *Forensic Science International*, *134*, 109–114. doi:10.1016/S0379-0738(03)00137-3

Thali, M. J., Yen, K., Vock, P., Ozdoba, C., Kneubue, W. B. P., & Sonneschein, M. (2003). Image guided virtual autopsy findings of gunshot victims performed with multislice computed tomography (MSCT) and magnetic resonance imaging (MRI) and subsequent correlation between radiology and autopsy findings. *Forensic Science International*, *138*, 8–16. doi:10.1016/S0379-0738(03)00225-1

Wallace, S. K., Cohen, W. A., Stern, E. J., & Reay, D. T. (1994). Judicial hanging: Postmortem radiographic CT, and MR imaging features with autopsy confirmation. *Radiology*, *193*(1), 263–267.

Yen, K., Lovblad, K. O., Scheurer, E., Ozdoba, C., Thali, M. J., & Aghayev, E. (2007). Post-mortem forensic neuroimaging: Correlation of MSCT and MRI findings with autopsy results. *Forensic Science International*, *173*, 21–35. doi:10.1016/j.forsciint.2007.01.027

Yen, K., Thali, M. J., Aghayev, E., Jackowski, C., Schweitzer, W., & Boesch, C. (2005). Strangulation signs: Initial correlation of MRI, MSCT, and forensic neck findings. *Journal of Magnetic Resonance Imaging*, *22*, 501–510. doi:10.1002/jmri.20396

Yen, K., Vock, P., Tiefenthaler, B., Ranner, G., Scheurer, E., & Thali, M. J. (2004). Virtopsy: Forensic traumatology of the subcutaneous fatty tissue. Multislice computed tomography (MSCT) and magnetic resonance imaging (MRI) as diagnostic tools. *Journal of Forensic Sciences*, *49*(4), 799–806. doi:10.1520/JFS2003299

Zamora, G., Sari-Sarraf, H., & Long, L. R. (2003). Hierarchical segmentation of vertebrae from X-ray images. In. *Proceedings of SPIE Medical Imaging*, *5032*, 631–642.

zur Nedden, D., Knapp, R., Wicke, K., Judmaier, W., Murphy, W. A., & Seidler, H. (1994). Skull of a 5,300-yearold mummy: Reproduction and investigation with CT-guided stereolithography. *Radiology*, *193*, 269–272.

KEY TERMS AND DEFINITIONS

Computer Aided Diagnosis: It's a procedure in medicine that assist doctors in the interpretation of medical images. CAD is a relatively young interdisciplinary technology combining elements of artificial intelligence and digital image processing with radiological image processing.

Forensic Radiology: Usually comprises the performance, interpretation and reportage of those radiological examination and procedures that have to do with the courts and/or the law.

Statistical Shape Models: It's a useful tools to study variation in anatomical shapes. The method is applicable to any problem in which explicit shape features are not easily identifiable and is based on the iterative closet point algorithm.

Vertebral Fractures: Correspond to an alteration in the shape and size of the vertebral body, with a reduction in vertebral body height as a wedge, and-plate (mono or biconcave) or collapse vertebral deformity.

Vertebral Morphometry: Is a quantitative method to identify osteoporotic vertebral fractures that relies on the measurement of distinct vertebral dimensions, calculating relative changes. May be performed on conventional spinal radiographs (MRX) or on images obtained from dual X-ray absorptiometry (DXA) scans (MXA).

Vertebral Shape Analysis: Numeric scores are assigned to vertebral deformities according to their shape or type and their severity in a definable and reproducible manner without making direct measurements.

ENDNOTES

[1] The SQ method is based on evaluation of conventional radiographs by radiologists or experienced clinicians in order to identify and then classify vertebral fractures. Vertebrae T4-L4 are graded by visual inspection and without direct vertebral measurement as normal (grade 0), mild but "definite" fracture (grade 1 with approximately 20–25% reduction in anterior, middle, and/or posterior height, and 10–20% reduction in area), moderate fracture (grade 2 with approximately 25–40% reduction in any height and 20–40% reduction in area), and severe fracture (grade 3 with approximately 40% or greater reduction in any height and area) Additionally, a grade 0.5 was used to designate a borderline deformed vertebra that is not considered to be a definite fracture. Incident fractures are defined as those vertebrae that show a higher deformity grade on the follow-up radiographs.

[2] Since radiographs are still the preferred imaging modality in the detection of vertebral deformities, a new statistical model-based vision system called MorphoXpress has been developed by Image Metrics for Procter & Gamble Pharmaceuticals (MorphoXpress, P&G Pharmaceuticals, Rusham Park, Egham, UK) for semi- automated 6-point morphometry (Edmondston et al., 1999). The MorphoXpress operates as follows: original lateral vertebral radiographs are digitised using a TWAIN scanner (UMAX Power Look 1000, Techville, Inc., Dallas, USA). Analysis is then initialised by the manual targeting of the centres of the upper and lower vertebrae to be analyzed. The software then automatically finds the positions of landmarks for a standard 6-point morphometry measurement. The software then allows these points to be moved by the operator, if deemed necessary, before the points are confirmed as being correct. The positions of the confirmed points are then used by the software to calculate anterior, middle and posterior vertebral heights, which may also be used for the determination of deformity shape. There are two elements to the MorphoXpress software application. The first one is a one-time 'development'

phase that includes model building and the second one is the run-time 'use' phase where the model is matched in an image to obtain the 6-point morphometry. To build the model, a set of representative images of the anatomy to be modelled is manually marked by an expert using a set of points placed along the anatomical boundaries. This set of 'training' images effectively captures the expert's knowledge of how the anatomy of interest is presented in the chosen modality. The marked objects are aligned in scale and rotation before a form of statistical decomposition is applied to describe the variation of the aligned shapes. This decomposition results in an anatomical shape parameterization that is referred to as a model.

3   Minne (Minne et al., 1988) developed the Spine Deformity Index to quantify spinal deformity and assess progression of vertebral deformation during follow-up. Other authors introduced new morphometric indices to quantify the spinal deformity, namely, sums of anterior, middle, and posterior heights (AHS, MHS, PHS) of the respective 14 vertebral body heights from T4 to L5. Irregularity in the curvature of the spine can be quantified as the integrated average of the ratios of the anterior to posterior vertebral heights of adjacent vertebrae. This Spinal Curvature Irregularity Index (SCII) is a measure of the 'smoothness' of the spinal curvature, and a large SCII is correlated with the presence of vertebral deformities.

Chapter 5
Facial Reconstruction as a Regression Problem

Maxime Berar
Université de Rouen, France

Françoise Tilotta
Université Paris Descartes, France

Joan A. Glaunès
Université Paris Descartes, France

Yves Rozenholc
Université Paris Descartes, France

Michel Desvignes
GIPSA-LAB, France

Marek Bucki
Laboratoire TIMC-IMAG, France

Yohan Payan
Laboratoire TIMC-IMAG, France

ABSTRACT

This chapter presents a computer-assisted method for facial reconstruction. This method provides an estimation of the facial outlook associated with unidentified skeletal remains. Current computer-assisted methods using a statistical framework rely on a common set of points extracted form the bone and soft-tissue surfaces. Facial reconstruction then attempts to predict the position of the soft-tissue surface points knowing the positions of the bone surface points. This chapter proposes to use linear latent variable regression methods for the prediction (such as Principal Component Regression or Latent Root Root Regression) and to compare the results obtained to those given by the use of statistical shape models. In conjunction, the influence of the number of skull landmarks used was evaluated. Anatomical skull landmarks are completed iteratively by points located upon geodesics linking the anatomical landmarks. They enable artificial augmentation of the number of skull points. Facial landmarks are obtained using a mesh-matching algorithm between a common reference mesh and the individual soft-tissue surface meshes. The proposed method is validated in terms of accuracy, based on a leave-one-out cross-validation test applied on a homogeneous database. Accuracy measures are obtained by computing the distance between the reconstruction and the ground truth. Finally, these results are discussed in regard to current computer-assisted facial reconstruction techniques, including deformation based techniques.

DOI: 10.4018/978-1-60960-483-7.ch005

INTRODUCTION

In forensic medicine, craniofacial reconstruction refers to any process that aims to recover the morphology of the face from skull observation (Wilkinson, 2005). Otherwise known as facial approximation, it is usually considered when confronted with an unrecognisable corpse and when no other identification evidence is available. This reconstruction may hopefully provide a route to a positive identification. Forensic facial reconstruction is more of a tool for recognition, than a method of identification [Wilkinson]: it aims to provide a list of names from which the individual may be identified by accepted methods of identification. Since its conception in the 19th century, two schools of thought have developed in the field. To answer the question "will only one face be produced from each skull", facial "approximators" claim that many facial variations from the same skull may be produced, whereas practitioners of the other school of thought attempt to characterised the individual skull morphology to make the individual recognisable. In recent years, computer-assisted techniques have been developed following the evolution of medical imaging and computer science. As presented in the surveys in Buzug (2006), Clemens (2005), DeGreef (2005), and Wilkinson (2005), computerised approaches are now available with reduced performance timeline and operator subjectivity.

The first machine-aided methods were inspired by manual methods. Manual reconstruction follows four basic steps, (according to Helmer, 2003): Examination of the Skull, Development of a Reconstruction Plan, Practical Sculpturing and Mask Design. Translated into a computer-assisted framework, these steps are according to Buzug (2006): Computed Tomography Scan of the skull, Matching of a Soft Tissue Template, Warping of Template onto Skull Find and Texture Mapping/ Virtual Make-Up. The first step aims to extract structural characteristics: for example key skull dimension for manual methods or crest-lines (Quatrehomme, 1997) for computer assisted ones. Another example is the location, automatically or by an expert of cephalometric points. Skulls and facial surfaces have been collected using a variety of 2- and 3-D methods such as photography (Stratomeier, 2005), video (Evison 1996), laser scanning (Claes, 2006), magnetic resonance imaging (Paysan, 2009; Mang, 2006; Michael, 1996), holography (Hirsch, 2005; Hering, 2003), mobile digital ultrasound scanner (Claes, 2006), computed tomography scanning (Jones, 2001; Bérar, 2006; Tu, 2007) .The second step consists in compiling all the data obtained during the investigation and listing soft-tissue depths for specified points of the face in accordance with the individual 's gender and type of constitution. This is the equivalent of the "Matching of a Soft Tissue Template" step, which aims at identifying an appropriate soft-tissue template from a database or inject in the model the estimated age, body mass index, gender or ancestry.

The third step is either the modeling of the muscles using wax, followed by the embedding of eye glass, then by the modeling of the nose, mouth and eyelids, ... or the deformation of the face template in order to fit the set of virtual dowels placed on the virtual skull on given landmarks. Interactive correction of individual parts of the face was usually necessary in the computerized reconstruction and, similarly, the wax face is re-worked to achieve a natural appearance. The last step consists in achieving of a natural-looking face. In summary, the first machine-aided techniques fitted a skin surface mask to a set of interactively placed virtual dowels on the digitized model of the remains (Evenhouse, 1992; Vanezis, 2000; Shahrom, 1996). These techniques did not try to learn the relationships between bone surfaces and soft-tissue surfaces but to use the relationships described in soft-tissue depth tables (Rhine, 1980, 1984). Moreover, skilled operators were necessary in the choice of facial templates, features or sculptural distortions, thus creating a dependency on the practitioner training and subjectivity (Wilkinson, 2005).

Later techniques have moved away from the manual techniques and use the relationships between soft-tissue and bone surfaces. Two kinds of methods can be distinguished based on the representation of the bone and soft-tissue volumes. The first type of techniques aims to keep the continuous nature of the skull and soft-tissue surfaces. Estimates of the face are obtained by applying deformations of the space to couples of known bone and soft tissue surfaces, called reference surfaces. These deformations are learned between the surface of the dry skull and the surfaces of the reference skulls and then applied on the surfaces of the reference faces. They can be parametric (e-g B-splines) (Kermi 2007; Vandermeulen 2006), implicit using variational methods (Mang, 2006; Mang, 2007) or volumetric (Nelson, 1998; Quatrehomme, 1997). Depending on the method, the final estimated face can be either the deformed face whose reference skull is the nearest of the dry skull (Nelson, 1998; Quatrehomme, 19970 or a combination of all the deformed soft-tissue surfaces (Vandermeulen, 2006; Tu, 2007). Here, the relationships between the surfaces are not learned but conserved through the deformation fields. To a single dry skull corresponds as many deformed faces as subjects in the database, and all the combinations possible between them (the more common combination being the mean). The generic deformations applied to the templates are not face-specific, but only "smooth" in a mathematical sense. No problem arises when the differences between the model and the target skull-based surfaces are small. However, if these differences are relatively large, the required deformation will be more pronounced, resulting in a possibly unrealistic or implausible facial reconstruction.

The second type of approaches chooses to represent individuals using a common set of points, like soft-tissue depths were originally measured. As the position of the corresponding points for all the individuals can be summarised as variables

in a table, the main idea is then to use statistics to decipher the relation between the skull and the soft-tissue. The common set of points can either be anatomical landmarks (Claes, 2006; Vanezis, 2000) or semi-landmarks located following a point correspondence procedure (Berar, 2006; Kähler, 2003: Paysan, 2009). Semi-landmarks are defined as points that do not have names but that match across all the samples of a data set under a reasonable model of deformation (Bookstein, 1997). Usually, a small set of anatomical landmarks is used to represent the bone surface whereas a larger set of points is used to represent the soft-tissue surface. The larger the set, the more this representation of the surface approaches a real surface. Apart from the practical constraint of the number of anatomical landmarks that an expert can define and extract, there is no justification of a chosen number of points used to represent the skull surface. Indeed, the information given by the position of skull anatomical landmarks is double. First, there is geometric information given by the coordinates of the points. Then, "anatomic" information is given by the measures of tissue thickness made on this points. This information is available for a limited number of points. However, the geometric information given by the position of the point can be completed by automatic methods of landmark extraction. The second part of the data analysis framework consists in learning the relationships between the soft-tissue variables and the bone variables. In current techniques, a linear model of the common variability of the positions of the points is learned -following the works made in statistical atlas, medical or audiovisual speech- called a statistical shape model (Cootes, 1995). Either the variability of the points of the soft-tissue surface (Claes, 2006; Basso, 2005; Tu, 2007), or each set of points of each surface (Paysan, 2009), or a set containing the points of both surfaces (Berar, 2006; Mang, 2006) can be learned. Statistical shape models describe the shape as a mean shape and a set of linear variations around it. Each of these variations is controlled by the modes of the model, and any individual can be described by a set of values of the variations modes, also called variability parameters. Statistical shape models are an attempt to characterized the individual skull morphology to make the individual recognizable by the value of the variability parameters. For facial reconstruction, the predicted soft-tissue surface will be the instance of the shape model the nearest to the measured skull landmarks or analogous face points, depending on which of those points are included in the model.

However, the prediction of the positions of the soft-tissue points knowing the positions of the set of skull landmarks is a regression problem. The skull points will then be considered as entries of a regression model and the face points will be considered as the outputs of the model. Several regression methods have been developed, some sharing the ideas behind the statistical shape models. Principal Component Regression will build a statistical shape model of the shape of the skull and use the variability parameters of the model, also known as latent variables, as predictors for the regression problem. Another example of a latent variable regression method is Latent Root regression (Gunst, 1976; Vigneau, 2002). Designed to take into account the presence of co-linearity in the variables, in our case the positions of the skull landmarks and of the face semi-landmarks, it shares the use of Principal Component Analysis (Joliff, 1986) like the statistical shape model and indeed builds a joint statistical shape model of all the points, bone and soft-tissue alike.

For all facial reconstruction methods, the assessment of the accuracy, reliability and re-producibility of the computer-based systems is of paramount importance. Practitioners have relied for a long time on examples of success-ful forensic cases or subjective assessment of resemblance. Databases of surfaces enable us to obtain quantitative measures of the proximity between the shape of the predicted and validation samples. However, as each database is different, so are each digitalization and point correspondence

procedures. Comparison of methods is therefore difficult and the quantitative measures of the proximity of surfaces do not translate well into a success rate for identification. Simplified face-pool tests have been used in order to estimate the identification success rate, established generating 2D images from the 3D models and showing them to human observers (Claes, 2006). In the same vein, correspondences between facial landmarks on the predicted surface and photographies can be researched (Tu 2007) as a short cut for a pos-sible recognition.

In this chapter, we propose facial reconstruction techniques using linear regressions methods and compare the results obtained to those given by a statistical shape model. The deformation algorithm -used to build the database of soft-tissue meshes-provides one last facial reconstruction method-ology, where the deformation field computed between the surface of the dry skull and a bone surface of the learning database will be applied to the corresponding face surface of the base to obtain a facial reconstruction. The same error criteria will be used to quantitatively compare all the obtained reconstructed faces. In conjunction, we inter-rogate the number of skull landmarks necessary. Basing our first experimentation on anatomical skull landmarks extracted by an expert, we will iteratively add supplementary mathematical skull landmarks following the point correspondence technique described in Wang (2000), which relies on the geodesic paths between the landmarks to define new landmarks. Regression methods will be used to predict the new points given by each iteration and those results compared to those of the facial reconstruction methods.

The chapter is organized as follows. The mate-rial and method are presented in a first section, which presents the material on which this study has been done. The following sections focus on resolving the point correspondence problem, describing the two methods used to obtain the two subject-shared descriptions of the bone and soft-tissue surfaces. Next, statistical methods are discussed: the building and use of a statistical shape model, the Principal Component Regression and the multivariate Latent Root Regression method. Following this, the results obtained by the different models are shown and the influence of the number of skull landmarks and of the statistical method chosen is discussed.

MATERIAL AND METHODS

This study was performed using whole head and skull surface meshes extracted from whole head CT scanners acquired for a project on facial reconstruction of University Paris Descartes. In the framework of this study, we focus on a group of 47 women aged from 20 to 40 years. Soft-tissue and bone surface meshes have been obtained following mathematical and computational processes described in Tilotta (2009). Anatomical skull landmarks were also manually located on each CT Scan according to classical methods of physical anthropology (13 midpoints and two sets of 13 lateral points). In order to artificially augment the size of the database, the entries of the database will consist of left or right halves of each surface meshes. The skull and the face do not have symmetric shapes, but the relationships between these face and skull shapes do not depend on the side of the head. The plan minimizing the distances to the anatomical midpoints has been chosen as an artificial boundary between the right and left part of the shapes.

The next step is to establish correspondences between the shapes of each subject in order to quantify the anatomical differences between subjects. It is a common step of the building of statistical shape models or of statistical atlases. According to the nature of the representation of the shape in the statistical model (surface, lines, points), this problem is reduced to a problem of correspondence between sets of points, lines or surfaces. Points correspondence procedures extract points which correspond to the same places on the different individuals. In consequences, each skull or face shape mesh shares the same mesh structure with the same number of vertices. For example, anatomical landmarks located by the expert establish a rough mesh for each subject with a shared structure between the subjects, whereas the variability of the position of the vertices reflects the anatomical characteristics of each subject. In the opposite, deforming a common mesh on all the subjects meshes will too share the structure of the deformed mesh. The location of the vertices of each deformed mesh will too reflect the anatomical characteristics of each subject. According to the point correspondence procedures used, the surfaces have to be cut in two at different steps of the procedures. The surfaces will be either cut following the boundary plan as a pre-processing step (soft-tissue surfaces) or cut as a post-processing step (bone surfaces). The automatically extracted points respect this symmetry constraint. The points shared between the left and right entries will be located on the boundary plan.

Building Normalised Shapes: Point Correspondence Procedure for the Bone Surfaces

The anatomical landmarks located by the expert (Figure 1A) establish a first correspondence between the skulls. Following the scheme presented in Wang (2000), we define a set of triangular connections between these anatomical landmarks. For each pairs of connected points, we can extract a set of geodesic curbs between these points. Geodesics are defined to be the shortest path between points on the curved spaces of the shape surfaces (see Figure 1B). As the shape surface between two landmarks is different from a sphere, these geodesics are unique. At this step, a gross template of curbs on the surface between the landmarks is build. We then can define new landmarks as the midpoints of each geodesics and decompose each triangle into four new triangles. A more dense triangulation is then derived as seen Figure 1C.

Figure 1. Iterative extraction of skull landmarks

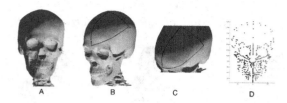

Figure 2. Skull shape meshes generated for iteration 0 to 5

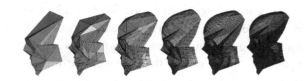

As the iterative process is repeated, the structure is refined to denser surface points and triangulation. The obtained structures form meshes, who share the same structure for each individual, and implicitly solve the point correspondence problem.

Moreover, the defined structure is symmetric: the two entries (left and right) of the database share a common substructure and set of midpoints (Figure 1D). Due to numerical instabilities, two methods of geodesics computation on surface meshes have been used: Surazhsky algorithm (Surazhsky, 2005) and Fast Marching Algorithm algorithm (Sethian, 1999), implemented by Peyre in the Geowave library. For two iterations of the procedure, it results in three sets of skull landmarks for each individual. A first set of points composed of the original landmarks: 13 midpoints and 13 lateral points. A second set composed of 54 points is added by the first iteration of the procedure (10 midpoints and 44 lateral points) and completed with 198 new landmarks by the second iteration (20 midpoints and 178 lateral points). The total number of points for each structure up to 5 iterations is shown Table 1.

Figure 2 shows skull meshes corresponding to successive iterations of the procedure. As more

points are extracted, new levels of details are obtained especially in the superior part of the skull. A limit of this procedure occurs for very small length of one or more side of the triangles. In this case, the triangle degenerates into a point or a segment and subsequent iteration will extract all supplementary points in the same location. Moreover, as the surface encompassed by each triangles becomes smaller, the triangles become planar. All supplementary points are then situated on the same plane and the information given by the supplementary points is less useful.

Building Normalised Shapes: Point Correspondence Procedure for the Soft-tissue Surfaces

For the soft-tissue surfaces, no landmarks are located. Moreover measures of tissue thickness are not provided: the number of skull landmarks corresponding to successive iterations of the former point correspondence procedure increases too much to allow manual measurements to be done. The quality of automatic extraction of tissue thickness on landmarks depends on the surface representation: the normal vectors on the surface meshes are sensitive to the triangulation used on the surfaces. Tissue thickness cannot be measured correctly and automatically on all possible landmarks (Tilotta, 2009).

Instead of facial points analogous to the anatomical skull points, we extract a set of semi-landmarks for each individuals neither really dense nor sparse. Working on the "half" surfaces previously defined, the point correspondence

Table 1. Number of points by iteration of the procedure

Iteration	0	1	2	3	4	5
Number of points	26	80	278	1034	3986	15650
Mid-points	13	23	43	83	163	323

procedure register a reference mesh (see Figure 3A) on the individual soft-tissue surface mesh (see Figure 3B) resulting on a deformed reference mesh (see Figure 3C). The registration is made computing an elastic deformation between the reference mesh and soft-tissue surface meshes of the database. The deformed meshes of each entry of the database have the same number of vertices (1741 for the mesh of an half face). The assumption of semi landmarks is then assumed: each vertex of the deformed reference meshes matches the same point for every individual. The 3D to 3D meshes matching algorithm used is a modified version of Szeliski algorithm (Szeliski, 1996). A first modification has been made to take into account the difference of density between the reference mesh and the high-density meshes of the soft-tissue surfaces. The second modification ensures that each vertex of the boundary of the deformed reference meshes is shared by the right and left meshes. The mesh used as the reference mesh correspond to the region of the face of head mesh modelled by F. Pighin (1999), where the density of vertices is greater in zones with high bending than in zones with low bending. This dissimilarity between the soft-tissue surface meshes and the reference meshes have consequences. The distances from the vertices of the deformed reference mesh to its associated soft-tissue surface mesh are null. However, the distances from the vertices of the soft-tissue mesh surface to the deformed reference mesh are not null.. The highest distances (superior to 3 mm) correspond to parts of the soft-tissue surfaces which do not have corresponding regions in the reference surface. Other distances correspond to regions like the forehead or the cheeks where the difference of the density of vertices is large. Vertices with no direct counterparts can be as far as 2 mm from the surface defined by the deformed reference mesh. A good measure of the error introduced during this point correspondence step is the median of the distances, which does not take into account the large distances generated by the lack of cor-

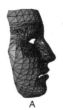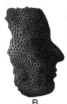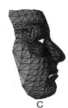

Figure 3. Establishing correspondences between the face: (a) reference mesh, (b) subject face surface mesh, (c) subject deformed reference mesh

A   B   C

respondence on the boundaries. Upon all samples of the database, the mean median of distances is 0.22 mm (with standard deviation of 0.04 mm). Individual correspondence error range from 0.17 mm to 0.34 mm, whereas the individual mean of the distances range from 0.54 mm to 2.66 mm.

STATISTICAL METHODS

The variables $\tilde{x}_i$ respectively, $\tilde{y}_i$ are obtained from the positions of the N skull points, respectively L soft-tissue points of subject i:

$$\tilde{x}_i = \left[S_x^1 S_y^1 S_z^1 \cdots S_x^N S_y^N S_z^N \right] \qquad (1)$$

$$\tilde{y}_i = \left[F_x^1 F_y^1 F_z^1 \cdots F_x^L F_y^L F_z^L \right] \qquad (2)$$

Two geometrically averaged templates $\overline{x}$ and $\overline{y}$ are computed and the data are centered:

$$x_i = \tilde{x}_i - \overline{x}_i \qquad (3)$$

$$y_i = \tilde{x}_i - \overline{x}_i \qquad (4)$$

The data tables X, respectively Y, of size n x N, respectively n x L, encompass the variables corresponding to the n centered samples x_i and y_i in the learning database. In the following paragraphs, the transposition of the matrix X will be noted X^T.

Principal Components Analysis

Principal Components Analysis (Joliff, 1986) performed on the data table X extracts a correlation-ranked set of statistically independent modes of principal variations from the set of subjects described in the data table X. These principal modes are vectors of 3D coordinates (of size 3N) defined as linear combinations of point positions. They capture the variations observed over all subjects in the database. The modes are sometimes also called variability parameters. These vectors are the eigenvectors of the covariance matrix $X^T X$ associated to the eigenvalues l_i sorted such as $l_1 > \dots > l_n \geq 0$. The eigenvectors are orthogonal.

$$l_i a_i = X^T X a_i . \tag{5}$$

Every entry x_i in the database can now be represented as a weighted linear combination of these eigenvectors:

$$x_i = \sum c_{ij} a_j \tag{6}$$

where c_{ij} is the weight attached to sample i and eigenvector j, also called the principal component of sample i on axis of variability j. As the modes are correlation-ranked, the first modes are responsible for the greatest part of the observed variance of the data. In most cases, only a small number of modes is necessary to represent most of the observed data. A classical criterion is to choose the number of modes t in order to represent 95% of the observed variance. A good approximation of each sample is then given using the first t components:

$$x_i = \sum c_{ij} a_j \tag{7}$$

For a new entry x_0, each weight can be extracted as the projection of the sample on each axis of variability:

$$c_{0j} = x_0^T a_j \tag{8}$$

A new sample can be build from these components and the variability axis.

$$\hat{x}_0 = \sum c_{0j} a_j$$

A measure of the generalisation power of the model is the reconstruction error, which we will call re-synthesis error to avoid confusion with (facial) reconstruction:

$$E_{0,s} = \left(x_0 - \hat{x}_0\right)^T \left(x_0 - \hat{x}_0\right) \tag{9}$$

which consists in the distance between the re-synthesised sample and the original.

Principal Components Regressions

Principal Components Regression (PCR) is a linear regression method. The multi-response linear regression model for centred data is defined as:

$$Y = XB + E \tag{10}$$

where B is 3N x 3L matrix of regression coefficients and E is a noise matrix of size n x 3L. The elements of the matrix E are assumed to be normally distributed with mean $E[E] = \sim 0$ and variance $var[E] = S$. Given a new sample x_0, an estimate of y_0 is:

$$y_0 = B^T x_0 . \tag{11}$$

The mean square estimation of the coefficients of B is given by

$$\hat{B} = \left(X^T X \right)^{-1} X^T Y \ . \qquad (12)$$

However, in case where the predictors (x) present a lot of co-linearity, this estimation is not optimal and a common way is to substitute the predictors by the first t principal components corresponding to the samples of the database, regrouped in matrix C. As the axis of variability are orthogonal, there are no co-linearity in the new predictors. A mean square estimation of the regression coefficients between the components C and Y is build:

$$\hat{G}_{PCR} = \left(C^T C \right)^{-1} C^T Y \qquad (13)$$

which can be used to estimate the regression coefficients B, (the matrix A regroup the t first axis of variability):

$$\hat{B}_{PCR} = A \left(C^T C \right)^{-1} C^T Y \qquad (14)$$

This kind of methods originates from chemiometrics were a small number of predictors must predict a great number of outputs. It is then particularly adapted to the ratio between a small number of skull landmarks and the great number of face points. However, the statistical model presented here will take into account only the skull data (X), and so will the regression model. How can we take into account the observed variability of the known face shapes (Y)?

A Common Statistical Shape Model

Consider the matrix Z formed by merging data tables X and Y and perform Principal Component Analysis on Z. The result of this PCA is still a correlation-ranked set of statistically independent modes of principal variations d_j , vectors of size 3(N+L). Each eigenvector d_i with positive eigenvalue obtained by PCA can be decomposed as the juxtaposition of two vectors $d_i = \left[v_i w_i \right]$, with v_i of size 3N and w_i of size 3L. Each part x_i and y_i of entry z_i can be expressed sharing the same weights b_{ij} and the vectors v_i and w_i :

$$x_i = \sum b_{ij} v_j \qquad (15)$$

$$y_i = \sum b_{ij} w_j \qquad (16)$$

For facial reconstruction, we search the best model fit: the instance $z_0 = \left[\hat{x}_0 y_0 \right]$ of the model the nearer from the measured skull landmarks x_0 . As z_0 can be represented using the parametric representation of the statistical model as a set of weights b_{0j} , the problem is resolved finding successively each weight b_{0j} for which the distance between the measured skull landmarks and the points of the model corresponding to skull landmarks is the smallest:

$$b_{0j} = argmin_{b_{0j}} \left(b_{0j} v_j - x_0 \right)^T \left(b_{0j} v_j - x_0 \right). \qquad (17)$$

The solution is given

$$b_{0j} = \left(\overline{x}_0^T v_j \right) / \left(v_j^T v_j \right) \qquad (18)$$

and the facial reconstruction is obtained by:

$$\hat{y}_0 = \overline{y} + \sum b_{0j} w_j \ . \qquad (19)$$

Latent Root Regression

Latent Root Regression (LRR) is a linear regression method. LRR is similar to Principal Component Regression (PCR) (and Partial Least Square (PLS) regression), with comparable results in the literature. Single response Latent Root Regression (Hawkins 73, Webster et al. 74) use the same vectors v_i as the common statistical shape model to estimate B. As these vectors are not necessary orthogonal, an iterative procedure build upon the first latent variable is necessary as in multi-responsee PLS (PLS2) (see Vigneau & Qannari, 2002 for details) for Multi-Response Latent Root Regression. It results in a sequence of orthogonal vectors $\tilde{v}_i$ which enables us to compute regression coefficients, following the formula:

$$\hat{B}_{LRR} = \sum \tilde{v}_i \left(\tilde{v}_i^T X^T X \tilde{v}_i \right)^{-1} \tilde{v}_i^T X^T Y \qquad (20)$$

RESULTS

Validation

The validation of the proposed statistical methods for craniofacial reconstruction is obtained by a leave-one-out cross-validation procedure. Each one in his turn, two couples, left and right, of skull and soft-tissue samples are removed from the database and used as test cases, the remaining entries are used to create the statistical model. The skull points of each couple are used as separate entries for the statistical model. The resulting location of the face points are then compared with their real location. However, the location of the face points is the result of the deformation of a common reference mesh. The distance between the location of each predicted face point and the original soft-tissue surface mesh of the test case -which is a better approximation of the ground truth- can be computed and is a more acurate measure.

How Many Skull Landmarks?

In order to assess the number of necessary skull landmarks, we can use the hierarchical nature of the extraction procedure presented in section 1.2 and the statistical methods presented in Section 2. Each landmark set of inferior level (containing less landmarks) can be used to predict the position of the landmarks of superior level. If one set can predict the positions of all points of all subjects of the following level with a very good accuracy, then there is no information added by the supplementary points. Therefore, it is not necessary to use more points for the description of the skull shape. However, we can first remark that the answer given by this experiment will be related but different to the answer to a question on the number of necessary skull landmarks to facial reconstruction. A common interrogation will be: is all the information given by the skull shape necessary to predict the shape of the face? Secondly, the techniques described here can be used when the skull is fragmented to predict missing fragments of the skull from the remaining parts.

For each set of landmarks, we build a PCA model. It gives us a linear model of the shape variations, as described by the set of landmarks. This model will be used to predict the position of the supplementary points in upper level sets, using Principal Components Regression. However, we first test the generalisation capacity of these models by projecting the landmarks of a test subject into the model, i.e. extracting its variability parameters, and then re-synthesising the landmarks using these variability parameters. If a model has a good generalisation capacity, then the location of the re-synthesised points will be very close to the location of the points of the test subject. These errors correspond to the accuracy of the prediction by model based upon N0 points of a shape described by N0 points, up to the accuracy of the prediction by model N5 of a N5-shape. These first results are shown in the diagonal of the Table 2.

Table 2. Accuracy of the prediction of landmarks (mm) (number of variability modes used)

Sets of points	N0 (26)	N1 (80)	N2 (278)	N3 (1034)	N4 (3986)	N5 (15650)
N0	0,04mm (43)	0,23mm (37)	2,55mm (18)	4,29mm (13)	4,56mm (10)	4.58 mm (12)
N1	–	0,16mm (43)	3,09mm (19)	4,47mm (14)	4,61mm (10)	4.58 mm (12)
N2	–	–	0,86mm (92)	1,44mm (79)	1,40mm (79)	4.60 mm (10)
N3	–	–	–	1,13mm (92)	1,16mm (92)	1.17 mm (92)
N4	–	–	–	–	1.13mm (92)	1.60 mm (92)

Next, we use principal components regression (PCR) to predict the location of the supplementary points. If the prediction of these points is accurate, then the supplementary points do not add any information that can't be extrapolated linearly using the previous set of points. Table 2 presents the mean prediction errors of the points introduced by each successive level of the procedure. For example, the model based on N1 points is used for the prediction of shapes described by N2, N3, N4 and N5 points.

First, the generalisation capacity of the different model as measured by the re-synthesis error decreases as the number of points increases (from 26 to 15650): the ratio between the number of points and subjects becomes unbalanced. For a N0, the model is built on 96 subjects for 3*26=78 coordinates, whereas for N5, the model is build on 92 subjects for 3*15650 coordinates. More subjects are necessary to take into account the variability of the data, as the optimal number of modes corresponds to the maximum number of modes. For N3, N4 and N5, the generalisation capacity of the models is not as good, but there are no significant differences between the errors (1.09 mm vs. 1.13 mm).

We can then observe that the model based on N0 points performs as well as the model based on N1 points, whatever the number of points describing the shape to predict, and uses the same number of principal components, even for shapes described by N1 points. Moreover, models based on N0 and N1 points are not sufficient to model the variability of the shapes of the upper levels, as shown by the large prediction errors. This seems to validate the use of a greater number of points than 100.

The models based on N2 and N3 points perform as well for re-synthesis than for the prediction of the supplementary points. It is particularly true in this experiment for the model based on N3 points, which perform as well on prediction than the models based on N4 and N5 points on re-synthesis (1.16 mm vs. 1.13 mm, 1.17 mm vs. 1.09 mm)). For the prediction of a really great number of points (N5), the model based on N2 points performs the same as the model based on less than a hundred of points.

Given our number of subjects in the database, one thousand points seems to be a sufficient number of points to model the shape of the skull. As such a number of points can't be located manually by an expert without being time consumptive, semi-automatic or fully automatic location methods for the landmarks are therefore necessary.

Facial Reconstruction: Results

The cross-validation procedure was performed on the available database resulting in 47 successive test cases. As the database is composed of half parts of the bone and skin surface, as much as 92 modes can be used for the prediction of the location of the points of the soft-tissue surface. The other limiting factor of the maximum number of modes is the number of known points per entries. For N0 = 26, the total number of components of the known points is 78 and is inferior to the size of the

Table 3. Accuracy of the prediction of the semi-landmarks (mm) (number of variability modes used)

	PCR	PCA JSSM	LRR
N0	3.09 + 0.68 mm (11)	4,09 +1.28 mm (4)	3,08 + 0.73 mm (13)
N1	3.08 + 0.67 mm (18)	3.93 + 1.12 mm (4)	3.17 + 0.72 mm (12)
N2	3.05 + 0.69 mm (19)	3.87 + 1.05 mm (4)	3,14 + 0.72 mm (12)
N3	3.07 + 0.69 mm (19)	3.69 + 0.94 mm (4)	3,13 + 0.70 mm (12)
N4	3.08 + 0.70 mm (19)	3.36 + 0.87 mm (6)	3.09 + 0.71 mm (14)

Figure 4. Example of facial reconstruction for LRR method. Left: Original face surface Reconstructed face. Right: distance card of the prediction of the left and right halves of the soft tissue surface

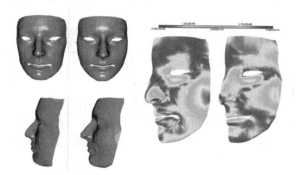

learning base. For the successive level, it won't be an issue as the total numbers of components is 3 times the number of points: the maximum number of modes is the number of learning samples (92).

For the three presented methods, the mean location error is given in Table 2. Figure 4 shows the evolution of the error for the first 25 modes. In a first time, we can observe that proper methods of regression (PCR, LRR) give better results for the task of prediction than the use of a joint statistical shape model. For this method (PCA JSSM), more points correspond to a better prediction of the location of the face semi-landmarks: from a mean prediction error of 4,09 mm with N0 points to a mean prediction error 3.19 mm with N5 points . However, even with N5 points, the prediction error is still higher than for the regression methods: 3.19 mm.

The results given by the regression methods are equivalent between each methods, and the benefits given by the number of points is less observable as the values of the mean prediction error are very close whatever the number of points: between 3.05 mm and 3.17 mm. The results given by the PCR method are consistent with the test realised to decipher the number of skull landmarks, with the best prediction given for N2 (then N3) points. Remember that for N5 points, most of the supplementary points locations can be

predicted using N3 points. The number of face points to be predicted (14616) is in the same range than N5, but the relationships between the points are not in these case concerning the interior of a triangle surface patch. For latent root regression, who shares a common scheme with the joint statistical shape model, the more points the more precise the prediction is, except for the N0 shape and N5 shape. N0 is influenced by the good prediction of one of the case, as the standard deviation (0.73mm) for N0 point is higher for any other results.

The results presented here plead for the use of a regression method, but which one choose. PCR performs slightly better than LRR and is less influenced by the number of skull points used in the model. For the moment, it seems that any latent variable linear regression can be chosen without great difference. The ideal number of points is in the range of a thousand.

This mean points location error is very influenced by the point correspondence procedure used for the soft-tissue surfaces. As the objective of facial reconstruction is to provide a prediction of the shape of the soft-tissue surface, a better measure would be the mean distance between the predicted points and the soft-tissue surface reconstructed from the original scan images. Moreover,

Table 4. Mean points-to-surface error (mm) (number of variability modes used)

	PCR	PCA JSSM	LRR
N0	1,31+0.28 mm (23)	1,89 + 0.50 mm (4)	1,33 + 0.26 mm (13)
N1	1,33+0.28 mm (19)	1,77 + 0.50 mm (4)	1,38 + 0.27 mm (13)
N2	1,30+0.26 mm (17)	1,74 + 0.41 mm (4)	1,36 + 0.25 mm (16)
N3	1,31+0.26 mm (18)	1,64 + 0.37 mm (8)	1,34 + 0.25 mm (16)
N4	1,32+0.26mm(17)	1,48 + 0.29 mm (9)	1,33 + 0.24 mm (15)

Figure 5. Mean error by points for N0 / LRR (left) and difference in mean error cards for subsequent level of number of points (right)

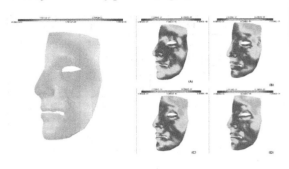

the points-to-surface error is the measure used in most works in facial reconstruction. Table 4 presents the results for the points-to-surface error. The results follow the same pattern than the points-to-points error and with a new order of magnitude of 1.4 mm, slightly modified by the projection operation on the surfaces.

An example of facial reconstruction is presented figure 4 for LRR method, with the associated distance cards. At each face landmark, a colour is associated following the prediction error giving us a spatial map of the reconstruction error. This reconstruction corresponds to the following global errors: 2.50 + 0.87 mm(P-P), 1.06 + 0.84 mm (P-S). The range of prediction error for a point is 0.007 mm to 4,81mm. The highest reconstruction errors are located on the side of the face in the masseter region. The others regions with high errors correspond to the nose and the lower eyelid. Note that the predictions and distance cards for each halve of the face is slightly different, as the face and the skull landmarks are not symmetric. However, each reconstructed half face shares many common features.

For each method, points number and components number, we can compute mean and standard deviation for each predicted point of the mask. The resulting spatial maps of the quality of the reconstruction procedure for the optimal number of parameters can be seen in figure 5 for the lo-

cal mean. The mean local errors range from 0.75 mm to 3 mm. Whatever the method, the facial areas with the highest reconstruction error are the outer limits of the surface and are for a part an artefact of the point correspondence step: there is no explicit correspondence to fix the limits of the surface in these zones. In the interior part of the face, the region with highest reconstruction error are the masseter region. These regions have few skull landmarks and the bones does not support the soft-tissue for a large part of the cheeks. The regions with the smallest errors (0.75 mm to 1 mm) are concentrated toward the middle of the face, a part where the number of skull landmarks is important and where the inter-subjects correspondence between the face meshes is more constrained. The effect of the increase of the number of skull landmarks can be observed in the difference in the error cards shown in Figure 5. The zones impacted by the increase are the nose and the side of the forehead above the temple.

The mesh-matching algorithm used to provide the point correspondence between the soft-tissue surfaces can be used in a facial reconstruction method by deformation. The deformation field computed between a source skull surface and a destination skull can be applied to the soft-tissue surface of the source. A couple of skull and soft-tissue surfaces can be chosen as the closest skull surface or each surfaces couple of the database

Table 5. Mean points-to-surface reconstruction error for deformation methods

	N0	N1	N2	N3	N4
Mean	2.61 mm	2.64 mm	2.78 mm	2.86 mm	2.88 mm

can be used and every deformed soft-tissue surface computed and considered. On a second time, a mean soft-tissue surface can be computed, merging all the deformed soft-tissue surfaces obtained by computing the mean location of the facial semi-landmarks. The accuracy of the deformation field depends on the number of points, as the criterion behind the computation of the deformation is the distance between the two surfaces.

Table 5 presents the mean points-to-surface error obtained using the different skull shapes for computing the deformation field. As we try to extrapolate the deformations fields for the deformation of the face surfaces, a very precise deformation field is not a benefit as seen with the increase of the error following a large increase in the number of points.

Comparison with Other Methods

We compare our results to those of Claes (2006) and Vandermeulen (2006). Among reconstruction techniques, the technique described in Claes (2006) is close to ours, with a supplementary deformation phase after the statistical prediction. The statistical step consists in finding the instance of a statistical face model coinciding with "dowels" of tissue thickness placed upon the skull landmarks. It corresponds to the joint statistical model method for a small number of skull landmarks (in the order of N1). The study is conducted on a database of 118 samples. The reconstruction error corresponds roughly to our point-to-surface errors. The mean reconstruction error is 1.14 mm with a standard deviation of 1.04 mm. The highest reconstruction errors (4 mm) are located in the chin and eyes regions, with errors for the region of the cheeks and the nose (except the tip) toward 2 mm. In regard to the smaller database and difference in the points correspondence step and artefacts generated, we seem to be able achieve similar results with a generally simpler methodology, i.e. without supplementary deformation phase with no phisicaly signifiance.

The technique developed in Vandermeulen (2006) is based on the use of continuous surface and the study conducted on 20 samples. The mean reconstruction error is 1.9 mm with a standard deviation of 1.7 mm. The largest reconstruction errors (2-3 mm on average) occurs on the nostrils and masseter region. We appear to outperform those results, however based on a smaller database. We can remark that the regions with large reconstruction errors coincide. Tilotta (2007) propose a local method of facial reconstruction combining prediction obtained on surface patches, delimited by landmarks. The study has been performed on two regions: the nose region and the chin region. For our methodology, the mean reconstruction error for the nose is 1.40 mm with a standard deviation of 0.25 mm. The mean reconstruction for the chin region is of 1.51 mm with 0.67 mm standard deviation. The results presented in this report outperform these estimations with a mean reconstruction error of 0.99 mm, which motivates us to consider more local procedure in the reconstruction process.

Statistical Shape Models and the Correction of the Shape of the Nose

As seen in the previous section, each of these statistical facial reconstructions are based on statistical shape models, either common or separated. For each model, we can observe the variations of the shape of the face caused by the variations upon each variability modes. For example, figure 6 presents the variations of the face shape according to the 7 first modes of LRR, PCA JSSM and PCR models for parameters of value 3 times standard

Figure 6. The variations of the face shape according to the 7 first modes of LRR, PCA JSSM and PCR models for parameters of value 3 times standard deviation. Top row: PCR model. Middle row: PCA JSSM model. Bottom row: LRR model

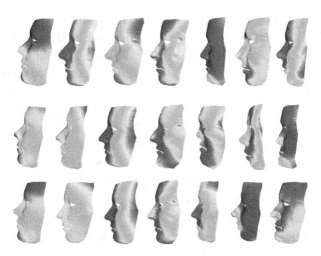

deviation. The strength of the variations is given by the color scheme and enables us to locate the parts of the face associated to each mode. The first parameter acts upon the shape of the lower part of the face, with the shape of the chin as the most influenced part of the face for both regression methods. For LRR and PCA JSSM, the second parameter models the higher part of the face, particularly the outer edge of the mask, whereas the third parameter influences variations of the skull width. For PCR, the second parameter models the difference between compressed and elongated faces along the anterior-posterior axis and these variations corresponds roughly to the third mode of the LRR model, whereas the third is linked to the height of the face. As LRR and PCA JSSM take into account the observed variability of the face points, the second parameter reproduces the large variability of the frontier of the face mask, a variability that cannot be observed in the skull points for the PCR model and thus not taken into account by the PCR model. The fourth parameter concerns the temporal region for all models. Beginning with fifth mode, each part of the model is described differently for each methods.

There are as much parameters than the minimum between the number of subjects or the number of points coordinates. However, as only the first parameters will be selected by the cross-validation procedure, if the parameters acting upon the variation of shape of the nose are later modes, no variation of the shape will be predicted for any test subject. All reconstructed faces will then share the same shape of the nose. Which parameters affect the shape of the nose and which skull landmarks correspond to the prediction of the shape of the nose, can be answered by the observation of the variations of the shape according to the modes. In the LRR case, the first parameter with consequences for the shape of the nose is the 6th parameter. The joint statistical shape model distributes variations on the shape of the nose between the 5th and the 6th parameters. PCR do not present any modes in the twenty first that influences only the shape of the nose.

As we know that our method performs badly for this region, we can offer several predictions with different shapes of nose, corresponding to different values of the "nose" parameters of the model. For example for the reconstructed test subject presented Figure 3 shows a very different shape of the nose than the original subject. Such modification on the value of a parameter will increase the facial reconstruction error as defined previously, but perhaps offer better recognition chances.

CONCLUSION

We proposed a statistical method for 3D computerised forensic facial reconstruction. It relies on the use of a common set of points for the description of the individuals. In this set of points, anatomical skull landmarks are completed by points located upon geodesic curbs linking the anatomical landmarks. Facial landmarks are obtained using a mesh-matching algorithm between a common reference mesh and the individual soft-tissue surface meshes. The facial reconstruction problem is resolved by the building of a linear regression model following either Latent Root regression method or Principal Component Regression method for equivalent results. The accuracy of the reconstructions made by the method was measured by leave-one-out cross-validation tests and compared to the use of a joint statistical shape model of both skull and face and a facial reconstruction method based on deformation fields. These results were discussed in regard to the results of other facial reconstruction methods on different databases and in regards to the problem of the shape of the nose. In conjunction, we have addressed the practical problem of the choice of the number of skull landmarks. Depending on the statistical method used and taking into account the size of the database and the limits of the extraction procedure, the necessary number ranges from two hundred to one thousand.

Some extensions can be proposed to the reconstruction method. First of all, having a larger database will increases the flexibility of the model. The more examples of the surfaces the model has, the better the relationships between the two surfaces are learned and the better the models based on a great number of skull landmarks will perform. Secondly, a better control of the point correspondence procedure for the soft-tissue meshes is necessary in order to soften the errors observed in the outer boundaries of the face mask. Then, an automatic extraction of the anatomical landmarks from the skull would make the complete reconstruction pipeline automatic. Lastly, to complete the computer-aided facial reconstruction procedure as a tool of generation of possible faces associated to an unknown skull, some graphic oriented computer applications must be added. A first one is the use of textures for the skin and the integration in the generated meshes of artificial eyes and hairs -which corresponds to the fourth step of reconstruction procedures (Mask Design / Virtual Make-Up). With these added features, a computerised facial reconstruction approach can compete with manual techniques. A second part would be the animation of the face using movements learned on example. The main principles applies for learning the movement of one face and for learning the variability of shapes observed between subjects. Numerous studies and data exist in the field of audiovisual speech (Bailly, 2003; Cohen, 2002; Lee, 1995; Pandzic, 2002; Turakate, 2003), where the main goal is to create "talking heads" of subjects. Other related and collaborative problems for facial reconstruction could also be found in maxillo-facial surgery (Marécaux, 2003; Payan, 2002; Schramm, 2006; Zachow, 2006), where one tries to predict the shape of face following an ablation of the jaw bones.

REFERENCES

Bailly, G., Bérar, M., Elisei, F., & Odisio, M. (2003). Audiovisual speech synthesis. *International Journal of Speech Technology*, *6*(4), 331–346. doi:10.1023/A:1025700715107

Basso, C., & Vetter, T. (2005). Statistically motivated 3D faces reconstruction . In Buzug, T. M., Sigl, K.-M., Bongartz, J., & Prüfer, K. (Eds.), *Facial reconstruction* (pp. 450–469). München: Wolters/Kluwer.

Berar, M., Desvignes, M., & Bailly, G. (2006). 3D semi-landmarks-based statistical face reconstruction. *Journal of Computing and Information Technology, 14*(1), 31–43. doi:10.2498/cit.2006.01.04

Bérar, M., Desvignes, M., Bailly, G., & Payan, Y. (2004). *3D meshes registration: Application to statistical skull model* (pp. 100–107). Berlin, Heidelberg: Springer.

Bookstein, F. L. (1997). Landmark methods for forms without landmarks: Morphometrics of group difference in outline shape. *Medical Image Analysis, 1*, 225–243. doi:10.1016/S1361-8415(97)85012-8

Buzug, T. (2006). Special issue on computer assisted craniofacial reconstruction and modelling [Editorial]. *Journal of Computing and Information Technology, 14*(1), 1–6. doi:10.2498/cit.2006.01.01

Claes, P., Vandermeulen, D., De Greef, S., Willems, G., & Suetens, P. (2006). Craniofacial reconstruction using a combined statistical model of face shape and soft tissue depths: Methodology and validation. *Forensic Science International, 159*, 147–158. doi:10.1016/j.forsciint.2006.02.035

Clement, J. G., & Marks, M. K. (2005). *Computer-graphic craniofacial reconstruction*. Boston: Academic Press.

Cohen, M. M., Massaro, D. W., & Clark, R. (2002). Training a talking head. In *Proceedings of IEEE Fourth International Conference on MultiModal Interfaces,* (pp. 499–504).

Cootes, T. F., Taylor, C. J., Cooper, D., & Graham, J. (1995). Active shape models-their training and application. *Computer Vision and Image Understanding, 61*(1), 38–59. doi:10.1006/cviu.1995.1004

De Greef, S., & Willems, G. (2005). Three-dimensional craniofacial reconstruction in forensic identification: Latest progress and new tendencies in the 21st century. *Forensic Science International, 50*(1), 12–17.

Evenhouse, R., Rasmussen, M., & Sadler, L. (1992). Computer-aided forensic facial reconstruction. *The Journal of Biocommunication, 19*(2), 22–28.

Evison, M. P. (1996). Computerized three dimensional facial reconstruction. Retrieved from www.shef.ac.uk/assem/1/evison.html

Frangi, A., Rueckert, D., Schnabel, J., & Niessen, W. (2002). Automatic construction of multiple object three-dimensional statistical shape models: Application to cardiac modeling. *IEEE Transactions on Medical Imaging, 21*(9), 1151–1166. doi:10.1109/TMI.2002.804426

Gunst, R., Webster, J., & Mason, R. (1976). A comparison of least squares and latent root regression estimator. *Technometrics, 18*, 75–83. doi:10.2307/1267919

Helmer, R. P., Buzug, T. M., & Hering, P. (2003). Plastic facial reconstruction on the skull-a transition in Germany from a conventional technique to a new one. *Proceedings of the First International Conference on Reconstruction of Soft Facial Parts.* (pp. 75–90). Wiesbaden: Bundeskriminalamt.

Hierl, T., Wollny, G., Peter, F., Scholz, E., Schmidt, J.-G., & Berti, G. (2006). CAD-CAM implants in esthetic and reconstructive craniofacial surgery. *Journal of Computing and Information Technology, 14*(1), 65–70. doi:10.2498/cit.2006.01.07

Hutton, T. J., Cunningham, S., & Hammond, P. (2000). An evaluation of active shape models for the automatic identification of cephalometric landmarks. *European Journal of Orthodontics, 22*(5), 499–508. doi:10.1093/ejo/22.5.499

Jolliffe, I. T. (1986). *Principal component analysis*. Berlin: Springer Verlag.

Jones, M.W. (2001). *Facial reconstruction using volumetric data.*

Kähler, K., Haber, J., & Seidel, H.-P. (2003). Re-animating the dead: Reconstruction of expressive faces from skull data. In *ACM Transactions on Graphics (SIGGRAPH 2003 Conference Proceedings), 22*(3), 554–561.

Kermi, A., Bloch, I. & Laskri, M.T. (2007). A non-linear registration method guided by b-splines free-form deformations for three-dimensional facial reconstruction. *International Review on Computers and Software, 20.*

Kuratate, T., Vatikiotis-Bateson, E., & Yehia, H. (2003). Cross-subject face animation driven by facial motion mapping. In Proceedings of *CE2003: Advanced Design, Production, and Managements systems,* (pp. 971–979).

Lee, Y., Terzopoulos, D., & Walters, K. (1995). *Realistic modeling for facial animation* (pp. 55–62).

Mang, A., Müller, J., & Buzug, M. T. (2005). Soft-tissue segmentation in forensic applications . In Buzug, T. M., Sigl, K.-M., Bongartz, J., & Prüfer, K. (Eds.), *Facial reconstruction* (pp. 62–67). München: Wolters/Kluwer.

Mang, A., Müller, J., & Buzug, T. M. (2006). A multi-modality computer-aided framework towards postmortem identification. *Journal of Computing and Information Technology, 14*(1), 7–19. doi:10.2498/cit.2006.01.02

Marécaux, C., Sidjilani, B. M., Chabanas, M., Chouly, F., Payan, Y., & Boutault, F. (2003). A new 3D cephalometric analysis for planning in computer aided orthognatic surgery. *Computer Aided Surgery, 8*(4), 217.

Michael, S. D., & Chen, M. (1996). The 3-D reconstruction of facial features using volume distortion. *Proceedings of 14th Annual Conference of Eurographics,* (pp. 297-305).

Nelson, L. A., & Michael, S. D. (1998). The application of volume deformation to three dimensional facial reconstruction: A comparison with previous techniques. *Forensic Science International, 94,* 167–181. doi:10.1016/S0379-0738(98)00066-8

Pandzic, I. S., & Forchheimer, R. (2002). *MPEG-4 facial animation. The standard, implementation, and applications.* Chichester, UK: John Wiley & Sons. doi:10.1002/0470854626

Payan, Y., Chabanas, M., Pelorson, X., Vilain, C., Levy, P., & Luboz, V. (2002). Biomechanical models to simulate consequences of maxillofacial surgery. *Comptes Rendus Biologies, 325,* 407–417. doi:10.1016/S1631-0691(02)01443-9

Paysan, P., Luthi, M., Albrecht, T., Lerch, A., Amberg, B., & Santini, F. (2009). Face reconstruction from skull shapes and physical attributes. In . *Proceedings of DAGM-Symposium, 2009,* 232–241.

Pighin, F., Szeliski, R., & Salesin, D. H. (1999). Resynthesizing facial animation through 3D model-based tracking. In . *Proceedings of International Conference on Computer Vision, 1,* 143–150. doi:10.1109/ICCV.1999.791210

Quatrehomme, G., Cotin, S., Subsol, G., Delingette, H., Garidel, Y., & Ollier, A. (1997). A fully three-dimensional method for facial reconstruction based on deformable models. *Journal of Forensic Sciences, 42*(3), 649–652.

Rhine, J. S., & Campell, H. R. (1980). Thickness of facial tissue in American blacks. *Journal of Forensic Sciences, 25*(4), 847–858.

Rhine, J. S., & Moore, C. E. (1984). *Facial reproduction: Tables of facial tissue thickness of American caucasoids in forensic anthropology. Technical series 1.* Albuquerque: University of New Mexico.

Schramm, A., Schön, R., Rüker, M., Barth, E.-L., Zizelmann, C., & Gellrich, N.-C. (2006). Computer assisted oral and maxillofacial reconstruction. *Journal of Computing and Information Technology, 14*(1), 71–77. doi:10.2498/cit.2006.01.08

Sethian, J. (1999). *Level sets methods and fast marching methods*. Cambridge University Press.

Shahrom, A. W., Vanezis, P., Chapman, R. C., Gonzales, A., Blenkinsop, C., & Rossi, M. L. (1996). Techniques in facial identification: Computer-aided facial reconstruction using a laser scanner and video superimposition. *International Journal of Legal Medicine, 108*, 194–200. doi:10.1007/BF01369791

Stratomeier, H., Spee, J., Wittwer-Backofen, U. & Bakker, R. (2005). *Methods of forensic facial reconstruction*.

Surazhsky, V., Surazhsky, T., & Kirsanov, D. (2005). Fast, exact, and approximate geodesics on meshes. In *Proceedings of ACM SIGGRAPH 2005, 24*(3).

Szeliski, R., & Lavallee, S. (1996). Matching 3-D anatomical surfaces with non-rigid deformation using octree splines. *International Journal of Computer Vision, 18*(2), 171–186. doi:10.1007/BF00055001

Tilotta, F., et al. (2007). Statistical facial reconstruction by tree functional regression on surfaces. *Proceedings of the Third Mediterranean Academy of Forensic Sciences Congress, Porto, Portugal*.

Tilotta, F., Richard, F., Glaunès, J., Bérar, M., Gey, S., & Verdeille, S. (2009). Construction and analysis of a head CT-scan database for craniofacial reconstruction. *Forensic Science International, 191*(1), 112–118. doi:10.1016/j.forsciint.2009.06.017

Tu, P., Book, R., Liu, X., Krahnstoever, N., Adrian, C., & Williams, P. (2007). Automatic face recognition from skeletal remains. In *IEEE Computer Society Conference on Computer Vision and Pattern Recognition (CVPR 2007)*, Minneapolis.

Vandermeulen, D., Claes, P., Loeckx, D., De Greef, S., Willems, G., & Suetens, P. (2006). Computerized craniofacial reconstruction using CT-derived implicit surface representations. *Forensic Science International, 159*, S164–S174. doi:10.1016/j.forsciint.2006.02.036

Vanezis, P., Vanezis, M., McCombe, G., & Niblett, T. (2000). Facial reconstruction using 3-D computer graphics. *Forensic Science International, 108*(2), 81–95. doi:10.1016/S0379-0738(99)00026-2

Vigneau, E., & Qannari, M. (2002). A new algorithm for latent root regression analysis. *Computational Statistics & Data Analysis, 41*, 231–242. doi:10.1016/S0167-9473(02)00071-3

Wang, Y., Peterson, B., & Staib, L. (2000). Shape-based 3D surface correspondence using geodesics and local geometry. *IEEE Conference on Computer Vision and Pattern Recognition, 2*, 644-651.

Wilkinson, C. (2005). Computerized forensic facial reconstruction: A review of current systems. *Forensic Science, Medicine, and Pathology, 1*(3), 173–177. doi:10.1385/FSMP:1:3:173

Zachow, S., Hege, H.-C., & Deuflhard, P. (2006). Computer assisted planning in cranio-maxillo-facial surgery. *Journal of Computing and Information Technology, 14*(1), 53–64. doi:10.2498/cit.2006.01.06

KEY TERMS AND DEFINITIONS

Landmark: An anatomical structure used as a point of orientation in locating other structures.

Regression: A: functional relationship between two or more correlated variables that is often empirically determined from data and is used especially to predict values of one variable when given values of the others <the regression of y on x is linear>

Template: A template can be thought of as an exemplary instance of the object, containing all the information required to measure and analyze the object. The most common dataset in orthodontics is related to analysis of a lateral cephalogram and contains the conventional cephalometric points and measurements. However, templates are completely user-definable, so they can be created for whatever purpose is desired. Examples include templates for measuring dental casts, facial photographs, osseous structures from CTs, etc.

Section 2
Basic Research:
A Bridge to Digital Forensics

Chapter 6
Monitoring the Trascriptome

Stilianos Arhondakis
Biomedical Research Foundation of the Academy of Athens, Greece

Georgia Tsiliki
Biomedical Research Foundation of the Academy of Athens, Greece

Sophia Kossida
Biomedical Research Foundation of the Academy of Athens, Greece

ABSTRACT

The technologies monitoring the transcriptome are under a continuous status of development and implementation, producing high amounts of expression data which require reliable and well structured databases. This chapter provides a general overview and a reliable guide of these technologies, as developed from the early '90s until today, and of the most important available expression databases. The first part aims at introducing to the reader the fundamental functional aspects of these technologies, which are under a continuous development in order to obtain a more accurate description of the transcriptome. The second part offers the necessary information to those who are interested in further exploiting expression data in their research.

INTRODUCTION: FROM THE GENOME TO THE TRANSCRIPTOME

After the complete sequencing of the human genome, and that of other organisms (Venter et al., 2001; Lander et al., 2001, 2002) there was an unavoidable increase of genomic information which allowed the development of different technologies, in order to achieve a complete use of this large information, and a faithful identification of the transcriptome, i.e. the combined variability of all transcripts produced by the genome. Since the official announcement from the International Human Genome Sequence Consortium (IHGSC) in 2001 that there are only 32,000 genes in the human genome, new sequences are still being added into the chromosome maps and their relative locations are being adjusted (Kidd et al., 2008; The ENCODE project Consortium, 2007; Jobling et al., 2004). Furthermore, the overall gene fragmentation has rapidly decreased the number of genes originally identified. For example, the number of genes located by Ensembl genome annotation system (http://www.ensembl.org/index.

DOI: 10.4018/978-1-60960-483-7.ch006

Figure 1. Transciptome techniques

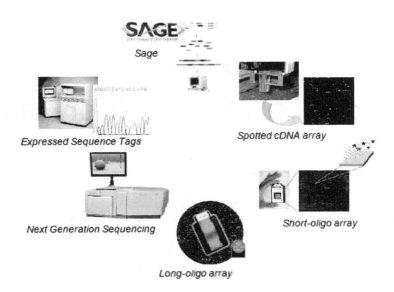

Sage

Expressed Sequence Tags

Next Generation Sequencing

Long-oligo array

Spotted cDNA array

Short-oligo array

html) decreased from the initial 29,700 to 22,800 in one year.

Unlike the 'genome', the profiles of the counts of the human genes' transcripts will vary not only among cell types, but also among the state of a cell, and from the stimuli on that cell. Consequently, the transcriptome will therefore vary both spatially and temporally within an individual. Indeed, one could define 'transcriptome' as a dynamic entity which is spatially and temporally changing (formed by pooling transcripts from all cell types at all times), and an experiment would provide a snapshot of this dynamic entity. Alternatively, one might define the term 'transcriptome' as the transcripts (mRNA species and their levels) at the particular time and place in the history of the individual when the snapshot was taken (see, e.g., the National Human Genome Research Institute's definition; http://www.genome.gov/13014330; Stearns et al., 2003). However, in both cases the snapshot is in practice ex vivo and often obtained only after experimental manipulation of the cells or tissue samples. In order to assess how such a picture corresponds to the in vivo situation, cautious samples manipulation, verified experimental procedures,

and reproducibility is necessary. This latter bias became the major force driving the development and improvement through time, of several technologies monitoring the transcriptome (Figure 1). These technologies can be divided mainly in two major types: sequencing- and hybridization-based techniques. The first include Expressed Sequence Tags (ESTs), Serial Analysis of Gene Expression (SAGESAGESAGE: Velculescu et al., 1995), the Massively Parallel Signature Sequencing (MPSSMPSSMPSS: Brenner et al., 2000a, MPSS2000b; Meyers et al., 2004a, 2004b), and the Next Generation Sequencing techniques, i.e., 454 (http://www.454.com; Margulies et al., 2005) and the Solexa system (http://www.illumina.com). The second category, named hybridization-based techniques, is mainly referred to the microarray technology. Microarray technology can be classified based on different attributes such as, commercial or custom made arrays, probes' length arrays, spotted or in situ synthesized, glass or membrane based, one- or two-colour arrays. Here, arrays will be classified in two major categories, the 3'-based arrays and the recently developed exon arrays. The former arrays will be examined in this chapter,

Figure 2. General schematic representation of ESTs (Expressed Sequence Tags) construction

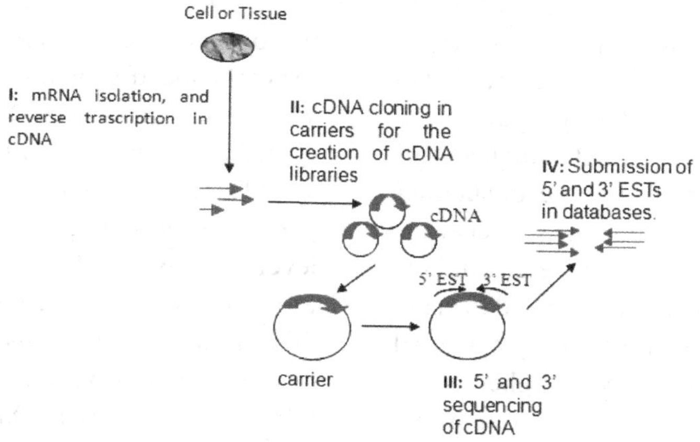

given their probes' length, particularly, we can distinguish three principal types: spotted cDNA arrays (Schena et al., 1995), long-oligonucleotide arrays (50-80 mer: Blanchart et al., 1999, Hughes et al., 2001), and short-oligonucleotides (25-30 mer: Lockhart et al., 1996).

TRANSCRIPTOME TECHNOLOGIES

Sequencing-Based Techniques

The first sequencing-based technique, ESTs (Expressed Sequence Tags) is based on the rapid generation of short sequences in a single sequencing pass (Figure 2). Originally they were proposed in the late 80s', under different criticisms until their first successful application at the beginning of 90s' (Adams et al., 1991). Since EST data are generated in a single sequencing pass, they are characterized by a higher error (3%; Boguski et al., 1993) than that of sequences generation, and they often contain substitutions, insertions/deletions, bacterial, mitochondrial or vector sequence contamination. Despite their limited fidelity, related to sample preparation, i.e., experimental procedures such as cloning of cDNA and reverse transcription of cDNA clones, those short, single strand

reads of transcribed sequences (ESTs) generated from cDNA clones (Adam et al., 1991, 1992) still represent a powerful tool for gene discovery and prediction in genomic studies (Boguski et al., 1994; Bailey et al., 1998; Gibson & Muse, 2002). ESTs also provide an instrument for assessing the transcripts' levels and/or differences in gene expression between different conditions (different samples, different pathological stages).

One widely used tool, available by UniGene (see below for details) allowing the comparison of expression profiles obtained from ESTs among the various libraries or pools of libraries, is the Digital Differential Display (DDD; http://www. ncbi.nlm.nih.gov/UniGene/ddd.cgi). In summary this tool allows to identify those genes that differ among libraries of different conditions (condition-specific genes) or those differentially expressed. The output includes, for each gene, the frequency of its transcript in each library and results are sorted by significance ($p \leq 0.05$, Fisher Exact test).

As far as the cDNA libraries are concerned, there are mainly two different types: non-normalized and normalized. The non-normalized libraries best reflect the population of mRNA sequences in a tissue, giving better estimations of the transcripts' expression profiles and of their differential expression among different conditions (Audic & Claverie, 1997; Schmitt et al., 1999). The redundancy of the highly expressed transcripts and the scarcity of the rare ones led to the development of experimental procedures, such as normalization, which reduces the frequency of the mRNA species to a narrow range, or subtractive hybridization, where a pool of sequences is removed in order to leave only sequences unique to that library (Soares et al., 1994; Bonaldo et al., 1996). Those procedures provide only a general picture of those genes expressed at higher levels, without allowing detailed quantitative analyses.

The two following sequencing-based techniques, SAGE and MPSS, are based on the generation of short sequence tags derived from an mRNA population and the mapping of these tags to transcript databases.

The SAGE represents a widely used experimental technique, ranging from gene discovery to quantitative gene expression analysis (Velculescu et al., 1995; Madden et al., 2000) through the isolation of short unique sequence tags (9-14 bp) from a specific location, within a transcript (Figure 3). Those short sequences (tags) are concatenated, cloned and sequenced, where the frequency and abundance of a tag sequence within a sequence population, provides an estimation of expression levels. As with all transcriptomic techniques, efficient bioinformatic tools are required for a faithful quantitative transcription profiling, particularly, the custom tool SAGE Software Suite (Genzyme Molecular Oncoloogy, Framington, MA, USA) was properly designed to handle and process tag data from SAGE experiments, in a three step procedure: extraction and count of tag sequences, comparison of tag abundance among projects, and matching to reference sequences.

An advantage of this technique is that it does not require an a priori knowledge of the expres-

Figure 3. Schematic diagram of SAGE method

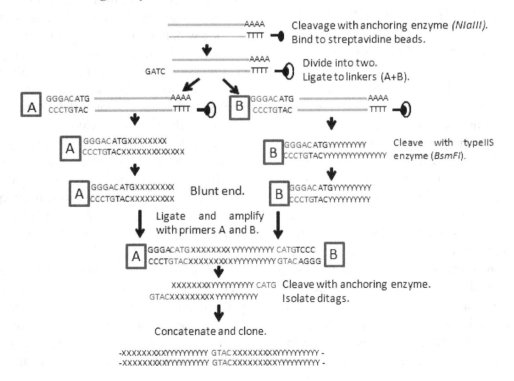

sion pattern of an mRNA source, allowing the application of the same procedure to any sample. However, the generation of tags sequences often lead to complications on their assignment to distinct genes (tag-to-gene ambiguity; Lash et al., 2000; Stollberg et al., 2000), reduced by the use of longer tag sequences such as, the 21-base LongSAGE tags (Saha et al., 2002), or the 26-base SuperSAGE tags (Matsumura et al., 2003). Another disadvantage is the requirement of a large amount of sequencing, not always particularly sensitive, often leading to the necessity of high amounts of mRNA. Finally, an important improvement upon SAGE technique was achieved by the detection of an experimental GC-bias (Margulies et al., 2001) related to a variety of tag protocols.

The other sequencing-based technique, MPSS, was developed and commercialized by Lynx Therapeutics (Hayward, CA) and is based on methods of cloning individual cDNA molecules on microbeads and sequence, in parallel, short tags (signatures) from these cDNAs (Brenner et al., 2000a, 2000b) representing a high-throughput technique on estimating the concentration of mRNA transcripts in a sample.

There are two basic MPSS methods, the original one called Classic MPSS, and the more recent, called Signature MPSS method. The difference between these methods is that in the first, the entire fragment from the Sau3A (GATC, or DpnII) site to the poly(A) is cloned and loaded onto the beads for sequencing. In the Signature method, during cloning a MmeI enzyme recognition site is added to cut 21 or 22 bp from the recognition site for sequencing, intending to remove any bias during the bead loading or sequencing reactions (Meyers et al., 2004a, 2004b). One of the main advantages of MPSS is that it measures the transcript abundance by counting signature sequences, and, unlike SAGE, there is no need of identifying in advance the target transcripts. That reduces the number of misleading annotations due to sequence database updates, contrary to microarray technology during the probes' selec-

tion (Stolovinsky et al., 2005; Chen & Rattray, 2006). However, MPSS technique is also associated with different deficiencies such as the lack of Sau3A (DpnII) site in some genes, whereas in humans they have been estimated to represent near the 7% of the total number of genes, and as the unusual long distance (e.g. > 800 bp) between the 3' end of the transcript (poly(A) site) and the first Sau3A (DpnII) site, leading to a tag-position bias for some genes (Jongeneel et al., 2005), which they will appear as absent at transcriptome level. Chen and Rattray (2006) studied and confirmed the existence of a tag-position bias in both MPSS methods (Classic and Signature) which affects a faithful detection, and measurement of transcripts abundance. More precisely, for the Classic MPSS it was found that those tags far from 3' end, are associated to low tag-counts (lowly expressed), and as this distance increases they tend to have lower or zero counts. On the other hand, for both MPSS methods, it was found that the transcripts having a tag near the 3' end tend to increase their expression.

Finally, the very recently developed sequencing technologies, named Next Generation Sequencing techniques, comprehend several commercially available types, such as the 454 (http://www.454.com; Margulies et al., 2005) and the Solexa system (http://www.illumina.com). These two NGS techniques, mentioned above, are based on sequencing, with the former using a pyrosequencing technology and the latter one using detection fluorescence signals. These new techniques are able to execute millions of sequencing reactions in parallel, and produce a vast amount of data, allowing to conduct a variety of experimental approaches in order to characterize a transcriptome. Their applications range from detection to quantification (Bainbridge et al., 2006; Weber et al., 2007), such as single-end and paired-end cDNA sequencing, tag profiling (3' end sequencing; for estimating expression level), methylation assays, and splice variant analyses. Despite their wide applications, and their prominent future upon the biomedical field, there are several challenges that they still need to be addressed, such as, their high cost, the high demands for storage and analysis.

The above mentioned sequencing-based techniques, from EST to NGS, despite their large differences, still play a fundamental role to the study of several biological processes. Indeed, the knowledge and understanding of the specific limitations and caveats of each technique, is fundamental for a complete detection of the transcriptome, and their combination may enhance detailed viewing of the snapshot within a tissue/cell in a certain condition of a certain organism.

Hybridization-Based Techniques

The hybridization-based techniques (Schena et al., 1995; Lockhart et al., 1996) are well-known since the mid of 80s' and are able to identify and quantify with a single hybridization the expression level of thousand of genes, or even of the entire genome. Such techniques can be also seen as a miniaturized gene-hybridization assay (Barrett & Kawasaki, 2003). During the previous year's this technology represented one of the greatest scientific achievements, and allowed molecular biology to move from the study of few related genes towards a global investigation of entire cellular activities. Hybridization-based techniques exhibit a wide range of applications ranging from transcriptional profiling (Schena et al., 1995; Lockhart et al., 1996) to the identification of allelic differences between individuals (CGHCGHCGH: Pinkel et al., 1998), localization of binding-sites of DNA binding proteins (ChiP: Ren et al., 2000), single nucleotide polymorphism (SNP) and re-sequencing (Guo et al., 1994; Drmanac et al., 1998; Hacia, et al.,1998; Hacia & Collins, 1999).

Microarrays consist of a solid surface on which poly-nucleotides are attached in specific positions, named probes, each representing a gene, and they are characterized by different manufacture, design, hybridization and data handling (Mirnics et al., 2000; Okamoto et al., 2000; Van Hal et al., 2000).

Their main functional principle is based on labeled targets that bind to probes, which they measure the intensity of the label bound to each probe, providing an estimation of the expression level of the corresponding mRNA in a cell or sample (Barrett & Kawasaki, 2003). Here, as it was previously mentioned, microarrays are divided in 3'-based expression arrays and exon arrays. The former are further sub-divided based on their probes' length measured in bases, into spotted cDNA arrays (Schena et al., 1995), long-oligonucleotide arrays (50-80 mer; Blanchart et al., 1999; Hughes et al., 2001), and short-oligonucleotide arrays (25-30 mer; Lockhart et al., 1996; see Figure 4).

The spotted cDNA arrays consist of cDNA probes of several hundred bases long, which are mostly robotically printed into a slide (Brown et al., 1999). Then, mRNA samples of two tissues are extracted, separately reverse transcribed into cDNA and labelled with different colours (Cy3 and Cy5). The mixture of labelled cDNA is co-hybridized onto the microarray, competing to bind to their complementary cDNA. Finally, the slide is scanned at different wavelengths of a laser to obtain numerical intensities of each dye (Speed 2003). The spotted cDNA arrays are used to estimate the differential expression level of genes between two different conditions (normal versus pathological states). Often the second sample (the Cy5 dye for example) represents a specimen of biological interest, or a reference sample used among all arrays, in order to detect experimental quality related to the first. Those arrays do not require sequence information, and the large size of the PCR product enables a more stringent hybridization and limits cross-reactivity. However, several technical challenges had arisen during robotic printing, often increasing signal variation, related to perturbations in spot structure (Dielh et al., 2001; McQuain et al., 2003), hybridization efficiency across the slide (Yang et al., 2002) and dye bias during labeling (Tseng et al., 2001; Dobbin et al., 2003a, 2003b; Liang et al., 2003).

Figure 4. Schematic representation of the three array types divided based on their probes' length: a) spotted cDNA, b) short-oligo arrays and c) long-oligo arrays

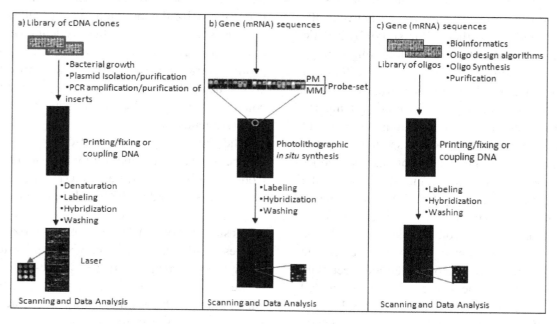

There are several steps to be followed until the image analysis: gridding, segmentation, foreground intensity extraction and background correction. After those necessary adjustments, statistical analysis usually relies on the log-ratios of the two dyes (R) to assess the expression level of each spot,

$$R = \log 2 \frac{\text{(FR-BR)}}{\text{(FB-BG)}}$$

where R (sometimes denoted by M-values) is the differential expression level of a gene in the two samples, each labeled with different fluorescent dyes, i.e. red (Cy3) and green (Cy5). The FR and FG are the foreground mean or median intensities of the red and green channels respectively, and BR and BG the background mean or median intensities. It is common to use base 2 in the logarithm because the intensities usually range from 0 to 2^{16}. On this scale, R=0 represents equal expression, R=1 represents a 2-fold change between samples, R=2 represents a 4-fold change, and so on.

Despite the various normalization procedures available, the Print-tip Loess is one of the common techniques followed in this case. It corrects the R values both for sub-array spatial variation and for intensity-based trends, particularly each R value is normalized by subtracting from it the corresponding value of the tip group loess curve. Then, the normalized log-ratios R, are the residuals from the tip group loess regression (Smyth & Speed, 2003). The purpose of normalization is to adjust for effects which arise from variation in the microarray technology rather than from biological differences between the RNA samples or between the printed probes. The dye-bias, the position on the slide, artifacts on the surface of the array, differences between print-tips on the array printer, any changes on the scanner settings are some reasons to consider normalization between as well as within arrays.

The second array type, long oligonucleotide arrays (Kane et al., 2001), was introduced and implemented as an alternative to the spotted cDNA arrays and short oligonucleotide arrays (see below). Their probes have a length, between 40-80 mer, and are synthesized in situ or by robotic printing. An advantage of the long-oligo arrays is the possibility to design in silico customized arrays, bypassing database updates that may affect annotations, with very similar melting temperature (T_m) and GC level, containing an exon and without repetitive- or hairpin sequences. Here, despite the high number of companies producing long-oligo arrays, we mainly focus on the two-colour arrays by Agilent (http://www.home. agilent.com/agilent/home.jspx?cc=US&lc=eng; for details see also Wolber et al., 2006). Those are constructed via an in situ synthetic scheme based on inkjet printing of nucleotide precursors and common chemical processing of each added nucleotide layer (Blanchard et al., 1996; Hughes et al., 2001; Kronick, 2004). The probe design (standard length of 60-mer) is initially performed in silico using similar techniques to the methods for designing long oligomer probes (Shannon et al., 2001; Chou et al., 2004; Gordon & Sensen, 2004; Rimour et al., 2005). Additionally, in the two-colour arrays, similarly with the cDNA spotted arrays mentioned above, the main interest is placed on the R values and similar normalization techniques are applied.

Agilents' long-oligo arrays, have different application areas, from gene expression profiling, to comparative genomic hybridization (aCGH), and chromatin immunoprecipitation mapping of transcription factor-binding sites (location analysis/ LA or "ChIP on Chip"). The first one measures the relative levels of gene expression in two different samples on a gene-by-gene basis. In the Agilent's two-colour system, the two samples are labelled with distinct fluorophores (Cy3 and Cy5) and hybridize to a single microarray. The final labelled sample, either single-stranded cDNA or linearly amplified, single-stranded cRNA, is produced from the mRNA component of total cellular RNA. After hybridization, scanning, and data extraction the arrays yield a list of hybridization intensities (denoted by I) in each channel and a list of normalized expression ratios (denoted by R). It is worth mentioning, that Agilent recently, developed and introduced a one-colour expression profiling array, similar to Affymetrix short-oligo arrays, using the same arrays employed by two-colour applications and samples labelled with Cy3 only (Agilent, 2005h).

The third array type, short-oligonucleotide arrays, is represented mainly by two platforms: CodeLink (GE Healthcare formerly Amersham Biosciences, Chandler, AZ), and GeneChip (Affymetrix, Santa Clara, CA; http://www.affymetrix. com/estore/index.jsp). Those are characterized by a series of differences, for example GeneChip uses multiple probes as opposed to the one pre-validated probe per gene of CodeLink, GeneChip is a 2-D surface array, whereas there is a 3-D surface in CodeLink, and GeneChip involves in situ synthesized probes, whereas CodeLink consists of pre-synthesized probes. This reduction of length to 25-mer reduces sequencing errors and fabrication expenses. In order to achieve a sufficient binding strength of such short oligos, hybridization conditions must be less stringent than those of cDNA or long-oligo arrays, increasing cross-hybridization. To deal with co-hybridization effects, each probe set is constructed from multiple probe pairs (16-20) for each target (Lockhart et al., 1996). A probe pair consists of a 25-mer oligonucleotide perfectly complementary to a sequence of a gene (Perfect Match: PM), and a 25-mer oligonucleotide that differs from the perfect match probe by a single mismatched nucleotide at the central position (13th position; Mismatch: MM). This combination of a 25-mer pair, PM and MM, offers a highest sensitivity (fluorescence intensity) and specificity (ratio), especially for the lowly expressed transcripts, and partially solves co-hybridization problems related to their length.

The average of the (PM - MM) differences for all probe pairs in a probe set, called Average Difference or Signal (see below for more details), is used as the expression index for the target gene. Contrary to long-oligo, and cDNA arrays the intensities measured by Affymetrix are considered to be absolute expression levels. The less efficient hybridization of the MM probe to the target, allows the (PM - MM) difference for each probe to offer a better estimation of intensity, due to hybridization of the true target.

For the Affymetrix platforms, the GeneChip™ software is readily used to analyze the image data file, perform background correction of intensities and compute a single intensity value for each probes set. The Affymetrix's Micro Array Suite (MAS) developed two widely used algorithms, MAS 4.0, and MAS 5.0, for the estimation of hybridization signals (absolute expression levels), based on intensity differences of (PM - MM). The first one, MAS 4.0, calculates a weighted average of the probe-pair differences (PM – MM) for each probe pair representing a gene, named AD, through the following formula:

$$AD = \frac{1}{n} \sum (PMi - MMi)$$

where n denotes the total number of probe pairs for a probes set (or gene), PMi and MMi indicate the corresponding perfect and mismatch probe intensities after background correction for the ith probe pair for the probe set (or gene).

The above algorithm frequently produced negative AD values and consequently led to a new upgraded version, MAS 5.0 (and recently MAS 5.1) An added advantage of this algorithm is the inclusion of statistical significance (p-value) associated with detection and comparison calls of every gene. The MAS 5.0 algorithm uses the One-Step Tukey's Biweight Estimate to compute the "Signal Log Value" for each probe set (Hubbell et al., 2002; Liu et al., 2002). The algorithm uses normalization and scaling techniques to correct for variations between two arrays. This absolute

expression for a probe set is called "Signal Log Value", and is given by the following formula:

SLVk = Biweight [log$_2$ (PMi,k – CTi,k): i=1,…,n],

where CT is the contrast value of the ith probe pair for the kth probe set, and equals MM if PM>MM or else it is a function of PM and MM.

Together with absolute expression values, given by the algorithms described previously, a detection call (DC) is also estimated, using a detection algorithm. Particularly, they employ a Wilcoxon signed-ranked test between PM and MM probe intensities, and based on the p-values of the tests as well as pre-specified p-value cut-offs, they classify transcript calls of a sample to present (P), marginal (M) or absent (A).

However, alternative methods for estimating expression levels have been developed for Affymetrix arrays, for example the robust multi-array average (RMA) method (Bolstad et al., 2003; Irizzary et al., 2003a, 2003b) and its successor, the GC-RMA algorithm (Wu et al., 2004; Naef & Magnasco, 2003; Irizzary et al., 2006). RMA estimates are based upon a robust average of background corrected PM intensities, quantile normalization and linear modeling are then applied to estimate the log-scale expression levels. Finally, intensity values are combined via 'median polish' to get a single intensity value for each gene. While RMA accounts for background effects, the GC-RMA accounts for nucleotide-specific affinities during hybridization. The affinity modelling used by GC-RMA is based on observations (Naef & Magnasco, 2003; Wu et al., 2004) that when one takes labelling into account, effective hybridization to 25-mers is especially strong for C and weak for A bases in the sequence, especially near the middle.

Recently another array type has been developed, the exon arrays. These arrays were developed in order to study the important role that alternative splicing mechanism has in several biological pathways and processes. In particular, approximately 74% of all human multi-exon genes (approximately ½ of human genes) are predicted to be alternatively spliced (Modrek & Lee, 2003; Johnson et al., 2003). This event is of fundamental importance in several conditions, and despite of deficits in its machinery it has been shown to be implicated in many diseases (Venables, 2006; Faustino & Cooper, 2003).

More precisely, Affymetrix Exon arrays, compared to the previous array generations, are characterized by several technical changes, starting from the removal of the MM probes, the reduction of number of probes within a probe set (from 11 to 4), the increase of the total probe set count (~1.4 million), and the positioning of the probe sets along the full length of each gene (see: http://www.affymetrix.com, and Dalma-Weiszhausz et al., 2006). However, such changes would unavoidably have effects on the study of the transcriptome, as seen until now, even if most of the protocols remain almost invariant. In particular, the same normalization procedures previously mentioned, such as RMA, are applied, although there are not MM probes in exon arrays. Other similar algorithms, such as the Probe Logarithmic Intensity Error (PLIER) algorithm, remain valid with exon arrays. Nonetheless, there are differences in the Detection call algorithms, which they remove those poorly performing probe sets. In the Exon arrays, in which paired MM probe sets are absent, a separate pool of 25,000 background probes, designed not to perfectly match, are used in order to allow detection of present or absent genes. Once significant probe sets are identified, multiple statistical tests are necessary in order to assess how likely changes in differential expression are real or have occurred by chance, with most easy and popular strategy being that of the detection of a differential expression threshold.

Summarizing, within this section we provide a brief though concrete description of the most fundamental functional aspects of hybridization-based techniques. Of course, length restrictions limit possibilities for a detailed description of all available arrays, and an extension on their limitations and deficits, although those still represent an important subject of study.

DATABASES AND WEB RESOURCES

The development and the wide use of both sequencing- and hybridization-based technologies resulted in a huge amount of detailed transcriptomic data. These data are largely freely available, from numerous web resources. Given the high number of available expression web resources, specific to organisms, diseases or type of techniques, in this section we briefly describe few pioneering web resources of Table 1. However, at the end of this section we provide a wide list of expression databases, reflecting the extended application of these technologies.

As far as ESTs are concerned, still representing a widely used sequencing-based technique, they are submitted into different international databases such as, NCBI (database of Expressed Sequence Tags: dbEST; www.ncbi.nlm.nih.gov/dbEST/; Boguski et al., 1993), EMBL (http://

Table 1. Names and corresponding links of web-resources described in the text

Databases
1- Sequencing-Based Techniques
Unigene: http://www.ncbi.nlm.nih.gov/sites/entrez?db=unigene
TIGR Gene Indices: http://compbio.dfci.harvard.edu/tgi/tgipage.html
STACKdb: http://www.sanbi.ac.za/resources/tools-for-downloading/the-stack-project/
Body Map: http://bodymap.ims.u-tokyo.ac.jp
SAGEmap: http://www.ncbi.nlm.nih.gov/projects/SA
ArabidopsisMPSS database: http://mpss.udel.edu/at
2- Hybridization-Based Techniques
Gene Expression Omnibus: http://www.ncbi.nlm.nih.gov/geo/
Array Express: http://www.ebi.ac.uk/microarray-as/ae/
Gene Expression Atlas: http://www.ebi.ac.uk/gxa

www.ebi.ac.uk/embl/) and DDBJ (http://www. ddbj.nig.ac.jp/). In the mid 2000, human ESTs reached to be approximately 2.0 million, and such a high number was impossible to represent a unique sequence (gene), leading to the necessity of grouping those sequences representing the same gene. Different resources of clustering human EST data were developed, among them the most important and widely used are the following: UniGene (, TIGR (Quackenbush et al., 2000), STACK (and BodyMap (Okubo et al., 1991; Hishiki et al., 1999; see Table 1 for the links corresponding to each database). Unigene, is a resource of NCBI that clusters ESTs, and other mRNA sequences, with coding sequences using MegaBlast (Boguski & Schuler, 1995), and each cluster is made up of sequences produced by a single gene, including alternative spliced transcripts, where each gene may be represented by more than one cluster. The TIGR database, represents another important resource of EST handling, and consists of Tentative Consensus sequences (TC; for human THC or Tentative Human Consensus) producing the Gene Indices (Quackenbush et al., 2000) which are assemblies of ESTs, rather than simple clusters as in UniGene, and each transcript is represented only once with alternative splicing transcripts grouped independently. STACK resource (SANBI; South African National Bioinformatics Institute) uses a combination of clustering and assembly, compared to UniGene and TIGR, where in a first step EST data are separated by tissue/sample type, then clustered (d2_cluster: Burke et al., 1999) and finally assembled (PHARPPHARP: Green et al., 1999). Finally, BodyMap resources a collection of 3'-ESTs from non-normalized cDNA libraries constructed at the Osaka University, and provide three distinct in silico mRNA experiments: estimation of the sample/source mRNA composition, genes' expression pattern, and the detection of genes with high tissue specificity for human and mice.

For the other two sequencing-based techniques, SAGE and MPSS, repositories for online data access and analysis are also available. For SAGE data the SAGEmap (Table 1) was originally constructed, aiming to archive SAGE data produced by the Cancer Genome Anatomy Project (CGAP; http://www.ncbi.nlm.nih.gov/cgap), which was afterwards extended including also SAGE sequence data from different studies. For MPSS data, some study specific databases are available like the Plant MPSS Databases (Nakano et al., 2009) i.e.,the Arabidopsis MPSS database (see link in Table 1). Additionally, the produced data from both SAGE and MPSS techniques are also included within the Gene Expression Omnibus repository (see Table 1) of NCBI (http://www. ncbi.nlm.nih.gov/; see below for details).

As for the widely used microarrays hybridization-based technique, there is a vast amount of data produced by studies of bio-medical interest, developmental biology or genome-wide analyses. Thus, accurate databases were necessary, not only for storing the data but also for clarifying the experimental and statistical procedures followed in each case. One such resource is the Gene Expression Omnibus (see Table1; Edgar et al., 2002; Barrett et al., 2009) of NCBI, which contains data from more than 6,000 different microarray experiments including a high mount of samples. However, as anticipated above, this resource also includes non-array techniques such as serial analysis of gene expression (SAGE; 73 experiments) and quantitative sequence data (MPSS; 16 experiments). Similarly, microarray data recourse is also the ArrayExpress (see Table 1; Parkinson et al., 2009) of EMBL-EBI (http:// www.ebi.ac.uk/) which includes data from more than 10,000 experiments derived from nearly 200,000 samples. Based on ArrayExpress, the Gene Expression Atlas (see Table 1; Kapushesky et al., 2009) has been developed, which is an archive of approximately 1,200 experiments re-annotated, and offers the possibility for individual gene expression query under different biological conditions across experiments (meta-analyses). These databases contain information concerning the type of study, the array type, the experimental protocol, as well as algorithms and normalization procedures. Moreover, raw data are also available in order to allow meta-analyses approaches (see Table 1).

The creation of such databases from studies upon the transcriptome, using sequencing- or hybridization-based techniques, allowed not only the collection of several biological observation concerning diseases or biological processes, but also the improvement of those technologies, within and amongst them. These latter studies, aimed to improve limitation of these techniques in order to obtain an accurate detection and estimation of expression of the transcriptome. The subject of limitations and deficits of each of the above mentioned techniques still presents an important scientific challenge, which continuously evolves but nonetheless it is beyond the scope of this chapter.

Additional List of Expression Databases

- Maize Oligonucleotide Array Project: http://www.maizearray.org/
- Mouse Gene Expression Database (GXD http://www.informatics.jax.org/expression.shtml)
- Stanford Microarray Databases http://smd.stanford.edu/resources/
- Center for Information Biology Gene Expression Database http://cibex.nig.ac.jp/index.jsp
- RNA Abundance Database http://www.cbil.upenn.edu/RAD/php/index.php
- Pancreatic Expression Database http://www.pancreasexpression.org/index.html
- Riken Expression Array Database (READ): http://read.gsc.riken.go.jp/
- Plant Expression Database: http://www.plexdb.org/
- Xenopus Database: http://xenbase.org/common/

- Filamentous Fungal Gene Expression Database: http://bioinfo.townsend.yale.edu/index.jsp
- E. coli Community's Gene Expression Database (GenExpDB): http://genexpdb.ou.edu/
- Pig Expression Data Explorer: http://pede.dna.affrc.go.jp/
- Tomato Functional Genomics Database: http://ted.bti.cornell.edu/
- Ludwig Institute for Cancer Research: http://mpss.licr.org/
- Chip DB: http://staffa.wi.mit.edu/chipdb/public/index.html
- Gene Expression Atlas/Bio GPS (The Gene Port Hub): http://biogps.gnf.org/#goto=welcome

REFERENCES

Adams, M. D., Dubnick, M., Kerlavage, A. R., Moreno, R., Kelley, J. M., & Utterback, T. R. (1992). Sequence identification of 2,375 human brain genes. *Nature*, *355*(6361), 632–634. doi:10.1038/355632a0

Adams, M. D., Kelley, J. M., Gocayne, J. D., Dubnick, M., Polymeropoulos, M. H., & Xiao, H. (1991). Complementary DNA sequencing: Expressed sequence tags and human genome project. *Science*, *252*(5013), 1651–1656. doi:10.1126/science.2047873

Audic, S., & Claverie, J. M. (1997). The significance of digital gene expression profiles. *Genome Research*, *7*(10), 986–995.

Bailey, L. C. Jr, Searls, D. B., & Overton, G. C. (1998). Analysis of EST-driven gene annotation in human genomic sequence. *Genome Research*, *8*(4), 362–376.

Bainbridge, M. N., Warren, R. L., Hirst, M., Romanuik, T., Zeng, T., & Go, A. (2006). Analysis of the prostate cancer cell line LNCaP transcriptome using a sequencing-by-synthesis approach. *BMC Genomics, 7*, 246. doi:10.1186/1471-2164-7-246

Barrett, J. C., & Kawasaki, E. S. (2003). Microarrays: The use of oligonucleotides and cDNA for the analysis of gene expression. *Drug Discovery Today, 8*(3), 134–141. doi:10.1016/S1359-6446(02)02578-3

Barrett, T., Troup, D. B., Wilhite, S. E., Ledoux, P., Rudnev, D., & Evangelista, C. (2009). NCBI GEO: Archive for high-throughput functional genomic data. *Nucleic Acids Research, 37*(Database issue), D5–D15. doi:10.1093/nar/gkn764

Blanchard, A. P., Kaiser, R. J., & Hood, L. E. (1996). High density oligonucleotide arrays. *Biosensors & Bioelectronics, 11*(6/7), 687–690. doi:10.1016/0956-5663(96)83302-1

Boguski, M. S., Lowe, T. M., & Tolstoshev, C. M. (1993). dbEST-database for expressed sequence tags. *Nature Genetics, 4*(4), 332–333. doi:10.1038/ng0893-332

Boguski, M. S., & Schuler, G. D. (1995). Establishing a human transcript map. *Nature Genetics, 10*(4), 369–371. doi:10.1038/ng0895-369

Boguski, M. S., Tolstoshev, C. M., & Bassett, D. E. Jr. (1994). Gene discovery in dbEST. *Science, 265*(5181), 1993–1994. doi:10.1126/science.8091218

Bolstad, B. M., Irizarry, R. A., Astrand, M., & Speed, T. P. (2003). A comparison of normalization methods for high density oligonucleotide array data based on bias and variance. *Bioinformatics (Oxford, England), 19*(2), 185–193. doi:10.1093/bioinformatics/19.2.185

Bonaldo, M. F., Lennon, G., & Soares, M. B. (1996). Normalization and subtraction: Two approaches to facilitate gene discovery. *Genome Research, 6*(9), 791–806. doi:10.1101/gr.6.9.791

Brenner, S., Johnson, M., Bridgham, J., Golda, G., Lloyd, D. H., & Johnson, D. (2000a). Gene expression analysis by massively parallel signature sequencing (MPSS) on microbead arrays. *Nature Biotechnology, 18*(6), 630–634. doi:10.1038/76469

Brenner, S., Williams, S. R., Vermaas, E. H., Storck, T., Moon, K., & McCollum, C. (2000b). In vitro cloning of complex mixtures of DNA on microbeads: Physical separation of differentially expressed cDNAs. *Proceedings of the National Academy of Sciences of the United States of America, 97*(4), 1665–1670. doi:10.1073/pnas.97.4.1665

Brown, P. O., & Botstein, D. (1999). Exploring the new world of the genome with DNA microarrays. *Nature Genetics, 21*(Suppl. 1), 33–37. doi:10.1038/4462

Burke, J., Davison, D., & Hide, W. (1999). d2_cluster: A validated method for clustering EST and full-length cDNA sequences. *Genome Research, 9*(11), 1135–1142. doi:10.1101/gr.9.11.1135

Chen, J., & Rattray, M. (2006). Analysis of tag-position bias in MPSS technology. *BMC Genomics, 7*, 77. doi:10.1186/1471-2164-7-77

Chou, H. H., Hsia, A. P., Mooney, D. L., & Schnable, P. S. (2004). Picky: Oligo microarray design for large genomes. *Bioinformatics (Oxford, England), 20*(17), 2893–2902. doi:10.1093/bioinformatics/bth347

Dalma-Weiszhausz, D. D., Warrington, J., Tanimoto, E. Y., & Miyada, C. G. (2006). The Affymetrix GeneChip platform: An overview. *Methods in Enzymology, 410*, 3–28. doi:10.1016/S0076-6879(06)10001-4

Diehl, F., Grahlmann, S., Beier, M., & Hoheisel, J. D. (2001). Manufacturing DNA microarrays of high spot homogeneity and reduced background signal. *Nucleic Acids Research, 29*(7), E38. doi:10.1093/nar/29.7.e38

Dobbin, K., Shih, J. H., & Simon, R. (2003a). Questions and answers on design of dual-label microarrays for identifying differentially expressed genes. *Journal of the National Cancer Institute*, *95*(18), 1362–1369.

Dobbin, K., Shih, J. H., & Simon, R. (2003b). Statistical design of reverse dye microarrays. *Bioinformatics (Oxford, England)*, *19*(7), 803–810. doi:10.1093/bioinformatics/btg076

Drmanac, S., Kita, D., Labat, I., Hauser, B., Schmidt, C., & Burczak, J. D. (1998). Accurate sequencing by hybridization for DNA diagnostics and individual genomics. *Nature Biotechnology*, *16*(1), 54–58. doi:10.1038/nbt0198-54

Edgar, R., Domrachev, M., & Lash, A. E. (2002). Gene expression omnibus: NCBI gene expression and hybridization array data repository. *Nucleic Acids Research*, *30*(1), 207–210. doi:10.1093/nar/30.1.207

Faustino, N. A., & Cooper, T. A. (2003). Pre-mRNA splicing and human disease. *Genes & Development*, *17*(4), 419–437. doi:10.1101/gad.1048803

Gibson, G., & Muse, S. V. (2004). *A primer of genome science* (2nd ed.). Sunderland, MA: Sinauer Associates.

Gordon, P. M., & Sensen, C. W. (2004). Osprey: A comprehensive tool employing novel methods for the design of oligonucleotides for DNA sequencing and microarrays. *Nucleic Acids Research*, *32*(17), e133. doi:10.1093/nar/gnh127

Green, P. (1999). Phrap. Retrieved from http://phrap.org

Guo, Z., Guilfoyle, R. A., Thiel, A. J., Wang, R., & Smith, L. M. (1994). Direct fluorescence analysis of genetic polymorphisms by hybridization with oligonucleotide arrays on glass supports. *Nucleic Acids Research*, *22*(24), 5456–5465. doi:10.1093/nar/22.24.5456

Hacia, J. G., Brody, L. C., & Collins, F. S. (1998). Applications of DNA chips for genomic analysis. *Molecular Psychiatry*, *3*(6), 483–492. doi:10.1038/sj.mp.4000475

Hacia, J. G., & Collins, F. S. (1999). Mutational analysis using oligonucleotide microarrays. *Journal of Medical Genetics*, *36*(10), 730–736.

Hishiki, T., Kawamoto, S., Morishita, S., & Okubo, K. (2000). BodyMap: A human and mouse gene expression database. *Nucleic Acids Research*, *28*(1), 136–138. doi:10.1093/nar/28.1.136

Hubbell, E., Liu, W. M., & Mei, R. (2002). Robust estimators for expression analysis. *Bioinformatics (Oxford, England)*, *18*(12), 1585–1592. doi:10.1093/bioinformatics/18.12.1585

Hughes, T. R., Mao, M., Jones, A. R., Burchard, J., Marton, M. J., & Shannon, K. W. (2001). Expression profiling using microarrays fabricated by an ink-jet oligonucleotide synthesizer. *Nature Biotechnology*, *19*(4), 342–347. doi:10.1038/86730

Irizarry, R. A., Bolstad, B. M., Collin, F., Cope, L. M., Hobbs, B., & Speed, T. P. (2003). Summaries of Affymetrix GeneChip probe level data. *Nucleic Acids Research*, *31*(4), e15. doi:10.1093/nar/gng015

Irizarry, R. A., Hobbs, B., Collin, F., Beazer-Barclay, Y. D., Antonellis, K. J., & Scherf, U. (2003). Exploration, normalization, and summaries of high density oligonucleotide array probe level data. *Biostatistics (Oxford, England)*, *4*(2), 249–264. doi:10.1093/biostatistics/4.2.249

Irizarry, R. A., Wu, Z., & Jaffee, H. A. (2006). Comparison of Affymetrix GeneChip expression measures. *Bioinformatics (Oxford, England)*, *22*(7), 789–794. doi:10.1093/bioinformatics/btk046

Jobling, M. A., Hurles, M. E., & Tyler-Smith, C. (2004). *Human evolutionary genetics: Origins, people and disease*. Garland Science, Taylor & Francis Group.

Johnson, J. M., Castle, J., Garrett-Engele, P., Kan, Z., Loerch, P. M., & Armour, C. D. (2003). Genome-wide survey of human alternative pre-mRNA splicing with exon junction microarrays. *Science, 302*(5653), 2141–2144. doi:10.1126/science.1090100

Jongeneel, C. V., Delorenzi, M., Iseli, C., Zhou, D., Haudenschild, C. D., & Khrebtukova, I. (2005). An atlas of human gene expression from massively parallel signature sequencing (MPSS). *Genome Research, 15*(7), 1007–1014. doi:10.1101/gr.4041005

Kane, M. D., Jatkoe, T. A., Stumpf, C. R., Liu, J., Thomas, J. D., & Madore, S. J. (2000). Assessment of the sensitivity and specificity of oligonucleotide (50 mer) microarrays. *Nucleic Acids Research, 28*(22), 4552–4557. doi:10.1093/nar/28.22.4552

Kapushesky, M., Emam, I., Holloway, E., Kurnosov, P., Zorin, A., & Malone, J. (2010). Gene expression atlas at the European Bioinformatics Institute. *Nucleic Acids Research, 38*(Database issue), D690–D698. doi:10.1093/nar/gkp936

Kidd, J. M., Cooper, G. M., Donahue, W. F., Hayden, H. S., Sampas, N., & Graves, T. (2008). Mapping and sequencing of structural variation from eight human genomes. *Nature, 453*(7191), 56–64. doi:10.1038/nature06862

Kronick, M. N. (2004). Creation of the whole human genome microarray. *Expert Review of Proteomics, 1*(1), 19–28. doi:10.1586/14789450.1.1.19

Lander, E. S. (2001). Initial sequencing and analysis of the human genome. *Nature, 409*(6822), 860–921. doi:10.1038/35057062

Lander, E. S. (2002). Initial sequencing and comparative analysis of the mouse genome. *Nature, 420*(6915), 520–562. doi:10.1038/nature01262

Lash, A. E., Tolstoshev, C. M., Wagner, L., Schuler, G. D., Strausberg, R. L., & Riggins, G. J. (2000). SAGEmap: A public gene expression resource. *Genome Research, 10*(7), 1051–1060. doi:10.1101/gr.10.7.1051

Liang, M., Briggs, A. G., Rute, E., Greene, A. S., & Cowley, A. W. (2003). Quantitative assessment of the importance of dye switching and biological replication in cDNA microarray studies. *Physiological Genomics, 14*(3), 199–207.

Liu, W. M., Mei, R., Di, X., Ryder, T. B., Hubbell, E., & Dee, S. (2002). Analysis of high density expression microarrays with signed-rank call algorithms. *Bioinformatics (Oxford, England), 18*(12), 1593–1599. doi:10.1093/bioinformatics/18.12.1593

Lockhart, D. J., Dong, H., Byrne, M. C., Follettie, M. T., Gallo, M. V., & Chee, M. S. (1996). Expression monitoring by hybridization to high-density oligonucleotide arrays. *Nature Biotechnology, 14*(13), 1675–1680. doi:10.1038/nbt1296-1675

Lu, J., Lal, A., Merriman, B., Nelson, S., & Riggins, G. (2004). A comparison of gene expression profiles produced by SAGE, long SAGE, and oligonucleotide chips. *Genomics, 84*(4), 631–636. doi:10.1016/j.ygeno.2004.06.014

Madden, S. L., Wang, C. J., & Landes, G. (2000). Serial analysis of gene expression: From gene discovery to target identification. *Drug Discovery Today, 5*(9), 415–425. doi:10.1016/S1359-6446(00)01544-0

Margulies, E. H., Kardia, S. L., & Innis, J. W. (2001). Identification and prevention of a GC content bias in SAGE libraries. *Nucleic Acids Research, 29*(12), E60–E0. doi:10.1093/nar/29.12.e60

Margulies, M., Egholm, M., Altman, W. E., Attiya, S., Bader, J. S., & Bemben, L. A. (2005). Genome sequencing in microfabricated high-density pico-litre reactors. *Nature, 437*(7057), 376–380.

Matsumura, H., Reich, S., Ito, A., Saitoh, H., Kamoun, S., & Winter, P. (2003). Gene expression analysis of plant host-pathogen interactions by SuperSAGE. *Proceedings of the National Academy of Sciences of the United States of America, 100*(26), 15718–15723. doi:10.1073/pnas.2536670100

McQuain, M. K., Seale, K., Peek, J., Levy, S., & Haselton, F. R. (2003). Effects of relative humidity and buffer additives on the contact printing of microarrays by quill pins. *Analytical Biochemistry, 320*(2), 281–291. doi:10.1016/S0003-2697(03)00348-8

Meyers, B. C., Tej, S. S., Vu, T. H., Haudenschild, C. D., Agrawal, V., & Edberg, S. B. (2004a). The use of MPSS for whole-genome transcriptional analysis in Arabidopsis. *Genome Research, 14*(98), 1641–1653. doi:10.1101/gr.2275604

Meyers, B. C., Vu, T. H., Tej, S. S., Ghazal, H., Matvienko, M., & Agrawal, V. (2004b). Analysis of the transcriptional complexity of Arabidopsis thaliana by massively parallel signature sequencing. *Nature Biotechnology, 22*(8), 1006–1011. doi:10.1038/nbt992

Mirnics, K., Middleton, F. A., Marquez, A., Lewis, D. A., & Levitt, P. (2000). Molecular characterization of schizophrenia viewed by microarray analysis of gene expression in prefrontal cortex. *Neuron, 28*(1), 53–67. doi:10.1016/S0896-6273(00)00085-4

Modrek, B., & Lee, C. J. (2003). Alternative splicing in the human, mouse and rat genomes is associated with an increased frequency of exon creation and/or loss. *Nature Genetics, 34*(2), 177–180. doi:10.1038/ng1159

Naef, F., & Magnasco, M. O. (2003). Solving the riddle of the bright mismatches: Labeling and effective binding in oligonucleotide arrays. Physical review. E, Statistical, nonlinear, and soft matter physics. *E (Norwalk, Conn.), 68*(1 Pt 1), 011906.

Nakano, M., Nobuta, K., Vemaraju, K., Tej, S. S., Skogen, J. W., & Meyers, B. C. (2006). Plant MPSS databases: signature-based transcriptional resources for analyses of mRNA and small RNA. *Nucleic Acids Research, 34*(Database issue), D731–D735. doi:10.1093/nar/gkj077

Okamoto, T., Suzuki, T., & Yamamoto, N. (2000). Microarray fabrication with covalent attachment of DNA using bubble jet technology. *Nature Biotechnology, 18*(4), 438–441. doi:10.1038/74507

Okubo, K., Hori, N., Matoba, R., Niiyama, T., & Matsubara, K. (1991). A novel system for large-scale sequencing of cDNA by PCR amplification. *DNA Sequence, 2*(3), 137–144. doi:10.3109/10425179109039684

Parkinson, H., Kapushesky, M., Kolesnikov, N., Rustici, G., Shojatalab, M., & Abeygunawardena, N. (2009). ArrayExpress update-from an archive of functional genomics experiments to the atlas of gene expression. *Nucleic Acids Research, 37*(Database issue), D868–D872. doi:10.1093/nar/gkn889

Pinkel, D., Segraves, R., Sudar, D., Clark, S., Poole, I., & Kowbel, D. (1998). High resolution analysis of DNA copy number variation using comparative genomic hybridization to microarrays. *Nature Genetics, 20*(2), 207–211. doi:10.1038/2524

Quackenbush, J., Liang, F., Holt, I., Pertea, G., & Upton, J. (2000). The TIGR Gene Indices: reconstruction and representation of expressed gene sequences. *Nucleic Acids Research, 28*(1), 141–145. doi:10.1093/nar/28.1.141

Ren, B., Robert, F., Wyrick, J. J., Aparicio, O., Jennings, E. G., & Simon, I. (2000). Genome-wide location and function of DNA binding proteins. *Science, 290*(5500), 2306–2309. doi:10.1126/science.290.5500.2306

Rimour, S., Hill, D., Militon, C., & Peyret, P. (2005). GoArrays: Highly dynamic and efficient microarray probe design. *Bioinformatics (Oxford, England)*, *21*(7), 1094–1110. doi:10.1093/bioinformatics/bti112

Saha, S., Sparks, A. B., Rago, C., Akmaev, V., Wang, C. J., & Vogelstein, B. (2002). Using the transcriptome to annotate the genome. *Nature Biotechnology*, *20*(5), 508–512. doi:10.1038/nbt0502-508

Schena, M., Shalon, D., Davis, R. W., & Brown, P. O. (1995). Quantitative monitoring of gene expression patterns with a complementary DNA microarray. *Science*, *270*(5235), 368–371. doi:10.1126/science.270.5235.467

Schmitt, A. O., Specht, T., Beckmann, G., Dahl, E., Pilarsky, C. P., & Hinzmann, B. (1999). Exhaustive mining of EST libraries for genes differentially expressed in normal and tumour tissues. *Nucleic Acids Research*, *27*(21), 4251–4260. doi:10.1093/nar/27.21.4251

Shannon, K. W., Wolber, P. K., Delenstarr, G. C., Webb, P. G., & Kincaid, R. H. (2001). *Method for evaluating oligonucleotide probe sequences*. Palo Alto, CA: Agilent Technologies Inc.

Smyth, G. K., & Speed, T. P. (2003). Normalization of cDNA microarray data. *Methods (San Diego, Calif.)*, *31*, 265–273. doi:10.1016/S1046-2023(03)00155-5

Soares, M. B., Bonaldo, M. F., Jelene, P., Su, L., Lawton, L., & Efstratiadis, A. (1994). Construction and characterization of a normalized cDNA library. *Proceedings of the National Academy of Sciences of the United States of America*, *91*(20), 9228–9232. doi:10.1073/pnas.91.20.9228

Speed, T. (2003). *Interdisciplinary statistics: Statistical analysis of gene expression microarray data*. Chapman & Hall/CRC.

Stearns, S. C., & Magwene, P. (2003). American Society of Naturalists. The naturalist in a world of genomics. *American Naturalist*, *161*(2), 171–180. doi:10.1086/367983

Stollberg, J., Urschitz, J., Urban, Z., & Boyd, C. D. (2000). A quantitative evaluation of SAGE. *Genome Research*, *10*(8), 1241–1248. doi:10.1101/gr.10.8.1241

Stolovitzky, G. A., Kundaje, A., Held, G. A., Duggar, K. H., Haudenschild, C. D., & Zhou, D. (2005). Statistical analysis of MPSS measurements: Application to the study of LPS-activated macrophage gene expression. *Proceedings of the National Academy of Sciences of the United States of America*, *102*(5), 1402–1407. doi:10.1073/pnas.0406555102

The ENCODE Project Consortium et al. (2007). Identification and analysis of functional elements in 1% of the human genome by the ENCODE pilot project. *Nature*, *447*(7146), 799–816. doi:10.1038/nature05874

Tseng, G. C., Oh, M. K., Rohlin, L., Liao, J. C., & Wong, W. H. (2001). Issues in cDNA microarray analysis: Quality filtering, channel normalization, models of variations and assessment of gene effects. *Nucleic Acids Research*, *29*(12), 2549–2557. doi:10.1093/nar/29.12.2549

van Hal, N. L., Vorst, O., van Houwelingen, A. M., Kok, E. J., Peijnenburg, A., & Aharoni, A. (2000). The application of DNA microarrays in gene expression analysis. *Journal of Biotechnology*, *78*(3), 271–280. doi:10.1016/S0168-1656(00)00204-2

Velculescu, V. E., Zhang, L., Vogelstein, B., & Kinzler, K. W. (1995). Serial analysis of gene expression. *Science*, *270*(5235), 484–487. doi:10.1126/science.270.5235.484

Venables, J. P. (2006). Unbalanced alternative splicing and its significance in cancer. *BioEssays*, *28*(4), 378–386. doi:10.1002/bies.20390

Venter, J. C. (2001). The sequence of the human genome. *Science, 291*(5507), 1304–1351. doi:10.1126/science.1058040

Weber, A. P., Weber, K. L., Carr, K., Wilkerson, C., & Ohlrogge, J. B. (2007). Sampling the Arabidopsis transcriptome with massively parallel pyrosequencing. *Plant Physiology, 144*(1), 32–42. doi:10.1104/pp.107.096677

Wolber, P. K., Collins, P. J., Lucas, A. B., De Witte, A., & Shannon, K. W. (2006). The agilent in situ-synthesized microarray platform. *Methods in Enzymology, 410*, 28–57. doi:10.1016/S0076-6879(06)10002-6

Wu, Z., Irizarry, R. A., Gentleman, R., Martinez-Murillo, F., & Spencer, F. (2004). A model based background adjustment for oligonucleotide expression arrays. *Journal of the American Statistical Association, 99*(468), 909–917. doi:10.1198/016214504000000683

Yang, I. V., Chen, E., Hasseman, J. P., Liang, W., Frank, B. C., & Wang, S. (2002). Within the fold: Assessing differential expression measures and reproducibility in microarray assays. *Genome Biology, 3*(11), 62.

ADDITIONAL READING

454 (http://www.454.com)

Affymetrix, Santa Clara, CA (http://www.affymetrix.com/estore/index.jsp)

Agilent. http://www.home.agilent.com/agilent/home.jspx?cc=US&lc=eng

Cancer Genome Anatomy Project. CGAP; http://www.ncbi.nlm.nih.gov/cgap

Digital Differential Display. (DDD; http://www.ncbi.nlm.nih.gov/UniGene/ddd.cgi

Ensembl. http://www.ensembl.org/index.html

MAS. http://media.affymetrix.com/support/technical/whitepapers/sadd_whitepaper.pdf

National Human Genome Research Institute. http://www.genome.gov/13014330

PLIER. http://media.affymetrix.com/support/technical/technotes/plier_technote.pdf

Solexa system. http://www.illumina.com

UniGene. http://www.ncbi.nlm.nih.gov/sites/entrez?db=unigene

KEY TERMS AND DEFINITIONS

Differential Expression: Differential expression relies on assessing which genes have expression values which differ significantly between two conditions (cancer versus normal, adult versus development) or between two or more groups of patients, and confers a direction to the expression changes of genes (up- or down-regulation). The estimation of differential expressed genes has many biomedical applications, including the identification of biomarkers, which allow a better understanding and diagnosis of a disease or a biological process.

Expression Databases: The biological databases are an integrated collection of biology-related expression data, either elaborated or raw data, and of detailed experimental protocols, under a common structural format for multiple uses.

Gene Expression: Genes store information and their expression is required to produce functional RNA and protein molecules in a cell. The process of gene expression is divided in two major stages, transcription and translation. During the first stage, a gene is copied to produce a primary transcript (RNA molecule) with essentially the same sequence to that of the gene, subsequently most of the genes are processed (splicing) to generate messenger RNA (mRNA).

Hybridization-Based Techniques: Hybridization-based techniques rely on measuring the magnitude of hybridization of a probe to its target in a background, relative to the signal from the background or the control probes. These techniques are also known as microarrays, which through a single hybridization are able to identify and quantify thousand transcripts in a collection of cells or samples (transcriptome).

Sequencing-Based Techniques: Sequencing-based techniques rely on obtaining direct information about the order of nucleotides of an RNA molecule, by involving sequencing methods and generating short tags or randomly primed cDNAs, able to provide information on the expressed transcripts and their level in a collection of cells or samples (transcriptome).

Transcritptome: The transcriptome is a dynamic "entity" spatially and temporally changing, representing a snapshot of the transcripts at a particular time and place in the history of an individual or collection of cells or samples.

Chapter 7
Resolving Sample Traces in Complex Mixtures with Microarray Analyses

George I. Lambrou
University of Athens, Greece

Eleftheria Koultouki
University of Athens, Greece

Maria Adamaki
University of Athens, Greece

Maria Moschovi
University of Athens, Greece

ABSTRACT

High throughput technologies have facilitated the study of thousands of factors simultaneously. A well-known method that has been utilized throughout recent years is microarray technology. Since their advent, microarrays have been used to discover differences between samples, such as those on the level of gene expression or polymorphism detection. This technique has found applications in many areas of life sciences, including forensics. Despite its usefulness, the microarray method is not flawless. Microarray experimentation contains a lot of bias, which makes the use of sophisticated statistical techniques necessary in order to overcome these problems. One basic assumption made from the very first microarray experiments, concerning expression studies, was that samples are homogeneous. This assumption was based on the fact that the biggest part/percentage of a biological sample consists of cells of the same type. For example, tumor biopsies, although considered to be homogeneous, are infiltrated with many other cell types such as macrophages, surrounding fibroblasts and even normal, healthy tissue surrounding tumor cells. As a consequence, forensic samples may consist of tissue mixtures that need to be distinguished.

This chapter reviews the microarray technology and deal with the majority of aspects regarding microarrays. It focuses on today's knowledge of separation techniques and methodologies of complex signal, i.e. samples. Overall, the chapter reviews the current knowledge on the topic of microarrays and presents

DOI: 10.4018/978-1-60960-483-7.ch007

the analyses and techniques used, which facilitate such approaches. It starts with the theoretical framework on microarray technology; second, the chapter gives a brief review on statistical methods used for microarray analyses, and finally, it contains a detailed review of the methods used for discriminating traces of nucleic acids within a complex mixture of samples.

INTRODUCTION

High throughput technologies have facilitated the study of thousands of factors simultaneously. A well-known method that has been utilized throughout the recent years is microarray technology. Microarrays are based, mainly, on the well known trait of nucleic acid sequences to hybridize with their complement chains. One of the best known techniques in science is hybridization which is based on the 'simple' property of nucleic acids (i.e. DNA and RNA) to bind to their complementary sequence. In the 1970s *Edward Southern* invented the technique, known as *Southern Blotting* (Southern, 1975, 1992) for DNA hybridization. *Northern Blotting* is the equivalent technique used for RNA hybridization. Microarrays could be regarded as the successor or the continuation of the *Southern* and *Northern* techniques. Microarrays, as the name implies, consist of arrayed series of genes ranging from a few hundreds to the complete transcriptome. The first arrayed DNA sequences were reported back in 1987 (Kulesh, Clive, Zarlenga, & Greene, 1987), spotted on filter paper. In the mid 90's, the first dense, small scale spotting was reported by *Schena, Brown* and *Botstein et al. (1995)* at Stanford University (Schena, Shalon, Davis, & Brown, 1995). Although invented elsewhere, Stanford has been regarded as the main developer of microarray technology. Since then, microarrays have evolved both in the number of spotted genes or oligonucleotides (Figure 1) they contain and in the methods of its analysis. In other words, we can say that microarray technology exploits the property of DNA to hybridize to its complementary sequence but *a contrario* to the classical techniques; it allows the hybridiza-

tion of thousands to tens of thousands of genes simultaneously.

Since their advent, microarrays have been used to discover differences between biological samples. For example, on the level of gene expression, a sample is compared to a reference, in order to discover differences in the gene expression profile. Similarly, microarrays have been used for the detection of polymorphisms. During the past few years, microarray technologies have attracted a major deal of interest from the scientific community due to their potential in screening thousands of factors simultaneously.

Microarrays consist of glass slides or membranes printed with oligonucleotides or cDNA fragments. Later on this chapter we will describe the dynamics of microarray hybridization, since this plays an important role in the analysis and evaluation of microarray data. Based on this property and the progress of high fidelity robotic technologies, microarrays have proven extremely valuable for the detection of literally, tens of

Figure 1. The evolution of printed chips. The first chips used had a few hundred spots i.e. genes. With time chip densities have increased dramatically, reaching today over 2M spots on a single slide

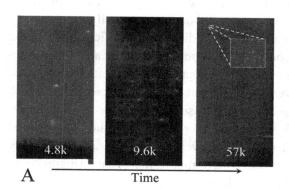

thousands of targets within one experiment. For this reason alone, this particular method has found applications in many areas of life sciences, including forensics.

In time, microarrays expanded to various types of high-throughput experimentations. Examples of these include *methylation studies*, *SNP* (*Single Nucleotide Polymorphism*) detection, *CGH* (*Comparative Genomic Hybridization*) microarrays and *CHIP-chip* (*Chromatin Immunoprecipitation Chip*) microarrays. Microarray applications include experiments for comparing gene expressional profile of biological samples or detection of genetic polymorphisms in forensic samples. Furthermore, protein and tissue microarrays have been developed, but it is outside the scope of this chapter to deal with this topic.

Therefore, the aim of the present work is to review the major aspects of microarray methodology and its applications, which include the dynamics and kinetics of nucleic acid hybridization, the microarray platforms, microarray experimentation design issues and data analysis: *data filtering, normalization, clustering* and *Principal Component Analysis.*(*PCA*) Special emphasis will be given to the known up-to-date methods for microdissecting the complex signal, received from microarray experiments, to its constituents. The aspects we will be dealing with are a brief introduction to microarray methodologies and the references to the known applications of microarrays in life sciences, including forensic sciences. In addition, we refer to the platforms used today in microarray methodologies. Also, as an important part of microarray methodology, we will discuss known aspects of hybridization dynamics, either in the context of competitive hybridization or single-stranded, one sample hybridization dynamics. A very important aspect of microarrays, which should be discussed in a separate section since it influences further analysis, is the experimental design. Another very important issue of microarray analysis is the normalization of data. This probably includes the most important aspect of microar-

ray methodology, since it is the component that influences all further decisions and conclusions. Following this, we will discuss the methods used for classification and clustering. Finally, we will discuss the relatively novel and intriguing topic of sample signal microdissection. This involves the separation of a sample signal (in the case of microarrays it is the spot) into further small signals, which several smaller samples have contributed.

Microarray Principle and Methodology

At this point we need to define the types of nucleic acids that are utilized in microarray analyses. The first and most abundantly used molecules were cDNAs. The *in vitro* reversely transcribed total RNA yields the respective cDNAs of all expressed exons at a certain time point under investigation. This method usually requires large amounts of total RNA as starting material, which ranges from 20-50ug per sample. Since this is not always the case, i.e. samples could be rare or difficult to obtain or of low quantity, other alternatives should be considered. A solution to aforementioned problems came with the methodology of RNA amplification. It was first described by *Van Gelder et al.* in 1990 (Van Gelder et al., 1990). This methodology is based on the linear amplification of dsDNA transcribed to cRNA with use of the *T4 DNA Polymerase, T3 RNA Polymerase* and *T7 RNA Polymerase*. It is a very successful technique since it can amplify 20ng to 2ug of total RNA yielding an approximately 5000-fold amplification. This means that samples of 200ng could yield 40ug of cRNA or samples of 2ug of total RNA could yield up to 100ug of *cRNA. cRNA* (complementary RNA) is also called *aaRNA* (*anti-sense amplified RNA*). Finally, when the desired molecules have been extracted and sample quality has been tested, nucleic acids have to be labeled with fluorochromes and let to hybridize (Figure 2). The basic and decisive step in microarray methodology is the sample selection and nucleic acid extraction, with RNAs or DNAs.

Figure 2. The main principle of microarray labeling (http://en.wikipedia.org/wiki/DNA_microarray, 2010)

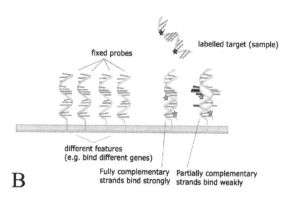

Figure 3. The basic microarray experiment consists of two samples co-hybridized on a microarray chip. Each sample is labeled with a different fluorescent dye and genes (cDNAs or cRNAs) bind antagonistically on the complementary spot (http://en.wikipedia.org/wiki/DNA_microarray, 2010)

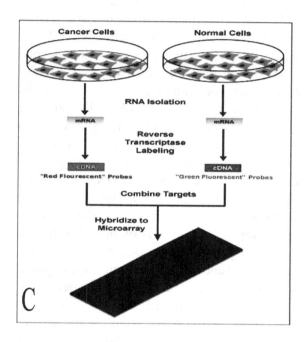

In order to define the expression profile of genes at specific time points, one needs to "capture" the cell's RNA or DNA at that specific time point. DNA and RNA quality is the most important step as it actually defines the output.

Microarray Applications

Gene Expression Profiling Microarrays

The first use of microarray technology was for detecting differences between two samples at the mRNA level. Samples that are treated differently, for example a drug treatment against no treatment or normal cells against tumor cells (Figure 3), are used for RNA extraction and hybridized, either as cDNAs or as cRNAs (*complementaryRNAs* or also mentioned as *anti-sense amplified RNAs*). The result is the 'snap-shot" of the transcriptome at a given time point. Usually, in order to obtain more useful information, it is necessary to perform multiple experiments at different time points or conditions and then one speaks of a *functional genomic assay*. Although this type of microarray application has been used extensively for research purposes, its use has also been recently reported in forensics (Sakurada et al., 2009; Zehner, Amendt, & Boehme, 2009).

Single Nucleotide Polymorphisms (SNPs) Microarrays

The human genome is known to have differences among individuals at specific gene sites at the level of one nucleotide. Previously it was possible to detect one such polymorphism at a time. Microarray technology has revolutionized the aspect of polymorphism detection. *SNP* microarrays can facilitate the discovery of millions of *SNP*s in a single sample within one experiment. Nowadays, there are chips that contain almost over 2 million sequences on a single glass slide. However, because the alleles differ by only one nucleotide, it is difficult to obtain optimal conditions for hybridization. The DNA fragments under investigation can give mismatches with the resulting false-positive signals. This can be resolved by adding to such an array many oligos, with the polymorphism at different sites and with mismatch positions for the *SNP* itself. Although this approach has less sensitivity and selectivity as compared to classical methods, the vast amount of data it produces makes it extremely attractive. This method has found applications to almost all areas of life sciences, including forensics (Homer et al., 2008; L. Li et al., 2006), since the detection of polymorphisms is considered to be a regional or better national trait characterizing a particular population. It provides a tool for investigating "lost" or "suspect" samples at a glance and in more detail. Furthermore, it can be applied to old, buried or fossilized samples, as long as the extraction of trace amounts of DNA is possible, providing evidence for the history of a finding, whether this is recent or ancient. For example, three very interesting reports have highlighted the use of genetic information in unraveling the mysteries of ancient secrets, such as the origin of smallpox (Y. Li et al., 2007), and the interactions of Asian populations with the Western civilization by studying the *SNP*s in the mitochondria of human bone fossils in Central Asia (Lalueza-Fox et al., 2004). Finally, a very interesting example of the use of molecular techniques for forensic purposes is the attempt to detect the *SNP*s in the *Mycobacterium leprae,* the parasite responsible for leprosy (Watson & Lockwood, 2009).

Comparative Genomic Hybridization (CGH Microarrays)

CGH or *Chromosomal Microarray Analysis* (*CMA*) is a method for detecting mainly gene copy amplifications, but also deletions and chromosomal abnormalities in general. The same principle applies here as in the previous microarray applications. The sample under investigation is treated in a way such that the end product would be a fragmented DNA; in concordance the reference sample is treated similarly. Both samples

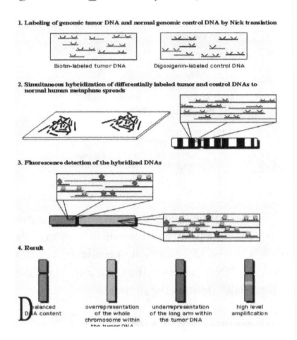

Figure 4. The principle of CGH microarrays. It is a method for the detection of gene copy numbers or chromosomal abnormalities (http://en.wikipedia. org/wiki/DNA_microarray, 2010)

are labeled and hybridized on a microarray chip spotted with all known gene sequences (Figure 4). Similarly to the *SNP* microarrays, this method has also found applications in all fields of life sciences, especially in diagnosis, with emphasis on cancer. Surprisingly, the use of this type of microarray application has also been reported for forensic purposes (Salama et al., 2007; L. Zhang et al., 2009).

CHIP-Chip Microarrays

This is the last application involving microarrays on the genomic level. As with the previous applications, chromatin immunoprecipitation was initially considered to be a powerful technique for the detection of DNA-specific proteins and binding motifs. However, the limitation was the number of DNA-binding proteins that could be identified at a given time-point. As a consequence,

Figure 5. The principle of the CHIP-chip microarray. A very useful technique for the detection of gene regulatory/expression factors, as it detects on high-throughput scale transcription factors binding on DNA sites (http://en.wikipedia.org/wiki/DNA_microarray, 2010)

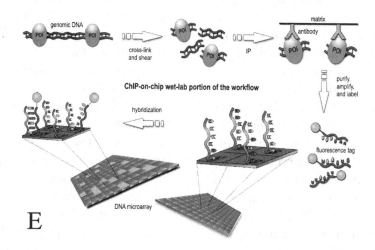

the method of *CHIP-chip* microarrays was applied to microarray technology (Buck & Lieb, 2004). This follows a similar work-flow (Figure 5) to the previous applications, since it is based on the hybridization of DNA fragments on printed oligonucleotides, with the difference that these fragments are specific for DNA-binding proteins. There are no known reports on uses of *CHIP-chip*

applications on forensic issues. In Figure 6, the uses of nucleic acids and subsequent applications are presented.

Microarray Technology

Microarray Slide (Chip) Printing

The main principle of microarray technology is the 'printing' of the microarray slides. The cDNAs are collected from cDNA banks amplified by Polymerase Chain Reaction (PCR). The amplicons, also known as *probes* or *reporters*, are dissolved in *dimethyl sulfoxide (DMSO)* which acts as a soft denaturant and prevents the cDNAs from dehydrating. The cDNAs are then transferred to a robot for printing. The robot is equipped with pins that absorb the cDNAs, by capillary forces, printing them on the slides by gently touching the slides' surface, generating the so-called 'spot'. Slides are covered with an amino acid sheath which assists the binding of the cDNAs or oligonucleotides on the biochip. In standard microarrays the *probes* are attached to a chemical matrix on the surface by covalent bonding. Approximately 50 μl of each cDNA is required for a spot to be printed.

Figure 6. An overview of the sample extracts used for respective microarray applications. The first nucleic acids utilized were cDNAs, transcribed from the sample's mRNA. A more modern alternative has been the hybridization of cRNA as far as expressional analysis is concerned

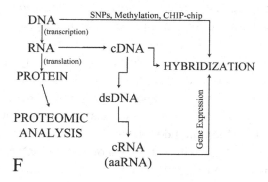

Of the 50 µl, 30 µl is essentially DMSO. Such a printed slide is called a '*biochip*'. The procedure is roughly described by the following steps: (a) pins are cleaned-up by ultrasound in a hydrous solution, (b) excess water is absorbed by vacuum, and (c) a wash step proceeds the vacuum step. Steps (b) and (c) are repeated three times before the pins can absorb the cDNAs to print them on the slide. Depending on the potential of the robot and the number of pins, approximately 50 slides can be printed within 3 days. However, the more complicated the robotic system, the more problems may occur. There are several robots for slide printing and the most sophisticated ones have an automatization method for controlling the whole process from PCR implementation to chip printing. This procedure refers to the older methods for printing. Since the beginning of microarray spotting, technological progress has allowed the spotting of multiple thousands of *probes* on a surface. Today it is possible for several thousands of genes, or even millions in the case of *SNP* microarrays, to be printed on a slide. Last but not least, there is the photolithographic oligonucleotide synthesis or *in-situ synthesis*. This is a technique where light sensitive *MAS*king agents build an oligonucleotide sequence, one nucleotide at a time. This method is more efficient than the spotting methods in terms of density, as it allows the spotting of more sequences per surface unit.

Microarray Technological Platforms

Whilst getting into the details of microarray platforms, we should mention the main categories of the microarray methodology. We could distinguish them into two main categories. *Dual-Channel* and *Single-Channel* platforms. Both types of platform are based on the same principle, which is the property of fluorescence-bearing nucleic acids to hybridize with their complementary structures/ sequences (Figure 2). However, there is a major difference in the way that these nucleic acids are applied on the respective slides. *Dual-Channel* platforms use the simultaneous hybridization of two samples on the same slide, as opposed to *Single-Channel* platforms that use one sample per slide. This has the advantage of making feasible the comparison of two samples under the same conditions and therefore reduces bias. However, one disadvantage is that comparison between different slides becomes laborious, i.e. increases bias and further algorithms for *cross-slide* normalization are needed. Usually, in this type of experiments (*Dual-Channel*, dual comparison), and for purposes of gene expression profiling, cDNAs are used. However, cRNAs (or aaRNAs) can also be utilized.

On the other hand, the alternative and more up-to-date microarray platforms are *Single-Channel* platforms. These are based on the same hybridization principle as the *Dual-Channel* ones but in this case the molecules to be hybridized are almost exclusively cRNAs. The reason for this is the abundance of starting material, as we described at the beginning of this section.

In the case of *SNP*, *Methylation* and *CHIP-chip* microarrays both types of platforms have been utilized. There are examples for both *Dual-Channel* (e.g. *Nimblgene*) and *Single-Channel* applications (e.g. *CodeLink*, *Affymetrix*).

We will now discuss the *Single-Channel* platforms into more detail, since these find applications in almost every microarray use, ranging from research to diagnosis and forensics. On the level of gene expression there are two main platforms: *CodeLink* and *Affymetrix*.

CodeLink arrays use a novel method for printing. They use a *piezoelectric deposition* of oligonucleotide probes onto a 3D polyacrylamide aqueous gel surface. This produces a *donut-shaped* spot which takes such morphology, probably due capillary phenomena, that it transports solutes to the periphery of an evaporating solution. *CodeLink* arrays contain several positive and negative controls, which include bacterial RNAs as internal *spikes*. Approximately 1-5% of the total RNA is the mRNA of a cell at given time point. This varies with the cell type, cell condition or phenotype. For this reason internal spikes are used in order to detect *minimal detection limits* and *bioarray performance*.

On the other hand, *Affymetrix* arrays have probes which are lithographically synthesized directly on the chip and which are by far more homogeneous than those present in cDNA arrays. The reduction of the length to 25-mer, reduces synthesis errors and fabrication costs. In order to achieve a sufficient binding strength with such short oligos, hybridization conditions must be less stringent than those utilized with cDNA, which increase cross-hybridization phenomena (Simon, Mirlacher, & Sauter, 2004). In order to deal with the cross-hybridization effects, each probe is actually a set of multiple probe pairs (16-20) corresponding to each target (Lockhart et al., 1996). A probe pair consists of a 25-mer oligonucleotide perfectly complementary to the sequence of a gene (*Perfect Match: PM*), and a 25-mer oligonucleotide that differs from the perfect match probe by a single mismatched nucleotide at the central position (13th position; *Mismatch: MM*). This combination of a 25-mer pair, *PM* and *MM*, offers the highest sensitivity and specificity, while it solves, in part, co-hybridization problems.

The difference between *PM* intensities minus *MM* intensities averaged across the probe pairs gives an estimation of the hybridization intensity. The intensities measured using *Affymetrix* arrays are considered to be the absolute expression levels: the less efficient hybridization of the *MM* probe to the target, allows the PM intensity minus the MM intensity of the probe to offer a better estimation of intensity. Background correction (*BC*) on the intensities is done automatically (GeneChipTM software) using a regionalized method, i.e. dividing the array in several rectangular zones. Within each zone, background intensities are estimated averaging the lowest 2% of probe cell intensities, and background values are smoothed across the number of zones, to obtain the cell specific background. The *Affymetrix' Micro Array Suite* (*MAS*)

developed two widely used algorithms, *MAS* 4.0, and *MAS* 5.0, for the estimation of hybridization signals (absolute expression levels), based on intensity differences between *PM* and *MM*. The first approach, implemented in *MAS* 4.0, uses an empirical algorithm to estimate the hybridization intensity, named *Average Difference* (*AD*), and is based in the following formula:

$$AD = \frac{1}{n}\sum(PM_i - MM_i) \tag{1}$$

Where n is the total number of probe pairs for a probe set/gene, and PM_i and MM_i indicate the perfect and mismatch probe intensities after background correction (BC) for the ith probe pair for the probe set/gene. The above algorithm has frequently produced negative values of expression (AD) in the past. In order to avoid this, a new statistical algorithm (*MAS* 5.0.) was developed, where the *MM* value was higher than the *PM* value. A new MM value was introduced (called the *Contrast Value* or *CT*), based either on the average ratio between *PM* and *MM* for all the probe pairs of that probe set or a slightly higher value than the *PM*. This absolute expression for a probe set is called *Signal Log Value* (SLV_k), and is described as follows:

$$SLV_k = BiWeight\{\log_2(PM_{i,k} - CT_{i,k}) : i = 1,...,n\} \tag{2}$$

Where a one-step *Tukey biweight function* is applied to the logarithms of the pair-wise intensity differences between the *PM* and *MM* probe pairs of all the *n* probe pairs in the probe set *k*. Together with the absolute expression values, a *detection call* (*DC*) is also estimated, using a detection algorithm. This defines whether a transcript is present (*P*), marginal (*M*) or absent (*A*) in a sample, and associates a *p*-value, based on a *Wilcoxon signed-ranked test* between *PM* and *MM* probe intensities. More precisely, only if the number of *PM* probes have higher intensity than the *MM* within a probe set, this probe set will be considered as present (Simon, et al., 2004). Nonetheless, alternative methods for estimating expression levels have been developed for *Affymetrix* arrays, and are still under continuous academic research. Two of the most widely used methods, other than *MAS*, that have been proposed for processing the raw intensities observed during a single array experiment, are: the *Robust Multiarray Average* or *RMA* method (Bolstad, Irizarry, Astrand, & Speed, 2003; Irizarry, Bolstad et al., 2003; Irizarry, Hobbs et al., 2003), which subtracts background effects, and its successor, the *GC-RMA* algorithm (Irizarry, Hobbs, et al., 2003; Irizarry, Ooi, Wu, & Boeke, 2003; Naef, Hacker, Patil, & Magnasco, 2002; Naef & Magnasco, 2003), which has an additional goal, namely to account for nucleotide-specific affinities during hybridization. The affinity modeling used by *GC-RMA* is based on observations (Naef, et al., 2002; Naef & Magnasco, 2003; Naef, Socci, & Magnasco, 2003) that when one takes labeling into account, effective hybridization to 25-mers is especially strong for *C*'s and weak for *A*'s in the sequence, especially near the middle.

Design Issues of Microarray Experiments

The microarray scanner produces a vast amount of data, which is meaningless unless some parameters are considered. The simplest form of a microarray experiment is presented in Figure 3, and it refers to the comparison between two biological samples in order to detect differentially expressed genes. The experiment presented in Figure 3, refers to the comparison between two samples in order to detect differentially expressed genes. There are several drawbacks to this approach, which include the detection of false positives or false negatives or the rejection of spots (genes) as poor. In order to avoid these problems, several additional techniques have been applied to the main method. One of them is the printing of the same gene on different but usually adjacent spots on the chip,

or on every two spots. This provides investigators with the certainty that the hybridization observed is correct and it gives more statistical significance to the measured intensities. Even this technique, however, has some drawbacks, especially in the first printed chips: it reduces the spot count at least by half (it is preferable to obtain the maximum number of genes on a slide) since older chips have a limited amount of genes that could be spotted on a chip. Therefore, alternative techniques have been developed for dual-channel experiments, such as the '*sandwich*' technique: with this technique, the printed chip does not entail a large amount of gene doublings, but instead a collection of genes that are printed three or four times on the chip at different positions on the grid. Secondly, instead of covering the slide with the special cover slips, one can cover it with another slide, thus obtaining two hybridizations of the samples simultaneously (*sandwich*). The intensity of the spots scanned on one slide should be identical to the intensities of the spots on the other slide and in that way cross-slide bias can be filtered. Another way to reduce noise is the expansion of the *sandwich* method, the so-called '*flipped-color sandwich*', where a total of four slides is hybridized; the first two contain the samples stained with the fluorescent stains and hybridize as mentioned above, i.e. as a '*sandwich*', and the other two contain the same samples but are stained reversely.

In the case of single-channel chips, the aforementioned problems have been resolved, firstly, by the fact that the number of spots that can be printed on a slide exceeds by far the number of genes in the genome. Secondly, by the usage of spikes in the experimentation procedure, which offers an internal control for both effectiveness and detection. Last but not least, the effects of dye bias, which is attributed to the intensity measured in particular due to the chemical structure or affinities of the dyes, is bypassed since only one fluorescent dye is used.

If, however, one wishes to compare multiple samples or multiple situations, then more sophis-

Figure 7. Experimental design issues have been of great importance in microarray methodology. Two main design are presented here were (A) is the Reference Design and (B) is Loop Design. Each of these two designs has its advantages and disadvantages. One of the most important characteristics is that the reference design is simpler in its application and analysis while the loop design is more complicated. Not many tools have still developed for the analysis of loop experiments

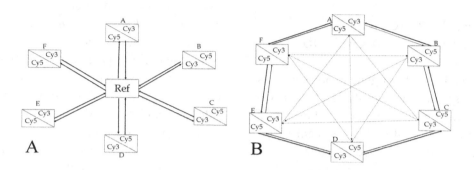

ticated experimental designs must be applied. As microarray technology goes more mature, many design, analysis and normalization approaches have been developed to successfully address more complicated questions (Butte, 2002; Townsend, 2003). Experimental design issues have been addressed by *Kerr* and *Churchill* (Churchill, 2002; Kerr & Churchill, 2001). The first and most simple design applied was the *reference design*, which is presented in Figure 7A. The advantage of the reference design is that it is simple in its application, easy to evaluate and to analyze. The disadvantage is that, unless the control or reference sample is in the main question, it gives a significant statistical evaluation of the reference since it is performed multiple times, as compared to the samples under investigation, which are analyzed once or twice. To address this issue, an alternative design has been proposed, the *loop design* (Figure 7B), where more than two fluorescent dyes can be used (Churchill, 2002; Kerr & Churchill, 2001; Townsend, 2003; Vinciotti et al., 2005; Woo, Krueger, Kaur, & Churchill, 2005). Other investigations have focused on the comparison of the two methodologies i.e. *loop designs vs. reference designs* (Vinciotti, et al., 2005). There are *pros* and *cons* for every design. The *reference*

design, albeit simple to the point of being self-evident, has the disadvantage that the reference sample is used multiple times, thus minimizing noise variation for itself, while the other samples are measured only once, thus exposed in heavier impact of noise. In this sense, the superiority of the *loop* compared to the *"reference"* design, in terms of reliability and robustness, has been suggested by several authors (Altman & Hua, 2006; Townsend, 2003). However, the disadvantage of using *loop design* is its complexity and the lack of methods to render channel ratios comparable among experiments (Dobbin & Simon, 2002; Townsend, 2003). An alternative methodology to *loop design* analyses has been proposed by *Lambrou et al. (2009)* using vectorial approaches, in an attempt to set a rational framework for the analysis of *loop* designed microarray experiments, exploiting the vectorial nature of microarray sample instances (Lambrou et al., 2009).

Design issues are considered of major importance regardless of the application of microarray technology. Despite the progress in technological aspects, there is still a lot of work to be done in matters of statistical analysis and microarray data evaluation. Decision-making, based on microarray data, still relies on the available methodologies for analysis. For example, the choice of *reference* vs. *loop designs* is crucial, especially in cases where *dual-channel* platforms are utilized to investigate a sample or answer specific questions.

A BRIEF INTRODUCTION TO MICROARRAY DATA ANALYSIS

Until recently, the study of gene expression was limited to the simultaneous study of 2 to 4 genes. The analysis of such an amount of data limited the *"angle"* of perception of biologic systems. This was accompanied by the immediate consequence of not facing biological phenomena as systems but rather as "*snapshots*", even though biological research was always considered to study systems biology. In addition, analysis of the produced data was easy. One had only to consider the time point and the gene's function at that certain point. On the contrary, the analysis of the data produced by a single microarray chip is immense. A relatively small-scale microarray chip of 1.2k produces at least 1.2×4 thousand numbers (which equals to 4.8k numbers). The first step in the analysis of microarray data is the definition of data distribution. Scattering techniques are utilized for this purpose (Figure 8A, 8B). Scatter plots are not however a reliable means for the evaluation of gene expression. Another statistical tool used for microarray visualization are *M-A Plots* (Figure 8C, 8D). *M* is the intensity ratio and *A* is the average intensity of each spot. *M-A Plots* are used to visualize intensity-dependent ratios of raw microarray data. It is assumed that the majority of genes should not manifest differential expression and this should be apparent on an *M-A Plot*. As it is shown in Figure 8 this is indeed the case. Also, many normalization methodologies assume relative stable expression in order to be successful. However, in our opinion, no assumptions should be made for gene expression. Biological systems are dynamical systems and gene expression, whether a sample has been taken in real-time or

whether it has been biopsied, is the stationary image of the specific moment that genes have been investigated. There are, though, algorithms that make no previous assumptions on the raw data. Further on, other processing tools exist in order to filter microarray data, such *z-score* (Figure 8E) estimation and *gene flagging* (Figure 8F). Gene flagging is a filtering process, which can also be considered as a pre-processing procedure and rules out genes of low quality. There is a lot of debate on which spots on a microarray chip should be ruled out and which shouldn't but we will not analyse this subject further.

In order to have a more precise image of the expression profile, normalization and classification methods are required. There is a variety of normalization methods for microarray data. Such algorithms include *Global Median, Lowess* (Figure 8G-8K), *Loess, Rank Invariant* and others. As we have mentioned above, raw microarray data entail a lot of bias, which makes microarray experiments difficult to process and evaluate. Therefore, methods for filtering, background correction, normalization and classification are required.

Basic Transformations

The basis of gene expression in microarrays is the ratio of intensities. Absolute quantification is almost impossible in microarrays, at least not without the help of secondary methodologies (for example Real-Time PCR), which confirm the microarray findings. Therefore, relative quantification is in the heart of microarray analyses. An exception to this are the SNP and CGH microarrays, where the question is the detection or not of certain genomic abnormalities.

$$x_{ij} = \log_2 \frac{Cy5_{ij}}{Cy3_{ij}}, \qquad (3)$$

Figure 8. Some of the basic analysis tools for microarray include scatter plots, M-A plots and log2 transformations. In (A) and (B) the scatter plots of two chips is presented from 4.8k and 9.6k genes respectively. In (C) and (D) the M-A plots of the same chips is presented. Further analysis includes a z-score estimation (E) and gene flagging (F) which is the out-ruling of low quality spots. Further data can be normalized with different algorithms and in (G-H) the normalization of 5 experiments is presented, normalized with the Lowess algorithm. Images are from in-house experiments (not published data)

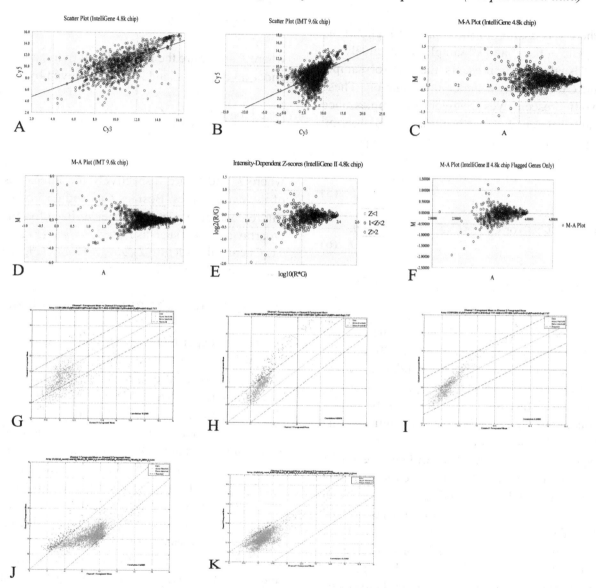

is the basic mathematical formulation of gene expression.

Where *Cy5* is an example of one fluorescent stain and *Cy3* (Figure 10, Chemical Structure 1)

is an example of a second fluorescent stain, x_{ij} is the log_2 of the expression ratio of the ith gene in the jth sample as measured by the j array. The same applies to the case of single-channel microarrays, only it is formulated as:

$$x_i = \log_2 \frac{Cy5_{ij}}{Cy5_{ik}}, \qquad (4)$$

where x_j is the log_2 of the expression ratio of the ith gene in the jth and k^{th} samples respectively.

Usually, $Cy3$ represents the control sample and $Cy5$ the sample under investigation. These two fluorescent dyes are given as examples since many different dyes can be utilized in microarray experiments, yet these two are the most popular.

If $Cy5_{i,j} > Cy3_{i,j}$ or $Cy5_{i,j} > Cy5_{i,k}$ then $x_{i,j}, x_i > 0$,

$$\qquad (5)$$

If $Cy5_{i,} < Cy3_{i,j}$ or $Cy5_{i,j} < Cy5_{i,k}$ then $x_{i,j}, x_i < 0$,

$$\qquad (6)$$

If $Cy5_{i,} = Cy3_{i,j}$ or $Cy5_{i,j} = Cy5_{i,k}$ then $x_{i,j}, x_i = 0$,

$$\qquad (7)$$

In other words, if $x_{i,j} > 0$, the ith gene in the jth experiment is over-expressed, if $x_{i,j} < 0$, then the ith gene in the jth experiment is under expressed. Finally, if $x_{ij} = 0$ (which is mostly NOT the case), then there is an equal expression of the two genes. Equation 4 can be represented, theoretically, in a graphical pattern for an infinitesimal number of experiments. The use of logarithms is essential because, if a gene is 2-fold over-expressed, then the raw data will give as a result $Cy5/Cy3 = 2$. On the other hand, if a gene is 2-fold under expressed, then $Cy5/Cy3 = 0.5$. Accordingly, for a 4-fold induction, $Cy5/Cy3 = 4$ and for a 4-fold reduction $Cy5/Cy3 = 0.25$. It is obvious that a graph of these values shows a great difference between the induced vs. the reduced genes. However, logarithmically these differences minimize and become: for the 2-fold induction $log_2(Cy5/Cy3) = 1$, for the 2-fold reduction $log_2(Cy5/Cy3) = -1$, for the 4-fold induction $log_2(Cy5/Cy3) = 2$ and for the 4-fold

reduction $log_2(Cy5/Cy3) = -2$. So, a graph of these results gives an equivalent picture of the expression profiles of genes. A very good estimator of microarray data quality is the *M-A* plot. It outlines the relations between *M* which is given by:

$$M = \log R - \log G, \qquad (8)$$

where R and G are the intensities of two samples under investigation. and A which is given by:

$$A = \left(\frac{\log_2 R + \log_2 G}{2} \right) = \log_2 \sqrt{R \cdot G}, \qquad (9)$$

where R and G are respectively the intensities of the two samples. Besides $Cy3$ and $Cy5$ other fluorescent molecules have been utilized for microarray analyses such as *Phycoerythrin* (Figure 11, Chemical Structure 2), *Alexa Fluors* (Figure 12, Chemical Structure 3) and others.

Background Subtraction, Correction

Microarray experiments are subject to many factors of bias. Background signal is one of these factors which can influence array quality and data evaluation. Briefly we refer to the methodologies that deal with background correction.

In general, background correction is applied before normalization. One of the main methods used is the subtraction of background signal either locally or globally. Local background subtraction is measured from the mean or median intensities of the surrounding pixels of a spot. It is considered to be a robust measure of background intensity (Ritchie et al., 2007). However, several disadvantages have been described, such as negative spot values, missing values, or spots with undesirable statistical properties. These properties have also been described previously (Beissbarth et al., 2000; Bilban, Buehler, Head, Desoye, & Quaranta, 2002; Finkelstein et al., 2002). Global background subtraction methods include the calculation of the total noise along the whole chip and subtraction from the mean or median signal of spot intensities. Other methods also have been proposed, such as the *Robust Multichip Analysis (RMA)* (Irizarry, Hobbs, et al., 2003; Irizarry, Ooi, et al., 2003).

Interestingly, an approach to background correction claims that the probability of no subtracting background should be considered as a possible method for microarray data handling. This has been reported previously by *Yang et al. (2002)* and *Quackenbush et al. (2001)* (Quackenbush, 2001; Yang & Speed, 2002). It is considered that with no background correction, measured intensities of minimal amplitude can be evaluated, something which is impossible when background subtraction is performed.

However, the choice for background subtraction or not, and consequently the method of subtraction, rely mainly as a factor of personal choice, without any given global guidelines on what is the most proper thing to do.

In Figure 9 we present several microarray experiments with low and high background intensities. The effect of background can be devastating. Due to this fact, background intensity can affect the estimation of differentially expressed genes.

Data Normalization

The next and most critical procedure that should take place is the normalization of data. Data normalization has evolved through time. One of the first and most simple methods is the reduction of noise levels and other bias through division or subtraction with *Global Mean* or *Global Median*.

So, let $y_{norm,ij}$ be the normalized value of $x_{i,j}$. and let

$$x_{new,ij} = x_{ij} - \bar{x}_{ij} , \tag{10}$$

Where $\bar{x}_{ij}$ is the mean or median value of the intensity $x_{i,j}$ of the ith gene in the jth sample and is equal to:

$$\bar{x}_i = \frac{1}{n} \sum_{j=1}^{n} x_{ij} , \tag{11}$$

The normalized value is given by:

$$y_{norm,ij} = \frac{x_{new,ij}}{\sigma_i} , \tag{12}$$

where (*Sigma*) is the standard deviation of the intensity of gene *I*,

$$\sigma_i = \sqrt{\frac{1}{n-1} \sum_{j=1}^{n} (x_{ij} - \bar{x}_i)^2} , \tag{13}$$

In time, since more sophisticated algorithms were needed in order to analyze the increasing complexity of experimental designs and questions under investigation, several more robust methodologies were developed. Such algorithms include *Lowess, Robust Lowess, Loess, Rank Invariant* and others. As we have mentioned before, for background correction methodologies, there are no global rules, at least up-to-date, on whether one should apply certain algorithms to noise subtraction. The same applies to normalization methods. There is no global rule on deciding which algorithms should be used, since this is an aspect of data distribution, of the question under investigation, and so on. We are not going to get into more depth on this topic, since it is outside of the scope of this chapter, yet it is an aspect of outmost importance and therefore worth mentioning. As a general rule, however, the choice of normalization methodology affects the final interpretation of data. In some cases, the discrimination between an up-regulated or a

Figure 9. Spot intensity of a dual-channel experiment is visualized in the form of a 3D diagram. A relatively good hybridization for Cy3 (A) and Cy5 (C) with relatively low background intensities (B, D) for the two dyes respectively. Division with the background median reduces the signals' intensities but the expression profiles are still visible. In contrast to a bad hybridization (G, H) where spot intensities are barely visible due to high background intensity (I, J). As a consequence, division of signals with the median background intensities produces a low quality expression image (K, L). Notice that Cy3 background intensity (B, I) is higher that Cy5 (D, J), something expected, since Cy3 is considered to be more fluorescent and long-lasting that Cy5, yet it produces higher background signals. Fluorescent dye variations accounts for a lot of bias in microarrays. This difference in fluorescence intensities due to dyes chemistry is one of the reasons that normalization is imperative. These images are from in-house microarray experiments (not published data) and have been produced with the ARMADA microarray software (National Hellenic Research Foundation, Athens Greece) (Chatziionannou et al. 2009)

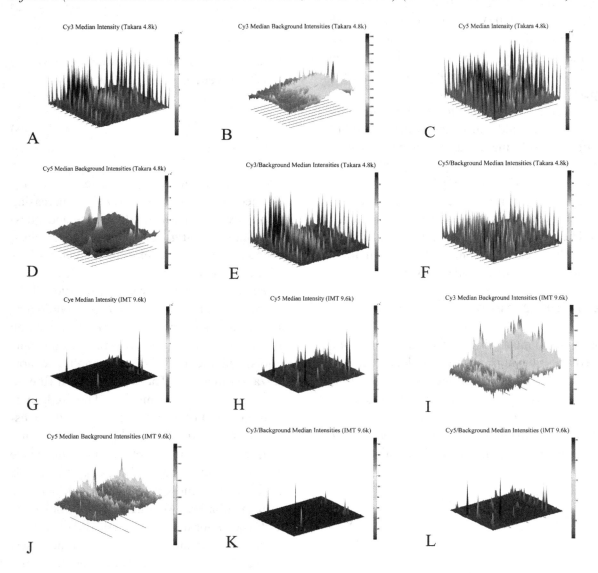

down-regulated gene, or between the presence or absence of a polymorphism, is dependent on the normalization method.

Data Classification

Last but not least, we refer to data classification. This is the final step in microarray analysis, since it is the part that gives the information on the functional and relational classification of data. This type of analysis is known as *clustering*. A large amount of algorithms has been proposed for the purpose of *clustering*, with the most popular being the *hierarchical clustering* with *Euclidian distance*.

The first step is similarity measurement between expression patterns. A common way to measure this is by using the *Pearson correlation (r)*. If *x* and *y* are the *n*-component vectors for which we want to calculate the similarity in the expression pattern, then the correlation coefficient is given by the similarity measurement with *Pearson Correlation*:

$$r = \frac{\sum_{i=1}^{n}(\mathbf{x} - \bar{\mathbf{x}})(\mathbf{y}_i - \bar{\mathbf{y}})}{\sqrt{\sum_{i=1}^{n}(\mathbf{x}_i - \bar{\mathbf{x}})^2}\sqrt{\sum_{i=1}^{n}(\mathbf{y}_i - \bar{\mathbf{y}})^2}}, \qquad (14)$$

where $\bar{x}$ and $\bar{y}$ are the means of vectors *x* and *y* respectively. The value of *r* varies between -1 and 1, with 1 meaning that the two series are identical, 0 meaning they are completely independent and -1 meaning they are perfect opposites. In other words, if two genes are found to have an *r* of 0,9, or even better if they can be considered as having a similar expression pattern, they can be clustered together. There are several techniques for calculating the correlation coefficients of genes, such as: *uncentered Pearson correlation, coefficient, squared correlation coefficient, averaged dot product, cosine correlation coefficient, covariance, Euclidian distance, Manhattan distance mutual formation, Spearman Rank-Order correlation* and *Kendall's Tau*

Finding similarities between expression patterns is the first step in *clustering*. The second step is taking the two genes most alike and putting them together as a cluster. One starts from a number *n* of *objects*, where each object represents one gene, and assimilates them to 1 (n→1). This is called *hierarchical clustering* since it is based on clustering according to a hierarchy set by the similarity patterns of genes, with those most alike on top of the hierarchy and those less similar at the bottom of the hierarchy.

The hierarchical clustering process can be summarized in a *dendrogram*. The *dendrogram* sorts genes according to similarities in expression patterns, by setting related genes closely. If a cluster of genes equals another cluster of genes then these two clusters create a *branch* in the *tree* a level higher. As an alternative to hierarchical clustering other methodologies are used, namely called *non-hierarchical clustering,* which include *Self Organizing Maps (SOMs), k-Means Clustering, Support Vector Machines, Principal Component Analysis* and *Correspondence Analysis*.

Some New Tools for Microarray Data Analysis

As mentioned earlier, the progress in life sciences research is immense. Yet, the new data produced by microarray technology is becoming increasingly complicated and therefore new bioinformatics tools are needed to unlock the secrets. The first efforts focused on the area of managing the amount of data. At first, techniques such as *neural networks* and *artificial intelligence* were used. Later on, new techniques, such as *Support Vector Machines (SVM)*, were developed. All of these techniques had a common characteristic, they all had the ability to '*learn*'. Because microarray data is not as concise as it is theoretically considered to be, one needs "smart" machines that would have the ability to distinguish between "*false*" and "*real*" values and come up with the correct result. In addition to the learning capability of neural networks or *SVM*, another characteristic they shared was the ability to be trained to learn. In general, certain methodologies have been developed for the analysis and *interpretation* of microarray data. These can be divided into five areas: a) image optimization, b) selection of genes which play an important role in the pathogenesis of cancer, c) gene interaction definitions, i.e. expression pathways, d) determination of subtypes of the samples, e) which sample type or subtype is impossible to determine with classical methods, i.e. achievement of diagnosis by using supervised (or unsupervised) pattern recognition.

HYBRIDIZATION DYNAMICS OF NUCLEIC ACIDS ON SOLID SURFACES

After our brief presentation of the microarray analysis fundamentals, we should get into more detail and discuss the aspects that are considered to influence microarray experimentation and data interpretation thereafter.

Differential Expression of Genes

As mentioned before, the key point to microarray methodology is the fact that it makes it possible to examine multiple genes of a sample at the same time, exploiting the hybridization property of nucleic acids. In dual-channel experiments, each spot has two samples, each with a different dye bound to it. Depending on the abundance of the genes of the control sample and of the genes of the sample under investigation, each binds antagonistically to its complementary cDNA on the spot of the chip. In the case of a single-channel microarray experiment, there is one dye which does not have to antagonize with a second dye, yet there are dynamics, which participate in this process.

How can we be certain that the binding of the genes is antagonistic and not accidental? First of all, one has to assume that the mixture applied to a biochip is homogeneous. Second, that the dynamics of hybridization may not be homogeneous, since the abundance of genes varies according to their expression, and third, that many of the genes may hybridize accidentally on the spots forming *mismatches,* thus giving the wrong impressions about the expression profile of the samples. The latter is probably due to capillary effects, where the samples do not diffuse equally on the biochip's surface. As the field of microarray experimentation has matured, research has gone into more depth and has been occupied with questions regarding the nature of binding and the accuracy of measured concentrations (Y. Zhang, Hammer, & Graves, 2005). In several tests performed on commercially available platforms, such as *CodeLink* microarrays and *Affymetrix*, different results were obtained when dilutions of samples were used in microarray experiments (Relogio, Schwager, Richter, Ansorge, & Valcarcel, 2002). For example, several statistical errors were detected with the *CodeLink* platform when the hybridization of dilutions of samples was attempted, and at the same time it was observed that the discrimination between a perfect match (*PM* and a Mismatch (*MM)* was not possible when hybridization times were prolonged in the *Affymetrix* platforms (Y. Zhang, et al., 2005).

The Thermodynamics and Kinetics of Microarray Hybridization

A previous report by *Chan V et al. (1995)* (Chan, Graves, & McKenzie, 1995) referred to the thermodynamics of nucleic acid hybridization, and it was mentioned that efforts were being made for the development of technologies for high-throughput detection of nucleic acids. That particular work focused on the kinetics of the reactions, i.e. the patterns of hybridization. Before that time, the question had already been posed on how nucleic acids, and especially DNAs, can bind to a solid surface and to immobilized DNA molecules (Adam & Delbruck, 1968). One particular problem that was addressed at the time was how the *Reduction of Dimentionality (RD)* enhances the rate of capture on a surface and how the subsequent 2D diffusion of the capture site can enhance the overall capture rate (Adam & Delbruck, 1968). Several approaches to that problem have been made which can be distinguished into three main categories:

1) the maximum capture rate to a surface that is uniformly reactive and a perfect sink (Berg & Purcell, 1977), 2) capture by a surface with dispersed small capture sites which act as perfect sinks (Berg & Purcell, 1977; D. Wang, Gou, & Axelrod, 1992), 3) capture by a surface with dispersed small capture sites with intrinsic reaction limitation (Axelrod & Wang, 1994). In those physical situations with dispersed small capture sites, the presence or absence of surface diffusion, mediated by nonspecific adsorption to non-capture site regions of the surface, can be explicitly included in the predicted reaction rate. *Axelrod and Wang (1994)* developed a combined *reaction-diffusion* rate-limited model for *ligand-receptor* interactions that occur on a cell surface. They based their theory on the *Brownian* nature of a ligand's motion.

Therefore, the main attempts to model the events describing hybridization kinetics relied on the ligand-receptor and the reaction-diffusion dynamics. The idea behind these attempts can be summarized into the following: free DNA in solution with a known concentration *C* diffuses in a 3D space towards a solid surface with immobilized DNA molecules. One possible explanation for this could be that the DNAs hybridize complementarily to their sister-chromatin fragments or that they bind to the solid surface non-specifically. At this point a second reaction-diffusion takes place but this time on the 2D level, pushing unbound molecules towards their complementary sequence.

We refer to the previous work by *Zhang et al (2005)* (Y. Zhang, et al., 2005) to describe the basic model of hybridization dynamics, as it is one of the most recent ones addressing the subject. In addition, this work addresses the problem of microarray quality from the thermodynamics point of view and indeed gives some interesting results as far as microarray experimentation is concerned.

The idea is simple in its conception. Let *S* be the soluble part of nucleic acids to be hybridized. Let *I* be the immobilized part of the nucleic acids attached to a solid surface. Then it is true through the *Kinetics Law* that:

$$S + I \underset{k_2}{\overset{k_1}{\rightleftharpoons}} SI, \tag{15}$$

where k_1 and k_2 are the forward and reverse rate constants of the reaction. Hence, we can define the total rate constant of the reaction K_r which would be equal to:

$$K_r = \frac{k_1}{k_2}, \tag{16}$$

K_r is equal to 1 when $k_1 = k_2$. With these considerations the events resulting in a hybridization can be formulated as:

$$\frac{d[SI]}{dt} = \frac{1}{vN} \{k_1[S][I] - k_2[SI]\}, \tag{17}$$

and when solved for initial concentrations it can be formulated:

$$\frac{d[SI]}{dt} = \frac{1}{vN} \{k_1[S_0]([I_0] - [SI]) - k_2[SI]\}, \tag{18}$$

Where *N* is the *Avogadro Number* and S_0 and I_0 are the initial concentrations of the soluble and immobilized DNA molecules respectively.

$$\frac{d[SI]}{dt} = \frac{1}{vN} \{k_1[S_0]([I_0] - [SI]) - k_2[SI]\}$$

reported by *Zhang et al* is identical to the receptor-ligand interaction dynamics reported by *Lauffenburger* and *Lindermann (1987)* (Lauffenburger, Linderman, & Berkowitz, 1987; Linderman & Lauffenburger, 1986, 1988). It is worth referring to the estimations of the magnitude of the term $1/vN$. A typical microarray slide might have 10ul of solution in contact with 1cm² of spot surface area. Therefore, $1/vN$ would be on the order of 10^{-18}cm²×mole×liter^{-1}×molecule^{-1}. A monolayer of DNA in a surface spot could contain up to ~10^{12} molecules×cm^{-2} (although it is often-considerably less; (Graves, 1999) Microarrays: powerful tools for genetic analysis). The equivalent of this concentration in liquid phase units would thus be ~10^{-6} mole×liter^{-1} or less, not an unreasonable figure in comparison with what is likely to be present in the liquid phase.

The above model describes the hybridization of one molecule to one substrate. This, as reported, can also be solved for two or probably multiple species (DNAs) competing for a substrate. In the work of *Zhang et al (2005)* (Y. Zhang, et al., 2005) the next solution presented is the one that describes the dynamics between a *perfect match* (*PM*) and a *mismatch* (*MM*). So, let us assume that there is one DNA sequence of concentration C, which binds to two immobilized molecules (I_a and I_b) to form the complexes of molecules $I_{C,a}$ and $I_{C,b}$ respectively. Equation 18 can be rewritten for the two differential equations.

The differenti*al equation for the PM*:

$$\frac{d[I_{C,p}]}{dt} = k_{1,1}[S_c][I_a] - k_{2,1}[S_c I_{C,a}], \qquad (19)$$

The differenti*al equation for the MM*:

$$\frac{d[I_{C,p}]}{dt} = k_{1,1}[S_c][I_b] - k_{2,2}[S_c I_{C,b}], \qquad (20)$$

which forms a system of differential equations to be solved computationally and represents the *PM* and *MM* hybridization of a species on a solid substrate. If we define the rate constant of the reactions in Equations 19 and 20 as $K_{d,1}$ and $K_{d,2}$ respectively and we also assume that $K_{d,1} = 10 \cdot K_{d,2}$, which means that the PM binds to its target 10 times stronger and with more affinity as compared to the mismatch. In solving the systems of differential equations a surprising result appears. It would also be expected that the concentration of I_a would be 10 times higher than that of I_b, but this does not appear to be the case. Computational approach has shown that the difference in concentrations is only on the scale of 3-fold, something which brings two irrelevant spots or genes or targets close to the statistical error or insignificance. In other words, when a DNA sequence is immobilized on an incorrect spot, it is highly unlikely that it would remobilize and find the correct complementary sequence to hybridize. This is an important aspect to be taken into consideration for the types of microarrays that utilize such approaches. Of course, it is only to be expected that, since this is shown on an idealized system, things would be much more complicated in a real experiment. Some other important factors which are not taken into account in the present model, are the time of hybridization, the temperature and the molecules' free energy, or the required energy for the hybridization to take place.

The final step in this analysis is the consideration of multiple samples antagonizing for one target and multiple samples hybridizing on multiple targets.

So, let us assume that the immobilized molecules I_a and I_b are two DNA sequences of two separate genes. Let two species (or genes or cDNAs or cRNAs) S_A and S_B be the nucleic acids in solution and $S_{A,Cy3}$ $S_{A,Cy5}$ and $S_{B,cy3}$, $S_{B,Cy5}$ be the sequences of these species but with different fluorescent labels. The reaction between those species and the respective immobilized targets would give the complexes $I_{a,A,Cy3}$ and $I_{b,B,Cy3}$ and the respective complexes for the *Cy5* labeled species. Then these reactions could be described by the following system of differential equations

$$\frac{d[S_{A,Cy3}I_{a,A,Cy3}]}{dt} = k_{1,1}[S_{A,Cy3}][I_a] - k_{2,1}[S_{A,Cy3}I_{a.A,Cy3}]$$

$$\frac{d[S_{A,Cy5}I_{a,A,Cy5}]}{dt} = k_{1,2}[S_{A,Cy5}][I_a] - k_{2,2}[S_{A,Cy5}I_{a.A,Cy5}]$$

$$\frac{d[S_{B,Cy3}I_{b,B,Cy3}]}{dt} = k_{1,2}[S_{B,Cy3}][I_b] - k_{2,2}[S_{B,Cy3}I_{b.B,Cy3}]$$

$$\frac{d[S_{B,Cy5}I_{b,B,Cy5}]}{dt} = k_{1,2}[S_{B,Cy5}][I_b] - k_{2,2}[S_{B,Cy5}I_{b,B,Cy5}]$$

(21)

this is a system of equations that better describes a real experiment where two different species antagonize to hybridize on two immobilized sequences. This analysis includes both the correct (perfect matches) hybridization dynamics as well as the incorrect (mismatches). This system is used to describe the kinetics of a reaction with equal quantities of the soluble species, equally available concentrations of immobilized targets and different k rate constants. To simplify this analysis we could concentrate on the hypothesis that there is one species, i.e. one gene, but contributed differentially from two different populations. This makes all constant rates equal but it changes the initial concentrations with which each participates in the reaction. Therefore, in the case of dual-channel experiments, the systems of equations becomes exactly as in Equation 21, the only difference being that the immobilized species is the same for both gene species, so we obtain:

$$\frac{d[S_{A,Cy3}I_{a,A,Cy3}]}{dt} = k_{1,1}[S_{A,Cy3}][I_a] - k_{2,1}[S_{A,Cy3}I_{a.A,Cy3}]$$

$$\frac{d[S_{A,Cy5}I_{a,A,Cy5}]}{dt} = k_{1,2}[S_{A,Cy5}][I_a] - k_{2,2}[S_{A,Cy5}I_{a.A,Cy5}]$$

$$\frac{d[S_{B,Cy3}I_{b,B,Cy3}]}{dt} = k_{1,2}[S_{B,Cy3}][I_b] - k_{2,2}[S_{B,Cy3}I_{b.B,Cy3}]$$

$$\frac{d[S_{B,Cy5}I_{b,B,Cy5}]}{dt} = k_{1,2}[S_{B,Cy5}][I_b] - k_{2,2}[S_{B,Cy5}I_{b,B,Cy5}]$$

$$\frac{d[S_{B,Cy5}I_{a,B,Cy5}]}{dt} = k_{1,2}[S_{B,Cy5}][I_b] - k_{2,2}[S_{B,Cy5}I_{b,B,Cy5}]$$

(22)

and in the case of *Single-Channel* experiment we get:

$$\frac{d[S_{A,Cy5}I_{a,A,Cy5}]}{dt} = k_{1,2}[S_{A,Cy5}][I_a] - k_{2,2}[S_{A,Cy5}I_{a,A,Cy5}]$$

$$\frac{d[S_{B,Cy5}I_{a,A,Cy5}]}{dt} = k_{1,2}[S_{B,Cy5}][I_a] - k_{2,2}[S_{B,Cy5}I_{a,A,Cy5}]$$

(23)

where we obtain a system of two differential equations and four unknowns if we consider the complex between species S and immobilized target I to be of unknown concentration.

As it has been shown previously, in solving the above systems computationally, the proportion of fluorescence of the complexes of the soluble species with the immobilized targets is directly proportional to the initial concentrations of the soluble species. In other words, the more of the gene being present, the more fluorescence would be measured in the *[SI]* complex.

From these analyses we can understand that, given the constant rates and the fluorescent intensities of an experimental set-up, it is possible to obtain valuable information in real experiments on the fraction of genes/species that participate on a given spot.

THE MICRODISSECTION OF MICROARRAY DATA OR "SEARCHING NEEDLES IN THE HAYSTACK"

As we have mentioned throughout this chapter, despite its usefulness, the microarray method is not flawless. Microarray experiments contain a lot of bias, which makes necessary the use of sophisticated statistical techniques, in order to overcome such flaws. The assumption that samples are homogeneous is based on the fact that the biggest part/percentage of a sample consists of cells of the same type. For example, tumor biopsies, although considered to be homogeneous, are infiltrated with many other cell types. Accordingly, forensic or other samples of various forms may consist of cell or tissue mixtures that need to be further distinguished. In the previous section we discussed an approach which could probably discriminate the fraction of species participating in the fluorescent intensity of a microarray spot.

Methods for distinguishing between traces of samples within biological mixtures were elucidated a few years after the appearance of microarray methodology. Only a few groups have been occupied with such approaches (Braun, Rowe, Schaefer, Zhang, & Buetow, 2009; Ghosh, 2004; Lahdesmaki, Shmulevich, Dunmire, Yli-Harja, & Zhang, 2005). It is of high significance to be able to estimate the percentage which a certain cell type contributes to a microarray spot, i.e. a gene. Such knowledge would change radically the way of examining and interpreting microarray data. However promising and sophisticated these methods may seem, still a question comes to mind: how can these results be validated and how accurate can these estimations be? Not many research groups have managed to answer that question. It is indeed very complicated, laborious and sometimes of debatable performance to do such a meta-analysis. However, such approaches open avenues of discovery towards pioneering fields which remain challenging due to their complexity.

Forensic science has embraced the use of DNA molecular biology tools for diagnostic purposes more than any other scientific field. Although forensic science did not initially seem ready to give up on older, solid methodologies, or to embrace newer methodologies such as microarray technologies, this changed gradually with time, since the new tools started to become more and more attractive (Budowle & van Daal, 2009). In general, the discipline of Forensics has been guided by the need for high-resolution human identity testing techniques. Over the past 20–25 years, forensic science has developed and implemented various robust and reliable DNA technologies (Budowle, Adamowicz et al., 2005; Budowle & van

Daal, 2008). Technological and methodological progress have enabled the reliable identification of extremely minute quantities of DNA, with an immense resolving power such that, in many cases, the number of evidence-sample contributors can be reduced to a few individuals, if not just one source. In addition, forensic molecular biology tools are very reliable because of the well-defined validation requirements (Budowle et al., 1991).

In a recent report by *Budowle* and *van Daal (2009)*, it is nicely presented how new molecular techniques find applications in forensic sciences. So, we briefly refer to this report in order to get a better idea of these applications. The first use is *phenotypic information from a DNA sample,* which refers to the detections of genetic traces such as *SNPs* or other phenotypic characteristics. In forensics, when there is no *suspect*, it is probably crucial to approach one through a series of eliminations i.e. by narrowing down the target population from which suspects could be pooled. The second use is *expression analysis for tissue type determination.* We could say that this is a direct application of microarray technology in forensics, as the need for discriminating between sample contributions is of major importance. In forensics, more than any other discipline, the tissues or samples for testing usually consist of a mixture of cells or tissues or other material. For example, in cases where the samples come from *post mortem* specimens, there is huge variation in sample constitution. This can vary from tissues in mixture with surrounding mixtures, along with bacterial or fungal genomes. More specifically, the RNA content is sometimes the only factor which can determine the tissue of origin. To this, two molecular methodologies can be of use. Microarray analysis would be the first method of choice, since it would be the only one to offer high throughput screening, and secondly, *Real-Time PCR.* Finally, and with increasing attention to it, is the discovery of *pharmacokinetic information* from a DNA sample. In many cases where drug-related information must be drawn, it is of great importance to use nucleic acid screening methods. As it is reported by specialists in the field, in cases where death is considered to be suicide or heart failure and drug usage is involved, it can be detected whether death has been due to physiological drug malfunction or deliberate administration of poisonous substances. Finally, something very crucial in this field of science is terrorism. Forensics could provide a highly valuable tool for the detection of traces in samples of bio-terror attacks. The threat of criminal use of microorganisms and their toxins is of great concern for biosecurity worldwide (Budowle, Schutzer et al., 2005; Budowle et al., 2003; Schutzer, Budowle, & Atlas, 2005). The *anthrax-letters attack* of 2001 not only demonstrated the public's vulnerability to such attacks, but also showed governmental inability to forensically investigate the evidence for investigation purposes (Morse & Budowle, 2006). This resulted in the birth of the field of microbial forensics. Microbial forensics is an evolving sub-discipline of forensic science for analyzing evidence from a terrorist act, or crime (Budowle, et al., 2003; Morse & Budowle, 2006). In many ways, we could not refer to microbial forensics as a new field, since its fundamentals derive from similar approaches established in public health and epidemiology (Morse & Budowle, 2006). The difference between microbial forensics and epidemiology is that the first desires to further individualize a sample. Nonetheless, microbial forensic analyses must encompass sample handling, collection, preservation, method selection, work analysis, interpretation of results, validation, and quality assurance. Molecular genetics, genomics and bioinformatics will be crucial to microbial species identification, virulence determination, pathogenicity characterization, and source investigation. The ultimate in source investigation is the ability to identify a sample as unique, such that it can be traced to a unique source.

Although the field of microarray applications in forensic science is still in its infancy, we are in agreement with the notion that microarrays offer an opportunity for new endeavors in forensics, hence our current report on the progress performed up-to-date on the field of finding trace contributions of samples in a given microarray spot.

Although microarrays are a relatively recent methodology, such questions have been addressed since its advent. We have already reported in this chapter that one of the approaches made to microarray analyses concerned the kinetics and dynamics of microarray hybridization, with applications to both dual-channel and single-channel platforms.

In this section we will refer to the historical progress performed until today on the discrimination of traces of samples in a microarray spot.

Estimating the Number of Contributors in a DNA Sample

The statistical interpretation of forensic DNA mixtures is mentioned and analyzed in previous reports (Evett, Buffery, Willott, & Stoney, 1991; Fukshansky & Bar, 1998; Weir, 1995; Weir et al., 1997). A general approach to the question of whether a sample is essentially a mixture of samples is dealt by *Egeland et al. (2003)* (Egeland, Dalen, & Mostad, 2003).. Their approach is mainly based on the assumption that a sample can have three variations as far as the presence of an allele is concerned. Let B be a variant, with B_f being the most frequent and B_r being the less frequent (rare). Let p_i denote the frequency of B at locus I, where i takes the values 0, 1, 2 where 0 denotes the presence of B_f only, 1 denotes the presence of B_r only and 2 denotes the presence of both. For example, for a homogeneous sample we could form a vector n which would be $n=\{1,...k\}$ where k is equal to the number of alleles investigated. For a non-homogeneous sample, the vector n would take the same values as equal to the number of alleles investigated but with the difference that each allele can take values between 0, 1 and 2, depending on the presence of alleles in the sample.

Continuing with this formulation, the probability of observing the different combinations of alleles would be:

$$\left.\begin{cases} p_{0,i} = p_i^{2x} \\ p_{1,i} = (1 - p_i)^{2x} \\ p_{2,i} = 1 - p_i^{2x} - (1 - p_i)^{2x} \end{cases}\right\}, \qquad (24)$$

The probability functions assume independence between the two alleles whether they come from one person or from multiple persons. Therefore, the probability of observing a phenotype z of $z = (0, 0, 1, 1, 2, 2)$ is $p_{o,1}p_{0,2}p_{1,3}p_{1,4}p_{2,5}p_{2,6}$.

Furthermore, to the question of whether the sample under investigation is a mixture or not, two approaches are being used: a *frequentist* and a *Bayesian*. In the *frequentist* approach the parameter x can be considered fixed but unknown and two hypotheses can be formulated:

H_0: One person contributed, i.e. x=1
H_1: More than one person contributed i.e. x>1
  H_0 can be rejected when:

$$K = \frac{\max_{j=1,2,3,...,n} P(data \mid x = j)}{P(data \mid x = 1)} > c, \qquad (25)$$

Where c can be estimated by simulating K under H_0.

On the other hand the *Bayesian approach* gives:

$$P(x = i \mid data) = \frac{P(data \mid x = i)\alpha(i)}{\displaystyle\sum_{j=1}^{\infty} P(data \mid x = j)\alpha(j)}, \qquad (26)$$

where $P(x=j)=\alpha(j)$ is the prior distribution. The posterior odds for a sample to be a mixture are:

$$\frac{P(x > 1 \mid data)}{P(x = 1 \mid data)} = \sum_{j=2}^{\infty} \frac{P(x = j \mid data)}{(x = 1 \mid data)} = \sum_{j=2}^{\infty} \frac{P(data \mid x = j)\alpha(j)}{P(data \mid x = 1)\alpha(1)}$$
$$, \qquad (27)$$

This approach consists of statistical tools for the detection of contributors in a sample. Further, more analyses have been proposed which we present below. For further details see the work of *Egeland et al.* (2003).

Interpreting DNA Mixtures

In a crime situation where a stain is collected from the scene and the reference sample is gathered from a suspect, through a profiling system, the suspect cannot be excluded as a contributor to the stain if the reference sample matches the crime stain. Usually, a series of hypotheses will be raised in the attempt to explain who the contributors might be, and the likelihood ratio (*LR*) is an effective tool to assess the strength of the evidence. It is usually common case that the DNA material from a crime scene is contributed by more than one person, meaning the victim and the perpetrator (Hu & Fung, 2003). *Weir et al. (1997)* (Weir, et al., 1997) derived a general formula for the evaluation of the *LR*, with regards to the interpretation of DNA mixtures; *Curran et al. (1999)* (Curran, Triggs, Buckleton, & Weir, 1999) and *Fung and Hu (2000a)* (Fung & Hu, 2000a) further extended the formula to the point where the relation (relation could be defined here, as more the presence of kinship) between persons is described by the formula given by *Balding and Nichols (1994)* (Balding & Nichols, 1994). The model of *Balding and Nichols (1994)* is general and the formulae are simple to apply. *Harbison and Buckleton (1998)* (Harbison & Buckleton, 1998) applied the *Balding-Nichols* formula to a simple mixed sample case. Expressions of *Likelihood Ratios* for six common cases are reported in *Fung and Hu (2002a)* where the contributors to a DNA mixture belonged to different ethnic groups. *Fung and Hu (2000b,2002b)* discussed the evaluation of match probability in single and multiple racial groups. Previously, *Fukshansky and Bär (2000)* (Fukshansky & Bar, 2000) constructed a formula for the evaluation of *Likelihood Ratio* in situations where the suspect is not tested but the relatives are. In addition, *Najarian et al. (2004)* proposed a *Mixture Model Method* utilizing the *Likelihood Ratio* with applications on the determination of differentially expressed genes (Najarian, Zaheri, Rad, Najarian, & Dargahi, 2004).

Therefore, this model can be applied for general discrimination of contributors to a complex sample. We present here the theory from *Hu and Fung (2003),* which has also been used by *Najarian et al. 2004,* and the general part of the model addresses the question of contributors in the mixed sample (Hu & Fung, 2003).

Likelihood Ratio

Suppose that the mixed sample taken from a crime scene and some persons, e.g. the victim and the suspect, are tested with the aim of identifying the true perpetrator(s). The likelihood ratio, would be:

$$LR = \frac{P(Evidence | H_p)}{P(Evidence | H_d)}, \qquad (28)$$

which is usually used to evaluate the weight of the evidence, regarding whether the suspect has contributed to the mixed sample, where H_p and H_d are the prosecution and defense positions, and the evidence is the genetic information obtained from the mixed sample and the investigated person(s). Following *Fung and Hu (2000a,2001)* (Fung & Hu, 2000a; Fung & Hu, 2001), let K denote the collection of genotypes (not necessarily distinct) of the typed person(s) and M denote the (distinct) genetic profile of the mixed stain. Expressing the evidence as (M,K), we have:

$$LR = \frac{P(M,K | H_p)}{P(M,K | H_d)} = \frac{P(M | K, H_p)}{P(M | K, H_d)} \cdot \frac{P(K | H_p)}{P(K | H_d)} = \frac{P(M | K, H_p)}{P(M | K, H_d)},$$
$$\qquad (29)$$

from the third law of probability. The latter equation stands true because both hypotheses H_p and H_d contain no different assumptions about the relationship (and origin) of the persons with known genotypes (K), and so $P(K|H_p)=P(K|H_d)$. Thus the evaluation of *LR* is induced to the evaluation of the conditional probability $P(M|K,H)$ for some hypothesis *H*. Under *H*, let x be the number of unknown contributor(s) and X be their genetic profile. Since the mixture M is contributed by the known and unknown contributors, we have $U \subset X \subset M$, where set U comprises the alleles present in mixture M but not in the genetic profile of the known contributor(s) declared by H, i.e., the alleles in set U have to be contributed by the x unknown contributor(s). Following this, we use the notation $P_x(U,M|K)$, instead of $P(M|K,H)$, to express the conditional probability $P(UX \subset M \mid K)$, and the evaluation of *LR* becomes the evaluation of $P_x(U,M|K)$. Without loss of generality, assume $M=\{1,2,...,m\}$ and the corresponding allele frequencies be $p1,p2,...,pm$. By the principle of inclusion and exclusion, we have:

$$\left| \begin{aligned} &P_x(U,M | K) = P(U \subset X \subset M | K) = \\ &= P(X \subset M | K) - P(U_{i \in U}(X \subset M \setminus \{i\}) | K) = \\ &= \sum_{M \setminus U \subset C \subset M} (-1)^{\left| \frac{M}{C} \right|} W(C) = \\ &= W(M) - \sum_{i \in U} W(M \setminus \{i\}) + \sum_{i,j \in U} W(M \setminus \{i,j\}) - ... + (-1)^{|U|} W\left(\frac{M}{U}\right) \end{aligned} \right|$$
$$\qquad (30)$$

where:

$$W(C) = P(X \subset C | K), \qquad (31)$$

is defined for arbitrary subset C of M satisfying $M \setminus U \subset C \subset M, |U||$ is the cardinality of set U with $|U| \leq 2x$. It is now clear that the kernel of the evaluation of *LR* is converted into the evaluation of $W(C)$. Under the *Hardy-Weinberg (HW)* law, we obtain:

$$W(C) = \left(\sum_{i \in C} p_i \right)^{2x}, \qquad (32)$$

and points out to the formula reported in *Weir et al. (1997)* and *Fukshansky and Bär (1998)* (Fukshansky & Bar, 1998; Weir, et al., 1997):

$$P_x(U, M) = s^{2x} - \sum_{i \in U}(s - p_i)^{2x} + \sum_{i,j \in U}(s - p_i - p_j)^{2x} -, \dots \qquad (33)$$

where:

$$s = p_1 + p_2 + \dots + p_m, \qquad (34)$$

For the other types of $W(C)$ regarding dependence and ethnicity, see the work by *Fukshansky and Bär (1999,2000)* (Fukshansky & Bar, 2000), *Fung and Hu (2000a,2000b,2001,2002b)* (Fung & Hu, 2000a, 2000b; Fung & Hu, 2001, 2002a, 2002b). Based on the formula of the right side of Equation 33, the subset U of M, and the sum s for the allele frequencies in M, the following function is defined:

$$Q(r, U, s) = s^r - \sum_{i \in U}(s - p_i)^r + \sum_{i,j \in U}(s - p_i - p_j)^r - \dots, \qquad (35)$$

where r is an integer, and introduce (Fukshansky & Bar, 2000):

$$\begin{bmatrix} L(r, u, s) \equiv L_\phi(r, u, s) = Q(r, \{1, 2, \dots, u\}, s) \\ L_i(r, u-1, s) \equiv L_{\{i\}}(r, u-1, s) = Q(r, \{1, 2, \dots, u\} \setminus \{i\}, s) \\ L_{i,j}(r, u-2, s) \equiv L_{\{i,j\}}(r, u-2, s) = Q(r, \{1, 2, \dots, u\} \setminus \{i, j\}, s) \end{bmatrix}, \qquad (36)$$

for every distinct $1 \leq i, j \leq u$. It is noted that the computational calculation of $Q(r,U,s)$ is straightforward and so are the calculations of $L(r,u,s)$, $L_i(r,u-1,s)$, and $L_{ij}(r,u-2,s)$.

Mixture Models for Assessing Differential Expression in Complex Tissues

As we have mentioned before, the main purpose of microarray technology is the screening of multiple nucleic acid targets simultaneously. This principle has found applications in every field of life science and it has been known from the beginning of microarray experimentation that samples of human or animal origin consist of a mixture of cells and therefore are not homogeneous. This question has been addressed experimentally by *Staal et al (2003)* (Staal et al., 2003) and efforts have been made to incorporate this question into the microarray analysis *Venet et al (2001)* (Venet, Pecasse, Maenhaut, & Bersini, 2001). In general, in microarray analyses the samples are treated as homogeneous. When it comes to differential gene expression, final analysis for example, is dependent on the fractions of cells contributing to a sample. The estimations one can make on the heterogeneity of the sample under investigation, vary from experimental set-up to set-up and depend on the questions posed. For example, when the samples under investigation are tissue samples, an anatomist's or pathoanatomist's estimation is not meaningless in describing the types of cells that make up the particular tissue. On the other hand, when cell culture models are used for the discovery of more basic puzzles, cell population is considered homogeneous, but here too it is in essential fact not. Cells can be treated or not treated, they can be in different phases of the cell cycle or entering apoptosis or necrosis. To this, *Gosh (2004)* has proposed a *mixture model* for defining sample traces in complex mixtures (Ghosh, 2004). This model deals mainly with the discrimination between tumor samples but the approach can be extended to any sample that is a mix of variant genomic profiles. Below we present the model proposed by *Ghosh (2004)*.

Let an observation of random samples $(X_1^t,...X_n^t)$ and $(Y_1^c,...Y_n^c)$, where X_i^t is the p-dimensional gene expression profile for the ith sample under investigation, and Y_j^c is the corresponding profile for the jth control or reference sample, $i = (1,...,n)$ and $j=(1,...,m)$. In addition, we observe $\pi \equiv (\pi_1,..., \pi_n)$, where π_i represents the proportion of the ith sample representing the sample's cells $i=(1,...,n)$. The assumption made here is that there are two cell types: the sample under investigation and the reference sample. In addition, it has been mentioned that this approach refers to *Dual-Channel* experimentation. Therefore, $(1-\pi_i)$, $(i=1,...,n)$ will represent the percentage of the ith sample. It is assumed that the data have been appropriately pre-processed and normalized. Again, the methods for assessing differential expression reported previously in the literature have made the assumption that $\pi_i=1$, $i=(1,...,n)$.

Before describing the model formulations, we need to make some assumptions on the design of the study. When the sample under investigation and the reference samples are of different origin, for example, from different individuals, comparisons between the two samples are treated as statistically independent, and it will not necessarily be the case that $m=n$. In other experiments, the sample under investigation and the reference samples come from the same source, for example, from the same individual, and in this case we can assume that $m=n$. Following this, we briefly describe the model specifications.

Model for Unpaired Study Design

The first step in the model's implementation is to consider the gene expression profiles for the reference samples. Let us define $Y_{i,g}^c$ to be the expression measurement for the gth gene using the ith reference sample, $g=(1,...,G)$; $i=(1,..., m)$. Similarly, $Y_{i,g}^c$ is the gth component of Y_i^c. Then,

the model for gene expression in reference samples is:

$$Y_{1,g}^c,...,Y_{m,g}^c \sim f_g^c(y), \tag{37}$$

$$f_1^c(y),...,f_G^c(y)^{iid} \sim f^c(y), \tag{38}$$

Thereafter, for tumor samples the model can be formulated as:

$$X_{1g}^t,...,X_{mg}^t \sim (1-\pi_i)f_g^c(x) + \pi_i f_g^t(x)$$
$$f_g^t(x)_-^{iid} p_+ f_+^t(x) + p_- f_-^t(x) + (1 - p_- - p_+)f^c(x) \tag{39}$$

Model for Paired Study Design

The formulation of the probability model for samples under investigation and reference samples in the case of paired specimens is as follows:

$$\binom{X_{g,i}^t}{Y_{g,i}^c} \bigg| \mu_i \sim \begin{bmatrix} (1-\pi_i)f_g^c(x)+\pi_i f_g^t(x) \\ f_g^c(x) \end{bmatrix}, \tag{40}$$

$$\binom{f_g^c(x)}{f_g^t(x)} \sim \begin{bmatrix} f^c(x) \\ p+f_+^t(x)+p-f_-^t(x)+(1-p_--p_+)f^c(x) \end{bmatrix}, \tag{41}$$

$$\mu_1,...,\mu_n \sim M, \tag{42}$$

This model takes into account the pairing of samples. In Equation 37, it is assumed that the reference and sample under investigation expression measurement for the gth gene from the ith sample, conditional on a gene effect, is a random sample from a bivariate distribution, where the first part involves the heterogeneity of the sample under investigation, and the second component is a gene-specific density for reference samples. The second part of the model is given in Equation 38 and Equation 39, where the densities are a random sample from a bivariate distribution. The density for f_g^t corresponds to that given in Equation 37. Finally, a model formulation is also needed for the sample effects $\mu_1,...,\mu_n$; the distribution of these effects is given by M in Equation 33. While there is a multi-stage formulation in both models, the latter model is bivariate, while the former model models the distributions of the gene expression profiles for control and tumor samples separately. Both models are examples of mixture models. It should also be noted that these models imply that there is dependence in gene expression measurements between genes. This is because of the two-stage hierarchical formulation adopted by *Ghosh (2004)* which is also implied by the models of *Newton et al. (2001)* (Newton, Kendziorski, Richmond, Blattner, & Tsui, 2001), *Efron et al. (2001)* (Efron, Tibshirani, Storey, & Tusher, 2001), *Ibrahim et al. (2002)* (Ibrahim, Chen, & Gray, 2002) and *Parmigiani et al. (2002)* (Ghosh, 2004; Parmigiani, Garret, Andazhagan, & Gabrielson, 2002). However, these methods assume that $\pi_i=1$ for $i=1,...,n$. Thinking about probabilistic specifications for the models described previously, the proposed model incorporates the fact that the number of samples *(n, m)* will be much smaller than the number of genes *(G)* in gene expression studies. What this implies is that it has to be parametric in the first stage and less parametric in the second stage of the models. This approach was also incorporated by other authors, such as *Newton et al. (2001)*, *Efron et al. (2001)* and *Parmigiani et al. (2002)* (Efron, et al., 2001; Parmigiani, et al., 2002). However, they did not deal with the complex sample scenario addressed by *Ghosh (2004)*.

In Silico **Microdissection of Microarray Data**

Succeeding the work of *Ghosh (2004)*, the report by *Lähdesmäki et al. (2005)* proposed a computational method for the microdissection of microarray data (Lahdesmaki, et al., 2005).

More specifically, they proposed a linear model for discriminating differentially expressed genes in a mixture of RNAs from tumor and normal cells. This model could probably be applied to other types of cells or tissue mixtures. We present the proposed model as follows:

Two samples, S_1 (which represents *RKO* colon cancer cells in their model) and S_2 (which represents normal lymphocytes) have been mixed at the RNA level. Therefore, the model is assumed to be linear. Let x_i^c and x_i^l be the expression level of the ith gene in the S_1 and S_2 samples, respectively. Assuming only two different cell types are mixed, the sample heterogeneity is modeled by a linear model:

$$\gamma_i^k = a_k x_i^c + (1 - a_k)x_i^l, \qquad (43)$$

where y_i^k is the expression value of the ith gene in the kth heterogeneous sample, and $0 \leq a_k \leq 1$ denotes the fraction of the S_1 cells in the kth mixture. In Equation 43 it is assumed that the expression level is fixed and does not change between heterogeneous measurements.

The first step is to invert the mixing effect shown in Equation 43, that is, to obtain estimates for the expression values of the pure S_1 cells and the pure S_2 cells. By making some distributional assumptions, one could use standard model-based estimation methods. However, in order to avoid making additional modeling assumptions, it is more preferable to use a general least squares method to estimate the gene expression levels corresponding to the pure samples. Let the number of genes be n and assume that one has measured the expression values for K different heterogeneous mixtures. Thus, one has measurements, $1 \leq i \leq n$, $1 \leq k \leq K$. Let also that the mixing percentages are known or have been measured. For the ith gene the sample heterogeneity can be expressed as:

$$
\begin{pmatrix} a_1 & \cdots & 1-a_1 \\ \vdots & \ddots & \vdots \\ a & \cdots & 1-a_k \end{pmatrix} \begin{pmatrix} x_i^c \\ x_i^l \end{pmatrix} = \begin{pmatrix} \gamma_i^1 \\ \vdots \\ \gamma_i^K \end{pmatrix} \Leftrightarrow \mathbf{A} x_i = y_i,
\tag{44}
$$

when including all *n* genes, the above model can be written as:

$$
\begin{pmatrix} A & 0 & \cdots & 0 \\ 0 & A & \cdots & 0 \\ \vdots & \vdots & \ddots & \vdots \\ 0 & 0 & \cdots & A \end{pmatrix} \begin{pmatrix} x_1 \\ x_2 \\ \vdots \\ x_n \end{pmatrix} = \begin{pmatrix} y_1 \\ y_2 \\ \vdots \\ y_n \end{pmatrix},
\tag{45}
$$

where $\mathbf{0}$ denotes the *K*-by-2 zero matrix. Let the matrix in Equation 45 above be denoted as $\tilde{A}$. Assuming the column rank of A is full, the least squares solution is given by:

$$
\hat{x} = (\tilde{\mathbf{A}}^T \tilde{\mathbf{A}})^{-1} \tilde{\mathbf{A}}^T y,
\tag{46}
$$

where $y = (y_1^T y_2^T \cdots y_n^T)^T,$

$$\tag{47}$$

Due to the structure of the matrix $\tilde{A}$, the least squares solution can be obtained gene wise as:

$$
\hat{x} = (\mathbf{A}^T \mathbf{A})^{-1} \mathbf{A}^T y_i,
\tag{48}
$$

The *Gauss-Markov theorem* states that the standard least squares solution is the best linear unbiased estimate if the noise in the measurements is additive and with constant variance. However, a common observation is that the *homoscedasticity* does not always apply to microarray data but instead, the noise variance depends on the underlying signal intensity. Such *heteroscedasticity* may decrease the power of the inversion method shown in Equation 48. The structure of the matrix $\tilde{A}$ ensures that the inversion can also be performed for each gene separately. Consequently, it is not necessary for the *homoscedasticity* to hold globally. Indeed, all that needs to be assumed is that the noise variance is approximately constant for each gene separately. Also, in this two-cell type model, no prior knowledge about the expression values of either of the two cell types is needed, since the method estimates the expression values for both cell types. The same also applies to more general models that include more cell types, assuming the model is sufficiently over-determined.

Identification and Separation of DNA Mixtures Using Peak Area Information

Another interesting approach to the analysis of complex mixtures has been proposed by *Cowell et al. (2007)* (Cowell, Lauritzen, & Mortera, 2007). Their approach is based on two main methodologies: *Probabilistic Expert Systems* and *Peak Area Information* through regular *Gaussian* analysis. *Probabilistic Expert Systems* (*PES*) for evaluating DNA evidence were introduced by *Dawid et al. (2001)* (Dawid, Mortera, & Pascali, 2001). As it is reported by *Cowell et al. (2007)* in a general review of the analysis of DNA evidence, *Foreman et al.(2003)* (Foreman, Champod, Evett, Lambert, & Pope, 2003) include several applications of *PES* and emphasize their potential by predicting that this methodology "will offer solutions to DNA mixtures and many more complex problems in the future". In general, the work of *Cowell et al. (2007)* is concerned with the analysis of mixed traces, where several individuals may have contributed to a DNA sample. *Mortera et al. (2003)* (Mortera, Dawid, & Lauritzen, 2003) have reported how to construct a *PES* using information about which alleles were present in a mixture, and reference to their work is used as a general description of the problem and for genetic background information. Other earlier contributions based on the presence of alleles in a mixture came from *Evett et al. (1991)* (Evett, et al., 1991), *Weir et al. (1997)* (Weir, et al., 1997) and *Curran et al. (1999)* (Curran, et al., 1999).

In this model it is assumed that the usual *Mendelian* genetic model applies for the allele composition of the mixture traces with known gene frequencies of single (*Short Tandem Repeats*) *STR* alleles, using those reported in *Evett et al. (1998)* (Evett, Gill, & Lambert, 1998) and *Butler et al. (2003)* (Butler, Schoske, Vallone, Redman, & Kline, 2003) for U.S. Caucasians (Cowell, et al., 2007). The latter has been used by *Cowell et al. (2007)*, for analyzing data (taken from *Wang et al. (2006)*) (T. Wang, Xue, & Birdwell, 2006). *PES* is a probabilistic model for relating the pre-amplification and post-amplification relative amounts of DNA in a mixture sample. This model is idealized, since it ignores complicating artifacts such as stutter, drop-out alleles and so on, and assumes that the mixture comprises of DNA from two people, who are referred to as p_1 and p_2. Prior to amplification, and provided that the mixture sample has not been degraded, the sample put into the amplification procedure will consist of an unknown number of cells from p_1 and a further unknown number of cells from p_2. Then, with every cell containing exactly two alleles from each gene, the fraction or proportion of cells from p_1 is also a common measure across the genes of the amount of DNA from p_1. This common fraction, or proportion, is symbolized by θ. In an ideal amplification methodology, during each amplification cycle the proportion of alleles of each allelic type would be preserved without error. -Deviations from this ideal are modeled as random variation using the *Gaussian* distributions as in Equation 51, whose mean for each allele is its pre-amplification proportion for the marker system it belongs to. The variance has a dependence on the mean for the two limiting cases: (i) the pre-amplification proportion is zero, or (ii) the pre-amplification proportion is unity. In the case where (i) stands true, it means that if there is no specific allele in the mixture prior to amplification, there is none post-amplification. In the case

where (ii) stands true, it means that for a given marker there is only one allelic type present in the mixture pre-amplification, and only that type is present in that marker post-amplification. The proposed model introduces an additional variance term, represented by v_2. The post-amplification fractions of alleles for each marker are represented in the peak area information, which is included in the analysis through the relative peak weight. The (absolute) peak weight w_a of an allele with repeat number a is defined by scaling the peak area with the repeat number as:

$$w_a = aa_a, \tag{49}$$

where a_a is the peak area around allele a. Multiplying the peak area with the repeat number is a crude way of correcting for the fact that alleles with a high repeat number tend to be less amplified than alleles with a low repeat number. Further on, it is assumed that a) the pre-amplification mixture proportion θ is constant across genes, b) the peak weight for an allele is approximately proportional to the amount of DNA of that allelic type and c) the peak weight for an allele possessed by both contributors equals to the sum of the corresponding weights for the two contributors.

To avoid arbitrariness in scaling, the observed relative peak weight r_a is considered, obtained by scaling with the total peak weight as:

$$\left\{ \begin{array}{l} r_a = \dfrac{w_a}{w_+} \\ w_+ = \sum_a w_a \end{array} \right\}, \tag{50}$$

So, then:

$$\sum_a r_a = 1$$

This simple model for the relative peak weight, denoted by the random variable R_a, assumes a *Gaussian* error distribution such as:

$$R_a \sim N(\mu_a, \tau_a^2)$$
$$\mu_a = \frac{\{\theta n_a^{(1)} + (1-\theta)n_a^{(2)}\}}{2}, \qquad (51)$$

where θ is the proportion, or fraction, of DNA in the mixture originating from the first contributor, $n_a^{(i)}$ is the number of alleles with repeat number a possessed by person i. The error variance τ_a^2 is obtained by:

$$\tau_a^2 = \sigma^2 \mu_a (1 - \mu_a) + \omega^2, \qquad (52)$$

where σ^2 and ω^2 are factors of variance for the contributions to the variation from the amplification and measurement processes. The model can be considered as a second order approximation to a more sophisticated model, based on *gamma distributions* for the absolute scaled peak weights. In addition, the correlation between weights due to the fact that they must add up to unity should be considered. If this is the only source of correlation, its inferential effect can be taken correctly into account by using the variance structure:

$$\tau_a^2 = \sigma^2 \mu_a + \omega^2, \qquad (53).$$

and considering, as observed evidence, the complete set of observed peak weights.

In general, the variance factors may depend on the genes in the sample and on the amount of DNA analyzed, but for simplicity reasons the values above are usually used. The proposed *PES* model is robust to small changes in these parameter estimates. The simple model presented seems sufficiently accurate and adequate for the purposes of mixture separation, and has the advantage that the calculations needed may be performed

quickly using any available *Bayesian network* software that implements evidence propagation for *conditional-Gaussian* networks.

Resolving Individuals Contributing Trace Amounts of DNA to Complex Mixtures with *SNP* Microarrays

The resolution of an individual's genomic DNA, whether it is present or absent in a complex mixture, is a field that really involves many disciplines, as we have seen throughout this chapter. In forensics, in order to determine whether a person contributes to a DNA mixture, it is essential to use a manual process that requires extensive experience and training. This is a laborious procedure which, in some cases, is also questionable, due to the bias obtained from laboratory experience, i.e. different laboratories can give different results. In particular, in the field of forensics, as well as in the field of genetics, it is often the basic assumption that it is not possible to identify individuals using pooled *SNP* data. We have mentioned above several works that deal with this aspect (Balding, 2003; Egeland, et al., 2003; Hu & Fung, 2003). Several of the reported techniques include the use of *STRs* on the Y chromosome. These are, however, of limited power when the sample under investigation consists of heavily degraded DNA -. In addition, sequencing of the *hypervariable region* of *mtDNA* has been used for detection purposes due to the its improved stability. Nonetheless, *mtDNA* also has its weakness since it follows a uniparental mode of inheritance (Homer, et al., 2008). The approach reported by *Homer et al. (2008)* (Homer, et al., 2008), which we present in this section, resulted in the rapid and sensitive detection of a trace amount of DNA, which consists of less than 1% of the total DNA content.

Experimentally, their approach included the formation of eight pooled genomic DNA complex mixtures. These pooled sample mixtures have been screened with two known commercial microarray platforms: *Illumina* and *Affymetrix*.

Current microarray technology can assay millions of SNPs. Genotypes are expected to result from such assays and data have attained the form of **AA**, **AB**, **BB**, or **NoCall** where **A** and **B** symbolically represent the two alleles for a biallelic *SNP* (Homer, et al., 2008). The first step is to define the ratios of normalized data. Hence, the ratio of transformation is given by:

$$Y_i = \frac{A_i}{(A_i + kB_i)},\qquad (54)$$

where A_i is the probe intensity for the **A** allele and B_i is the probe intensity for the **B** allele on the ith SNP respectively. Numerous studies have shown that Y_j transformation approximates allele frequency, where k_j is the SNP specific correction factor accounting for experimental bias and is easily calculated from individual genotyping data (Homer, et al., 2008; Macgregor et al., 2008; Pearson et al., 2007). Therefore, with this transformation, Y_i is an estimate of allele frequency, called p_A, for each SNP. Since there are two copies in each individual of the genome for autosomal *SNPs*, values for the **A** allele frequency (p_A) in a single individual may be 0%, 50%, or 100% for the **A** allele at **AA**, **AB**, or **BB**, respectively. Therefore, Y_i will be approximately 0, 0.5, or 1, with a certain variation from these values due to noise. For example, as it is stated by *Homer et al.,* if $k_j= 1$, intensity measurements of $\underline{A}j= 450$ and $B_j= 550$ would yield $Y_j =0.45$ and this SNP would be called **AB**. For a single individual, it is a case of a three-mode distribution for *Y* across all SNPs, since only **AA**, **AB**, or **BB** genotype calls are expected. However, when a mixture of multiple individuals is present, the assumptions of the algorithm are invalid, since only **AA**, **AB**, **BB**, or **NoCall** are given, regardless of the number of pooled chromosomes. Nonetheless, it is still possible to extract information from the relative probe intensity data. In this proposed approach,

allele frequency estimates from the mixture (*M*) are compared, where:

$$M_i = \frac{A_i}{(A_i + k_iB_i)},\qquad (55)$$

to the mean allele frequencies of a reference population. It is assumed that the samples consist of similar population distribution as far as substructures, ethnicity, or ancestral components are concerned, and it is possible to define similar ancestral components for an individual or mixture from similar allele frequencies across all SNPs. Hence, let $Y_{i,j}$ be the allele frequency estimate for the ith individual and the jth SNP, with an example measurement of $Y_{i,j}M\{0,0.5,1\}$, from a SNP assay. The absolute values for the two differences are compared. The first difference $|Y_{i,j}-M_j|$ measures how the allele frequency of the mixture M_j at the jth SNP is different from the allele frequency of the individual $Y_{i,j}$ for the jth SNP. The second difference, stated as $|Y_{i,j}-Pop_j|$, measures how the reference population's allele frequency Pop_j is different from the allele frequency of the individual $Y_{i,j}$ for the jth SNP. The values for Pop_j can be determined from an array of equimolar pooled samples or from databases containing genotype data of various populations. By calculating the difference between these two differences, we obtain the distance measure used for individual Yi:

$$D(Y_{i,j}) - \left|Y_{i,j} - Pop_j\right| - \left|Y_{i,j} - M_j\right|,\qquad (56)$$

In the case where the null hypothesis is true, i.e. that the individual is not part of the mixture, $D(Y_{i,j})$ approaches zero since the mixture and reference population are assumed to have similar allele frequencies. In the case where the alternative hypothesis is true, $D(Y_{i,j})>0$ since the M_j diverges from the reference population by Y_i's contribution to the mixture. In the case where $D(Y_{i,j})<0$, Y_i is more similar to the reference population than to the mixture, and thus less likely to be in the mixture. Consistent with Equation 56, $D(Y_{i,j})$ is positive when $Y_{i,j}$ approaches M_j and $D(Yi,j)$ is negative when $Y_{i,j}$ approaches Pop_j. By screening 500k SNPs, it would be expected that $D(Y_{i,j})$ would follow a normal distribution due to the *central limit theorem*. In this type of analysis, *Homer et al. (2008)* use a one-sample *t-test* for the particular individual, sampled across all SNPs, and thus obtain:

$$T(Y_i) = \frac{E(D(Y_i)) - \mu_0}{SD(D(Y_i)) \Big/ \sqrt{s}}, \qquad (57)$$

In Equation 57 it is assumed that μ_0 is the mean of $D(Y_k)$ over individuals Y_k not present in the mixture, $SD(D(Y_i))$ is the standard deviation of $D(Yi,j)$ for all the jth *SNPs* and individual Y_i, and s is the number of *SNPs*. It is also assumed that μ_0 is zero since a random individual Y_k should be equally distant from the mixture and the mixture's reference and therefore:

$$T(Y_i) = \frac{E(D(Y_i))}{SD(D(Y_i)) \Big/ \sqrt{s}}, \qquad (58)$$

If the null hypothesis is true $T(Y)$ is zero, and if the alternative hypothesis is true then it is $T(Y_i) > 0$. In order to consider for differences in ancestry between the individual, mixture, and reference populations among other biases, allele frequency data is normalized by using a reference population.

The above model was proposed by *Homer et al. 2008*. A response to this came from *Braun et al. (2009)* (Braun, et al., 2009), who claimed that the model proposed by *Homer et al. (2008)* uses the assumption that only independent loci are chosen and that the *z*-score of D_i across all loci follows a normal distribution such as:

$$T(Y_i) = \frac{\langle D_i \rangle - \mu_0}{\sqrt{Var(D_i)} \Big/ s} = T(Y_i) = \frac{\langle D_i \rangle}{\sqrt{Var(D_i)} \Big/ s} \sim N(0,1)$$

$$(59)$$

where $\langle D_i \rangle$ is the average over all *SNPs* and i, s are the number of *SNPs*. The main point of the work by *Braun et al. (2009)* is that the assumptions made in the model presented in this section are difficult to control in practice and therefore they (Braun, et al., 2009) investigated the effect of deviations from the assumptions of *Homer et al. (2008)* (Homer, et al., 2008). Summarizing the response, the authors (Braun, et al., 2009) conclude that, even though the proposed model has certain disadvantages, it is able to perform good separations for the positive and null samples. However, the classification of samples with the proposed model is subject to the underlying assumptions, such as that null samples do not follow a normal distribution.

When it comes to applying the proposed model (Homer, et al., 2008) to positively identify the presence of a particular individual in a mixed pool of genetic data of unknown size and composition, it is difficult to achieve the desired results.

Let g_i be a sample from forensic evidence and a suspect genotype be y_i. To apply the above method, one would need to take into account 1) the assumption that Y and G are indeed samples of the same population P; 2) a sample F which would also be a sample of the underlying population P, well-matched in size and composition to G; 3) an estimate of the sample size of G such that sample-size effects can be appropriately discounted and 4) the assumption that the *p*-values are accurate. The high false-positive rates which result from violations of these criteria make it probable that an innocent individual will be wrongly identified as suspicious; this is also likely to be the case for a relative of an individual whose DNA is present in G (Braun, et al., 2009).

Nonetheless, even though the proposed model has its disadvantages, it is still considered as pioneering work that opens new avenues to the field of discrimination of samples in a complex mixture, with applications not only to forensic disciplines but in life sciences in general.

Reinterpretation of Microarray Data and Resolving Cell Population Heterogeneity

Expression Deconvolution and Reinterpretation of Microarray Data

In this last section we will discuss two reports which deal with the aspect of gene expression and the separation of cell subpopulations within complex mixtures.

In the work presented by *Lu et al. 2003*, a modelling approach was used for re-interpreting microarray expression data from asynchronous yeast cells, as far as the cell cycle distribution is concerned (Lu, Nakorchevskiy, & Marcotte, 2003). This is an interesting approach since it uses a method applied to engineering and signal transduction for analysis of biological data/phenomena. Briefly, the *deconvolution* method is concerned with finding the solution of the convolution equation defined as:

$$f * g = h, \qquad (60)$$

where, h is a recorded signal, f is the signal to be recovered but has been convolved by another signal g. In general real measurements are of the form:

$$(f * g) + \varepsilon = h, \qquad (61)$$

where ε is the *noise* that enters the recorded signal.

The reference to gene expression is essential for two reasons: methodologies that can discriminate the fraction of contributors to a microarray signal are useful for both the life sciences as well as for the forensic sciences. In the work of *Lu et al. 2003*, a deconvolution approach is used, the so-called *expression deconvolution*, in order to resolve cell population dynamics. The basic idea is that gene expression from growing populations, and at this point we could include complex populations, is a mixture of mRNAs with different patterns of expression, depending on the cell cycle distribution of the cell population. This could probably be applied to a variety of samples that are mixtures of cells in different phases of the cell cycle or even different types of cells. It would probably be a matter of definition on what is differential or asynchronous.

Hence, the model proposed by *Lu et al. (2003)* has the following formulation:

Let e_n be the expression of the nth gene of the fraction f of cells in a specific cell cycle phase named, $f_{G1}, f_{G2}, f_S, f_M, f_{M/G1}$ for the fraction of cells in G_1, G_2, S, M and M/G_1 phases respectively. This is formulated mathematically as shown in Box 1.

In the proposed work by *Lu et al.*, as shown in Equation 62, a system is produced of 696 equations and only 5 unknowns: $f_{G1}, f_{G2}, f_S, f_M, f_{M/G1}$. The authors (Lu, et al., 2003), have used microarray datasets in order to validate and interpret these assumptions.

Expression deconvolution provides a theoretical framework for the analysis of expression data, which in turn opens new avenues for the interpretation of biological phenomena. In addition, the application of such algorithms and approaches could be extremely valuable to forensic science, where expression profiles of mixture samples are essential.

Resolving Cell Population Heterogeneity with Real-Time PCR

As we proceed to more recent reports on the detection of individual samples in complex mixtures, we should mention the study by *Diercks et al. (2009)*, regarding the detection of population heterogene-

Box 1.

$$
\left[
\begin{array}{l}
e_{1,population} \cong (f_{G1} \times e_{1,G1}) + (f_s \times e_{1,s}) + (f_{G2} \times e_{1,G2}) + (f_M \times e_{1,M}) + (f_{M/G1} \times e_{1,M/G1}) \\
e_{2,population} \cong (f_{G1} \times e_{2,G1}) + (f_s \times e_{2,s}) + (f_{G2} \times e_{2,G2}) + (f_M \times e_{2,M}) + (f_{M/G1} \times e_{2,M/G1}) \\
e_{3,population} \cong (f_{G1} \times e_{3,s}) + (f_s \times e_{3,s}) + (f_{G2} \times e_{3,G2}) + (f_M \times e_{3,M}) + (f_{M/G1} \times e_{3,M/G1}) \\
\qquad\qquad \vdots \\
e_{n,population} \cong (f_{G1} \times e_{n,s}) + (f_s \times e_{n,s}) + (f_{G2} \times e_{n,G2}) + (f_M \times e_{n,M}) + (f_{M/G1} \times e_{n,M/G1})
\end{array}
\right]
\tag{62}
$$

ity with the technique of Real-Time PCR (Diercks, Kostner, & Ozinsky, 2009). Real-Time PCR is a very sensitive technique which can detect, or better, amplify, the presence of a gene from minimum copies of mRNA. In this work, it is highlighted that the method offers high sensitivity, since it can detect as low as 30 copies of any given gene in a sample. The proposed methodology is based on the principle that mixed cell populations manifest a gene expression pattern that is averaged through most available methods. More specifically, by using standard techniques, it is possible to average the responses of cell populations, and therefore mask the cell-cell heterogeneity. In this way, the ability to distinguish between the individual responses of different cells within a sample is diminished (Bar-Even et al., 2006; Colman-Lerner et al., 2005; Elowitz, Levine, Siggia, & Swain, 2002; McAdams & Arkin, 1997; Newman et al., 2006; Ozbudak, Thattai, Kurtser, Grossman, & van Oudenaarden, 2002; Ramsey et al., 2006; Vilar, Guet, & Leibler, 2003). In other words, what has been proposed here is that the measurements of genes should be taken from the small fractions of cells that have been isolated by flow cytometric techniques. Even though the authors do not propose a model for separating cell populations, they reach out to the subject of heterogeneity from the reverse point of view. They point out that, even in almost homogeneous populations, as in the case of the mouse *macrophages* used, where over 99% were expressing CD11[b+] and F4/80[+] markers, there was an inherent heterogeneity in gene expression,

and more specifically in cytokine expression. They also report that the heterogeneity was not due to cell size factors, since cells were filtered for uniformity in size and granulation with filters set in *Forward* and *Side Scatters* of the cytometer.

A very interesting finding of their work was the fact that, even though all cells were found to express IκBα, a smaller percentage (60%) of the cells expressed measurable levels of IL1β. More interestingly, the fraction of cells expressing the protein was around 40%. This indicates a regulated mechanism from mRNA to protein expression, since the expression values do not coincide. As we mentioned earlier, this work does not present a model for the discrimination of complex populations, but it proposes a methodology through which an apparent problem is highlighted. All measurements in experimental procedures, or even diagnostic procedures, do measure the average expression levels of a target gene, therefore they could underestimate the contribution of certain cell populations that regulate molecular functions independently. It is in actual fact quite surprising that such approaches could revolutionize the view we have on biological phenomena. Being able to distinguish between signals and "dissect" through them to extract smaller differential ones would probably provide more insight on the mechanisms governing biological phenomena.

CONCLUSION

In this work we have reviewed the knowledge on the topic of algorithms and methodologies for the discrimination of sample traces in complex mixtures. We have described the mathematical formulations governing those models and, -in our point of view, we have given a spherical view of the areas of sample separation within a microarray experiment, ranging from expressional studies to genetic analysis. We provide the theoretical framework, first of all, on microarray technology; second, a brief review on statistical methods used for microarray analyses and finally, a detailed review of the methods used for discriminating traces of nucleic acids within a complex mixture of samples.

-Surprisingly enough, not many studies have been made regarding this subject. This - opens the door for further investigation and literally opens new avenues of discovery. Thousands of microarray experiments have been performed up to date. The analyses that come from such experiments, in their majority, have considered samples to be homogeneous. If this view changes, there are uncountable possibilities for further meta-analyses which will give a new angle to the way we have been looking at biological phenomena. In general, the study of gene expression, DNA mutation or *SNP* detection, assumes the homogeneity of the population under investigation. However, what happens in reality is that from conventional measurements we have the *average* image of the sample. It is known that tissues, and even cell culture cell populations, which are considered to be homogeneous, are characterized by exceptional heterogeneity. We have reported in a previous section the work of *Diercks et al (2009)* (Diercks, et al., 2009) who outlined exactly this aspect i.e. the heterogeneity of phenomenically homogeneous populations, and we have presented the analyses and techniques which facilitate such approaches.

REFERENCES

Altman, N. S., & Hua, J. (2006). Extending the loop design for two-channel microarray experiments. *Genetical Research, 88*(3), 153–163. doi:10.1017/S0016672307008476

Axelrod, D., & Wang, M. D. (1994). Reduction-of-dimensionality kinetics at reaction-limited cell surface receptors. *Biophysical Journal, 66*(3 Pt 1), 588–600. doi:10.1016/S0006-3495(94)80834-3

Balding, D. J. (2003). Likelihood-based inference for genetic correlation coefficients. *Theoretical Population Biology, 63*(3), 221–230. doi:10.1016/S0040-5809(03)00007-8

Balding, D. J., & Nichols, R. A. (1994). DNA profile match probability calculation: How to allow for population stratification, relatedness, database selection, and single bands. *Forensic Science International, 64*(2-3), 125–140. doi:10.1016/0379-0738(94)90222-4

Bar-Even, A., Paulsson, J., Maheshri, N., Carmi, M., O'Shea, E., & Pilpel, Y. (2006). Noise in protein expression scales with natural protein abundance. *Nature Genetics, 38*(6), 636–643. doi:10.1038/ng1807

Beissbarth, T., Fellenberg, K., Brors, B., Arribas-Prat, R., Boer, J., & Hauser, N. C. (2000). Processing and quality control of DNA array hybridization data. *Bioinformatics (Oxford, England), 16*(11), 1014–1022. doi:10.1093/bioinformatics/16.11.1014

Berg, H. C., & Purcell, E. M. (1977). Physics of chemoreception. *Biophysical Journal, 20*(2), 193–219. doi:10.1016/S0006-3495(77)85544-6

Bilban, M., Buehler, L. K., Head, S., Desoye, G., & Quaranta, V. (2002). Defining signal thresholds in DNA microarrays: Exemplary application for invasive cancer. *BMC Genomics, 3*(1), 19. doi:10.1186/1471-2164-3-19

Bolstad, B. M., Irizarry, R. A., Astrand, M., & Speed, T. P. (2003). A comparison of normalization methods for high density oligonucleotide array data based on variance and bias. *Bioinformatics (Oxford, England)*, *19*(2), 185–193. doi:10.1093/bioinformatics/19.2.185

Braun, R., Rowe, W., Schaefer, C., Zhang, J., & Buetow, K. (2009). Needles in the haystack: Identifying individuals present in pooled genomic data. *PLOS Genetics*, *5*(10), e1000668. doi:10.1371/journal.pgen.1000668

Buck, M. J., & Lieb, J. D. (2004). ChIP-chip: Considerations for the design, analysis, and application of genome-wide chromatin immunoprecipitation experiments. *Genomics*, *83*(3), 349–360. doi:10.1016/j.ygeno.2003.11.004

Budowle, B., Adamowicz, M., Aranda, X. G., Barna, C., Chakraborty, R., & Cheswick, D. (2005). Twelve short tandem repeat loci Y chromosome haplotypes: Genetic analysis on populations residing in North America. *Forensic Science International*, *150*(1), 1–15. doi:10.1016/j.forsciint.2005.01.010

Budowle, B., Giusti, A. M., Waye, J. S., Baechtel, F. S., Fourney, R. M., & Adams, D. E. (1991). Fixed-bin analysis for statistical evaluation of continuous distributions of allelic data from VNTR loci, for use in forensic comparisons. *American Journal of Human Genetics*, *48*(5), 841–855.

Budowle, B., Schutzer, S. E., Ascher, M. S., Atlas, R. M., Burans, J. P., & Chakraborty, R. (2005). Toward a system of microbial forensics: From sample collection to interpretation of evidence. *Applied and Environmental Microbiology*, *71*(5), 2209–2213. doi:10.1128/AEM.71.5.2209-2213.2005

Budowle, B., Schutzer, S. E., Einseln, A., Kelley, L. C., Walsh, A. C., & Smith, J. A. (2003). Public health. Building microbial forensics as a response to bioterrorism. *Science*, *301*(5641), 1852–1853. doi:10.1126/science.1090083

Budowle, B., & van Daal, A. (2008). Forensically relevant SNP classes. *BioTechniques*, *44*(5), 603–608, 610. doi:10.2144/000112806

Budowle, B., & van Daal, A. (2009). Extracting evidence from forensic DNA analyses: Future molecular biology directions. *BioTechniques*, *46*(5), 339–340, 342–350. doi:10.2144/000113136

Butler, J. M., Schoske, R., Vallone, P. M., Redman, J. W., & Kline, M. C. (2003). Allele frequencies for 15 autosomal STR loci on U.S. Caucasian, African American, and Hispanic populations. *Journal of Forensic Sciences*, *48*(4), 908–911.

Butte, A. (2002). The use and analysis of microarray data. *Nature Reviews. Drug Discovery*, *1*(12), 951–960. doi:10.1038/nrd961

Chan, V., Graves, D. J., & McKenzie, S. E. (1995). The biophysics of DNA hybridization with immobilized oligonucleotide probes. *Biophysical Journal*, *69*(6), 2243–2255. doi:10.1016/S0006-3495(95)80095-0

Chatziioannou, A., Moulos, P., & Kolisis, F. N. (2009). Gene ARMADA: An integrated multi-analysis platform for microarray data implemented in MATLAB. *BMC Bioinformatics*, *10*, 354. doi:10.1186/1471-2105-10-354

Churchill, G. A. (2002). Fundamentals of experimental design for cDNA microarrays. *Nature Genetics*, *32*, 490–495. doi:10.1038/ng1031

Colman-Lerner, A., Gordon, A., Serra, E., Chin, T., Resnekov, O., & Endy, D. (2005). Regulated cell-to-cell variation in a cell-fate decision system. *Nature*, *437*(7059), 699–706. doi:10.1038/nature03998

Cowell, R. G., Lauritzen, S. L., & Mortera, J. (2007). Identification and separation of DNA mixtures using peak area information. *Forensic Science International*, *166*(1), 28–34. doi:10.1016/j.forsciint.2006.03.021

Curran, J. M., Triggs, C. M., Buckleton, J., & Weir, B. S. (1999). Interpreting DNA mixtures in structured populations. *Journal of Forensic Sciences, 44*(5), 987–995.

Dawid, A. P., Mortera, J., & Pascali, V. L. (2001). Non-fatherhood or mutation? A probabilistic approach to parental exclusion in paternity testing. *Forensic Science International, 124*(1), 55–61. doi:10.1016/S0379-0738(01)00564-3

Diercks, A., Kostner, H., & Ozinsky, A. (2009). Resolving cell population heterogeneity: Real-time PCR for simultaneous multiplexed gene detection in multiple single-cell samples. *PLoS ONE, 4*(7), e6326. doi:10.1371/journal.pone.0006326

Dobbin, K., & Simon, R. (2002). Comparison of microarray designs for class comparison and class discovery. *Bioinformatics (Oxford, England), 18*(11), 1438–1445. doi:10.1093/bioinformatics/18.11.1438

Efron, B., Tibshirani, R., Storey, J. D., & Tusher, V. (2001). Empirical Bayes analysis of a microarray experiment. *Journal of the American Statistical Association, 96*, 1151–1160. doi:10.1198/016214501753382129

Egeland, T., Dalen, I., & Mostad, P. F. (2003). Estimating the number of contributors to a DNA profile. *International Journal of Legal Medicine, 117*(5), 271–275. doi:10.1007/s00414-003-0382-7

Elowitz, M. B., Levine, A. J., Siggia, E. D., & Swain, P. S. (2002). Stochastic gene expression in a single cell. *Science, 297*(5584), 1183–1186. doi:10.1126/science.1070919

Evett, I. W., Buffery, C., Willott, G., & Stoney, D. (1991). A guide to interpreting single locus profiles of DNA mixtures in forensic cases. *Journal - Forensic Science Society, 31*(1), 41–47. doi:10.1016/S0015-7368(91)73116-2

Evett, I. W., Gill, P. D., & Lambert, J. A. (1998). Taking account of peak areas when interpreting mixed DNA profiles. *Journal of Forensic Sciences, 43*(1), 62–69.

Finkelstein, D., Ewing, R., Gollub, J., Sterky, F., Cherry, J. M., & Somerville, S. (2002). Microarray data quality analysis: Lessons from the AFGC project. Arabidopsis Functional Genomics Consortium. *Plant Molecular Biology, 48*(1-2), 119–131. doi:10.1023/A:1013765922672

Foreman, L. A., Champod, I. W., Evett, J. A., Lambert, S., & Pope, S. (2003). Interpreting DNA evidence: A review. *International Statistical Review, 71*(3), 473–495. doi:10.1111/j.1751-5823.2003.tb00207.x

Fukshansky, N., & Bar, W. (1998). Interpreting forensic DNA evidence on the basis of hypotheses testing. *International Journal of Legal Medicine, 111*(2), 62–66. doi:10.1007/s004140050116

Fukshansky, N., & Bar, W. (2000). Biostatistics for mixed stains: The case of tested relatives of a non-tested suspect. *International Journal of Legal Medicine, 114*(1-2), 78–82. doi:10.1007/s004140000155

Fung, W. K., & Hu, Y. Q. (2000a). Interpreting forensic DNA mixtures: Allowing for uncertainty in population substructure and dependence. *Journal of the Royal Statistical Society. Series A (General), 163*, 241–254.

Fung, W. K., & Hu, Y. Q. (2000b). *Interpreting DNA mixtures based on the NRC-II recommendation 4.1.* Forensic Science Communications.

Fung, W. K., & Hu, Y. Q. (2001). The evaluation of mixed stains from different ethnic origins: General result and common cases. *International Journal of Legal Medicine, 115*(1), 48–53. doi:10.1007/s004140100205

Fung, W. K., & Hu, Y. Q. (2002a). Evaluating mixed stains with contributors of different ethnic groups under the NRC-II Recommendation 4.1. *Statistics in Medicine, 21*(23), 3583–3593. doi:10.1002/sim.1313

Fung, W. K., & Hu, Y. Q. (2002b). The statistical evaluation of DNA mixtures with contributors from different ethnic groups. *International Journal of Legal Medicine, 116*(2), 79–86. doi:10.1007/s004140100256

Ghosh, D. (2004). Mixture models for assessing differential expression in complex tissues using microarray data. *Bioinformatics (Oxford, England), 20*(11), 1663–1669. doi:10.1093/bioinformatics/bth139

Graves, D. J. (1999). Powerful tools for genetic analysis come of age. *Trends in Biotechnology, 17*(3), 127–134. doi:10.1016/S0167-7799(98)01241-4

Harbison, S. A., & Buckleton, J. S. (1998). Applications and extensions of subpopulation theory: A caseworkers guide. *Science & Justice, 38*(4), 249–254. doi:10.1016/S1355-0306(98)72119-7

Homer, N., Szelinger, S., Redman, M., Duggan, D., Tembe, W., & Muehling, J. (2008). Resolving individuals contributing trace amounts of DNA to highly complex mixtures using high-density SNP genotyping microarrays. *PLOS Genetics, 4*(8), e1000167. doi:10.1371/journal.pgen.1000167

Hu, Y. Q., & Fung, W. K. (2003). Interpreting DNA mixtures with the presence of relatives. *International Journal of Legal Medicine, 117*(1), 39–45.

Ibrahim, J. G., Chen, M.-H., & Gray, R. J. (2002). Bayesian models for gene expression with DNA microarray data. *Journal of the American Statistical Association, 97*, 88–99. doi:10.1198/016214502753479257

Irizarry, R. A., Bolstad, B. M., Collin, F., Cope, L. M., Hobbs, B., & Speed, T. P. (2003). Summaries of Affymetrix GeneChip probe level data. *Nucleic Acids Research, 31*(4), e15. doi:10.1093/nar/gng015

Irizarry, R. A., Hobbs, B., Collin, F., Beazer-Barclay, Y. D., Antonellis, K. J., & Scherf, U. (2003). Exploration, normalization, and summaries of high density oligonucleotide array probe level data. *Biostatistics (Oxford, England), 4*(2), 249–264. doi:10.1093/biostatistics/4.2.249

Irizarry, R. A., Ooi, S. L., Wu, Z., & Boeke, J. D. (2003). Use of mixture models in a microarray-based screening procedure for detecting differentially represented yeast mutants. *Statistical Applications in Genetics and Molecular Biology, 1*(1), 2.

Kerr, M. K., & Churchill, G. A. (2001). Experimental design for gene expression microarrays. *Biostatistics (Oxford, England), 2*(2), 183–201. doi:10.1093/biostatistics/2.2.183

Kulesh, D. A., Clive, D. R., Zarlenga, D. S., & Greene, J. J. (1987). Identification of interferon-modulated proliferation-related cDNA sequences. *Proceedings of the National Academy of Sciences of the United States of America, 84*(23), 8453–8457. doi:10.1073/pnas.84.23.8453

Lahdesmaki, H., Shmulevich, L., Dunmire, V., Yli-Harja, O., & Zhang, W. (2005). In silico microdissection of microarray data from heterogeneous cell populations. *BMC Bioinformatics, 6*, 54. doi:10.1186/1471-2105-6-54

Lalueza-Fox, C., Sampietro, M. L., Gilbert, M. T., Castri, L., Facchini, F., & Pettener, D. (2004). Unravelling migrations in the steppe: Mitochondrial DNA sequences from ancient central Asians. *Proceedings. Biological Sciences, 271*(1542), 941–947. doi:10.1098/rspb.2004.2698

Lambrou, G. I., Chatziioannou, A., Sifakis, E. G., Prentza, A., Koutsouris, D., Koultouki, E., et al. (2009). *Setting a rational framework for experimental design and analysis of high-throughput DNA microarray experiments and data.* Paper presented at the 9th International Workshop on Mathematical Methods in Scattering Theory and Biomedical Engineering, Patras, Greece.

Lauffenburger, D. A., Linderman, J., & Berkowitz, L. (1987). Analysis of mammalian cell growth factor receptor dynamics. *Annals of the New York Academy of Sciences, 506*, 147–162. doi:10.1111/j.1749-6632.1987.tb23816.x

Li, L., Li, C. T., Li, R. Y., Liu, Y., Lin, Y., & Que, T. Z. (2006). SNP genotyping by multiplex amplification and microarrays assay for forensic application. *Forensic Science International, 162*(1-3), 74–79. doi:10.1016/j.forsciint.2006.06.010

Li, Y., Carroll, D. S., Gardner, S. N., Walsh, M. C., Vitalis, E. A., & Damon, I. K. (2007). On the origin of smallpox: Correlating variola phylogenics with historical smallpox records. *Proceedings of the National Academy of Sciences of the United States of America, 104*(40), 15787–15792. doi:10.1073/pnas.0609268104

Linderman, J. J., & Lauffenburger, D. A. (1986). Analysis of intracellular receptor/ligand sorting. Calculation of mean surface and bulk diffusion times within a sphere. *Biophysical Journal, 50*(2), 295–305. doi:10.1016/S0006-3495(86)83463-4

Linderman, J. J., & Lauffenburger, D. A. (1988). Analysis of intracellular receptor/ligand sorting in endosomes. *Journal of Theoretical Biology, 132*(2), 203–245. doi:10.1016/S0022-5193(88)80157-7

Lockhart, D. J., Dong, H., Byrne, M. C., Follettie, M. T., Gallo, M. V., & Chee, M. S. (1996). Expression monitoring by hybridization to high-density oligonucleotide arrays. *Nature Biotechnology, 14*(13), 1675–1680. doi:10.1038/nbt1296-1675

Lu, P., Nakorchevskiy, A., & Marcotte, E. M. (2003). Expression deconvolution: A reinterpretation of DNA microarray data reveals dynamic changes in cell populations. *Proceedings of the National Academy of Sciences of the United States of America, 100*(18), 10370–10375. doi:10.1073/pnas.1832361100

Macgregor, S., Zhao, Z. Z., Henders, A., Nicholas, M. G., Montgomery, G. W., & Visscher, P. M. (2008). Highly cost-efficient genome-wide association studies using DNA pools and dense SNP arrays. *Nucleic Acids Research, 36*(6), e35. doi:10.1093/nar/gkm1060

McAdams, H. H., & Arkin, A. (1997). Stochastic mechanisms in gene expression. *Proceedings of the National Academy of Sciences of the United States of America, 94*(3), 814–819. doi:10.1073/pnas.94.3.814

Morse, S. A., & Budowle, B. (2006). Microbial forensics: Application to bioterrorism preparedness and response. *Infectious Disease Clinics of North America, 20*(2), 455–473. doi:10.1016/j.idc.2006.03.004

Mortera, J., Dawid, A. P., & Lauritzen, S. L. (2003). Probabilistic expert systems for DNA mixture profiling. *Theoretical Population Biology, 63*(3), 191–205. doi:10.1016/S0040-5809(03)00006-6

Naef, F., Hacker, C.R., Patil, N. & Magnasco, M. (2002). Characterization of the expression ratio noise structure in high-density oligonucleotide arrays. *Genome Biology, 3*(1), 01.

Naef, F., & Magnasco, M. O. (2003). Solving the riddle of the bright mismatches: Labeling and effective binding in oligonucleotide arrays. *Physical Review E: Statistical, Nonlinear, and Soft Matter Physics, 68*(1 Pt 1), 011906. doi:10.1103/PhysRevE.68.011906

Naef, F., Socci, N. D., & Magnasco, M. (2003). A study of accuracy and precision in oligonucleotide arrays: Extracting more signal at large concentrations. *Bioinformatics (Oxford, England)*, *19*(2), 178–184. doi:10.1093/bioinformatics/19.2.178

Najarian, K., Zaheri, M., Rad, A. A., Najarian, S., & Dargahi, J. (2004). A novel mixture model method for identification of differentially expressed genes from DNA microarray data. *BMC Bioinformatics*, *5*, 201. doi:10.1186/1471-2105-5-201

Newman, J. R., Ghaemmaghami, S., Ihmels, J., Breslow, D. K., Noble, M., & DeRisi, J. L. (2006). Single-cell proteomic analysis of S. cerevisiae reveals the architecture of biological noise. *Nature*, *441*(7095), 840–846. doi:10.1038/nature04785

Newton, M. A., Kendziorski, C. M., Richmond, C. S., Blattner, F. R., & Tsui, K. W. (2001). On differential variability of expression ratios: Improving statistical inference about gene expression changes from microarray data. *Journal of Computational Biology*, *8*(1), 37–52. doi:10.1089/106652701300099074

Ozbudak, E. M., Thattai, M., Kurtser, I., Grossman, A. D., & van Oudenaarden, A. (2002). Regulation of noise in the expression of a single gene. *Nature Genetics*, *31*(1), 69–73. doi:10.1038/ng869

Parmigiani, G., Garret, E. S., Andazhagan, R., & Gabrielson, E. (2002). A statistical framework for molecular-based classification in cancer. *Journal of the Royal Statistical Society. Series B. Methodological*, *64*, 717–736. doi:10.1111/1467-9868.00358

Pearson, J. V., Huentelman, M. J., Halperin, R. F., Tembe, W. D., Melquist, S., & Homer, N. (2007). Identification of the genetic basis for complex disorders by use of pooling-based genomewide single-nucleotide-polymorphism association studies. *American Journal of Human Genetics*, *80*(1), 126–139. doi:10.1086/510686

Quackenbush, J. (2001). Computational analysis of microarray data. *Nature Reviews. Genetics*, *2*(6), 418–427. doi:10.1038/35076576

Ramsey, S., Ozinsky, A., Clark, A., Smith, K. D., de Atauri, P., & Thorsson, V. (2006). Transcriptional noise and cellular heterogeneity in mammalian macrophages. *Philosophical Transactions of the Royal Society of London. Series B, Biological Sciences*, *361*(1467), 495–506. doi:10.1098/rstb.2005.1808

(1968). Reduction of dimensionality in biological diffusion processes. In Adam, G., & Delbruck, M. (Eds.), *Structural chemistry and molecular biology*. San Francisco: W.H. Freeman and Company.

Relogio, A., Schwager, C., Richter, A., Ansorge, W., & Valcarcel, J. (2002). Optimization of oligonucleotide-based DNA microarrays. *Nucleic Acids Research*, *30*(11), e51. doi:10.1093/nar/30.11.e51

Ritchie, M. E., Silver, J., Oshlack, A., Holmes, M., Diyagama, D., & Holloway, A. (2007). A comparison of background correction methods for two-colour microarrays. *Bioinformatics (Oxford, England)*, *23*(20), 2700–2707. doi:10.1093/bioinformatics/btm412

Sakurada, K., Ikegaya, H., Fukushima, H., Akutsu, T., Watanabe, K., & Yoshino, M. (2009). Evaluation of mRNA-based approach for identification of saliva and semen. *Legal Medicine*, *11*(3), 125–128. doi:10.1016/j.legalmed.2008.10.002

Salama, N. R., Gonzalez-Valencia, G., Deatherage, B., Aviles-Jimenez, F., Atherton, J. C., & Graham, D. Y. (2007). Genetic analysis of Helicobacter pylori strain populations colonizing the stomach at different times post-infection. *Journal of Bacteriology*, *189*(10), 3834–3845. doi:10.1128/JB.01696-06

Schena, M., Shalon, D., Davis, R. W., & Brown, P. O. (1995). Quantitative monitoring of gene expression patterns with a complementary DNA microarray. *Science, 270*(5235), 467–470. doi:10.1126/science.270.5235.467

Schutzer, S. E., Budowle, B., & Atlas, R. M. (2005). Biocrimes, microbial forensics, and the physician. *PLoS Medicine, 2*(12), e337. doi:10.1371/journal.pmed.0020337

Simon, R., Mirlacher, M., & Sauter, G. (2004). Tissue microarrays. *Methods in Molecular Medicine, 97*, 377–389.

Southern, E. M. (1975). Detection of specific sequences among DNA fragments separated by gel electrophoresis. *Journal of Molecular Biology, 98*(3), 503–517. doi:10.1016/S0022-2836(75)80083-0

Southern, E. M. (1992). Detection of specific sequences among DNA fragments separated by gel electrophoresis. *Biotechnology, 24*, 122–139.

Staal, F. J., van der Burg, M., Wessels, L. F., Barendregt, B. H., Baert, M. R., & van den Burg, C. M. (2003). DNA microarrays for comparison of gene expression profiles between diagnosis and relapse in precursor-B acute lymphoblastic leukemia: Choice of technique and purification influence the identification of potential diagnostic markers. *Leukemia, 17*(7), 1324–1332. doi:10.1038/sj.leu.2402974

Townsend, J. P. (2003). Multifactorial experimental design and the transitivity of ratios with spotted DNA microarrays. *BMC Genomics, 4*(1), 41. doi:10.1186/1471-2164-4-41

Van Gelder, R. N., von Zastrow, M. E., Yool, A., Dement, W. C., Barchas, J. D., & Eberwine, J. H. (1990). Amplified RNA synthesized from limited quantities of heterogeneous cDNA. *Proceedings of the National Academy of Sciences of the United States of America, 87*(5), 1663–1667. doi:10.1073/pnas.87.5.1663

Venet, D., Pecasse, F., Maenhaut, C., & Bersini, H. (2001). Separation of samples into their constituents using gene expression data. *Bioinformatics (Oxford, England), 17*(1), S279–S287.

Vilar, J. M., Guet, C. C., & Leibler, S. (2003). Modeling network dynamics: The lac operon, a case study. *The Journal of Cell Biology, 161*(3), 471–476. doi:10.1083/jcb.200301125

Vinciotti, V., Khanin, R., D'Alimonte, D., Liu, X., Cattini, N., & Hotchkiss, G. (2005). An experimental evaluation of a loop versus a reference design for two-channel microarrays. *Bioinformatics (Oxford, England), 21*(4), 492–501. doi:10.1093/bioinformatics/bti022

Wang, D., Gou, S. Y., & Axelrod, D. (1992). Reaction rate enhancement by surface diffusion of adsorbates. *Biophysical Chemistry, 43*(2), 117–137. doi:10.1016/0301-4622(92)80027-3

Wang, T., Xue, N., & Birdwell, J. D. (2006). Least-square deconvolution: A framework for interpreting short tandem repeat mixtures. *Journal of Forensic Sciences, 51*(6), 1284–1297. doi:10.1111/j.1556-4029.2006.00268.x

Watson, C. L., & Lockwood, D. N. (2009). Single nucleotide polymorphism analysis of European archaeological M. leprae DNA. *PLoS ONE, 4*(10), e7547. doi:10.1371/journal.pone.0007547

Weir, B. S. (1995). DNA statistics in the Simpson matter. *Nature Genetics, 11*(4), 365–368. doi:10.1038/ng1295-365

Weir, B. S., Triggs, C. M., Starling, L., Stowell, L. I., Walsh, K. A., & Buckleton, J. (1997). Interpreting DNA mixtures. *Journal of Forensic Sciences, 42*(2), 213–222.

Woo, Y., Krueger, W., Kaur, A., & Churchill, G. (2005). Experimental design for three-color and four-color gene expression microarrays. *Bioinformatics (Oxford, England), 21*(1), i459–i467. doi:10.1093/bioinformatics/bti1031

Yang, Y. H., & Speed, T. (2002). Design issues for cDNA microarray experiments. *Nature Reviews. Genetics*, *3*(8), 579–588.

Zehner, R., Amendt, J., & Boehme, P. (2009). Gene expression analysis as a tool for age estimation of blowfly pupae. *Forensic Science International. Genetics Supplement Series*, *2*(1), 292–293. doi:10.1016/j.fsigss.2009.08.008

Zhang, L., Foxman, B., Drake, D. R., Srinivasan, U., Henderson, J., & Olson, B. (2009). Comparative whole-genome analysis of Streptococcus mutans isolates within and among individuals of different caries status. *Oral Microbiology and Immunology*, *24*(3), 197–203. doi:10.1111/j.1399-302X.2008.00495.x

Zhang, Y., Hammer, D. A., & Graves, D. J. (2005). Competitive hybridization kinetics reveals unexpected behavior patterns. *Biophysical Journal*, *89*(5), 2950–2959. doi:10.1529/biophysj.104.058552

KEY TERMS AND DEFINITIONS

Antisense Amplified RNA (aaRNA or Complementary RNA (cRNA): The RNA molecule that is produced from an *in vitro* transcription reaction. It was first described by *Van Gelder et al.* in 1990 (Van Gelder, et al., 1990). This methodology is based on the linear amplification of dsDNA transcribed to cRNA with use of the *T4 DNA Polymerase, T3 RNA Polymerase* and *T7 RNA Polymerase*. It is a very successful technique since it can amplify 20ng to 2ug of total RNA yielding an approximately 5000-fold amplification. This means that samples of 200ng could yield 40ug of cRNA or samples of 2ug of total RNA could yield up to 100ug of *cRNA* (complementary RNA) is also called *aaRNA* (*anti-sense amplified RNA*).

Average Difference (AD): This was first approach, implemented in *MAS* 4.0 from Affymetrix, which uses an empirical algorithm to estimate the hybridization intensity. It is based on the following formula:

$$AD = \frac{1}{n}\sum(PM_i - MM_i) \qquad (63)$$

where n is the total number of probe pairs for a probes set/gene, and PM_i and MM_i indicate the perfect and mismatch probe intensities after background correction (BC) for the ith probe pair for the probe set/gene. The above algorithm has frequently produced negative values of expression (AD) in the past. Point clouds are collections of 3D points.

Avogadro Number or Avogadro's Constant: The Avogadro's Number or Avogadro constant (symbols: L, N_A) is the number of "*elementary entities*" (usually atoms or molecules) in one mole, that is (from the definition of the mole). It is equal to

$$N_A = 6.02214179 \cdot 10^{23}\, elements \cdot mol^{-1}, \qquad (64)$$

cDNA: Also known as complementary DNA. It is the product of *in vivo* or *in vitro* reactions where RNA is reverse transcribed to DNA (cDNA). Usually, the parts of the RNA that are reversly transcribed are the exons or the protein-coding gene segments

Central Limit Theorem: The central limit theorem states conditions under which the mean of a sufficiently large number of independent random variables, each with finite mean and variance, will be approximately normally distributed. The central limit theorem also requires the random variables to be identically distributed, unless certain conditions are met. It also justifies the approximation of large-sample statistics to the normal distribution in controlled experiments.

Comparative Genomic Hybridization (CGH): Comparative genomic hybridization (CGH or Chromosomal Microarray Analysis (CMA) is a high throughput method for the analysis of copy number changes (gains/losses) in the DNA content of a given subject's DNA and often in tumor cells. CGH will detect only unbalanced chromosomal changes. Structural chromosome aberrations such as balanced reciprocal translocations or inversions can not be detected, as they do not change the copy number.

CHIP-chip (CHIP-on-chip) Microarrays: ChIP-chip (also known as ChIP-on-chip) is a high throughput technique that combines chromatin immunoprecipitation (*ChIP*) with microarray technology (*chip*). ChIP-on-chip is used to investigate interactions between proteins and DNA *in vivo*. Whole-genome analysis can be performed to determine the locations of binding sites for almost any protein of interest

Clustering: Clustering or Cluster analysis is the assignment of a set of observations into subsets (called *clusters*) so that observations in the same cluster are similar in some sense. Clustering is a method of unsupervised learning, and a common technique for statistical data. It is usually applied through the similarity measuremt of data. Methods for clustering, among others, include: *uncentered Pearson correlation coefficient, squared correlation coefficient, averaged dot product, cosine correlation coefficient, covariance, Euclidian distance, Manhattan distance, mutual formation, Spearman Rank-Order correlation* and *Kendall's Tau.*

Cy3 and Cy5 (Cyanines): Cyanine is a non-systematic name of a synthetic dye family belonging to polymethine group. Cyanines have many uses as fluorescent dyes, particularly in biomedical imaging. Depending on the structure, they cover the spectrum from IR to UV. Cyanines were first synthesized over a century ago, and there are a large number reported in the literature.

Deconvolution: Briefly, the *deconvolution* method is concerned with finding the solution of the convolution equation defined as: $f * g = h$, In text Equation 60 where, h is a recorded signal, f is the signal to be recovered but has been con-

volved by another signal g. In general real measurements are of the form: $(f * g) + \varepsilon = h$, In text Equation 61 where ε is the *noise* that enters the recorded signal.

Dendrogram: It is the a tree-like diagram or graph used to represent the arrangement of clusters, which are usually produced by hierarchical clustering.

Euclidian Distance: In general the Euclidian distance or Euclidian metric is the distance between two points and it is derived from the Pythagorian Theorem ($\alpha^2 = \beta^2 + \gamma^2$). Hence, the distance d between two points a and b with coordinates a($x_1, x_2, ..., x_n$) and b($y_1, y_2, ..., y_n$) is given by:

$$d(a,b) = \sqrt{(x_1 - y_1) + (x_2 - y_2) + ... + (x_n - y_n)} = \sqrt{\sum_{i=1}^{n}(x_i - y_i)^2}$$

(65)

Exons: Exons are nucleic acid sequences appearing in the RNA molecule after selective splicing. In many genes each exon contains a part from Open Reading Frames (ORFs), which code for the specific region of a protein.

Expression Deconvolution: *Expression deconvolution*, is a term proposed by *Lu et al. (2003)*, which includes a deconvolution approach, in order to resolve cell population dynamics. The basic idea is that gene expression from growing populations, and at this point we could include complex populations, is a mixture of mRNAs with different patterns of expression, depending on the cell cycle distribution of the cell population.

Fluorochromes: Fluorochrome or also known as fluorophore, in analogy to the chromophore, is the part of a molecule that attributes fluorescence to it. That is the emission of light after it has been stimulated by an energy source usually an electromagnetic wave.

γ (gamma) Distribution: Is a two parameter continuous probability distribution function. A random variable X is considered to have a gamma distribution with scale θ and shape k when:

$$X \sim \Gamma(k, \theta) \text{ or } X \sim Gamma(k, \theta), \qquad (66)$$

and with a probability density function:

$$f(x; k; \theta) = x^{k-1} \frac{e^{-\frac{x}{\theta}}}{\theta^k \Gamma(k)}, \text{ for } x > 0 \text{ and } k, \theta > 0, \qquad (67)$$

Gaussian: The term Gaussian refers to Gauss distribution, Gaussian error, Gaussian analysis and Gaussian networks. The Gauss distribution is also known as the normal distribution that cluster data around the mean. The Gauss error function (also called the error function) is a function of sigmoid shape which occurs in probability, statistics, materials science, and partial differential equations. It is defined as:

$$e(x) = \frac{2}{\sqrt{\pi}} \int_0^x \left[e^{-t^2} \right] dt, \qquad (68)$$

The Gaussian network model (GNM) is a representation of a biological macromolecule as an elastic mass-and-spring network to study, understand, and characterize mechanical aspects of its long-scale dynamics.

Gauss-Markov Model: In statistics, the Gauss–Markov theorem, states that in a linear model in which the errors have expectation zero, are uncorrelated and have equal variances, a best linear unbiased estimator of the coefficients is given by the ordinary least squares estimator. The errors are not assumed to be normally distributed, nor are they assumed to be independent (but only uncorrelated — a weaker condition), nor are they assumed to be identically distributed (but only having zero mean and equal variances) (source: www.wikipedia.org).

Hardy-Weinberg Theorem: The Hardy–Weinberg Theorem (also known as: Hardy-Weinberg principle HWP, Hardy–Weinberg equilibrium, Hardy–Weinberg, HWE, or Hardy–Weinberg law) states that both allele and genotype frequencies in a population remain constant. That is, they are in equilibrium, from generation to generation, unless specific disturbing influences are introduced. Those influences include non-random mating, mutations, selection, limited population size, "overlapping generations", random genetic drift and gene flow.

Hybridization: It is the process through which two complementary sequences, usually nucleic acids, attach to form a dimmer. It finds applications in many methodologies such as: Southern and Northern Blottings, all sorts od microarrays in-situ hybridization and others.

Kendall's Tau: Kendall rank correlation coefficient, more commonly referred to as Kendall's tau (τ) coefficient or a tau test, is a non-parametric statistic used to measure the association or statistical dependence between two measured quantities. It is defined as:

$$\tau_A = \frac{n_c - n_d}{\frac{1}{2} n(n-1)}, \qquad (69)$$

k-means Clustering: k-means is a method of cluster analysis, which partitions n observations into k clusters, in which each observation belongs to the cluster with the nearest mean. Given a set of observations $(x_1, x_2, ..., x_n)$, where each observation is a d-dimensional real vector, then k-means clustering aims to partition the n observations into k sets $(k < n)$ $S = \{S_1, S_2, ..., S_k\}$ so as to minimize the within-cluster sum of squares.

Likelihood Ratio: Suppose that the mixed sample taken from a crime scene and some persons, e.g. the victim and the suspect, are tested with the aim of identifying the true perpetrator(s). The likelihood ratio, would be:

$$LR = \frac{P(Evidence|H_p)}{P(Evidence|H_d)}, \qquad (70)$$

which is usually used to evaluate the weight of the evidence, regarding whether the suspect has contributed to the mixed sample, where H_p and H_d are the prosecution and defense positions, and the evidence is the genetic information obtained from the mixed sample and the investigated person(s).

M-A Plots: M-A plots are used for the comparison of data from one sample against another. This is the case for two channel DNA microarrays where both samples are hybridised on the same chip or with single channel arrays where each sample is hybridized on pairs of chips. M is, the intensity ratio and A is the average intensity for a dot in the plot. M-A plots are then used to visualize intensity-dependent ratio of raw microarray data. The M-A plot uses M as the y-axis and A as the x-axis. The M-A plot gives a quick overview of the data. The majority of the points on the y axis (M) would be located at 0, since $log_2(1)$ is 0. M and A are given by:

$$\begin{aligned} M &= \log_2 R - \log_2 G \\ A &= \frac{1}{2} \cdot (\log_2 R + \log_2 G) \end{aligned}, \qquad (71)$$

where, R and G are the intensities of the fluorescent dyes measured during an experiment.

Mismatch and Perfect Match: These terms have been utilized by Affymetrix microarray chips and methodology for data analysis. In particular, a probe pair consists of a 25-mer oligonucleotide perfectly complementary to the sequence of a gene (*Perfect Match PM* and a 25-mer oligonucleotide that differs from the perfect match probe by a single mismatched nucleotide at the central position (13th position; *Mismatch: MM).* This combination of a 25-mer pair, *PM* and *MM*, offers the highest sensitivity and specificity, while it solves, in part, co-hybridization problems. The difference between, *PM* intensities minus *MM*

intensities averaged across the probe pairs gives an estimation of the hybridization intensity. The intensities measured using *Affymetrix* arrays are considered to be the absolute expression levels: the less efficient hybridization of the *MM* probe to the target, allows the PM intensity minus the MM intensity of the probe to offer a better estimation of intensity. Background correction (*BC*) on the intensities is done automatically (GeneChipTM software) using a regionalized method, i.e. dividing the array in several rectangular zones.cDNA

Normalization: It is the process of removing statistical bias from measured data. It is applies to many forms of data and in many disciplines. Within this context it mainly refers to microarray data normalization. Since it is known that microarray data entail a lot of bias, methods have been developed in order to remove systematic errors. Such methods include, Global Median division, Lowess, Loess, Robust Lowess, Rank Invariant and others.

Polymorphism: It is described as the variation in the phenotypes of living organisms. In molecular biology and genetics it is used mainly with the term Single Nucleotide Polymorphism. This refers to the change in one nucleotide in the genome between two individuals resulting frequently in two different phenotypes. The existence of polymorphisms is an evolutionary process leading to adaptation and genetic variation.

Real-Time PCR: This is a variation of the Polymerase Chain Reaction, which uses fluorescent dyes in order to measure amplification and it does so in real time. In the classic technique a researcher had to wait for the reactions to end and then to visualize the amplified nucleic acids. In contrast, Real-Time PCR does amplification and visualization simultaneously.

Self Organizing Maps (SOMs): A self-organizing map (SOM) or self-organizing feature map (SOFM) is a type of artificial neural network that is trained using unsupervised learning to produce a low-dimensional (typically two-dimensional), discretized representation of the input space of the training samples, called a map. Self-organizing maps are different from other artificial neural networks in the sense that they use a neighborhood function to preserve the topological properties of the input space. This makes SOM useful for visualizing low-dimensional views of high-dimensional data, akin to multidimensional scaling. The model was first described as an artificial neural network by the Finnish professor Teuvo Kohonen, and is sometimes called a Kohonen map. Like most artificial neural networks, SOMs operate in two modes: training and mapping. Training builds the map using input examples. It is a competitive process, also called vector quantization. Mapping automatically classifies a new input vector. A self-organizing map consists of components called nodes or neurons. Associated with each node is a weight vector of the same dimension as the input data vectors and a position in the map space. The usual arrangement of nodes is a regular spacing in a hexagonal or rectangular grid. The self-organizing map describes a mapping from a higher dimensional input space to a lower dimensional map space. The procedure for placing a vector from data space onto the map is to find the node with the closest weight vector to the vector taken from data space and to assign the map coordinates of this node to our vector (source: www.wikipedia.org).

Single Nucleotide Polymorphism (SNP): See *Polymorphism(s)*.

Spearman Rank-Order Correlation: Spearman's rank correlation coefficient or Spearman's rho, denoted by the Greek letter ρ (rho) or as r_s, is a non-parametric measure of statistical dependence between two variables. It assesses how the relationship between two variables can be described using a monotonic function. If there are no repeated data values, a perfect Spearman correlation of $+1$ or -1 occurs when each of the variables is a perfect monotone function of the other. The n raw scores X_i, Y_i are converted to ranks x_i, y_i, and the differences $d_i = x_i - y_i$ between the ranks of each observation on the two variables

are calculated. If there are no tied ranks, then ρ is given by:

$$\rho = 1 - \frac{6\sum d_i^2}{n(n^2 - 1)}, \tag{72}$$

If tied ranks exist, Pearson's correlation coefficient between ranks should be used for the calculation:

$$r = \frac{\sum_{i=1}^{n}(\mathbf{x} - \bar{\mathbf{x}})(\mathbf{y}_i - \bar{\mathbf{y}})}{\sqrt{\sum_{i=1}^{n}(\mathbf{x}_i - \bar{\mathbf{x}})^2}\sqrt{\sum_{i=1}^{n}(\mathbf{y}_i - \bar{\mathbf{y}})^2}}, \tag{73}$$

Support Vector Machines (SVMs): Support vector machines (SVMs) are a set of related supervised learning methods used for classification and regression. Given a set of training examples, each marked as belonging to one of two categories, an SVM training algorithm builds a model that predicts whether a new example falls into one category or the other. A SVM model is a representation of the examples as points in space, mapped so that the examples of the separate categories are divided by a clear gap that is as wide as possible. New examples are then mapped into that same space and predicted to belong to a category based on which side of the gap they fall on. More formally, a support vector machine constructs a hyperplane or set of hyperplanes in a high or infinite dimensional space, which can be used for classification, regression or other tasks. Intuitively, a good separation is achieved by the hyperplane that has the largest distance to the nearest training datapoints of any class (so-called functional margin), since in general the larger the margin the lower the generalization error of the classifier (source: www.wikipedia.org).

T-test: A *t*-test is a statistical hypothesis test in which the test statistic follows a Student's *t* distribution if the null hypothesis is true. It is most commonly applied when the test statistic would follow a normal distribution. When the scaling term is unknown and is replaced by an estimate based on the data, the test statistic (under certain conditions) follows a Student's *t* distribution. Various forms of the *t*-test can be discriminated.

Independent one-sample t-test:

$$t = \frac{\overline{x} - \mu_0}{s/\sqrt{n}}, \tag{74}$$

Independent two-sample t-test, equal sample sizes, equal variance:

$$t = \frac{\overline{X_1} - \overline{X_2}}{S_{X_1 X_2} \cdot \sqrt{\frac{2}{n}}}, \tag{75}$$

Unequal sample sizes, equal variance:

$$t = \frac{\overline{X_1} - \overline{X_2}}{S_{X_1 X_2} \cdot \sqrt{\frac{1}{n_1} + \frac{1}{n_2}}}, \tag{76}$$

Unequal sample sizes, unequal variance:

$$t = \frac{\overline{X_1} - \overline{X_2}}{S_{\overline{X_1 - X_2}}}, \tag{77}$$

Dependent t-test for paired samples:

$$t = \frac{\overline{X_D} - \mu_0}{S_D/\sqrt{n}}, \tag{78}$$

APPENDIX

*Figure 10. Chemical Structure 1. The 2D structures of Cy3 (Cyanines) and Cy5 (Carbocyanines) (**A**) and the emission spectra of the two dyes (**B**). Cy3 PUBCHEM ID: CID 44154182, IUPAC: (2Z)-1-[6-(2,5-dioxopyrrolidin-1-yl)oxyhexyl]-2-[(E)-3-[1-[6-(2,5-dioxopyrrolidin-1-yl)oxyhexyl]-3,3-dimethyl-5-sulfoindol-1-ium-2-yl]prop-2-enylidene]-3,3-dimethylindole-5-sulfonate. MW:* **883.038460 g/mol.** *MF: $C_{43}H_{54}N_4O_{12}S_2$. Cy5 PubChem ID: NA, IUPAC NA, MW NA..(Source www.wikipedia.org)*

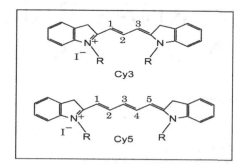 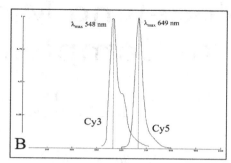

*Figure 11. Chemical Structure 2. The 2D structure of Phycoeryrthrin (**A**) and emission spectra (**B**)*

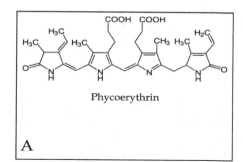 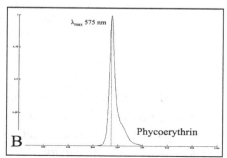

*Figure 12. Chemical Structure 3. The 2D structure of Alexa Fluor 488 (**A**) and emission spectra (**B**)*

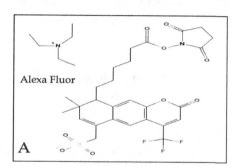 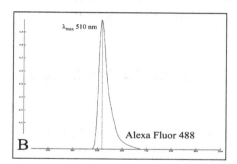

Chapter 8
Predictive Dynamical Modelling MicroRNAs Role in Complex Networks[1]

Elena V. Nikolova
Bulgarian Academy of Sciences, Bulgaria

Ralf Herwig
Max Planck Institute for Molecular Genetics, Germany

Svetoslav G. Nikolov
Bulgarian Academy of Sciences, Bulgaria

Valko G. Petrov
Bulgarian Academy of Sciences, Bulgaria

ABSTRACT

The aim of this chapter is to give an extended analytical consideration of mathematical modelling of the microRNA role in cancer networks. For this purpose, ordinary and partial differential equations are used for synthesizing and analyzing the models of gene, microRNAs and mRNAs concentration alterations as time-dependent variables related by functional and differential relations. The architecture of the models and the definitions of their components are inspired by the qualitative theory of differential equations. This chapter's analysis shows that it is able to ensure the authenticity and validity of the following qualitative conclusions: (a) the rates of protein production decrease with the increasing constant production rate of microRNA at microRNA-mediated target regulation on mRNAs; (b) time delay has a stabilizing role in the interaction between the miRNA-17-92 cluster and the transcription factors E2F and Myc.

INTRODUCTION TO THE SPECIFIED SCOPE

Dynamical modelling is an efficient *predictive* tool in the theory of microRNAs (cited as miRNAs to the end of this chapter) regulation of cancer networks. In this analytical review we widely use ordinary and partial differential equations for synthesis and analysis of gene, miRNAs and mRNA concentrations as time-dependent variables related by functional and differential relations between

DOI: 10.4018/978-1-60960-483-7.ch008

them. When we write differential equations, the main assumption is that concentrations of different substances are spatially homogeneous and vary continuously, which is not rigorously true for gene regulatory networks in principle and especially for cancer ones. Moreover, the deterministic behaviour of dynamical systems of differential equations is also not always exactly valid for the cases considered here. However, we often restrict our modelling to *qualitative* synthesis and analysis in terms of such named qualitative theory of dynamical systems, which notions and terms are very similar to those of molecular biology, so the *predictive* power of the models conserve their validity. In addition the method of differential equations allows very detailed description of the dynamical regulatory behaviour directly from the corresponding experimental biochemical diagrams containing full information about the network (or its module), which is difficult to obtain by another methods.

A principal problem toward complete understanding of miRNAs functions is to identify the target genes regulated by individual miRNAs. Most of them do not pair with perfect complementarity to their targets such that bioinformatical prediction is difficult and experimental validation is required. As a first movement toward target identification, global miRNA expression patterns are necessary to be reviewed, what is a main subject of our work in this specified scope.

Our goals are: (i) Considering the present insights into the miRNAs regulated functional modules of human cancers; (ii) Determining some computational approaches for modelling miRNAs role in cancerogenesis; (iii) Analysing the analogy (possibly inverse) between miRNAs roles in cancerogenesis and somitogenesis.

It is well-known that miRNA regulation is involved in many important biological processes such as cell proliferation, apoptosis and metabolism, the dysfunction of which state important hallmarks for human cancers. By considering connections of the miRNAs to target networks on different layers such as signalling, protein-protein interaction, metabolism and gene regulatory networks, we will be able to have some understanding how to identify and model the link between miRNA expression and cancer relevant read-outs on the molecular and cellular level.

At present, it is well established that gene expression in the human organism is post-transcriptionally regulated by miRNAs. MiRNAs are a class of small noncoding RNAs, typically ≈22nt size, that function is to modulate the activity of specific mRNA targets (Aguda et al., 2008). They are estimated to comprise 1-5% of animal genes (Khanin & Vinciotti, 2008), making them one of the most abundant classes of regulators. Their widespread and important role in animals is highlighted by recent estimates that up to approximately one-third of an organism's protein-coding genes are subject to miRNA-mediated control (Krek et al., 2005; Lewis et al., 2005; Stark et al., 2005). Current target-prediction computer programs (Watanabe et al., 2007; Maziere & Enright, 2007) predict that miRNAs play a central role in many biological (cellular) processes, including developmental timing, cell proliferation, apoptosis, metabolism, cell differentiation, somitogenesis and tumorgenesis (Alvarez-Garcia & Miska, 2006; Ambros, 2004; Gusev, 2008). In addition, miRNAs are a related class of short RNA molecules with an analogous functional role in Ribo Nucleic Acid interference (RNAi) (Bartel, 2004; Piriyapongsa & King Jordan, 2008). RNAi was elucidated for *Caenorhabditis elegans* (Fire et al., 1998) and according to (Plasterk, 2002; Waterhouse et al., 2001) each cell has a miniature "immune system" able to generate and amplify specific responses to a variety of gene transcripts. In other words, by RNAi, we can stop or significantly reduce the production of the specific protein encoded by the target gene.

It is seen from the literature, data sets are processed, normalised and statistically evaluated in order to identify defined, manually and pre-processed expression patterns for each available miRNA. These expression patterns can be correlated with gene expression patterns and sequence information in order to identify potential target sets of the miRNAs. An essential approach to the problem is such named statistical meta-analysis. It is based on a statistical Bootstrap approach and has been previously applied to the analysis of marker genes for type-2 diabetes mellitus. Meta-analysis includes quantitative data such as expression data as well as qualitative data such as reviews and publications. In each experiment (for example a case-control study) every miRNA will get a score that measures its disease relationship.

We hope that integrating miRNA and target expression data at specific stages of development will help to refine lists of possible targets for specific miRNAs. For example, it is of interest to design a sensitive microarray to expand expression analysis. Such an array can be utilized o study differences in miRNA expression during normal zebrafish development as well as in embryos treated with DAPT and cyclopamine and pharmacologic inhibitors of the Notch and Hedgehog signalling pathways.

RECENT STUDIES ON ANALYSING MODULES OF CANCER NETWORKS

MiRNAs have been implicated in various cancers, acting either as oncogenes or tumor suppressor genes. Biogenesis of miRNAs is likely to be regulated at both transcription and processing steps. MiRNAs are synthesized by RNA polymerase II (Lee et al., 2004, Cai et al, 2004), which also transcribes most mRNAs and is known to be highly regulated. Thus, it is conceivable that the transcription of miRNAs is regulated through mechanisms similar to those that have been elucidated for protein-coding genes. Regulation at the processing steps would provide a way to generate miRNA expression patterns distinct from those of the host genes (Faller et al, 2007). In (Mitchell et al, 2008), the authors hypothesized

that miRNAs could be an ideal class of blood-based biomarkers for cancer detection because: (i) miRNA expression is frequently dysregulated in cancer (Esquela-Kerscher & Clack, 2006); (ii) expression patterns of miRNAs in human cancer appear to be tissue-specific (Calin & Croce, 2006); and (iii) miRNAs have unusually high stability in formalin-fixed tissues (Xi et al., 2007).

Conceivably, regulation of miRNA biogenesis may occur at the level of Drosha processing, nuclear transport, or Dicer processing. In several studies have shown that miRNAs are present at the level of precursor but are not processed to the mature miRNA. The mature miRNA was detectable only in the normal colorectal tissue (Lee et al., 2008). By using published messenger RNA data to approximate the miRNA precursor expression encoded within introns, Thomson et al. (2006) widespread down-regulation of miRNA in cancer. This may due to the fact that the majority of miRNA studies have focused on quantifying the active mature miRNA and not the miRNA precursors. The first real-time RT PCR method (Thomson et al., 2006) to quantify miRNA was developed by the Schmittgen laboratory in 2004 (Schmittgen et al., 2004). This method quantified the miRNA precursors with the goal of predicting the expression of mature miRNA. By designing primers to the stem of the miRNA hairpin, the primary precursor and precursor miRNA were simultaneously quantified. Thus, this technology has been applied to profile the expression of over 200 miRNA precursors in a number of human cancer cell lines (Jiang et al., 2006). From the experimental results demonstrated in (Lee et al., 2008) it follows that unknown control processing mechanisms play a critical role in regulating the expression of the active mature miRNA.

Another unresolved issue is the mechanism by which miRNAs repress protein synthesis (Petersen et al., 2006). Recent experiments using in vitro translation systems have indicated that miRNAs can repress translation, at least in part, by inhibiting translation initiation (Nissan & Parker, 2008) although in some cases deadenylation of the mRNA might contribute to the observed repression (Wakiyama et al., 2007). For now, previous analysis revealed that mammalian miRNAs tend to cluster on chromosomes. However, the functional consequences of this clustering and conserved property remain unclear (Xu & Wong, 2008). For example, in (Dewis et al., 2006) the authors reported the first evidence of a cluster of miRNAs that could regulate functionality related proteins in cancer. They found that in *Myc* over expressing tumors, two anti-angiogenesis genes *Tsp1* and *Ctgf* are downregulated by one *Myc* activated miRNA cluster *miR-17-miR-92*. Noticeably, they confirmed that within the cluster, *miR-19* primarily responsible for *Tsp1* downregulation and *miR-18* for *Ctgf* downregulation in response to *Myc* activation.

The mechanism by which microRNAs regulate gene expression is post-transcriptional, possibly influencing the stability, compartmentalization and translation of mRNAs (Carthew, 2006). Most computational efforts to understand the post-transcriptional gene regulation by miRNAs have been focused on target prediction tools, as reviewed by Rajewsky (2006), while quantitative kinetic modeling of gene regulation by microRNAs has still had a pioneer character. There are only some ODE-based models of gene regulation by miRNAs to this end. (Aguda et al., 2008; Khanin &Vinciotti, 2008; Levine et al., 2007; Khanin & Higham, 2007; Xie et al., 2007; Nandi et al., 2009; Nissan & Parker, 2009). Generally speaking, the advantages of mathematical modeling are as follows: (i) the development of mathematical models leads to a decrease in the number of experiments using expensive biological material, and makes it possible to predict the results of many experiments with great precision; (ii) the use of dynamical systems theory leads to the creation of base models of complex biological processes such as gene regulation (transcription), gene expression, protein synthesis, interaction between various molecules, etc., and allows the

investigation of new mechanisms of miRNAs in qualitative ways; and (iii) the results of the modeling can be presented visually and used by biologists, biochemists, and immunologists in clinical practice and cancer therapy.

Max-Plank Institute for Molecular Genetics MPIMG has developed the ConsensusPathDB database (CPDB, http://cpdb.molgen.mpg.de/) that allows the storage and integration of information on biochemical reaction pathways, protein-protein interactions, signal transduction pathways and gene regulatory networks. CPDB is so far the only resource of integrated data that comes from different sources and in different formats. In addition, CPDB has a user-friendly web interface that offers many different ways of making use of the data. In the framework of CPDB, MiRNAs and the proteins derived from their associated RNAs can be integrated in the database and linked to the relevant reactions (Figure 1).

ON THE ROLE OF MICRORNAS IN SOMITOGENESIS

Somite Cell Polarization and the Role of Cell Polarity in Cancerogenesis

The somitogenesis correlates with the cycles of gene expression, which propagates from the embryon tail bud to the rostral end of PSM. Moreover the periods of gene oscillations and somite formations are equal. This fact is confirmed from many publications (Palmeirim et al., 1997; Aulehla & Pourquie, 2006). However it is not clear yet what is the mechanism (probably both biochemical and biomechanical) by which the temporal gene oscillations are transformed into spatial patterns (called somite segments or somites). The experimental investigations show that miRNAs can regulate gene expression by stimulating degradation of mRNA in some cases and /or repression in others. The somitogenesis presents a successive formation of pairs of somites from presomitic mesoderm

Figure 1. Integrated information on the protein expression of MYC and E2F1 involving the expression of two miRNAs annotated from literature. Display is created with the ConsensusPathDB web interface

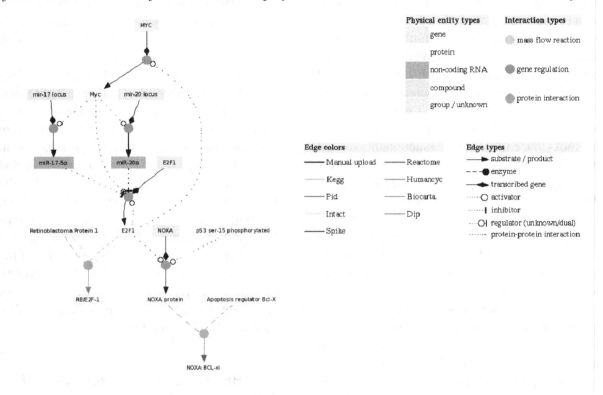

(PSM) at fixed time intervals. The formation is a periodic process controlled by a biological clock or an intracellular oscillator. It is established in several works that the periodicity of somitogenesis coincides with the periodic changes in the expression of certain genes in the cells of PSM (Hirata et al., 2002; Bessho et al., 2001). For example, in mouse embryos, the expression of the *Hes7* gene in the PSM oscillates with a cycle period of 2h, which is approximately equal to the formation time of a pair somites (Hirata et al., 2002; Bessho et al., 2001; Bessho et al., 2003).

In the PSM of zebrafish, the genes *Her1* and *Her7* exhibit periodic expression with a much shorter period of 30 min, which is also coincides with the formation time of a pair somites (Lewis, 2003). These genes are important components of the Notch signaling pathway (Lewis, 2003; Monk, 2003) and code for transcription factors. Some

authors consider the cycle expressions of *Hes7, Her1* and *Her7* is conditioned by delayed negative feedback loop in which the proteins repress the expression of their own genes by binding to their respective regulatory regions (Lewis, 2003; Monk, 2003). Recent mathematical models, built on experimental results (Lewis, 2003; Monk, 2003; Hirata, 2004) confirm such a mechanism. It is also known that miRNA can bind to mRNA to form an RNA Induced Silencing Complex (RISC), resulting in translational repression. On this basis we conclude that there is a need to incorporate miRNAs into recent mathematical models of gene expression during somitogenesis.

Once the miRNAs are bound to mRNA a set of molecular mechanisms are switched leading to remarkable phenomenon of PSM pre-pattern formation. In the paper of Goldbeter et al. (2007), a simple dependence between the *stable* steady state values of *fgf8* mRNA concentration in PSM and the positions along PSM of the lower and upper limits of the region of Retinoic Acid (RA) and Fibroblast Growth Factor (FGF) bistability is established. It is shown that, in order to prove the existence of bistability window in the PSM of the embryo, we have to consider the establishment of thresholds along morphogen gradients. Moreover, it is mathematically proven that mutually inhibitory gradients generate sharp morphogen thresholds in the PSM. For this purpose it is demonstrated that the antagonistic gradients of Retinoic Acid (RA) and Fibroplast Growth Factor (FGF) along PSM may lead to the coexistence of two stable states. Bistability results from the mutual inhibition of RA and FGF and provides a molecular mechanism for the "all-or-none" transitions and possibly more general cell polarization model of morphogenesis we intend to consider in this project. Recently, one of the authors of this project elaborated a continual approach to the problem of somitic cells polarization in a bistability window of embryonic mesoderm (Petrov & Timmer, 2009). The starting point is that the harmonization of biochemical and mechanical points of view has uncovered dynamical essence of somite formation such as transition from temporal gene oscillations to spatial pattern segmentations. Because the somitogenesis is a highly dynamic and coordinated process, this transition is subjected there to extensive theoretical modeling. The consideration is based on the understanding that somitic cells polarization in bistability window of embryonic (pre-somitic) mesoderm is a dynamical process. It occurs in the form of a polarization wave-front of somite cells spread in anterior-posterior direction of the embryonic mesoderm. It is assumed a macroscopic cell polarization has a bistable behavior corresponding to the molecular mechanism of bistability window formation. Moreover this type of polarization is supposed to be transmittable to the other cells by contact interaction.

By author's knowledge, at now the only experimental connections between miRNAs expression

and somitogenesis are in situ hybridisation studies where it is observed miRNA-206 expression in the mouse, fish, frog and chick to be restricted to somites (Wienholds et al., 2005; Wheeler et al., 2006; Sweetman et al., 2006; Darnell et al., 2006; Flynt et al., 2007; Wolff, et al., 2003). In paper of Wienholds et al. (2005) the temporal and spatial expression patterns of 115 conserved vertebrate miRNAs in zebrafish embryos by microarrays and by in situ hybridisations are determined by using locked-nucleic acid-modified oligonucledtide probes. Because of the fact that most miRNAs were expressed in a highly tissue-specific manner during segmentation and later stages, it is concluded that their role is not in tissue fate establishment but in differentiation or maintenance of tissue identity. The investigation of Wienholds et al. (2005) is the first comprehensive set of miRNA expression patterns in animal development. The patterns are found to be definitively specific and diverse, which is a reason to assume corresponding specific and diverse roles for miRNAs. It must be also noted that most miRNAs are expressed in a tissue-specific way in the process of segmentation and later developmental stages, but were not established in earlier development as it was done in Wheeler et al. (2006). Despite of the fact that authors do not exclude a role for undetectable early miRNAs, their observation suggest that: on one hand most miRNAs may not be essential for tissue fate establishment, but on the other one they may play decisive roles in differentiation of tissue identity.

In the paper of Wheeler et al. (2006), the authors describe two new miRNAs, cloned from brain tissue of mouse embryos. What is of interest in our case is that these two miRNAs are expressed mainly during embriogenesis. Additionally, the expression patterns of three recently identified miRNAs, available in authors RNA library, is also established. In the work of Sweetman et al. (2006), it is established that FGF-4 signaling is involved in mir-206 expression in developing somites of chicken embryos. Short RNAs from chicken embryos are cloned and five new chicken miRNA genes are identified. On the basis of sequence homology to previously characterized mouse miRNAs, 17 new chicken miRNAs genes are identified by genome analysis. Developmental Northern blots have also been applied to chick embryos. They show increased accumulation of most miRNAs analyzed from 1,5 days to 5 days, excepting the stem cell-specific mir-302, which was expressed at high levels at early stages and then declined. Restricted expression of mir-124 in the central nervous system and of miR-206 in *developing somites* are revealed by situ analysis. It is also investigated how miR-206 expression is controlled during somite development. As a result it is shown that Fibroplast Growth Factor (FGF) *negatively regulates* the initiation of mir-206 gene expression. In this way the effects of FGF on somite differentiation may be mediates miRNA expression, which is a demonstration that miRNA expression is influenced by FGF developmental signaling pathway. Authors obtain short RNA sequences, which are compared with all sequences in GenBank using BLAST Sequences matching rRNA, tRNA, sn/snoRNA and mRNA are removed, and the remaining sequences are compared with known miRNAs. Potential new miRNA sequences are localized in the chicken genome.

Further investigations on miRNA expression during chick embryo development are presented in paper of Darnell et al. (2006). There, high-throughput whole mount in situ hybridization is performed on chicken embryos to map expression of 135 miRNA genes including five miRNAs that had not been previously reported in chicken. It is established that from eighty-four miRNAs detected before day 5 of embryogenesis, 75 of them show differential expression. This study presents an important basis for further investigations of miRNA gene regulation in chick embryo development.

In the publication of Flynt et al. (2007) it is shown that miRNA-214 is expressed in skeletal muscle cell progenitors during zebrafish development and is demonstrated to specify muscle cell type during somitogenesis by modulating the response of muscle progenitors to Hedgehog signaling. The authors block miR-21 activity by injecting chemically-modified antisense oligonucleotides into zebrafish embryos. The last are decreased in the number of slow-muscle cell types present in the developing somites and distinctly changed the gross morphology of the somites in a way previously associated with attenuated Hedgehog signaling. This process is attributed to relief of miR-214- mediated inhibition of suppressor of fused expression (Flynt et al., 2007). It is some type of fine-tuner of Hedgehog essential for proper specification of muscle cell types during somitogenesis (Wolff et al., 2003). It is of interest to verify whether or not miR-214-plays a similar role in mammalian skeletal muscle development. Both studies (Flynt et al., 2007) and (Wolff et al., 2003) demonstrate that miRNAs function as regulators of gene expression are important for myoblast proliferation and differentiation and may play crucial roles in specifying cell types during development.

All developmental stages (including somitogenesis) are related with the fact that "cell to cell" signaling pathways are typically highly sensitive processes. For example, the Notch pathway in Drosophila contains three members (*Notch, Delta* and *Hartless*). Animal development relies upon a core set of cell signaling pathways: Notch (N), Hedgehog (Hh), Wnt/Wingless (Wg), TGF -β, Receptor Tyrosine Kinase (RTK), nuclear receptor, Jak/STAT, and Hippo pathways (Wolff et al., 2003; Flynt, et al., 2007). These pathways are abundant with components exhibiting genetic interactions in heterozygous state with other pathway components. This circumstance presents a basis of successful searches for new signaling genes dominantly suppressing or enhancing the pathway phenotype. As a result an all-or-nothing output may take place as it is for example considered in somitogenesis (Petrov & Timmer, 2009). The process of somite formation there is modeled as a result of epithelial cell polarization. However, the level of participations of miRNAs in epithelial cell differentiation was largely unknown until the paper (Tsuchiya et al., 2009) was published. There, the authors utilizing an epithelial differentiation model with T84 cells, demonstrate that miR-338-3p and miR-451 contribute to the formation of epithelial basolateral polarity by facilitating translocalization of β1 integrin to the basolateral membrane. It is established that, among 250 miRNAs screened, the expression levels of four miRNAs (miR-33a, 210, 338-3p and 451) are significantly elevated in the differentiated stage of T84 cells, when epithelial cell polarity is established. To order investigate the involvement of these miRNAs in terms of epithelial cell polarity, authors execute loss-of- and gain-of-function analyses of these miRNAs. It is shown that the blockade of endogenous miR-338-3p or miR-451 via each miRNA-specific antisense oligonucleotides inhibited the translocalization of β1 integrin to the basolateral membrane, whereas inhibition of miR-210 or miR-33a has no effect on it. An important circumstance is that, simultaneous transfection of synthetic miR-338-3p and miR-451 accelerate the translocalization of β1 integrin to the basolateral membrane, although the introduction of individual synthetic microRNAs exhibite no effect. Having in view this fact, authors conclude that both miR-338-3p and miR-451 are necessary for the development of epithelial cell.

Therefore, there are experimental evidences that some miRNAs play essential roles in somitogenesis by controlling "cell to cell" signaling during somite cell development and conditioning *cell polarity* by the mechanism of all-or-nothing output. On this basis in (Petrov & Timmer, 2009) the authors propose a mathematical consideration of somite formation process with an emphasis on insights gained from qualitative modeling. It is worth noting that the harmonization of biochemi-

cal and mechanical points of view has uncovered dynamical essence of somite formation such as transition from temporal gene oscillations to spatial pattern segmentations. Because the somitogenesis is a highly dynamic and coordinated process, this transition is subjected there to extensive theoretical modeling. The consideration is based on the understanding that somitic cells polarization in bistability window of embryonic (pre-somitic) mesoderm is a dynamical process. It occurs in the form of a polarization wave-front of somite cells spread in anterior-posterior direction of the embryonic mesoderm. It is assumed a macroscopic cell polarization has a bistable behavior corresponding to the molecular mechanism of bistability window formation. Moreover this type of polarization is supposed to be transmittable to the other cells by contact interaction. At the end, a volume of polarized cells is taken able to create mechanical tension in the volume of non-polarized neighbor cells and to inhibit their polarization. On this basis we explore the leading aspect of somitogenesis robustness by considering a simple wave-front model of polarization and analyzing its propagation in terms of the standard methods of qualitative theory of differential equations. The obtained theoretical results are interpreted in the context of their possible experimental verification. For this purpose an explicit formula for velocity segmentation front propagation is derived and proposed for experimental verification. The final discussion shows the experimental evidence to consider this possibility in the context of somitogenesis robustness.

The experimental observations of tumorogenesis suggest the most natural assumption that tumor cells polarization (or depolarization) wavefront looks like a moving plateau. If we use w to denote the wave front variable of polarization (depolarization), then in front of the wave, w is fixed at some low value, and behind the wave, w is fixed at higher value. A schematic diagram of such a wave front is presented in Figure 2. Such a wave is called *traveling front* (Keener et al., 1998).

Figure 2. Traveling wave front of tumor cells (polarization) depolarization

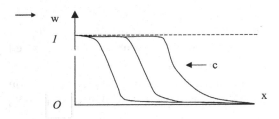

Figure 3. Graphical presentation of steady state points of Equation 1

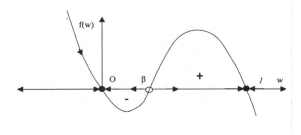

The observations show that the whole layer of tumor cells can be divided along the axis in three parts. The first one is a layer after the traveling front, where the polarization has a lower steady state value. The second is a layer of traveling front of polarization drop value. The third is a layer in front of the drop, where the polarization higher steady state value. The fact that relatively synchronous regions of two steady states are realized, means these states are stable, as otherwise they would not appear. So if we consider a tumor cells depolarization as synchronous process i.e. without diffusion, the corresponding dynamical system of ordinary differential equation should have two stable steady state solutions. We call such a system *bistable equation.*

One of the most well known forms of a bistable equation is

$$\frac{dw}{dt} = -\alpha w(w-1)(w-\beta), \qquad (1)$$

where $0 < \alpha$, $0 < \beta << 1$. This equation can be applied to describe the polarization (depolarization) of a single tumor cell with number i between its neighbors numbered $i-1$ and $i+1$. The right hand side of Equation 1 describes qualitatively the dynamical function of intracellular system for regulating polarization (or depolarization). In Figure 3, the well known "и-shaped" curve of the right side of Equation 1 is presented. The points $w_0=0$ and $w_2=1$ correspond to two stable steady state values of polarization – lower and higher

ones. The intermediate point $w_0 = \beta$ presents the unstable steady state. The type of the steady states w_0, w_1 and w_2, follows directly from the signs of function $f(w) = -\alpha w(w-1)(w-\beta)$, shown in Figure 3.

The corresponding *variation* equations centered at the steady state values w_0, w_1 and w_2 have the forms;

$$\frac{d\omega}{dt} = -\alpha\beta.\omega, \text{ for } w_0 = 0 \text{ (stable)} \qquad (2)$$

$$\frac{d\omega}{dt} = \alpha\beta(1-\beta).\omega, \text{ for } w_1 = \beta \text{ (unstable)}$$
$$\qquad (3)$$

$$\frac{d\omega}{dt} = -\alpha(1-\beta).\omega, \text{ for } w_2 = 1 \text{ (stable)}$$
$$\qquad (4)$$

Here the variation ω is an infinitesimal virtual deviation of the polarization variable w from the corresponding steady state value.

BISTABLE EQUATION WITH A DIFFUSION TERM

In (Petrov & Timmer, 2009) it is assumed the contact polarization between neighbour cells of a tumor is realised by the diffusion law of intracellular interactions from the higher to lower polarizations. In one-dimensional case, when the diffusion of interactions occurs along axial coordinate, the differential equation by accounting the diffusive term can be written in the form

$$\frac{\partial w}{\partial t} = f(w) + Q(x), \tag{5}$$

where the function $Q(x)$ defines dependence of the *cross* polarization w on the axial coordinate x, and the nonlinear function $f(w) = -\alpha w(w - 1)(w - \beta)$ in the right hand side of Equation 5 corresponds to a "point" model, i.e. the synchronous process considered in the previous section. The spatial distribution in the cell layer is presented by polarization-diffusion process of interaction between cells.

Let us assume that the solution of Equation 5 has the form

$$w = w(t, x). \tag{6}$$

In order to find in explicit form the function $Q(x)$ we consider the *competent* part of PreSomitic Mesoderm (PSM) as having the form of long narrow tube with a length L and cross section S (Figure 4). *Competent* means capability of PSM cells to be determined as polarized ones. Certainly, when somitogenesis finishes, cells at the end of PSM are not competent, because they remain non-polarized.

In the tube we separate an elementary volume ΔV with limiting coordinates x and $x + \Delta x$. Thus we have $\Delta V = S\Delta x$. The *quantity* ΔM_x of the polarization moving through the tube section with coordinate x is proportional to the gradient of polarization $\frac{\Delta w}{\Delta x}$ in direction x and to the time interval $[t, t + \Delta t]$ when the interactive diffusion occurs

$$\Delta M_x = -D\frac{\Delta w(x, t)}{\Delta x}S\Delta t, \tag{7}$$

where D is a diffusion coefficient, defined by the *ability* of cells to transmit polarization by contacting each the other.

Through the other limit of the volume with coordinate $x + \Delta x$, in the opposite direction and during the same time interval it diffuses a mass

$$\Delta M_{x+\Delta x} = D\frac{\Delta w(x + \Delta x, t)}{\Delta x}S\Delta t. \tag{8}$$

In this way, the total variation of polarization in the elementary volume ΔV at the expend of diffusion is

$$\Delta M = \Delta M_{x+\Delta x} + \Delta M_x = \frac{DS\Delta t}{\Delta x}\left[-\Delta w(x, t) + \Delta w(x + \Delta x, t)\right], \tag{9}$$

and the variation of polarization w is presented by

$$\Delta c_i = \frac{\Delta M}{\Delta V} = \frac{\Delta M}{S\Delta x} = \frac{D\Delta t}{\Delta x}\left[\frac{\Delta w(x + \Delta x, t)}{\Delta x} - \frac{\Delta w(x, t)}{\Delta x}\right]. \tag{10}$$

By limit transition to $\Delta x \to 0$ we obtain

$$\Delta w = D\Delta t\frac{\partial^2 w(x, t)}{\partial x^2}. \tag{11}$$

By definition, in the absence of cell polarization in correspondence with Equation 1 we have

$Q = \lim \frac{\Delta w}{\Delta t}$, when the limit transition $\Delta t \to 0$ takes place. Thus, at the same transition we can write

Figure 4. Scheme of spatial volume in tumour (A – anterior, P –posterior of tumour)

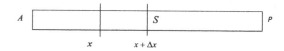

$$Q = D \frac{\partial^2 w(x,t)}{\partial x^2}, \qquad (12)$$

where the quantities Q have the same physical meaning as in Equation 5. Therefore, the distributed system of Equation 5 in case of one-dimensional diffusion has the form

$$\frac{\partial w}{\partial t} = f(w) + D \frac{\partial^2 w(x,t)}{\partial x^2}, \qquad (13)$$

where the nonlinear function

$$f(w) = -\alpha w (w - 1)(w - \beta)$$

corresponds as before to the point (synchronus) model and $D \dfrac{\partial^2 w(x,t)}{\partial x^2}$ corresponds to the diffusion transport between the neighbor cells volumes.

POLARIZATION (DEPOLARIZATION)-DIFFUSION MODEL WITH ELASTIC TENSION

In this section *fast* variables are the concentrations of Retinoic Acid (R), cyp26mRNA (M), CYP26 protein (C), and FGF protein (F) are considered. They are related by kinetic equations in the form

$$\frac{dR}{dt} = \nu - k_1.CR - k_5 R,$$

$$\frac{dM}{dt} = V_0 + V_1 \frac{F^n}{K^n + F^n} - k_3 M,$$

$$\frac{dC}{dt} = k_2 M_c - k_2 C, \qquad (14)$$

$$\frac{dF}{dt} = k_3 M_0 \frac{k_1{}^m}{k_1{}^m + R^m} - k_4 F,$$

where the coefficients have a meaning of kinetic constants. We accept that the only variable which steady state value parametrically defines the "all or none" cell behavior, is that of the fibroblast growth factor F. Following Belintsev et al. (1985, 1987), we take into account the inhibition of the elastic tension generated by the polarization (or depolarization) on its propagation. By analogy with the well-known activator-inhibitor interaction in the biochemical kinetics we just add a term proportional to elastic tension with negative sign to the right hand side of Equation 13. As a result we obtain

$$\frac{\partial w}{\partial t} = -\alpha w (w - 1)(w - \beta.F) + D \frac{\partial^2 w(x,t)}{\partial x^2} - \kappa\sigma, \qquad (15)$$

where σ is an *axial* elastic tension and κ is a coefficient of proportionality. When $\sigma > 0$, we say it is an axial *stretch* tension. For $\sigma < 0$ it is an axial *compression*. We use also the terms *positive* cross polarization when $w > 0$ and *negative* one for $w < 0$. (Figure 5).

As we already mentioned, the axial stretch tension σ not only inhibits the positive cross polarization w, but also depends on the polarization. The corresponding dependence is given by the equilibrium condition

$$\varepsilon \frac{\partial w}{\partial x} + \frac{\partial \sigma}{\partial x} = 0, \qquad (16)$$

Figure 5. Graphical presentation of polarization (depolarization) w and tension σ

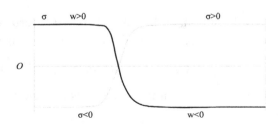

We call ε in Equation 16 a phenomenological coefficient of proportionality. To complete the consideration we also need to introduce the well-known Hook's law in the form

$$\sigma = E\frac{\partial u}{\partial x}, \qquad (17)$$

where u is an axial displacement as a result of the deformation.

Equation 16 and 17 present a system of non-linear partial differential equations for the unknown functions $w(t,x)$ and $\sigma(t,x)$ with partial derivatives. In order to analyze qualitatively these equations, it is necessary to fix some boundary conditions for the unknown *cross* polarization w at the tube ends $x=0$ and $x=L$ i.e.

$$\left.\frac{\partial w}{\partial x}\right|_{x=0,L} = 0, \quad u(0) = u(L). \qquad (18)$$

Further we integrate Equation 16 by taking into account Equation 17 and 18. The obtained result for σ we substitute in Equation 15 and as a result the following governing equation of polarization wavefront can be written:

$$\frac{\partial w}{\partial t} = -\alpha w(w-1)(w-\beta F) + D\frac{\partial^2 w(x,t)}{\partial x^2} - \kappa\varepsilon(w-\overline{w}), \qquad (19)$$

where

$$\overline{w} = \frac{1}{L}\int_0^L w(t,x)dx = \overline{w}(t) \qquad (20)$$

is a average (with respect to x) value of w, depending only on t.

Further we extend our consideration by introducing a second equation for the average polarization validating for arbitrary values of time in the form

$$\frac{d\overline{w}}{dt} = \delta f(w, \overline{w}), \qquad (21)$$

where $f(w, \overline{w})$ is unknown function, and δ is a small coefficient presenting the fact that the average polarization $\overline{w}$ is slow-varying with respect to the fast-varying w.

ON THE ROBUSTNESS OF POLARIZATION (DEPOLARIZATION) WAVE FRONT PROPAGATION IN A TUMOR

In this section we apply the qualitative and computational theory of differential equations to the dynamical system

$$\frac{\partial w}{\partial t} = -\alpha w(w-1)(w-\beta F) - \kappa\varepsilon(w-\overline{w}) + D\frac{\partial^2 w(x,t)}{\partial x^2}, \qquad (22)$$

$$\frac{d\overline{w}}{dt} = \delta f(w, \overline{w}) = \delta(w - \overline{w}). \qquad (23)$$

First of all we apply such named Quasi-Steady-State-Approximation (QSSA), Petrov et al. (2007). The essence of QSSA claims that the character of the solution for (22-23) does not change when the small parameter δ converges to zero. Thus we can assume $\delta = 0$ in Equation 23 and instead of differential equation to consider $\overline{w}$ is constant.

In this way the complete system of two equations (22-23) can be reduced to the degenerate system of Equation 23. Then the stationary values of the fast variable w depend only on the current values of the slow variable $\overline{w}$, but not on final stationary values. In this sense the variable $\overline{w}$ plays role of a *driver* of the *subordinated* variable w. The corresponding investigation of the dependence of Equation 22 solution behavior on the parameter $\overline{w}$, i.e. such named structural stability analysis (Nikolov et al. 2007), can be considered as a control analysis. Also in terms of QSSA, in the right hand side of Equation 23 we can replace w, by its zero solution from Equation 22, when $\overline{w}$ is considered as a constant. Moreover the experimental observations suggest that for sufficiently large time, $\overline{w}$ evidently tend to the stable steady state value of w, taken at fixed x. The simplest approximation of similar tending dynamics can be described by the differential equation 23 with linear function $f(w, \overline{w}) = \delta(w - \overline{w})$ in its right hand side. In this case at fixed x, the variable w approaches its steady state value very *fast* and then $\overline{w}$ (not depending of x) tends very *slow* to this value. If κ and ε are sufficiently small, in correspondence with QSSA the system (22-23) can be written in the form

$$\frac{\partial w}{\partial t} = -\alpha(w - w_0)(w - w_1 F)(w - w_2) + D\frac{\partial^2 w(x,t)}{\partial x^2},$$
(24)

$$\frac{d\overline{w}}{dt} = \delta(w - \overline{w}),$$
(25)

where $w_0, w_1 F$ and w_2 are positive roots of the cubic polynomial

$$\phi(w) = -\alpha w(w - 1)(w - \beta F) - \kappa\varepsilon(w - \overline{w})$$
(26)

in the right hand side of Equation 22. If $\delta = 0$ we have zero approximation $\overline{w} = const.$ and polynomial Equation 26 being a right hand side of Equation 22. Then the zero approximation for w can be found as a traveling front solution of Equation 24(1.4.3) at boundary conditions

$$\left.\frac{\partial w}{\partial x}\right|_{x=0,L} = 0$$
(27)

That means we search for solution in the form $w(x,t) = w(x \pm ct) = w(\eta)$, where $\eta = x \pm ct$. In the new variables, Equation 24 takes the form

$$\frac{dw}{d\eta} = v,$$
(28)

$$D\frac{dv}{d\eta} = \pm cv + \alpha(w - w_0)(w - w_1 F)(w - w_2).$$
(29)

The boundary conditions Equation 27 take the form

$$v(0) = v(L) = 0.$$
(30)

In this way Equation 27, 28-29 and 30 present an eigenvalue problem for the stationary traveling front.

In the phase plane v, w for the two-dimensional dynamical system (28-29) we obtain the following qualitative picture (phase portrait) of possible phase trajectories (Figure 6).

The fixed points 0, 1 and 2 correspond to the roots w_0, w_1 and w_2 respectively of the function $\phi(w)$. The separatrix going from saddle point 0 to saddle point 2 defines the form of traveling front and the stationary velocity c.

To find traveling front solutions we look for a solution of Equation 28 and 29 that connects the fixed points 0 and 2 in the v, w phase plane. Such a trajectory connects two different steady states and is called a heteroclinic trajectory. In

Figure 6. Phase portrait of system (28-29)

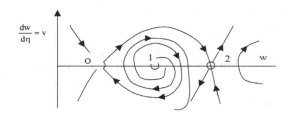

our case it is parametrized by η. The heteroclinic trajectory approaches the point 0 when $\eta \to -\infty$, and approaches 2 when $\eta \to +\infty$. The fixed points 0 and 2 are saddle ones. Our purpose is to define whether or not the velocity c can be chosen such that the trajectory leaving 0 for $\eta = -\infty$ can be made to connect with the saddle point 1 for $\eta = +\infty$.

As it is shown in the book of Keener et al. (1998), an unique velocity c of traveling front propagation exists. The corresponding analytical expression for the velocity c has the form

$$c = \pm\sqrt{D\alpha / 2}\left[w_0 + w_2 - 2w_1 F\right]. \tag{31}$$

The profile of the traveling front is defined by the formula

$$w(\eta) = \frac{w_0 + w_1 F}{2} - \frac{w_2 - w_0}{2} \, th \frac{\eta - \eta_0}{l_0}, \tag{32}$$

where $l_0 = \pm 2\sqrt{2 / \alpha}\,(w_2 - w_0)$, and η_0 is an arbitrary constant defined by the initial conditions.

The qualitative analysis shows that, if a traveling wave solution exists, then the sign of c is the same as the sign of the area under the curve $\phi(w)$ between the points 0 and 2. If this area is positive, then the traveling front propagates from the point 0 to 2, and the second point is called *dominant*. It is clear for sufficiently small β the fixed point 2 is dominant. For sufficiently large $\beta \cong 1$, the fixed point 0 is dominant. Thus in our case of tumor the depolarization front propagates from the point 2 to 0. In this way we can consider solved the problem of determining zero approximation ($\delta = 0$) of the depolarization wave front $w(x - ct)$.

The first approximation ($0 < \delta << 1$) can be qualitatively investigated by analogy with the above proposed phase analysis. For this purpose we transform the system Equation 22 in the form

$$\frac{dv}{d\eta} = \frac{\alpha}{D}(w - w_0)(w - w_1 F)(w - w_2) + \frac{k\varepsilon}{D}.\bar{w} + \frac{c}{D}.v,$$
$$\frac{dw}{d\eta} = v,$$
$$\frac{d\bar{w}}{d\eta} = \frac{\delta}{c}.(w - \bar{w}), \tag{33}$$

by accepting the specific form of solution $w = w(\eta), \bar{w} = \bar{w}(\eta), v = v(\eta), \eta = x + ct$. It is easy to show that for small κ, ε, the system in Equation 33 has three unstable fixed points in the three-dimensional phase space. The projections of these points in the phase plane v,w are positioned near the fixed points of the two-dimensional system (28-29) presented in Figure 6. The projections of the phase trajectories have similar behaviors as those in Figure 6. So we can assert that the fixed point $(w_0, 0, w_0)$ being analogous to point 0 plays role of *dominant* saddle point. Thus in this case the traveling front also propagates from the saddle point $(w_2, 0, w_2)$ to the dominant one $(w_0, 0, w_0)$.

CONCLUDING REMARKS ON THE POLARIZATION-DEPOLARIZATION MECHANISM OF CANCEROGENESIS

The main conclusion we can derive from the above considerations is the following: Despite the structural change of our model from the two-dimensional form (28-29) to the three-dimensional Equation 33, the saddle point with the lower value of polarization remains *dominant*. Moreover, the direction of traveling front propagation conserves the same too, i.e. - from small to the large length of the tumor. That means the model we constructed is *structurally stable* in sense analogous to the *robustness* property introduced in (Beloussov, 2001). We can consider the leading process of depolarization in tumorogenesis, being *robust* could play role of a scaffold of large number of other properties specifying different kinds of tumorogenesis. In this way our mathematical analysis supports the basic that tumorogenesis is a robust process based upon the mechanical relationship between a long-range tension forces stretching the cell tissue and short-range forces of presomitic cell cohesion. Indeed, this relationship postulated as a basis of the wavefront polarization (depolarization) model, presented here, leads to the above shown structurally stable or robust behavior.

In accordance with cancerogenesis robustness, the very dynamical process of the polarization (depolarization) front propagation is also stable in Lyapunov's sense, i.e. with respect to small disturbances of the initial conditions. As it is proved by Fife and McLeod (1977), the traveling wave solution of the bistable equation is stable in an asymptotic (i.e. very strong) way. Starting from arbitrary initial values lying between 0 and β in the limit $x \to -\infty$ and between βF and 1 in the limit $x \to \infty$, the solution approaches infinitesimally near to some phase displacement of the traveling front solution when time tends to infinity.

However, there is an essential exception of both structural and dynamical stability of the model, which is of crucial importance for its validation. Aronson and Weinberger (1975) proved that the initial value $w = \beta F$ is a threshold point for the bistable equation. It means, if the initial values are sufficiently small, then the solution of the bistable equation approaches zero, when $t \to \infty$. But for initial values lying between 0 and 1, the solution approaches 1 for $t \to \infty$. In this case we say that the initial values are *super-threshold*. In the threshold point the model is structurally and dynamically unstable, or non-robust. This threshold type exception from the robustness assures essential qualitative validation of the model, in sense that sufficiently large initial depolarization in the tissue is necessary in order to excite the propagation of a traveling front. For initial polarization larger than βF a traveling

front does not appear, thus tumorogenesis process does not start too.

We obtained realistic *qualitative* picture of polarization (depolarization) wave front propagation in cell tissue, in terms of dynamical model with distributed variables – functions of time and space coordinates, showing *robust* behavior. In order to confirm or reject *quantitatively* this robust model we could experimentally verify the relatively simple velocity formula

$$c = \pm \sqrt{D\alpha / 2} \left[w_0 + w_2 - 2w_1 F \right], \qquad (34)$$

where every parameter both in the right (morphogenetic) and left (cancerogenetic) hand side of Equation 34 could be in principle measured. In case of approximate validity of Equation 34 we will be able to conclude that model "seems to be" realistic. Certainly other versions of the model, for example with two space coordinates, would be of use to develop too. It depends on the results of experimental verification how this theory could be improved.

AN EXPERIMENTAL EVIDENCE OF THE CELL POLARIZATION ROLE IN TUMOROGENESIS

The plasma membrane of epithelial cells consists of two domains: basolateral domain being in contact with the internal environment and an apical domain faced to the external environment. These two plasma domains have different protein and lipid compositions (Deborde et al., 2008; Bruewer et al., 2003; Utech et al., 2005). Histological analysis of these domains reveals an extraordinary complex organization. Focal disruption or complete loss of this high-order structural organization as a rule accompanies neoplastic transformation. To understand disorganization in solid tumors, it is necessary to reveal the mechanisms that are responsible for normal tissue organization. It is established that the normal function requires the presence of cell polarity and maintenance of spatially organized intercellular adhesion. At present, the essential knowledge about the mechanisms of apical-basal cell polarity is contained in the studies (Bilder, 2004; Wodarz, 2005).

The biochemical mechanisms of cell polarity (polarization and depolarization) are rather complex. Nevertheless, it is established that three groups of proteins play a central role in the maintenance of apical-basal cell asymmetry. The protein complexes Crumbs-Pals1 (Stardust)-Patj and the Par3 (Bazooka)-Par6-aPKC localize to the apical membrane domain and promote apical-membrane-domain identity (Margolis & Borg, 2005; Suzuki & Ohno, 2006). The function of these proteins is antagonized by the basolterally placed Lethal giant larvae (Lgl), Scribble (Scrib) and Discs large (Dlg) proteins. All they together promote basolateral membrane identity (Bilder, 2004). It was revealed by epistatic genetic experiments that the apical aPKC-Par3-Par6 protein complex and the basolateral Lg1, Scrib and Dlg proteins are involved in a tug-of-war-type interaction. There a fine balance between their activities defines the boundary position and the sizes of the apical and basolateral membrane domains (Margolis & Borg, 2005; Suzuki & Ohno, 2006).

In the paper of Eric et al. (2008), it is shown that the protein Wnt plays role not only of universal regulator of embryon development by supplying its cells with polarity and ability to directional movement, but also controls cancer-genesis. The experiments demonstrate that, the protein Wnt conditions polarity of cell even in case of lack of intercellular contact and without being informed about the other cells in the embryon or tumor. Regulatory protein Wnt plays an important role in the individual development of animals. It is able to create polarity of cells in embryon development. The protein is necessary also for regeneration. It

defines the direction of anterior-posterior axis of *Caenorhabditis elegans* in the following way: one of the cells of embryon (blastomere P2) produces protein Wnt and forces the near cells to form the tail of the body. By distancing the blastomer P2, the other cell of embryon form amorphic body without anterior-posterior axis. But the minimal contact of blastomer P2 with every part of the embryon is enough to initiate tail formation.

Many efforts are applied to reveal the mechanism of protein Wnt function, but at now not everything is known yet. It is not clear, for example, whether or not it is sufficient for the cell polarization only the presence of protein Wnt in the surrounding media or the contact with other embryonal cells is also necessary to define cell position with respect to the other parts of the embryon. In order to answer this question in the study (Eric et al., 2008) a series of experiments have been accomplished on the influence of Wnt on isolated cells. Cells of human melanoma have been used. It was known before that the cells of malignant tumours actively synthesize the protein Wnt. So it was logically to suppose that the universal regulator of individual development would be able to control also the tumour growth and metastasis formation. It is established in (Eric et al., 2008), that under the influence of protein Wnt in separated, not contacted melanoma cells, an active redistribution of series of proteins occurs. These proteins participate in cell movements, intercellular interactions and malignant tumours. In order to observe the motion of different proteins, they were marked by fluorescing protein genes or by selecting marking them with antibodies. Certainly, not all proteins have been observed in this way. However some "prospective" candidates have been successfully checked. In this way – or step by step, the following picture has been drawn: Step by step, the following picture has been drawn. Under the influence of protein Wnt, at one of the ends of cell, only during several minits, a molecular complex is formed, called by W-RAMP (Wnt5a-mediated Receptor–Actin–Myosin Polarity structure). One of the participants of complex is the protein MCAM (Melanoma Cell Adhesion Molecule) – receptor from the family of immunoglobulins, playing important role in melanoma development. Similar receptors regulate intercellular contacts and interactions, and can take part, for example, in the metastasis of cancer cells through the organism. In the complex W-RAMP enter a series of other proteins, including structers formed by Actin and Myosin assuring cell motility. After forming complex W-RAMP at one of the cell poles, the cell membrane begins to short and as a result the nucleus goes together with the whole cell in a direction opposite to the place of W-RAMP formation.

In this way, it is demonstrated that under the influence of Wnt, the melanoma cell acquires polarity. Front and rear ends of the cell are formed and it begins to crawl away somewhere. Researchers noticed that the W-RAMP complexes are sometimes formed also in cells not treated with protein Wnt. This should be expected, since, as mentioned above, the cancer cells themselves synthesize a number of Wnt. Additional experiments showed that if in melanoma cells turn off the gene protein Wnt, "spontaneous" formation of complexes of W-RAMP stops completely - and start again, if the cell is processed with protein Wnt.

The study of Eric et al. (2008) represents an important step toward understanding the mechanism of action of protein Wnt - a key regulator of individual development, who also plays an important role in regeneration and carcinogenesis. It became clear that Wnt protein is able to polarize the cells and stimulate their direction of movement, even if the cells do not communicate with each other and therefore cannot do anything to "know" about its position relative to other cells of the embryo, the regenerating limb, or cancer.

SYNTHESIS OF DYNAMICAL MODEL OF MIRNA REGULATION OF A CANCER NETWORK

A Time Delay Model of MiRNA Regulation of a Cancer Network

In the paper of Aguda et al. (2008), a mathematical description of the miRNA regulation process is presented. Figure 9 shows a schematic outline of the basic elements comprising this model. Using the steps denoted in Figure 7, Aguda et al. (2008) obtain a dynamical system of two time delay equations, where the delay expresses the assumption that the rate of synthesis of the protein is not a function of its instantaneous concentration, but rather of its concentration at some time τ in the past.

Step 1 in Figure 7 represents the autocatalytic (positive feedback) growth of the protein module (Myc and E2Fs), which is inhibited by miRNA-17-92. Note that this step is an abstraction of all steps involved in protein expression- from transcription factor binding to DNA, gene transcription, to translation in ribosomes. Step 2 in the same figure depicts the protein-induced transcription of the miRNA cluster. The dynamics of concentrations of these two modules is described by the following system

Figure 7. Schematic diagram of the complex network which illustrate the mechanisms and conditions under which miRNA -17-92 operate

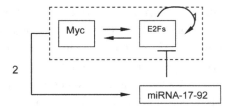

$$\frac{dp}{dt} = \alpha + \frac{k_1 \left[p\left(t - \tau\right)\right]^2}{\Gamma_1 + \left[p\left(t - \tau\right)\right]^2 + \Gamma_2 v\left(t - \tau\right)} - \delta p,$$

$$\frac{dv}{dt} = \beta + k_2 p - \gamma v,$$

$$(35)$$

where p and v are the protein module (Myc and E2Fs) and the miRNA cluster, α is the constant stands for constitutive protein expression due to signal transduction pathways stimulated by growth factors present in the extracellular medium, k_1 is the constant of protein expression, Γ_1 is the coefficient of protein expression, Γ_2 is a measure of the efficiency of miRNA inhibition of protein expression, δ is the fixed rate coefficient of a first order protein degradation, β is the constant represents p-independent constitutive transcription of v, k_2 is the rate constant and γ is the rate coefficient of degradation. Two component mechanisms with autocatalysis easily generate oscillations and bistability.

ANALYSIS OF DYNAMICAL MODEL OF MIRNA REGULATION OF A CANCER NETWORK

By using mathematical representation of the miRNA interaction cancer network Nikolov et al. (2010) derive explicit conditions on how the dynamics of a time delay model of the interaction between the miRNA-17-92 cluster and the transcription factors E2F and Myc depends on systems parameters. Their analysis reveals the complex behavior of the system. The authors compute the occurrence of a limit cycle after an Andronov-Hopf bifurcation for the time delay parameter, and show that the analytical results agree with numerical simulations, i.e. time delay has stabilization role.

The fixed points of the system Equation 1, $\bar{E}\left(\bar{p}, \bar{v}\right)$, can be analytically estimated and are defined by the following set of algebraic equations, including the constants of the model

$$\bar{p}^3 + a\,\bar{p}^2 + b\,\bar{p} + c = 0,$$

$$(36)$$

$$\bar{v} = \frac{\beta + k_2\,\bar{p}}{\gamma},$$

$$(37)$$

where

$$a = \frac{1}{\delta}\left(\frac{\delta k_2 \Gamma_2}{\gamma} - \alpha\right),$$

$$b = \frac{1}{\delta}\left(\delta \Gamma_1 + \frac{\Gamma_2\left(\delta\beta - \alpha k_2\right)}{\gamma}\right)$$

and $c = -\dfrac{1}{\delta}\left(\alpha \Gamma_1 + \dfrac{\alpha\beta\Gamma_2}{\gamma}\right)$.

Equation 36 has three physiologically feasible fixed points (real positive roots) if $a < 0$, $b > 0$, $c < 0$ and $K_3 < 0$, where

$$K_3 = 27c^2 + 4a^2c - 8abc - a^2b^2 + 4b^3.$$

$$(38)$$

Thus, the following necessary (but not sufficient) conditions for existence of three steady states of the system in Equation 35 are obtained:

$$\frac{\delta\beta}{k_2} < \alpha < \frac{\delta k_2 \Gamma_2}{\gamma}$$

$$(39)$$

Linearizing Equation 35 near the equilibrium solutions, i.e. $p = \bar{p} + x$, $v = \bar{v} + y$, the following variation equations are derived:

$$\frac{dx}{dt} = -\delta x + c_1 \ell^{-\chi\tau} x - c_2 \ell^{-\chi\tau} y + c_3 \ell^{-2\chi\tau} x^2 - c_4 \ell^{-2\chi\tau} xy - c_5 \ell^{-3\chi\tau} x^3 - $$
$$- c_6 \ell^{-3\chi\tau} x^2 y - c_7 \ell^{-4\chi\tau} x^4,$$
$$\frac{dy}{dt} = k_2 x - \gamma y,$$

(40)

where

$$c_1 = \frac{2\bar{p}k_1}{\Gamma_1}\left(1 - \frac{2\bar{p}^2 + \Gamma_2\bar{v}}{\Gamma_1}\right), \quad c_2 = \frac{k_1\Gamma_2\bar{p}}{\Gamma_1^2}, \quad c_3 = \frac{k_1}{\Gamma_1}\left(1 - \frac{6\bar{p}^2 + \Gamma_2\bar{v}}{\Gamma_1}\right),$$

$$c_4 = \frac{2k_1\Gamma_2\bar{p}}{\Gamma_1^2}, \quad c_5 = \frac{4k_1\bar{p}}{\Gamma_1^2}, \quad c_6 = \frac{k_1\Gamma_2}{\Gamma_1^2}, \quad c_7 = \frac{k_1}{\Gamma_1^2}.$$

(41)

Note, that function

$$\frac{1}{\Gamma_1 + \left[p\left(t-\tau\right)\right]^2 + \Gamma_2 v\left(t-\tau\right)}$$

is written in Maclaurin series and we take only the linear term. The associated transcendental characteristic equation of 40, where χ is a complex parameter, has the following form:

$$\chi^2 + \left(\gamma + \delta\right)\chi + \delta\gamma = \left(c_1\chi + c_1\gamma - k_2 c_2\right)\ell^{-\chi\tau}.$$

(42)

The stability of the equilibrium states depend on the sign of the real parts of the roots of 3.2.7). If both diagonal elements of the *Jacobian* (stability) matrix, i.e. $\left(-\delta + c_1\ell^{-\chi\tau}\right)$ and $-\gamma$, are always negative, then $tr(J)$ never changes sign and an Andronov-Hopf bifurcation cannot occur. If $\left(-\delta + c_1\ell^{-\chi\tau}\right)$ and $-\gamma$ are of opposite sign, then k_2 and $-c_2\ell^{-\chi\tau}$ must also be of opposite sign in order $\det\left(J\right)$ to be positive. Thus, in our case, the Jacobian matrix has the typically form that produce Andronov-Hopf bifurcation, i.e.

$$J = \begin{vmatrix} + & - \\ + & - \end{vmatrix}.$$

(43)

Note, that mechanisms like this one are called activator-inhibitor models.

Farther, in (nikolov et al., 2010) Andronov-Hopf bifurcation for the system Equation 35 is examined, using time delay as the bifurcation parameter. Equation 42 is rewritten in terms of its real and imaginary parts as

$$\begin{vmatrix} m^2 - n^2 + \left(\gamma + \delta\right)m + \delta\gamma = \ell^{-m\tau}\left[\left(c_1 m + c_1\gamma - k_2 c_2\right)\cos n\tau + c_1 n\sin n\tau\right], \\ 2mn + n\left(\gamma + \delta\right) = \ell^{-m\tau}\left[\left(c_1 m + c_1\gamma - c_2 k_2\right)\sin n\tau - c_1 n\cos n\tau\right]. \end{vmatrix}$$

(44)

To find the first bifurcation point Nikolov et al. (2010) look for purely imaginary roots $\chi = \pm in$, $n \in R$, of Equation 42, i.e. we set $m = 0$. This substitution reduces the above two equations in the form

$$\begin{vmatrix} -n^2 + \delta\gamma = \left(c_1\gamma - c_2 k_2\right)\cos n\tau + c_1 n\sin n\tau, \\ n\left(\gamma + \delta\right) = \left(c_1\gamma - c_2 k_2\right)\sin n\tau - c_1 n\cos n\tau, \end{vmatrix}$$

(45)

One can notice that if n is a solution of Equation 45, then so is $-n$. Hence, we the investigation only reduces to determination of the positive solutions n of Equation 45. Squaring both equations in 45 and adding, the following equation is obtained:

$$n^4 + \left(\gamma^2 + \delta^2 - c_1^2\right)n^2 - \left(c_1\gamma - c_2 k_2\right)^2 + \delta^2\gamma^2 = 0.$$

(46)

Because it is only considered the case when system in Equation 35 is unstable for $\tau = 0$, therefore the roots of the corresponding characteristic equation,

$$\chi^2 + (\gamma + \delta - c_1)\chi - (c_1\gamma - c_2 k_2) + \delta\gamma = 0, \tag{47}$$

must have positive real parts and from the Routh-Hurwitz conditions for a square polynomial

$$\delta\gamma - (c_1\gamma - c_2 k_2) > 0 \quad and \quad \gamma + \delta - c_1 < 0. \tag{48}$$

Then the left-hand side of Equation 47 is positive for large values of n and also positive for $n = 0$. On the other hand, for Equation 46 Nikolov et al. (2010) obtain

$$n_{\pm} = \sqrt{\frac{c_1^2 - \gamma^2 - \delta^2 \pm \sqrt{\Delta}}{2}}. \tag{49}$$

For both of these last expressions (Equation 46 and Equation 48) to be real positive valued, the discriminant

$$\Delta = \gamma^4 + 2(c_1^2 - \delta^2)\gamma^2 - 8c_1 c_2 k_2 \gamma + c_1^2(c_1^2 - 2\delta^2) + 4c_2^2 k_2^2 + \delta^2, \tag{50}$$

must be non-negative, and $c_1^2 > \gamma^2 + \delta^2 \mp \sqrt{\Delta}$. Hence, Equation 46 has at least one simple root and n^2 is the last positive simple root of this equation. Moreover, the following theorem in this situation is applied:

Theorem 1. Suppose that n_b is the last positive simple root of Equation 46. Then, $in(\tau_b) = in_b$ is a simple root of Equation 42 and $m(\tau) + in(\tau)$ is differentiable with respect to τ in a neighborhood of $\tau = \tau_b$.

To establish an Andronov-Hopf bifurcation at $\tau = \tau_b$, it is necessary to show that the following transversality condition $\left.\dfrac{dm}{d\tau}\right|_{\tau=\tau_b} \neq 0$ is satisfied.

Hence, if we denote

$$H(\chi, \tau) = \chi^2 + (\gamma + \delta)\chi + \delta\gamma - (c_1\chi + c_1\gamma - k_2 c_2)\ell^{-\chi\tau}, \tag{51}$$

then

$$\frac{d\chi}{d\tau} = -\frac{\partial H}{\partial\tau} \bigg/ \frac{\partial H}{\partial\chi} = \frac{-\chi(c_1\chi + c_1\gamma - k_2 c_2)\ell^{-\chi\tau}}{2\chi + \gamma + \delta - c_1\ell^{-\chi\tau} + \tau\ell^{-\chi\tau}(c_1\chi + c_1\gamma - k_2 c_2)}. \tag{52}$$

Evaluating the real part of this equation at $\tau = \tau_b$ and setting $\chi = in_b$ yield

$$\left.\frac{dm}{d\tau}\right|_{\tau=\tau_b} = \text{Re}\left(\frac{d\chi}{d\tau}\right)\bigg|_{\tau=\tau_b} = \frac{n_b^2\left[2n_b^2 + \gamma^2 + \delta^2 - c_1^2 - 2(\gamma+\delta)^2\right]}{L^2 + I^2}, \tag{53}$$

where $L = \gamma + \delta + \tau_b(-n_b^2 + \delta\gamma) - c_1\cos n_b\tau_b$ and $I = 2n_b + c_1\sin n_b\tau_b - n_b\tau_b(\gamma+\delta)$.

Let $\theta = n_b^2$. Then, Equation 46 reduces to

$$g = \theta^2 + (\gamma^2 + \delta^2 - c_1^2)\theta - (c_1\gamma - c_2 k_2)^2 + \delta^2\gamma^2. \tag{54}$$

Then, for $g'(\theta)$ we have

$$g'(\theta)\big|_{\tau=\tau_b} = \left.\frac{dg}{d\theta}\right|_{\tau=\tau_b} = 2\theta + \gamma^2 + \delta^2 - c_1^2. \tag{55}$$

If n_b is the least positive simple root of Equation 46, then $\left.\dfrac{dg}{d\tau}\right|_{\theta=n_b^2} > 0$. Hence,

$$\left.\frac{dm}{d\tau}\right|_{\tau=\tau_b} = \text{Re}\left(\frac{d\chi}{d\tau}\right)\bigg|_{\tau=\tau_b} = \frac{n_b^2\left[g' - 2(\gamma+\delta)^2\right]}{L^2 + I^2} < 0. \tag{56}$$

According to the Hopf bifurcation theorem, the main result of this investigation are defined in the form of the following theorem:

Theorem 2. If n_b is the least positive root of Equation 46, then an Andronov-Hopf bifurcation occurs as τ passes through τ_b if only if

$$g' < 2(\gamma + \delta)^2.$$

Corollary 2.1. When $\tau > \tau_b$, then the steady state $\bar{E}$ of system Equation 35 is locally asymptotically stable.

Next, the authors in (Nikolov et al., 2010) numerically analyze the time delay model constituted by system Equation 35 for the concentrations of the protein module p (Myc and E2Fs), and the miRNA cluster v at time t. The corresponding numerical values of the model parameters are taken from (Aguda et al., 2008), and in accordance with the condition Equation 39 the following expressions yield:

$$\Gamma_1 = 0.1\left[\mu M^2\right], \quad \Gamma_2 = 0.056\left[\mu M\right], \quad \alpha \in (0, 0.033)\left[\mu M h^{-1}\right], \beta = 0.01\left[\mu M h^{-1}\right],$$
$$\delta = 0.26\left[h^{-1}\right], \quad k_1 = 0.4\left[\mu M h^{-1}\right], \quad k_2 = 0.3\left[h^{-1}\right], \quad \gamma = 0.02\left[h^{-1}\right].$$
$$(57)$$

Since the exact values of time delay are unknown, Nikolov et al. (2010) set $\tau \in \left[0.05, 3\right]$ hours, which is feasible from a physiologically point of view,. The governing equations of the model were solved numerically using MATLAB (www.mathworks.com). In Figures 8a and 8b, the calculated one-parameter bifurcation diagrams of system Equation 35 are shown. As it can seen, when the bifurcation parameter τ decreases from 3, near the point $\tau = 2$ after an Andronov-Hopf bifurcation stable limit cycle with period one occur and the system Equation 35 shows periodic solutions (see Figure 8a). For time delay smaller than 2 hours, the system shows sustained oscillations with amplitude around 80% of the steady-state value reached for $\tau > 2$. Although there is not an all-nothing oscillation for v, the value in the minimum is below 40% of the steady-state value. Here it must note that $\alpha = 0.017$. Thus, it means that time delay amplifies the stability of steady states. In order words, as a result of the evidence obtained in Figure 8a, it may conclude that the time delay has a stabilization effect on the miRNA regulation process. This result is in exact accordance with the corresponding analytical results obtained above.

According to (Aguda et al., 2008), the system has very rich dynamical behavior when α (constant stands for constitutive protein expression due to signal transduction pathway) is bifurcation parameter. For example, at small values of α the system has three coexisting steady states, but only the lowest one is stable. When α is increased, only one steady state is available for the system and this steady state is asymptotically stable.

Figure 8. Bifurcation diagrams of system in Equation 35 when τ (a) and α (b) are bifurcation parameters

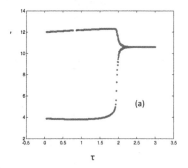
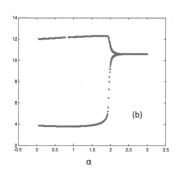

Figure 9. Periodic solutions of system (9.1) at different values of time delay, i.e. τ=0.05 (solid line) and τ=1.8 (dashed line). Parameter values are those from Equation 57 and α=0.017. The time is in hours

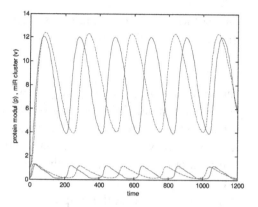

In Figure 8b the behavior of the system Equation 35 is shown when $\alpha \in \left[0.005, 0.023\right]$ and $\tau = 1$. For $\alpha \in \left[0.005, 0.0075\right]$ the system is stable. For smaller values, the system suddenly changes from stable to unstable regime and sustained oscillations occur. Finally, for α larger than 0.0185 the system is also in stable regime no matter whether the time delay has smaller or larger values. In figure 9 the dependence of the period and amplitude of oscillations from values of time delay is shown. It is seen that magnitude and period of oscillations increase with the increase of time delay for values smaller than the bifurcation point.

CONCLUSION

In conclusion of this section: we analyzed the dynamics of a time delay model of the interaction between miRNA-17-92 and the transcription factors Myc and E2F. The investigation is devoted to the use of the bifurcation analysis. Particularly, a Hopf bifurcation theorem. The basic view that

the time delay, τ, and the constant stands for constitutive protein expression due to signal transduction pathways stimulated by growth factors present in the extracellular medium, α, are a key factor in the dynamical behavior of system in Equation 35 has been confirmed by analytical and numerical calculations. It is obtained that time delay has a stabilization role under the regulation behavior of miRNA. Thus, the results obtained in (Aguda et al., 2008) have been extended. The model is from activator-inhibitor type. A species taking part in a stabilizing, respectively, destabilizing feedback loop, is called inhibitor, respectively, activator. Normally, an autocatalytic species is an activator. Usually, the dynamics of these models is to complicate. The rich dynamics arising from the interaction between two parameters, i.e. codimension-two bifurcation take place. In other words, occurrence of Takens-Bogdanov bifurcation, saddle-node bifurcation, pitchfork bifurcation and homoclinic orbits is possible. From the last one the emergence of Shilnikov chaos is possible.

AN APPLICATION OF QUASI-STEADY-STATE APPROXIMATION TO MIRNA ROLE IN CANCER NETWORKS

An Introduction to QSSA Theorem

The term Quasi-Steady-State Approximation (QSSA) is a mathematical method. We use it in a sense explained in the work of Schneider and Wilhelm (2000). The method find vast applications in many areas of systems biology, including studies related to cell proliferation, differentiation and the cell cycle (Petrov et al., 2004). A classical example of dimensionality reduction for nonlinear dynamic systems is the application to Michaelis–Menten type enzyme kinetics (Michaelis & Menten, 1913). Examples of reversible enzyme catalytic reactions that are well described by reversible kinetic scheme can be found in the literature (Alberty, 1959; Sellin & Mannervik, 1983; Duggleby,1994). An application of QSSA to the reversible case is presented in the work of Tzafriri and Edelman (2004). There, a QSSA for the reversible Michaelis–Menten equation is derived and its validity domain is delineated.

This section presents a more general approach to a QSSA, based on corresponding theorem proved in the work of Tichonov (1952). Some initial ideas of the present investigation were introduced in the work of Fall et al., (2002) and Petrov et al., (2007). The aim is to demonstrate the application of the method in this new form to the genetic processes and especially to miRNA target regulation (Nikolova et al., 2009a, Nikolova et al., 2009b). Towards this end, Nikolova et al., (2009) reduce dimensionality of the modified model mentioned above in order to show the specific feature of miRNA target regulation near its quasi-stationary state.

It is well known that biochemical interactions may occur in different time scales. In case of two scales that leads to dynamical system in the form:

$$\varepsilon \frac{d\vec{x}}{dt} = \vec{f}(\vec{x}, \vec{y}) \qquad (58)$$

$$\frac{d\vec{y}}{dt} = \vec{g}(\vec{x}, \vec{y}) \qquad (59)$$

where $\vec{x} \in R^m, \vec{y} \in R^n, 0 < \varepsilon << 1$. The QSSA theorem (Tichonov, 1952) claims that

*The solution of the **complete** system (58-59) tends to the solution of the **degenerate** system in Equation 59 at $\varepsilon \to 0$,* if the following conditions are satisfied:

a)   There is an isolated equilibrium (steady state) solution of the **attached** system in Equation 58 (i.e. there is not other solution in its neighborhood).

b)   *The existing equilibrium solution of the attached system is stable for every value of the**slow**variables $\vec{y}$.*

c)   The initial conditions (states) lie in a region of influence (a basin) of the equilibrium solution of the attached system.

d)   The solution of the complete system is single-valued and its right hand sides are continuous.

It therefore follows that in every concrete case we can find the equilibrium solution of the attached system and to replace it in the degenerate one. Moreover, we should demonstrate that all requirements of the formulated theorem are satisfied.

Consider in general case the simplest example of two differential equations ($m = 1, n = 1$) or $\vec{x} \equiv x, \vec{y} \equiv y$. Then the system (58-59) takes the form

$$\varepsilon \frac{dx}{dt} = f(x, y) \qquad (60)$$

$$\frac{dy}{dt} = g(x, y) \qquad (61)$$

The essence of QSSA theorem claims that the character of the solution of system (60-61) does not change when the small parameter ε tends to zero. Thus we can assume $\varepsilon = 0$ in Equation 60 and instead of differential equation obtain algebraic ones for the steady state value of fast variable x.

$$0 = f(x, y) \qquad (62)$$

$$\frac{dy}{dt} = g(x, y) \qquad (63)$$

From Equation 62 the fast variable x can be expressed as a function of y, i.e. $x = \phi(y)$ and substituted in Equation 63. As a result Equation 63 becomes

$$\frac{dy}{dt} = g[\phi(y), y] \tag{64}$$

In this way the complete system of two equations (60-61) is reduced to the degenerate system of Equation 64. Moreover the stationary values of the fast variable x depend only on the current values of the slow variable y, but not on final stationary values. In this sense the variable y plays role of a *driver* of the *subordinated* variable x. The number of initial conditions of the degenerate system (62-63) is smaller than that of the complete one (60-61). The initial condition of Equation 60 is not used in (62-63). In accordance with the QSSA theorem, when the stationary solution of the attached system is isolated and stable, then the solution of the degenerate system depends only on the initial values of the slow variables. Therefore, the presence of a small parameter is a necessary condition of dimensionality *reduction* of the complete system. A preliminary dimensionless procedure is necessary to apply on the corresponding system, however, in order to appear such parameter. The appropriate example for introduction of a similar procedure (We apply analogous to it in this paper) with application to enzyme kinetic reactions is given in (Romanovskii et al., 1975). The last one expresses rather in *normalization* (or scaling) of the terms in the right hand sides of the systems equations. In this way only ε is considered as a dimensionless parameter, drawing attention also that it has not any physical sense (as for example – concentration ratio of some conserved quantities, conservation sums, steady state values etc.) In more narrow sense it introduces in a pure mathematical way as an *order* ratio between measured data from on one hand, and *normalized* (i.e. reduced to unit order) ones on the other. As a result of similar scaling no contradiction between approximation procedure and total quantities conservation would arise. Moreover it is important to underline here that the conservation of total quantities is not related to this type of Quasi-Steady-State Approximation (QSSA), because the last concerns the estimation only of the rate of changes of the quantities, but not the very quantities. When estimating quantities, we are free to neglect or conserve small terms in correspondence to our purposes and without contradicting to the evaluation of the derivatives order.

A MODIFIED MINIMAL MODEL OF MIRNA-MEDIATED TARGET REGULATION

It is predicted that each miRNA regulates numerous (sometimes hundreds) different types target messenger RNAs (Krek et al., 2005). Therefore, in some cases the miRNA itself is likely to become a limiting factor and the potential competing binding sites on target mRNAs need to be taken into account (Doench & Sharp, 2004). In (Nikolova et al., 2009a) a minimal mathematical model presented in (Khanin & Higham, 2007) for the case of two targets $\{m_i\}_{i=1}^N$ is modified. According to Figure 10 each type of mRNA is being produced with a transcription rate q_i and decays with rate δ_i. The miRNA itself is being produced in the cell with a rate p_m and decays with a rate δ_m. In addition, mRNA and miRNA (reversibly) make complexes, miRNA & mi, with a forward rate β_i and a reverse rate β_i^-. The complex miRNA & mi decays with a rate δ_i^* .ie. Proteins, $\{p_i\}_{i=1}^N$ degrade at a rate δ_i^P and are being translated at a rate λ_i from free mRNAs, (mi), and with a rate λ_i^* from the complexes, miRNA & mi, which lead also to its decrease. MiRNA exerts its down-regulating effect on the targets by accelerating the degradation rate of the complexes or/and by slowing down the translation rate.

The key parameters that are believed to influence the extent of miRNA-mediated target down-regulation, are the fold-changes in mRNA degradation rate δ_i^* / δ_i, and translation rate λ_i^* / λ_i, that depend on specific target mRNA and miRNA base-pairing in and around the seed region. Here we assume that and translation rate $\lambda_i^* / \lambda_i \leq 0,001$, i.e, the translation rate of the proteins from the complexes miRNA & mRNAs is sufficiently slower than the translation rate from free mRNAs. MiRNA returns to the cytoplasm pool with the rate $q \sum_{i=1}^{N} \delta_i^*$ miRNA & mi, where q is the miRNA turnover rate (Levine et al., 2007). In this investigation we consider the case when $q = 1$ in the model, i.e. here the degradation of the miRNA & mRNA complex always results in the miRNA returning to the pool.

According to Figure 10 for two targets, N = 2, the model takes the form

$$\frac{dm_1}{dt} = q_1 - \delta_1 m_1 - \beta_1 m_1(miRNA) + \beta_1^-(miRNA \& m_1)$$
$$\frac{dp_1}{dt} = \lambda_1 m_1 - \delta_1^P p_1 - \lambda_1^*(miRNA \& m_1)$$
$$\frac{dm_2}{dt} = q_2 - \delta_2 m_2 - \beta_2 m_2(miRNA) + \beta_2^-(miRNA \& m_2)$$
$$\frac{dp_2}{dt} = \lambda_2 m_2 - \delta_2^P p_2 - \lambda_2^*(miRNA \& m_2)$$
$$\frac{d(miRNA)}{dt} = p_m - \delta_m(miRNA) - \beta_1 m_1(miRNA) + \beta_1^-(miRNA \& m_1)$$
$$-\beta_2 m_2(miRNA) + \beta_2^-(miRNA \& m_2) + \delta_1^* q(miRNA \& m_1) + \delta_2^* q(miRNA \& m_2)$$
$$\frac{d(miRNA \& m_1)}{dt} = \beta_1 m_1(miRNA) - \beta_1^-(miRNA \& m_1) - \delta_1^*(miRNA \& m_1)$$
$$\frac{d(miRNA \& m_2)}{dt} = \beta_2 m_2(miRNA) - \beta_2^-(miRNA \& m_2) - \delta_2^*(miRNA \& m_2)$$

$$(65)$$

Where m_1 and m_2 are two different types of mRNA molecules, targets of $miRNA$, p_1 and p_2 are proteins, produced by m_1 and m_2, and $miRNA \& m_1$ and $miRNA \& m_2$ are complexes between $miRNA$ and m_1 and m_2, respectively.

In (Khanin & Higham, 2007) the effects of m_1^{total} $(m_1^{total} = m_1 + (miRNA \& m_1))$ and p_1 levels are simulated as functions of transcription rate of the second target q_2, for three production rates for miRNA $(p_m = 5, 10, 15)$. For the simu-

Figure 10. Graphical representation of microRNA target regulation

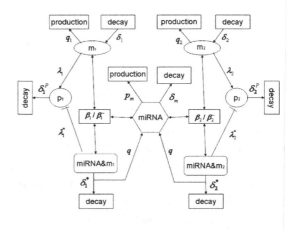

lations made in (Khanin & Higham, 2007) the following numerical values of coefficients of the original model are given:

$$q_1 = 5; \delta_1 = \delta_2 = 1; \beta_1 = \beta_2 = 50; \beta_1^- = \beta_2^- = 0,1;$$
$$\lambda_1 = \lambda_2 = 2; \delta_1^P = \delta_2^P = 1; \lambda_1^* = \lambda_2^* = 1; \delta_m = 1,1; \delta_1^* = \delta_2^* = 5;$$

$$(66)$$

Taking into account the last numerical values of the coefficients numerical simulations of the system in 65 at $p_m = 5$ show that there is complete coincidence between graphics of m_1 and m_2, p_1 and p_2, $(miRNA \& m_1)$ and $(miRNA \& m_2)$, respectively. This result supposes that difference between numerical values of the system coefficients, denoted by one and the same letters exists. In fact, from a biological point of view it is not possible the corresponding rate constants of two different mRNAs, the proteins, produced by them, and their complexes to have equal numerical values. By this reason Nikolova et al. (2009a) assume that the coefficients, denoted by one and the same letters have different numerical values but they are with one and the same order. For this investigation the authors take only the numerical values of $q_1, \delta_1, \beta_1, \beta_1^-$ and δ_1^P. Finally according their assumptions described above the numerical values of coefficients of the system in 65 are as it follows:

$$q_1 = 5; \quad \delta_1 = 1; \quad \beta_1 = 50; \quad \beta_1^- = 0,1; \quad \lambda_1 = 10; \quad \delta_1^P = 1; \quad \lambda_1^* = 0.01;$$
$$q_2 = 10; \quad \delta_2 = 2; \quad \beta_2 = 60; \quad \beta_2^- = 0,5; \quad \lambda_2 = 9; \quad \delta_2^P = 0,8; \quad \lambda_2^* = 0.02;$$
$$p_m = 10 \quad \delta_m = 1,1; \quad \delta_1^* = 5; \quad \delta_2^* = 6;$$

$$(67)$$

On the basis of the last values and taking into account data, given in (Khanin & Higham, 2007) numerical simulation of the model (13.1) is made at the following initial conditions:

$$m_1 = m_2 = 1; \quad p_1 = p_2 = 0; \quad miRNA = 0; \quad miRNA \,\&\, m_1 = miRNA \,\&\, m_2 = 0$$

$$(68)$$

Dynamics of mRNAs, proteins, miRNA and miRNA&mRNAs is presented in Figure 11. From Figure 11 the values near the settled (steady state) ones are selected in order to use them as characteristic values of state variables.

$$m_1^0 = 0,0263; \quad p_1^0 = 0.2731; \quad m_2^0 = 0,0664; \quad p_2^0 = 0.6972;$$
$$miRNA^0 = 4,5454; \quad (miRNA \,\&\, m_1)^0 = 0.9947; \quad (miRNA \,\&\, m_2)^0 = 1,6445;$$

$$(69)$$

The parameters and concentrations values, presented above are given here without units in view of the fact that we do not intend to compare them. What is of interest for us further is to compare neither parameters (some of them having different units) nor concentrations, but the terms in the equations in 65 (As it was explained in the previous section). In accordance with the scaling procedure each term in the right hand sides of the system equations mentioned must have an order of 1. For this purpose *scaling* substitutions are introduced for the model variables in the following manner:

$$m_1 = \varepsilon x_1; \quad p_1 = x_2; \quad m_2 = \varepsilon x_3; \quad p_2 = x_4;$$
$$miRNA = x_5 / \varepsilon; \quad (miRNA \,\&\, m_1) = x_6; \quad (miRNA \,\&\, m_2) = x_7 / \varepsilon;$$

$$(70)$$

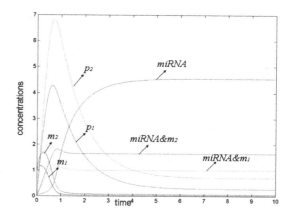

Figure 11. Graphs of all components of the complete system solution

where the small parameter $\varepsilon = 0.1$. Here the new variables xi $(i=1,2,..7)$ are not dimensionless. Nevertheless they have an order of 1 (i.e. they change in the interval between 0.1 and 1). The same approach is applied for scaling the model coefficients. The corresponding parameter substitutions have the following form:

$$q_1 = a_1 / \varepsilon; \quad \delta_1 = a_2; \quad \beta_1 = a_3 / \varepsilon^2; \quad \beta_1^- = a_4; \quad \lambda_1 = a_5 / \varepsilon;$$
$$\delta_1^P = a_6; \quad \lambda_1^* = \varepsilon a_7; \quad q_2 = a_8 / \varepsilon; \quad \delta_2 = a_9; \quad \beta_2 = a_{10} / \varepsilon^2;$$
$$\beta_2^- = a_{11}; \quad \lambda_2 = a_{12} / \varepsilon; \quad \delta_2^P = a_{13}; \quad \lambda_2^* = \varepsilon a_{14}; \quad p_m = a_{15} / \varepsilon;$$
$$\delta_m = a_{16}; \quad \delta_1^* = a_{17} / \varepsilon; \quad \delta_2^* = a_{18} / \varepsilon;$$

$$(71)$$

Here the new coefficients a_i $(i = 1,2,...,18)$ have also order of 1 conserving their physical dimensionality.

After replacing the variable and parameter transformation forms (70-71) in 65 the following system is obtained:

$$\varepsilon^3 \frac{dx_1}{dt} = \varepsilon a_1 - \varepsilon^3 a_2 x_1 - a_3 x_1 x_5 + \varepsilon^2 a_4 x_6$$

$$(72)$$

$$\frac{dx_2}{dt} = a_5 x_1 - a_6 x_2 - \varepsilon a_7 x_6$$

$$(73)$$

Figure 12. Behaviour of the fast variables m_1, m_2

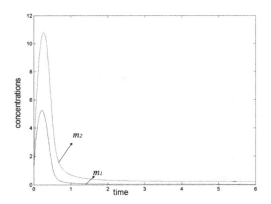

$$\varepsilon^3 \frac{dx_3}{dt} = \varepsilon a_8 - \varepsilon^3 a_9 x_3 - a_{10} x_3 x_5 + \varepsilon a_{11} x_7$$
(74)

$$\frac{dx_4}{dt} = a_{12} x_3 - a_{13} x_4 - a_{14} x_7$$
(75)

$$\varepsilon \frac{dx_5}{dt} = \varepsilon a_{15} - \varepsilon a_{16} x_5 - a_3 x_1 x_5 + \varepsilon^2 a_4 x_6 - $$
$$- a_{10} x_3 x_5 + \varepsilon a_{11} x_7 + \varepsilon a_{17} x_6 + a_{18} x_7$$
(76)

$$\varepsilon^2 \frac{dx_6}{dt} = a_3 x_1 x_5 - \varepsilon^2 a_4 x_6 - \varepsilon a_{17} x_6$$
(77)

$$\varepsilon \frac{dx_7}{dt} = a_{10} x_3 x_5 - \varepsilon a_{11} x_7 - a_{18} x_7$$
(78)

The presence of a small parameter ε in a part of system equations determines its order. This means in accordance with the terminology of QSSA theorem it can say that the five equations Equation 72, 74, 76, 77 and 78 form an *attached* system, and the other two form a *degenerate* one. Moreover it is seen that mRNAs m_1 and m_2 will chance faster than *miRNA* and *miRNA&mRNAs*. This result differs from the plausible assumption, made in (Khanin & Higham, 2007) that the

miRNA&mRNA complexes are being translated but at a slower rate than free mRNAs. The scaling system presented here shows that both free mRNAs and miRNA&mRNA complexes are fast variables. On the other hand $miRNA \& m_1$ chances faster than *miRNA* and $miRNA \& m_2$.

In order to support selection made here we numerical simulations of (13.8-13.14), which will directly demonstrate dynamical features of the both subsystems are presented. Figures 12, 13 and 14 show the behavior of the fast and slow variables, respectively for a period of 6 units. As it is seen, the obtained graphics completely confirm the conclusion made above on the basis of analytical results done in (Nikolova et al, 2009a).

Next, some properties of the attached, degenerate and complete systems following from the QSSA theorem are investigated.

APPLYING QSSA THEOREM TO DYNAMICAL SYSTEM (72-78)

Consider the attached system of equations Equation 72, 74, 76, (and 78 under condition that only the variables x_1, x_3, x_5, x_6, x_7 are unknown function of time. The system has a stationary (steady state) solution in the form

$$x_1^0 = \frac{\varepsilon^2 a_1}{\alpha_1^E}; \quad x_3^0 = \frac{\varepsilon^2 a_8}{\alpha_2^E}; \quad x_5^0 = \frac{a_{15}}{a_{16}};$$
$$x_6^0 = \frac{\varepsilon a_1 a_3 a_{15}}{\alpha_1^E a_{16}(\varepsilon a_4 + a_{17})}; \quad x_7^0 = \frac{\varepsilon^2 a_8 a_{10} a_{15}}{\alpha_2^E a_{16}(\varepsilon a_{11} + a_{18})};$$
(79)

where

$$\alpha_1^E = \varepsilon^3 a_2 + \frac{a_3 a_{15} a_{17}}{a_{16}(\varepsilon a_4 + a_{17})}; \quad \alpha_2^E = \varepsilon^3 a_9 + \frac{a_{10} a_{15} a_{18}}{a_{16}(\varepsilon a_{11} + a_{18})}.$$

In order to analyze the stability of the steady state (14.1) the following substitutions are introduced:

Figure 13. Behaviour of the fast variables $miRNA, miRNA \& m_1, miRNA \& m_2$

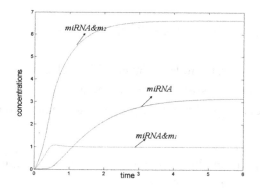

Figure 14. Slow variables behavior

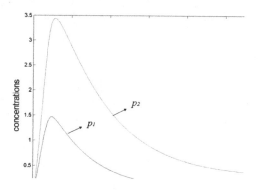

$$x_1 = x_1^0 + \xi_1; \quad x_3 = x_3^0 + \xi_2; \quad x_5 = x_5^0 + \xi_3; \quad x_6 = x_6^0 + \xi_4; \quad x_7 = x_7^0 + \xi_5;$$

(80)

in the attached system of equations Equation 72, 74, 76 and 77 and 78. As a result the variation equations are derived:

$$\varepsilon^3 \frac{d\xi_1}{dt} = -\varepsilon^3 a_2 \xi_1 - a_3 x_5^0 \xi_1 - a_3 x_1^0 \xi_3 + \varepsilon^2 a_4 \xi_4$$

$$\varepsilon^3 \frac{d\xi_2}{dt} = -\varepsilon^3 a_9 \xi_2 - a_{10} x_5^0 \xi_2 - a_{10} x_3^0 \xi_3 + \varepsilon a_{11} \xi_5$$

$$\varepsilon \frac{d\xi_3}{dt} = -\varepsilon a_{16} \xi_3 - a_3 x_1^0 \xi_3 - a_3 x_5^0 \xi_1 + \varepsilon^2 a_4 \xi_4 - a_{10} x_3^0 \xi_3$$
$$- a_{10} x_5^0 \xi_2 + \varepsilon a_{11} \xi_5 + \varepsilon a_{17} \xi_4 + a_{18} \xi_5$$

$$\varepsilon^2 \frac{d\xi_4}{dt} = a_3 x_5^0 \xi_1 + a_3 x_1^0 \xi_3 - \varepsilon^2 a_4 \xi_4 - \varepsilon a_{17} \xi_4$$

$$\varepsilon \frac{d\xi_5}{dt} = a_{10} x_5^0 \xi_2 + a_{10} x_3^0 \xi_3 - \varepsilon a_{11} \xi_5 - a_{18} \xi_5$$

(81)

Next we neglect the terms containing degrees of ε, higher than 1-rst one from variation equations Equation 81, in view of the fact they can be just neglected in comparison of the other terms in the right-hand sides, when estimating the order of derivatives. In this way the characteristic equation takes the form shown in Box 1.

In a polynomial form the same equation looks like

$$\mu^5 + p_1 \mu^4 + p_2 \mu^3 + p_3 \mu^2 + p_4 \mu + p_5 = 0,$$

(83)

where

$$p_1 = \varepsilon a_{11} + \varepsilon a_{16} + \varepsilon a_{17} + a_3 x_1^0 + a_3 x_5^0 + a_{10} x_3^0 + a_{10} x_5^0 + a_{18}$$

Box 1.

$$\begin{vmatrix} -a_3 x_5^0 - \mu & 0 & -a_3 x_1^0 & 0 & 0 \\ 0 & -a_{10} x_5^0 - \mu & -a_{10} x_3^0 & 0 & \varepsilon a_{11} \\ -a_3 x_5^0 & -a_{10} x_5^0 & -\varepsilon a_{16} - a_3 x_1^0 - a_{10} x_3^0 - \mu & \varepsilon a_{17} & \varepsilon a_{11} + a_{18} \\ a_3 x_5^0 & 0 & a_3 x_1^0 & -\varepsilon a_{17} - \mu & 0 \\ 0 & a_{10} x_5^0 & a_{10} x_3^0 & 0 & -\varepsilon a_{11} - a_{18} - \mu \end{vmatrix} = 0$$

(82)

$$p_2 = \varepsilon^2 a_{11} a_{16} + \varepsilon^2 a_{11} a_{17} + \varepsilon^2 a_{16} a_{17} + \varepsilon a_3 a_{11} x_1^0 + \varepsilon a_3 a_{11} x_5^0 +$$
$$+ \varepsilon a_3 a_{16} x_5^0 + \varepsilon a_3 a_{17} x_5^0 + + \varepsilon a_{10} a_{16} x_5^0 + \varepsilon a_{10} a_{17} x_3^0 + \varepsilon a_{10} a_{17} x_5^0 +$$
$$+ \varepsilon a_{16} a_{18} + \varepsilon a_{17} a_{18} + a_3 a_{10} x_1^0 x_5^0 + a_3 a_{10} x_3^0 x_5^0 + a_3 a_{10} (x_5^0)^2 +$$
$$+ a_3 a_{18} x_1^0 + a_3 a_{18} x_5^0 + a_{10} a_{18} x_5^0$$

$$p_3 = \varepsilon^3 a_{11} a_{16} a_{17} + \varepsilon^2 a_3 a_{11} a_{16} x_5^0 + \varepsilon^2 a_3 a_{11} a_{17} x_5^0 + \varepsilon^2 a_3 a_{16} a_{17} x_5^0 +$$
$$+ \varepsilon^2 a_{10} a_{16} a_{17} x_5^0 + \varepsilon^2 a_{16} a_{17} a_{18} + \varepsilon a_3 a_{10} a_{16} (x_5^0)^2 + \varepsilon a_3 a_{10} a_{17} (x_5^0)^2 +$$
$$+ \varepsilon a_3 a_{10} a_{17} x_3^0 x_5^0 + \varepsilon a_3 a_{16} a_{18} x_5^0 + + \varepsilon a_3 a_{17} a_{18} x_5^0 + \varepsilon a_{10} a_{16} a_{18} x_5^0 +$$
$$+ \varepsilon a_{10} a_{17} a_{18} x_5^0 + a_3 a_{10} a_{18} x_1^0 x_5^0 + a_3 a_{10} a_{18} (x_5^0)^2$$

$$(84)$$

$$p_4 = \varepsilon^3 a_3 a_{11} a_{16} a_{17} x_5^0 + \varepsilon^2 a_3 a_{10} a_{16} a_{17} (x_5^0)^2 + \varepsilon^2 a_3 a_{16} a_{17} a_{18} x_5^0 +$$
$$= \varepsilon^2 a_{10} a_{16} a_{17} a_{18} x_5^0 + \varepsilon a_3 a_{10} a_{16} a_{18} (x_5^0)^2 + \varepsilon a_3 a_{10} a_{17} a_{18} (x_5^0)^2$$

$$p_5 = \varepsilon^2 a_3 a_{10} a_{16} a_{17} a_{18} (x_5^0)^2$$

The Routh-Hurwitz coefficients have the following form:

$$D_1 = p_1; \quad D_2 = \begin{vmatrix} p_1 & 1 \\ p_3 & p_2 \end{vmatrix}; \quad D_3 = \begin{vmatrix} p_1 & 1 & 0 \\ p_3 & p_2 & p_1 \\ p_5 & p_4 & p_3 \end{vmatrix};$$

$$D_4 = \begin{vmatrix} p_1 & 1 & 0 & 0 \\ p_3 & p_2 & p_1 & 0 \\ p_5 & p_4 & p_3 & p_2 \\ 0 & 0 & p_5 & p_4 \end{vmatrix}; \quad D_5 = \begin{vmatrix} p_1 & 1 & 0 & 0 & 0 \\ p_3 & p_2 & p_1 & 0 & 0 \\ p_5 & p_4 & p_3 & p_2 & p_1 \\ 0 & 0 & 0 & p_4 & p_3 \\ 0 & 0 & 0 & 0 & p_5 \end{vmatrix}$$

$$(85)$$

From the formulas Equation 85 it is obvious that, p_1, p_2, p_3 are of one and the same order of 1, and p_4 is small of 1-rst degree of ε. Moreover, p_5 is of 2-nd degree of ε.

On the above basis for p_i orders, we can do the following considerations:

(1) The first coefficient of Routh-Hurwitz D_1 is *evidently positive*.

(2) It is seen that in the second coefficient D_2, all terms of p_3 can be cancelled with corresponding terms in $p_1 p_2$. Thus D_2 is also *positive* and has an order of 1.

(3) For the coefficient D_3, from its definition formula in the paper, we obtain

$$D_3 = p_3 D_2 + p_1 p_5 - p_1^2 p_4. \quad (86)$$

In this formula, the negative term has an order ε, so it is essentially smaller than $p_3 D_2$, having order of 1. Thus D_3 *is positive* and has also an order of 1.

(4) From the corresponding definition formula of D_4 we obtain

$$D_4 = p_4 D_3 - p_2 p_5 D_2 \quad (87)$$

where in the right hand side, the first term is of order of ε and the second one is of order of ε^2. Thus D_4 *is positive*.

(5) For D_5, from its definition formula we can obtain $D_5 = p_4 p_5 D_3$ $D_5 = p_5 D_4$, so we conclude that D_5 *is positive*.

In this way we have proved *all Routh-Hurwitz coefficients are positive*. According to the well-known Routh-Hurwitz theorem (Bautin, 1984), the steady-state solution Equation 79 will be stable, which allows us to apply QSSA theorem. Corresponding to this theorem In (Nikolova et al., 2009b) the formulas Equation 79 are replaced in the equations of the degenerate system Equation 73 and 75. As a result the system of two independent equations is obtained:

$$\frac{dx_2}{dt} = -a_6 x_2 + \frac{\varepsilon^2 a_1}{\alpha_1^E}\left(a_5 - \frac{\varepsilon a_3 a_7 a_{15}}{a_{16}(\varepsilon a_4 + a_{17})}\right)$$
$$\frac{dx_4}{dt} = -a_{13} x_4 + \frac{\varepsilon^3 a_8}{\alpha_2^E}\left(a_{12} - \frac{\varepsilon a_{10} a_{14} a_{15}}{a_{16}(\varepsilon a_{11} + a_{18})}\right)$$

$$(88)$$

The variations about the equilibrium of x_1 and x_2 evidently tend asymptotically to zero.

Figure 15. Coincidence of the graphs of complete (--) and reduced (o) system variables

Figure 15. Coincidence of the graphs of complete (--) and reduced (o) system variables

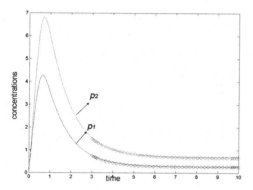

Figure 16. Growth of protein concentrations in a lack of miRNA production

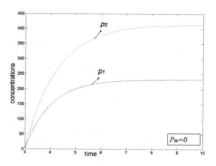

This means that the steady state solution of the degenerate system will be stable, too. Further, the substitutions (70-71) are replaced in Equation 88. As a result the original form of the reduced system is obtained:

$$\frac{dp_1}{dt} = -\delta_1^P p_1 + \frac{q_1 \delta_m (\beta_1^- + \delta_1^*)}{\delta_1 \delta_m (\beta_1^- + \delta_1^*) + \delta_1^* \beta_1 p_m}\left[\lambda_1 - \frac{\lambda_1^* \beta_1 p_m}{\delta_m (\beta_1^- + \delta_1^*)}\right]$$

$$\frac{dp_2}{dt} = -\delta_2^P p_2 + \frac{q_2 \delta_m (\beta_2^- + \delta_2^*)}{\delta_2 \delta_m (\beta_2^- + \delta_2^*) + \delta_2^* \beta_2 p_m}\left[\lambda_2 - \frac{\lambda_2^* \beta_2 p_m}{\delta_m (\beta_2^- + \delta_2^*)}\right]$$

$$(89)$$

Next the simulations of the complete and reduced systems are made. Figure 15 shows very good coincidence between both systems. after 3- th point, from the beginning of the process.

Finally it must mentioned, that from the last two equations, it follows a basic relationship: *The rates of protein production evidently decrease with the increasing constant rate production p_m of microRNA, what is not explicitly apparent in the kinetic system of equations in 65.* As it is seen from the right hand sides of Equation 89, in order to prove the last assertion it is essential to take into account that the inequalities $\lambda_i \gg \lambda_i^*$ $(i = 1, 2)$ are valid. As we already remembered, that means "the translation rate of the proteins from the complexes $miRNA \& m_i$

is sufficiently slower than the translation rate from free mRNAs (m_i)". From the relations in Equation 67 it also follows that such inequalities hold in our case indeed. So we can conclude that the applied QSSA reveals the basic property of the *miRNA* function in the context of model in 65.

The above formulated basic relationship is apparently demonstrated in the next Figures 16 and 17, where the time-behavior of protein synthesis is shown for two different values of *miRNA* production rate (p_m=0 and p_m=6). Namely at p_m=6 the proteins begin to decrease.

In order to reinforce the last results numerical simulations of protein dynamics are made at three different values of p_m. The Figures 18 and 19 show

Figure 17. Decay of protein concentrations in a presence of miRNA production

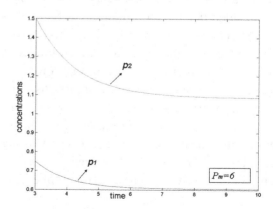

Figure 18. The behaviour of p_1 at three different values of p_m

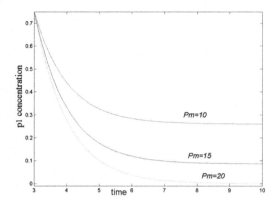

Figure 19. The behaviour of p_2 at three different values of p_m

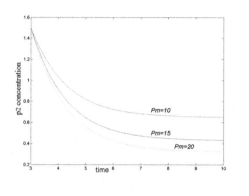

the rate of change of the concentrations of proteins p_1 and p_2, respectively at $p_m = 10, 15, 20$. It is evident that the protein concentrations essentially decrease with the increasing constant rate production p_m of miRNA, which confirms the theoretical conclusion made above. Moreover, as it can see from the Figure 7 at $p_m = 20$ the concentration of p_1 approaches zero values (about the 10-th time unit after beginning of the process). The last fact supposes that at such a value the miRNA target regulation will be the most successful.

CONCLUSION

The investigation in the last sections shows that, the considerations of time hierarchy in bimolecular interactions allow us to reduce the number of differential equations of a minimal model of miRNA target regulation, and to determine the independent (eventually - driving) reactions of the quasi-stationary genetic dynamics. For this purpose, the QSSA theorem for the quasi-stationary approximation (the replacement of fast varying variables by their steady state values in the equations for the slow varying ones) is applied. As

a result, the proteins, produced by mRNAs are identified to play an independent role in the dynamical behavior of the miRNA target regulation, but in post-initial (or quasi-stationary) stage as it was explained above. This independent role of protein synthesis is nevertheless parametrically controlled by the production rate of miRNAs in accordance with a basic relationship: *The rates of protein synthesis evidently decrease with the increasing constant rate production p_m of miRNA.* This conclusion is not explicitly included in the model [92], but can be derived by applying QSSA in the way shown in this investigation.

DISCUSSIONS AND UNRESOLVED PROBLEMS TO BE CONSIDERED IN THE FUTURE

To our knowledge, the biochemical pathway involving inhibitory mechanisms, feedback-loop control, cross-talk and threshold response are best investigated using the concepts and methodologies from dynamic systems theory. There are various examples in which a systems biology approach has been used to investigate the dynamical properties of the p53 pathway in context of tumor suppression and non-telomeric stress signals (Wienholds et al., 2005; Wheeler et al., 2006). However, there are no major efforts done in the mathematical modeling of the p16 pathway and the interaction between both pathways. The following questions will be considered in the future:

1. The first essential problem is to elucidate the critical intervals of values for the parameters of the models characterizing the response of the system under tumor suppression and tissue regeneration. These conditions in the proposal will be determined using elements of the systems theory, i.e. bifurcation analysis.

2. On the basis of the as made analysis of the art, the project includes investigation of microRNA regulation of cancer networks (for example, miRNA-17-92, E2F and Myc which is part of the mammalian G1-S regulatory network) and cell signaling of the link between cancer and aging with the development of methodologies for qualitative analysis of cell signaling models based on global sensitivity analysis, bifurcation analysis and mathematical controlled comparisons.

3. Concerning the somitogenesis, given the recent findings, it is necessary to argue the need of incorporating miRNAs into appropriate mathematical models of gene expression during embryo segmentation process, to explain how the temporal oscillations in PSM can be transformed into spatial formations of somites.

4. On the basis of miRNAs post-binding to mRNA bi-stability effects, connected with the mutual inhibition of RA and FGF and provided by molecular mechanism for the "all-or-none" transitions, a possibly more extended cell polarization model of morphogenesis needs to be elaborated and analysed in this project.

Our impression is that recently various mathematical models of a RNA silencing have been proposed with a goal to understand biological processes that are regulated by the dynamical properties of mRNA. To our knowledge, there are only a few published mathematical models of studies looking at the kinetics of the intracellular microRNAs processes. None of these models has combined the delivery process and the interaction with the RNAi machinery in mammalian cells. As most genetic regulatory networks of interest involve many components, an intuitive understanding of their dynamical behavior is hard to obtain. Nevertheless this difficulty, an enlightening the problems more in detail would be of use for the future development of this chapter.

ACKNOWLEDGMENT

This work was partially supported by ESF, OP Human Resources Development, grant No. BG051PO001/07/3.3–02–55/17.06.2008 and DAAD-Bulgarian National Science Fund project DOO02-23/05.03.2009

REFERENCES

Aguda, B., Kim, Y., Piper-Hunter, M., Friedman, A., & Marsh, C. (2008). MicroRNA regulation of a cancer network: Consequences of the feedback loops involving miR-17-92, E2F, and Myc. [PNAS]. *Proceedings of the National Academy of Sciences of the United States of America, 105*(50), 19678–19683. doi:10.1073/pnas.0811166106

Alberty, R. A. (1959). The rate equation for an enzymatic reaction. In Boyer, P. (Eds.), *Kinetics, thermodynamics, mechanisms and basic properties. The enzymes* (pp. 143–155). New York: Academic Press.

Alvarez-Garcia, I., & Miska, E. A. (2006). MicroRNA functions in animal development and human disease. *Development, 132*, 4653–4662. doi:10.1242/dev.02073

Ambros, V. (2004). The functions of animal microRNAs. *Nature, 431*, 350–355. doi:10.1038/nature02871

Aronson, D. G., & Weinberger, H. F. (1975). *Nonlinear diffusion in population genetics, combustion, and nerve pulse propagation*. New York: Springer–Verlag.

Aulehla, A., & Pourquie, O. (2006). On periodicity and directionality of somitogenesis. *Anatomy and Embryology, 211*(7), 3–8. doi:10.1007/s00429-006-0124-y

Bartel, D. (2004). MicroRNAs: Genomics, biogenesis, mechanism and function. *Cell, 116*, 281–297. doi:10.1016/S0092-8674(04)00045-5

Bautin, N. N. (1984). *Povedenie dinamichnih sistem v blizi granits oblasti ustoichivisti*. Nauka, Moskva.

Belintsev, B. N., Beloussov, L. V., & Zarayski, A. G. (1985). Model of epithelial morphogenesis basing on the elastic forces and contact polarization of cells. *Ontogenesis, 16*(1), 5–13.

Belintsev, B. N., Beloussov, L. V., & Zarayski, A. G. (1987). Model of pattern formation in epithelial morphogenesis. *Journal of Theoretical Biology, 129*, 369–394. doi:10.1016/S0022-5193(87)80019-X

Beloussov, L. V. (2001). Somitogenesis in vertebrate embryos as a robust macromorphological process. In Sanders, E. J. (Ed.), *The origin and fate of somites*. IOS Press.

Bilder, D. (2004). Epithelial polarity and proliferation control: Links from the Drosophila neoplastic tumor suppressors. *Genes & Development, 18*, 1909–1925. doi:10.1101/gad.1211604

Bruewer, M., Hopkins, A. M., & Nusrat, A. (2003). Proinflammatory cytokines disrupt epithelial barrier function by apoptosis-independent mechanisms. *Journal of Immunology (Baltimore, MD.: 1950), 171*, 6164–6172.

Cai, X., Hagedorn, C., & Cullen, B. (2004). Human microRNAs are processed from capped, polyadenylated transcripts that can also function as mRNAs. *RNA (New York, N.Y.), 10*, 1957–1966. doi:10.1261/rna.7135204

Calin, G., & Croce, C. (2006). MicroRNA signatures in human cancer. *Nature Reviews. Cancer, 6*, 259–269. doi:10.1038/nrc1997

Carthew, R. (2006). Gene regulation by microRNAs. *Current Opinion in Genetics & Development, 16*(2), 203–208. doi:10.1016/j.gde.2006.02.012

Chen, K., & Rajewsky, N. (2007). The evolution of gene regulation by transcription factors and microRNAs. *Nature Reviews. Genetics, 8*(2), 93–103. doi:10.1038/nrg1990

Deborde, S., Perret, E., Gravotta, D., Deora, A., Salvarezza, S., & Sch, R. (2008). Clathrin is a key regulator of basolateral polarity. *Nature, 452*, 719–723. doi:10.1038/nature06828

Doench, J., & Sharp, P. (2004). Specificity of microRNA target selection in translational repression. *Genes & Development, 16*(1), 504–511. doi:10.1101/gad.1184404

Duggleby, R. G. (1994). Product inhibition of reversible enzyme-catalized reactions. *Biochimica et Biophysica Acta, 1209*, 238–240. doi:10.1016/0167-4838(94)90190-2

Esquela-Kerscher, A., & Clack, F. (2006). Oncomirs: MicroRNAs with a role in cancer. *Nature Reviews. Cancer, 6*, 259–269. doi:10.1038/nrc1840

Fall, C. P., Marland, E. S., Wagner, J. M., & Tyson, J. J. (2002). *Computational cell biology*. New York: Springer-Verlag.

Faller, M., Matsunaga, M., Yin, S., Loo, J., & Guo, F. (2007). Heme is involved in microRNA processing. *Nature Structural & Molecular Biology, 14*(1), 23–29. doi:10.1038/nsmb1182

Fife, P. C., & McLeod, J. B. (1977). The approach of solutions of nonlinear diffusion equations to traveling front solutions. *Archive for Rational Mechanics and Analysis, 65*, 335–361. doi:10.1007/BF00250432

Fire, A., Hu, S., Mongomery, M. K., Kostas, S. A., Driver, S. E., & Mello, C. C. (1998). Potent and specific genetic interference by double-stranded RNA in Caenorhabditis elegans. *Nature, 391*, 806–811. doi:10.1038/35888

Flynt, A. S., Li, N., Thatcher, E. J., Solica-Krezel, L., & Patton, J. G. (2007). Zebrafish miR-214 modulates hedgehog signaling to specify muscle cell fate. *Nature Genetics, 39*(2), 259–263. doi:10.1038/ng1953

Goldbeter, A., Gonze, D., & Pourquie, O. (2007). Sharp developmental thresholds defined through bistability by antagonistic gradients of retinoic acid and FGF signaling. *Developmental Dynamics, 236*, 1495–1508. doi:10.1002/dvdy.21193

Gusev, V. (2008). Computational methods for analysis of cellular functions and pathways collectively targeted by differentially expressed microRNA. *Methods (San Diego, Calif.), 44*, 61–72. doi:10.1016/j.ymeth.2007.10.005

Hirata, H., Bessho, Y., Kokubu, H., Mazamizu, Y., Yamada, S., & Lewis, J. (2004). Instability of Hes7 protein is critical for the somite segmentation clock. *Nature Genetics, 36*, 750–754. doi:10.1038/ng1372

Hirata, H., Yoshiura, S., Ohtsuka, T., Bessho, Y., Harada, T., & Yoshikawa, K. (2002). Oscillatory expression of the bHLH factor Hes1 regulated by a negative feedback loop. *Science, 298*, 840–843. doi:10.1126/science.1074560

Jiang, J., Lee, E., & Schmittgen, T. (2006). Increased expression of microRNA-155 in Epstein-Barr virus transformed lymphoblastiodcell lines. *Genes, Chromosomes & Cancer, 45*, 103–106. doi:10.1002/gcc.20264

Keener, J., & Sneyd, J. (1998). *Mathematical physiology*. New York: Springer.

Khanin, R., & Higham, D. J. (2007). *A minimal mathematical model of post-transcriptional gene regulation by microRNAs.* Report to Glasgow University.

Khanin, R., & Vinciotti, V. (2008). Computational modelling of post-transcriptional gene regulation by microRNAs. *Journal of Computational Biology, 15*(3), 305–316. doi:10.1089/cmb.2007.0184

Krek, A., Grun, D., Poy, M. N., Woff, R., Roseberg, L., & Epstein, E. J. (2005). Combinatorial microRNA target predictions. *Nature Genetics, 37*, 495–500. doi:10.1038/ng1536

Lee, E., Myungwon, B., Gusev, Y., Brackett, D. J., Nuovo, G. J., & Schmittgen, T. D. (2008). Systematic evolution of microRNA processing patterns in tissues, cell lines, and tumors. *RNA (New York, N.Y.), 14*, 35–42. doi:10.1261/rna.804508

Lee, M., & Vasioukhin, V. (2008). Cell polarity and cancer-cell and tissue polarity as a non-canonical tumor suppressor. *Journal of Cell Science, 121*, 1141–1150. doi:10.1242/jcs.016634

Lee, Y., Kim, M., Han, J., Yeom, K. H., Lee, S., & Baek, S. H. (2004). MicroRNA genes are transcribed by RNA polymerase II. *The EMBO Journal, 23*(20), 4051–4060. doi:10.1038/sj.emboj.7600385

Levine, E., Ben Jacob, E., & Levine, H. (2007). Target-specific and global effectors in gene regulation by microRNA. *Biophysical Journal, 93*(11), L52–L54. doi:10.1529/biophysj.107.118448

Lewis, B., Burge, C., & Bartel, D. (2005). Conserved seed pairing, often flanked by adenosines, indicates that thousands of human genes are microRNA targets. *Cell, 120*, 15–20. doi:10.1016/j.cell.2004.12.035

Lewis, J. (2003). Autoinhibition with transcriptional delay: A simple mechanism for the zebrafish somitogenesis oscillator. *Current Biology, 19*, 1398–1408. doi:10.1016/S0960-9822(03)00534-7

Margolis, B., & Borg, J. P. (2005). Apicobasal polarity complexes. *Journal of Cell Science, 118*, 5157–5159. doi:10.1242/jcs.02597

Maziere, P., & Enright, A. (2007). Prediction of mictoRNA targets. *Drug Discovery Today, 12*, 452–458. doi:10.1016/j.drudis.2007.04.002

Mitchell, P., Parkin, R., Kroh, E., Fritz, B., Wimen, S., & Pogosova-Agadjanyan, E. (2008). Circulating microRNAs as stable blood-based markers for cancer detection. [PNAS]. *Proceedings of the National Academy of Sciences of the United States of America, 105*(30), 10513–10518. doi:10.1073/pnas.0804549105

Monk, N. A. (2003). Oscillatory expression of Hes1, p53, and NF-kappaB driven by transcriptional time delays. *Current Biology, 13*, 1409–1413. doi:10.1016/S0960-9822(03)00494-9

Nandi, A., Vaz, C., Bhattacharya, A., & Ramaswamy, R. (2008). MiRNA-regulated dynamics in circadian oscillator models. *RNA (New York, N.Y.), 14*, 1480–1491.

Nikolov, S., Vera, J., Herwig, R., Wolkenhauer, O. & Petrov, V. (2010). Dynamics of microRNA regulation of a cancer network, *Comptes rendus de l'Academie bulgare des Sciences, 63*(1), 61-70.

Nikolova, E., Herwig, R., & Petrov, V. (2009a). Quasi-stationary approximation of a dynamical model of microRNA target regulation. Part I. Establishment of time hierarchy in the model dynamics. *International Journal Bioautomation, 13*(4), 127–134.

Nikolova, E., Herwig, R., & Petrov, V. (2009b). Quasi-stationary approximation of a dynamical model of microRNA target regulation. Part II. Application of the QSSA theorem. *International Journal Bioautomation, 13*(4), 135–142.

Nissan, T., & Parker, R. (2008). Computational analysis of miRNA-mediated repression of translation: Implications for models of translation initiation inhibition. *RNA (New York, N.Y.), 14*, 1480–1491. doi:10.1261/rna.1072808

Palmeirim, I., Henrique, D., Ish-Horowicz, D., & Pourquie, O. (1997). Avian hairy gene expression identifies a molecular clock linked to vertebrate segmentation and somitogenesis. *Cell, 91*, 639–648. doi:10.1016/S0092-8674(00)80451-1

Petersen, C., Bordelean, M., Pelletier, J., & Sharp, P. (2006). Short RNAs repress translation after initiation in mammalian cells. *Molecular Cell, 21*, 533–542. doi:10.1016/j.molcel.2006.01.031

Petrov, V., Nikolova, E., & Timmer, J. (2004). Dynamical analysis of cell function models. A review. *Journal of Theoretical Applied Mechanics, 34*(3), 55–78.

Petrov, V., Nikolova, E., & Wolkenhauer, O. (2007). Reduction of nonlinear dynamic system with an application to signal transduction pathways. *IET Systems Biology, 1*, 2–9. doi:10.1049/iet-syb:20050030

Petrov, V., & Timmer, J. (2009). One-dimensional model of somitic cells polarization in a bistability window of embryonic mesoderm. *Journal of Mechanics in Medicine and Biology, 9*, 359–272. doi:10.1142/S0219519409003061

Piriyapongsa, J., & King Jordan, I. (2008). Dual coding of siRNAs and miRNAs by plant transposable elements. *RNA (New York, N.Y.), 14*, 814–821. doi:10.1261/rna.916708

Plasterk, R. (2002). RNA silencing: The genome's immune system. *Science, 296*(5571), 1263–1265. doi:10.1126/science.1072148

Rajewsky, N. (2006). MicroRNA target predictions in animals. *Nature Genetics, 38*, S8–S13. doi:10.1038/ng1798

Romanovskii, U. M., Stepanova, N. V., & Chernavskii, D. S. (1975). *Matematicheskoe modelirovanie v biofizike*. Nauka, Moskva.

Schmittgen, T., Jiang, J., Lin, Q., & Yang, L. (2004). A high-throughput method to monitor the expression of microRNA precursors. *Nucleic Acids Research, 32*, E43. doi:10.1093/nar/gnh040

Schneider, K. R., & Wilhelm, T. (2000). Model reduction by extended quasi-steady-state approximation. *Journal of Mathematical Biology, 40*, 443–450. doi:10.1007/s002850000026

Sellin, S., & Mannervik, B. (1983). Reversal of the reaction catalyzed by glyoxalase I: Calculation of the equilibrium constant for the enzymatic reaction. *The Journal of Biological Chemistry, 258*, 8872–8875.

Stark, A., Brennecke, J., Bushati, N., Russel, R. B., & Cohen, S. M. (2005). Animal microRNAs confer robustness to gene expression and have a significant impact on 3'UTR evolution. *Cell, 123*, 1133–1146. doi:10.1016/j.cell.2005.11.023

Suzuki, A., & Ohno, S. (2006). The PAR-aPKS system: Lessons in polarity. *Journal of Cell Science, 119*, 979–987. doi:10.1242/jcs.02898

Sweetman, D., Rathjen, T., Jefferson, M., Wheeler, G., Smith, T. G., & Wheeler, G. N. (2006). FGF-4 signaling is involved in mir-206 expression in developing somites of chicken embryos. *Developmental Dynamics, 235*, 2185–2191. doi:10.1002/dvdy.20881

Thomson, J., Newman, M., Parker, J., Morin-Kensicki, E. M., Wright, T., & Hammond, S. M. (2006). Extensive post-transcriptional regulation of microRNAs and its implications for cancer. *Genes & Development, 20*, 2202–2207. doi:10.1101/gad.1444406

Tichonov, A.N. (1952) Systemy differentsialnyh uravneniy, soderjashchie malye parametry pri proizvodnyh. *Matematicheskiy sbornik, 31*(3), 575-586.

Tsuchiya, S., Oku, M., Imanaka, Y., Kunimoto, R., Okuno, Y., & Terasawa, K. (2009). MicroRNA-338-3p and microRNA-451 contribute to the formation of basolateral polarity in epithelial cells. *Nucleic Acids Research, 37*(11), 3821–3827. doi:10.1093/nar/gkp255

Tzafriri, A. R., & Edelman, E. R. (2004). The total quasi-state-approximation is valid for reversible enzyme kinetics. *Journal of Theoretical Biology, 226*, 303–313. doi:10.1016/j.jtbi.2003.09.006

Utech, M., Ivanov, A. I., Samarin, S. N., Bruewer, M., Turner, J. R., & Mrsny, R. J. (2005). Mechanism of IFN-gamma-induced endocytosis of tight junction proteins: Myosin II-dependent vacuolarization of the apical plasma membrane. *Molecular Biology of the Cell, 16*, 5040–5052. doi:10.1091/mbc.E05-03-0193

Wakiyama, M., Takimoto, K., Ohara, O., & Yokoyama, K. (2007). Let-7 microRNA-mediated mRNA deadenylation and translational repression in a mammalian cell-free system. *Genes & Development, 21*, 857–1862. doi:10.1101/gad.1566707

Watanabe, Y., Tonita, M., & Kanai, A. (2007). Computational methods for microRNA target prediction. *Methods in Enzymology, 427*, 65–86. doi:10.1016/S0076-6879(07)27004-1

Waterhouse, P., Wang, M., & Lough, T. (2001). Gene silencing as an adaptive defence against viruses. *Nature, 411*, 834–842. doi:10.1038/35081168

Wheeler, G., Ntounia-Fousara, S., Granda, B., Rathjen, T., & Dalmay, T. (2006). Identification of new central nervous system specific mouse microRNAs. *FEBS Letters, 580*, 2195–2200. doi:10.1016/j.febslet.2006.03.019

Wienholds, E., Kloosterman, W., Miska, E., Alvarez-Saavedra, E., Berezikov, E., & de Bruijn, E. (2005). MicroRNA expression in zebrafish embrionic development. *Science, 309*, 310–311. doi:10.1126/science.1114519

Witze, E. S., Litman, E. S., Argast, G. M., Moon, R. T., & Ahn, N. G. (2008). Wnt5a control of cell polarity and directional movement by polarized redistribution of adhesion receptors. *Science, 320*, 365–369. doi:10.1126/science.1151250

Wodarz, A. (2005). Molecular control of cell polarity and asymmetric cell division in Drosophila neuroblasts. *Current Opinion in Cell Biology, 17*, 475–481. doi:10.1016/j.ceb.2005.08.005

Wolff, C., Roy, S., & Ingham, P. W. (2003). Multiple muscle cell identities induced by distinct levels and timing of hedgehog activity in the zebrafish embryo. *Current Biology, 13*(14), 1169–1181. doi:10.1016/S0960-9822(03)00461-5

Xi, Y., Nakajima, G., Gavin, E., Morris, K. K., Hayashi, K., & Ju, J. (2007). Systematic analysis of microRNA expression of RNA extracted from fresh frozen and formalin-fixed paraffin-embedded samples. *RNA (New York, N.Y.), 13*, 1668–1674. doi:10.1261/rna.642907

Xie, Zh., Yang, H., Liu, W., & Hwang, M. (2007). The role of microRNA in the delayed negative feedback regulation of gene expression. [BBRC]. *Biochemical and Biophysical Research Communications, 358*, 722–726. doi:10.1016/j.bbrc.2007.04.207

Xu, J., & Wong, Ch. (2008). A computational screen for mouse signalling pathways targeted by microRNA clusters. *RNA (New York, N.Y.), 14*, 1276–1283. doi:10.1261/rna.997708

KEY TERMS AND DEFINITIONS

Andronov-Hopf Bifurcation: From a mathematical point of view, the onset of sustained oscillations generally correspond to the passage through an Andronov-Hopf bifurcation point. Obviously, for a critical value of a control parameter (named bifurcation), the system displays damped oscillations and eventually reaches the steady state- stable focus. Beyond the bifurcation point, a stable solution arises in the form of a small-amplitude limit cycle surrounding the unstable steady state [Golbeter, A., Nature, 420:238-245, 2002]. This bifurcation is very typical for biological systems.

E2Fs: A group of genes that codifies a family of transcription factors (TF) in higher eukaryotes. Three of them are activators: E2F1,2 and E2F3a. Six others act as suppressors: E2F3b, E2F4-8. All of them are involved in the cell cycle regulation and synthesis of DNA in mammalian cells.

mRNA (Messenger RiboNucleic Acid): A molecule of RNA encoding a chemical "blueprint" for a protein product. mRNA is transcribed from a DNA template, and carries coding information to the sites of protein synthesis: the ribosomes.

microRNA: Short ~22 nucleotide RNA sequences that bind to complementary sequences in the 3' UTR of multiple target mRNAs, usually resulting in their silencing.

Myc: A gene encodes for a transcription factor that is believed to regulate expression of 15% of all genes, i.e. it codes for a protein that binds to the DNA of other genes. When Myc is mutated, or overexpressed, the protein doesn't bind correctly, and often causes cancer.

Polarization (Waves): Orientation of oscillations in the plane perpendicular to a transversal wave's direction of travel.

Somite: A division of the body of an animal. In vertebrates this is mainly discernible in the embryo stage, in arthropods it is a characteristic of a hypothetical ancestor.

Somitogenesis: A: process by which somites are produced. These segmented tissue blocks differentiate into skeletal muscle, vertebrae, and dermis of all vertebrates.

Time Delay: Past memory (history).

ENDNOTE

[1] This work was supported by DAAD-Bulgarian National Science Fund project DO02-23/05.03.2009 and by ESF, OP Human Resources Development grant No BG-051PO001/07/3.3-02.55/17.06.2008.

Chapter 9
Machine Learning for Clinical Data Processing

Guo-Zheng Li
Tongji University, China

ABSTRACT

This chapter introduces great challenges and the novel machine learning techniques employed in clinical data processing. It argues that the novel machine learning techniques including support vector machines, ensemble learning, feature selection, feature reuse by using multi-task learning, and multi-label learning provide potentially more substantive solutions for decision support and clinical data analysis. The authors demonstrate the generalization performance of the novel machine learning techniques on real world data sets including one data set of brain glioma, one data set of coronary heart disease in Chinese Medicine and some tumor data sets of microarray. More and more machine learning techniques will be developed to improve analysis precision of clinical data sets.

INTRODUCTION

Clinical data has increased dramatically with the rapid development of computing technology, which produces great need from intelligent techniques, especially novel machine learning techniques. During clinical data processing, there are great challenges to face for machine learning researchers:

- There are complex structures in the clinical data sets, e.g. for a patient, if he feel Stomachache, we need to record when, where and how he felt. In current data sets, we often ignore some of the elements like the exact occasion, which hurt the decision support from intelligent techniques, since different moments may imply different causes.
- The data set is in sparse representation, when there are many symptoms to describe

DOI: 10.4018/978-1-60960-483-7.ch009

one disease. We use some symptoms to describe some patients, while others to describe others. Sparse representation makes the features be high dimensional, while the samples be few, which hurts the modeling of machine learning techniques.

- The data sets are small sample due to the cost. Though support vector machines are developed to overcome this problem, but there is still a gap between the machine learning techniques with the human experience. Human doctors infer experience from only one or a few cases, while computer cannot. Computers make errors when there are only few cases due to the the law of large numbers.

- There are imbalanced problems between the positive class and the negative one. We often focus on positives, but they are often less than negatives. Computers often biases to the bigger class, i.e. the negative. This hurts the generalization performance and reduces the forecast accuracy of positive cases.

- There are noise and bias in the existing cases. We know different clinicians may produce different judgments on one patient, so what we collected may not objective, which also hurts the modeling of these applications.

- There are many classes or labels for one case, i.e. one patient may have two more diseases. This is also a challenge for machine learning techniques; the existing techniques are excellent on binary classification. Novel techniques are needed to develop to solve different problems.

- Understanding needs to be improved in the existing techniques, we not only need high forecast accuracy, we also want to know why the techniques produce such results, we need to interpret the results and the intrinsic principles behind the problem. Unfortunately, most of the popular ma-

chine learning techniques is black box; this may need further works for machine learning researchers after they developed good techniques with high performance.

To face the above challenges in clinical data processing, this chapter describes the novel techniques of support vector machines, ensemble learning, feature selection, multi-label learning and feature reuse by using multi-task learning. Applications include degree forecast of brain glioma, syndrome classification of inquiry diagnosis for coronary heart disease in Chinese medicine and tumor classification of microarray data sets.

Support vector machines (SVMs) are excellent in solving small sample problems (Boser, Guyon, & Vapnik, 1992; Vapnik, 1995). Since 1990s, they have developed rapidly and reached state-of-the-art performance in small sample problems (Cristianini & Shawe-Taylor, 2000; Chen, Lu, Yang, & Li, 2004). Compared to artificial neural networks (ANNs), SVMs have better generalization performance and can obtain a global optimal solution. At the same time, a type of feature selection algorithms based on SVMs named embedded algorithms has been proposed (Li, Yang, Liu & Xue, 2004; Lal, Chapelle, Weston & Elisseeff, 2006; Li, Meng, Yang & Yang, 2009) to solve the problems involving many irrelevant and redundant features such as symptom selection and tumor categorization. These embedded algorithms are designed to select features efficiently, but, compared to wrapper methods (Kohavi & George, 1997) the accuracy is sacrificed in some degree. Furthermore, subset generation methods used in most embedded algorithms are methods like sequential backward feature selection which cannot effectively handle combined features in the feature selection procedure.

In the literature, floating search (Pudil, Novovicova & Kittler, 1994) which is a heuristic feature subset generation algorithm, has been proved one of the best subset generation algorithms (Jain & Zongker, 1997; Kudo & Sklansky, 2000) when the training sample is comparatively small. At the same time, the wrapper method (Kohavi & George, 1997) which is optimal to specific learning machine can get better performance than filter methods and embedded methods such as recursive feature elimination. Since the medical data sets are comparatively small, combining floating search with wrapper based on SVMs is proper for clinical data processing, which are demonstrated on a glioma data set in this chapter.

Ensemble learning methods are excellent in processing the noise and bias in the data sets, which is popular in the present machine learning field. In general, an ensemble is built in two steps, that is, training multiple component learners and then combining their forecasts. According to the styles of training the component learners, current ensemble algorithms are roughly categorized into two classes, that is, algorithms where component learners could be trained in parallel, or algorithms where component learners must be trained sequentially. The representative of the first category is Bagging (Breiman, 1996), which utilizes bootstrap sampling to generate multiple training sets from the original training set and then trains a learner from each generated training set. The representative of the second category is AdaBoost (Bauer & Kohavi, 1999). It sequentially generates a series of component learners where the training instances that are wrongly forecasted by a component learner play a more important role in the training of its subsequent learner. It is worth mentioning that after obtaining multiple learners, most ensemble algorithms employ all of them to constitute an ensemble. Although such a scheme works well, recently Zhou, Wu, and Tang (2002) showed it may be better to ensemble some instead of all of them. They proposed an algorithm named GASEN, i.e. Genetic Algorithm based Selective ENsemble, which trains several individual neural networks and then employs genetic algorithm to select an optimum subset of individual neural networks to constitute an ensemble. Experiments

show the performance of GASEN is excellent by using different learning machines.

GASEN uses genetic algorithm as an individual selection method, whose computational complexity is $O(2^n)$, n is the number of individuals, therefore, GASEN need much computation capacity. In the model selection methods, clustering algorithm can effectively eliminate the redundancy individuals (Mitra, Murthy & Pal, 2002), whose computational complexity is $O(n^2)$. It is much lower than that of genetic algorithm. This chapter proposes a clustering algorithm based selective ensemble method (CLUSEN) and employ it to forecast the degree of malignancy in brain glioma.

Feature selection is excellent in treat data sets with high dimensional features, which chooses a subset of the original features according to the classification performance, whose optimal subset should contain relevant but non-redundant features. Feature selection helps to improve the generalization performance of classifiers, and to reduce learning time. There have been a great deal of works in machine learning and related areas to address this issue (H. Liu & Yu, 2005). In most practical cases, relevant features are selected and kept as input, while irrelevant and redundant features are removed. Although the removed features are redundant and weakly relevant, they contain useful information that may be used to improve forecast accuracy. Therefore, redundant feature reuse is proposed, where Multi-Task Learning (MTL) is a method of using the redundant information by selecting features from the discarded feature set to add to the target (Caruana & Sa, 2003). Although MTL achieves only limited improvement, it is nevertheless useful for real world cases like medical problems and multivariate calibration problems (Li, Yang, Lu, Lu & Chen, 2004; J. Y. Yang, Li, Meng & Yang, 2008).

Previous studies of search methods for multi-task learning mainly used heuristic methods (Caruana & Sa, 2003; Li, Yang, Lu, et al., 2004), where the number of features selected for the input and/or target is somewhat arbitrary. When the search method is regarded as a combinational optimization problem, random search may be used. The genetic algorithm (Goldberg, 1998) is a simple and powerful method which has obtained satisfactory results for feature selection (J. Yang & Honavar, 1998). Motivated by this, we proposed the random method GA-MTL (Genetic Algorithm based Multi-Task Learning) (Li & Liu, 2006), but GA-MTL did not consider irrelevant features in the data sets. Here we propose an enhanced version of GA-MTL (e-GA-MTL) which codes one feature with two binary bits. The e-GA-MTL algorithm and others are applied to tumor classification on microarray data sets, which will be presented in this chapter.

The degree of malignancy in brain glioma decides the treatment, because if it is grade I or II according to Kernohan, the success rate of operation is satisfactory; otherwise, if it is grade III or IV, there is a high surgical risk and poor life quality (Wang, Zhang, Liu, Sun, & Zhao, 2000) after surgery which must be taken into account before any further decision. Now, the degree of malignancy is forecasted mainly by Magnetic Resonance Imaging (MRI) findings and clinical data before operations. Some features obtained manually are fuzzy values; some features are redundant, even irrelevant, which makes the forecast of the degree of malignancy a hard task. Moreover, brain glioma is severe but infrequent and only a small number of neuroradiologists have the chances to accumulate enough experiences to make correct judgments. On this data set, Ye, Yang, Geng, Zhou, and Chen (2002) proposed a fuzzy rule extraction algorithm based on fuzzy min-max neural networks (FMMNN-FRE), although the rules are few and easy to understand, the accuracy of FMMNN-FRE was not better than that of ANNs. Furthermore, Li, Yang, Ye, and Geng (2006) employed SVMs to improve forecast accuracy, and obtained satisfactory results. Bagging of ANNs and SVMs has been combined with feature selection to solve degree forecast of brain glioma (Li, Liu, & Cheng, 2006;

T.-Y. Liu, Li, & Wu, 2006; J. Y. Yang, Li, Liu, & Yang, 2007; Li & Yang, 2008). This chapter will present the results by using SVMs and the novel algorithm CLUSEN.

Tumor classification is performed on microarray data collected by DNA microarray experiments from tissue and cell samples (Golub et al., 1999a; Alon, 1999; Dudoit, Fridlyand, & Speed, 2002). The wealth of such data for different stages of the cell cycle aids in the exploration of gene interactions and in the discovery of gene functions. Moreover, genome-wide expression data from tumor tissues gives insight into the variation of gene expression across tumor types, thus providing clues for tumor classification of individual samples. A lot of machine learning techniques have been employed to improve forecast accuracy of tumor classification including SVMs, ensemble learning (Li & Liu, 2006), feature extraction (Zeng, Li, Wu, Yang, & Yang, 2009b, 2009a; Li, Bu, Yang, Zeng, & Yang, 2008; Li & Zeng, 2009) and feature selection (Zeng, Li, Yang, Yang, & Wu, 2008). Here in this chapter, feature (gene) reuse by using multi-task learning to improve generalization performance of classification techniques will be described.

In this chapter we will introduce our works on medical data processing by using novel machine learning techniques; we focus on how to improve their generalization performance and partly to understand the medical problem. Support vector machines, ensemble learning, multi-label learning, feature selection and reuse will be described and demonstrated on brain glioma data sets and tumor data sets of microarray.

Support Vector Machines

Computational Methods

Support vector machines (SVMs) are state-of-arts techniques in handling small-sample data sets (Boser et al., 1992; Vapnik, 1995; Chen et al., 2004). So they are powerful tools to treat medical problems especially the clinical ones, which are often in limited cases due to the cost. In the medical data sets, there are irrelevant and redundant features, which hurt the generalization performance of learning machines. Therefore, the wrapper model based on SVMs and backward floating search are combined to select relevant features to perform tumor classification, the former is used as feature subset evaluation, and the latter is as feature subset generation (Li, Yang, et al., 2006).

We firstly introduce the techniques of SVMs. Denoting the training sample as $D = \{(\mathbf{x}, \mathbf{y})\} \subseteq \{R^n \times \{-1, 1\}\}^{\ell}$, SVMs discriminant hyperplane is written as

$$y = \text{sgn}(\langle \mathbf{w} \cdot \mathbf{x} \rangle + b)$$

where $\mathbf{w}$ is a weight vector, b is a bias. According to the generalization bound in statistical learning theory (Vapnik, 1995), we need to minimize the following objective function for a 2-norm soft margin version of SVMs

$$\text{minimize } \mathbf{w}, b \, \langle \mathbf{w} \cdot \mathbf{w} \rangle + C \sum_{i=1}^{\ell} (\xi_i)^2$$

$$\text{subject to } y_i(\langle \mathbf{w} \cdot \mathbf{x}_i \rangle + b) \geq 1 - \xi_i, i = 1, ..., \ell, \tag{1}$$

in which, slack variable ξ_i is introduced when the problem is infeasible. The constant $C > 0$ is a penalty parameter; a larger C corresponds to assigning a larger penalty to errors.

By building a Lagrangian and using the Karush-Kuhn-Tucker (KKT) complementarity conditions (Karush, 1939; Kuhn & Tucker, 1951), we obtain the value of optimization problem (1). Because of the KKT conditions, only those Lagrangian multipliers, α_is, which make the constraint active are non zeros, we denote these points corresponding to the non zero α_is as *support vectors* (sv). Therefore

we can describe the classification hyperplane in terms of α and b:

$$y = \text{sgn}\left(\sum_{i \in sv} \alpha_i \langle \mathbf{x}_i \cdot \mathbf{x} \rangle + b\right).$$

Though SVMs achieve high generalization performance, irrelevant and redundant features hurt their performance. Feature selection is needed to select relevant features for further classification. In this chapter, the wrapper model (Kohavi & George, 1997) which utilizes the forecast ability of specific learning machine is used to evaluate the feature subset. Compared to the filter (H. Liu & Yu, 2005) and embedded models (Li, Yang, Liu, & Xue, 2004; Li et al., 2009; Guyon, Gunn, Nikravesh, & Zadeh, 2006), the wrapper model tends to obtain a feature subset with higher accuracy measured by the used learning algorithm. It is defined as

$$W = R_{acc}(D_w)$$

where D_w is a feature subset candidate, and *Racc* is calculated by 10-fold cross validation. For the training sample D, *Racc* is defined as:

$$R_{acc} = \frac{1}{\ell} \sum_{j=1}^{\ell} (\tilde{y}_j == y_j)$$

where ℓ is the number of training examples, $\tilde{y}_j$ is the forecasted value by the used learning machines, like SVMs in this work. The feature subset corresponding to the largest W is the most significant one.

Backward floating search (BFS) (Pudil et al., 1994) is a feature subset generation method, and has been proved to be one of the best subset generation algorithms (Jain & Zongker, 1997; Kudo & Sklansky, 2000). In this work, we combine BFS with wrapper based on SVMs and name it

Algorithm 1. The SVM-BFS algorithm

1: **Begin**

2: *Initialization*, it uses SBS to reduce the least two important features and sets the value for the current number and the target number of features, since we want to eliminate the features from the maximum to 1, we set the target number is 1.

3: *Exclusion*, it uses the basic SBS method to remove the feature. In BFS this step is the main module.

4: *Conditional inclusion*, it finds the most significant feature among the excluded features, if it is not the feature just eliminated, the basic SFS method is used to add it.

5: *Continuation of conditional inclusion*. it continues to find the most significant feature among the excluded features with respect to the subset obtained in Step 4, if *Racc* of the subset is no higher than that of any other subset with the same number of features, then goto Step 3; otherwise, repeat Step 5.

6: *Display*, if the number of current subset is greater than the target number, go to Step 3; otherwise, display the optimal feature subset and the merit of subsets with different number of features.

7: **End**

---

as SVM-BFS. Motivation of this approach is to meet the need of high forecast accuracy and strong comprehensibility. SVM-BFS shown in Algorithm 1 is based on sequential backward search (SBS) and sequential forward search (SFS), of which SBS eliminates the least important feature one by one, while SFS adds the most important feature one by one.

Results on Brain Glioma

On the brain glioma data set we perform the SVM-BFS algorithm presented in the above subsection. Firstly, we compute the accuracy of forecast for two data sets with full features. Then, we select the most relevant feature subset by SVM-BFS, and compute the accuracy by different learning algorithms on the two data sets with the selected feature subset. At last, rules are generated to help the neuroradiologists forecast the degree of malignancy in brain glioma. The accuracy is compared with that of FMMNN-FRE on the whole training data set with the selected feature subset.

To compare the classification ability of the methods of SVMs, artificial neural networks, FMMNN-FRE on both the training data sets with the total features, we use the 10-fold cross validation method to produce the results in Table 1. The neural networks with weight decay in Bayesian learning frame (BNN) (Foresee & Hagan, 1997) are used. Because this type of neural network has a regularizing term whose coefficients are computed in Bayesian learning frame, the neural network which has been implemented in MATLAB (Demuth & Beale, 2001) overcomes the overfitting problem and is insensitive to the number of nodes in the hidden layer.

With the proposed algorithm SVM-BFS, the relevant feature subsets are selected on both data sets. Results of the forecast accuracy on the selected feature subset with different numbers are shown on Figure 1. From the results of feature selection on D280, it can be seen that a subset of six features gets the highest accuracy, though there are three subsets which contain different numbers of features get the same accuracy, we consider the subset which contains more than six features has redundant features, so the subset with six features is chosen as the selected feature subset on 280 cases, which contains *Gender, Age, Capsule of Tumor, Post-Contrast Enhancement, Blood Supply*, and *Hemorrhage*. Similarly, on 154 cases data set, we also select a subset with six features, which are *Gender, Age, Post-Contrast Enhancement, Blood supply, Necrosis/Cyst Degeneration*, and *Signal Intensity of the T2-weighted Image*. Totally, we select eight features on both data sets. It should be noted that the above two different feature subsets are evaluated as units on the classification accuracy of different data sets respectively. The points on Figure 1 are corresponding to subsets with different numbers of features and are not corresponding to different features. So we do not know which feature is the

Table 1. Results on Brain Glioma by using SVMs and related algorithms

Algorithm	Data set	Racc(%)	Std. Dev. (%)	High-grade(%)	Low-grade(%)
SVMs	Full-D280	85.70	6.52	96.43	71.43
	Full-D154	84.96	9.97	100.00	73.33
BNN	Full-D280	85.62	7.68	100.00	73.33
	Full-D154	84.00	7.76	100.00	73.33
FMMNN-FRE	Full-D280	83.21	5.31	89.29	75.00
	Full-D154	86.37	8.49	100.00	73.33
SVMs	SVM-BFS-D280	87.14	5.38	96.43	78.57
	SVM-BFS-D154	88.33	8.07	100.00	80.00
BNN	SVM-BFS-D280	86.07	6.61	96.42	78.57
	SVM-BFS-D154	84.75	9.28	100	68.75
SVMs	FMMNN-FRE-D280	85.36	8.66	96.43	64.28
	FMMNN-FRE-D154	84.37	9.44	93.75	66.67
BNN	FMMNN-FRE-D280	85.35	8.65	96.42	67.85
	FMMNN-FRE-D154	85.04	5.49	93.33	73.33
FMMNN-FRE	FMMNN-FRE-D280	83.21	5.31	89.29	75.00
	FMMNN-FRE-D154	86.37	8.49	100.00	73.33

most important one and list them in order. In the following, the classification accuracy and the rules are computed on different selected 6-feature subsets corresponding to different data sets of D280 or D154.

Accidentally, Ye et al. (2002) obtained six features for each data set, and totally 8 features. There are four features which are identical with ours, which are *Age, Post-Contrast Enhancement, Blood supply and Hemorrhage*. In addition, we use four features of the rest, which are *Gender, Capsule of Tumor, Necrosis/Cyst Degeneration* and *Signal Intensity of the T2-weighted Image*, while Ye et al. (2002) use other four different features, which are *Edema, Mass Effect, Calcification*, and *Signal Intensity of the T1-weighted Image*. It is also noted that it is the feature subsets of different data sets and not the individual features which yield the classification accuracy. So the classification accuracy on different data sets are computed on the selected 6-feature subsets respectively.

Figure 1. Forecast results on brain glioma with different numbers of features selected by SVM-BFS, of which a is on D280 and b is D154

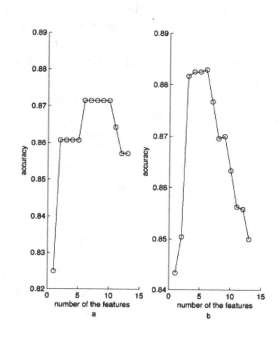

In fact, according to our experiences, all features are relevant to the degree of malignancy in brain glioma, but different combinations of features yield different forecast accuracy. Results of classification accuracy on the different 6-feature subsets corresponding to two data sets selected by SVM-BFS are calculated using SVMs and BNN with the 10-fold cross validation method, and shown in Table 1. At the same time, results on the 6-feature subset of two different data sets selected by FMMNN-FRE are shown in Table 1.

From Table 1, it can be seen that: (1) Accuracy by SVMs are comparable to that by FMMNN-FRE on two total data sets; (2) Results of classification accuracy by SVMs on the selected feature subsets of two different data sets by SVM-BFS are higher than that by SVMs on the feature subsets selected by FMMNN-FRE; (3) Accuracy by SVMs on the selected feature subset is higher than that on the total feature set; (4) Accuracy by BNN on the selected feature subset is slightly higher than that on the total feature set; (5) Accuracy by SVMs on the feature subsets of two different data sets selected by SVM-BFS are slightly higher than that by FMMNN-FRE on the feature subsets selected by FMMNN-FRE which are 87.14% for D280 and 88.33% for D154 by SVMs vs. 83.21% for D280 and 86.37% for D154 by FMMNN-FRE. (6) In total, SVM-BFS achieve slightly better results of classification accuracy than FMMNN-FRE does on the two data sets.

We train SVMs on the 6-feature subsets selected by SVM-BFS and obtain one rule for each data set. On all 280 cases, the rule is,

$$g = 4.0508 + [-0.5762 \; -1.7209, \; -0.1762, \\ -0.3244, \; -1.2274, \; -0.4096]*$$

[Gender, Age, Capsule of Tumor, Post −
Contrast Enhancement, Blood Supply, (2)

Hemorrhage]′ ,where a positive value means the degree is of low grade, while a negative one means it is of high grade, and *a′* means the trans-

pose of *a*. This rule is quantitative, and means that the tumor degree of *young* people with female *Gender*, intact *Capsule of Tumor*, absent *Post-Contrast Enhancement*, normal *blood Supply*, and absent *Hemorrhage* is of low grade, otherwise, it is of high grade.

On 154 cases, the rule is,

$$g = 5.1603 + [-0.4092, \; -2.9368, \; -0.9734, \\ -1.1179, \; -0.3506, \; 0.1928]*$$

[Gender, Age, Post −Contrast Enhancement,
Blood supply, (3)

Necrosis/Cyst Degeneration, Signal Intensity of the T2 −weighted Image]′ ,where a positive value means the degree is of low grade, while a negative one means it is of high grade. It means the tumor degree of *young* people with female *Gender*, absent *Post-Contrast Enhancement*, normal *blood Supply*, absent *Necrosis/Cyst Degeneration* and hypointense or hypointense accompanied by isointense *Signal Intensity of the T2-weighted Image* is of low grade, otherwise, it is of high grade.

These two rules are conducted from two related data sets, and they are unanimous. In a word, the two rules can be fused into one that the tumor degree of *young* people with female *Gender*, intact *Capsule of Tumor*, absent *Post-Contrast Enhancement*, normal *blood Supply*, absent *Necrosis/Cyst Degeneration*, absent *Hemorrhage* and hypointense or hypointense accompanied by isointense *Signal Intensity of the T2-weighted Image* tends to be low grade, otherwise it tends to be high grade.

Classification results of the above two rules are calculated on the respective selected feature subsets of data sets. Results are shown in Table 2, where SVM-BFS-D280 (D154) means this is the 6-feature subset of D280 (D154) selected by SVM-BFS, FMMNN-FRE-D280 (D154) is that by FMMNN-FRE. From Table 2, it can be seen that rules obtained by SVMs on the features selected by SVM-BFS obtain slightly higher accuracy than

Table 2. Results obtained by the rules (2) and (3) on their corresponding feature subsets.

Algorithm	Data set	Total (%)	High-grade (%)	Low-grade (%)
SVM-BFS	SVM-BFS-D280	88.21	86.98	90.09
	SVM-BFS-D154	88.96	88.41	89.41
FMMNN-FRE	FMMNN-FRE-D280	84.64	76.58	89.94
	FMMNN-FRE-D154	87.66	85.88	89.86

those by FMMNN-FRE do. Although we obtain higher accuracy than FMMNN-FRE and used different features, our rules have no conflicts with rules obtained by Ye et al. (2002).

Discussions

From the computation results, it can be seen that SVM-BFS yields slightly higher classification accuracy and more information than the FMMNN-FRE algorithm. This is due to support vector machines with better generalization ability and a different feature subset.

Compared with FMMNN-FRE, there are three distinct specialties of SVM-BFS. One is that with the concept of margin, SVMs can tolerate the noise and the fuzzy value in the data set, while FMMNN-FRE use the fuzzy set method to treat the fuzzy value in the data set. The former is easier to be implemented. The second specialty is that with the concept of margin, SVMs realize the principle of data dependent structure risk minimization, in which they make use of the relation between the target function and the data set, and do not depend on the dimension of data set. At the same time, they minimize the structure risk of both complexity and loss. All these greatly improve the generalization performance. The third specialty is that feature selection methods are used to select the most relevant feature subset. Compared with FMMNN-FRE, a rule extraction method, backward floating search method can eliminate the redundant features and handle the combined features efficiently which are more important in

forecast, to help the learning machine get better generalization performance.

In addition, although SVM-BFS does not take steps to treat the missing values in *Post-Contrast Enhancement*, accuracy on the data set of 280 cases is nearly equal to that on the data set of 154 cases. However, FMMNN-FRE treat the missing values using hyper box, but accuracy on the data set of 280 cases is 3% less than that on 154 cases. This advantage of SVM-BFS should be owed to the second specialty of SVM-BFS, the excellent generalization performance.

From the rules (2) and (3), it can be seen that the feature subset of *Age, Post-Contrast Enhancement, Blood supply, Hemorrhage, Gender, Capsule of Tumor, Necrosis/Cyst Degeneration and Signal Intensity of the T2-weighted Image*, seems to be more useful than other subsets even the full feature set for the degree forecast of malignancy in brain glioma. These features used in our subset have already been verified, i.e. *Gender* is in (Lopez Gonzalez & Sotelo, 2000), *Age* in (Ye et al., 2002; Lopez Gonzalez & Sotelo, 2000), *Capsule of Tumor, Hemorrhage* in (Ye et al., 2002), *Post-Contrast Enhancement* in (Ginsberg, Fuller, Hashmi, Leeds, & Schomer, 1998) *Blood supply* in (Ye et al., 2002), *Necrosis/Cyst Degeneration and Signal Intensity of the T2-weighted Image* in (Chow et al., 2000). The rules obtained in this work are also in accord with the experiences of human experts (Lopez Gonzalez & Sotelo, 2000; Wang et al., 2000). In fact, the combination of features but not the individuals are more important for the forecast, so the features need not be explained one by one from the point of statistics.

At last, we can conclude that (1) combining support vector machines and feature selection methods can get another different feature subset, based on which higher accuracy and qualitative information for the degree forecast of malignancy have been obtained, since this subset does not conflict with the results in (Ye et al., 2002), this chapter may be complementary to the research of Brain Glioma; (2) support vector machines with feature selection produce slightly higher classification accuracy with the additional benefits of rule extraction and redundancy feature elimination and therefore have the potential to be powerful tools in computer aided medical diagnosis problems like the degree forecast of malignancy in brain glioma.

Ensemble Learning

Computational Methods

Ensemble learning is a learning paradigm where many base learners are jointly used to solve a problem (Zhou et al., 2002; Li & Yang, 2008), which is presently a popular technique to treat the noise and bias in data sets in the machine learning and its applications community. It effectively improves stability of individual learners. In general, an ensemble model is constructed in two steps, i.e., training a number of component individuals and then combining the component forecasts. As for combining the forecasts of components, the most prevailing approaches are plurality voting or majority voting for classification tasks. As for training components, the most prevailing approaches are Bagging and Boosting. These ensemble approaches employ all of those individuals to constitute an ensemble. Zhou et al. (2002) reveals that using many of the available individuals may be better than using all of those individuals and an approach named GASEN (Genetic Algorithm based Selective ENsemble) is presented. But GASEN is low efficiency because it is based on genetic algorithm which is of high computation complexity in $O(2^n)$, n is the number of individual learners.

One of the approaches to eliminate redundant individuals differing from genetic algorithm is clustering algorithm (Mitra et al., 2002) which clusters the similar individual into different groups. If using the individuals nearest the cluster center to represent their group, the diversity is improved. Since the computational complexity of clustering algorithm in (Mitra et al., 2002) is $O(n^2)$, which is lower than that of genetic algorithm. Therefore, clustering algorithm based selective ensemble (CLUSEN) (Li, Yang, Kong, & Chen, 2004) is proposed to solve decision support in medical problems.

The CLUSEN algorithm is shown in Algorithm 2. Firstly, the whole data set is split into the training and test data sets. A validation data set for choosing the number of clusters is randomly sampling from the training data sets. Secondly, CLUSEN employs the training sets to generate many individual learners. Thirdly, CLUSEN clusters the output of all individuals and selects individuals of the cluster center to compose the ensemble in which the number of clusters is decided by the validation data set. When the selected individuals are obtained, the final ensemble model is generated by majority voting (Li, Yang, Kong, & Chen, 2004).

Results on Brain Glioma

On the brain glioma data set, we perform the CLUSEN algorithm to test its performance. In the experiments, 10-fold cross validation is employed. Back propagation based multi-layer neural works are used as the base learner in CLUSEN. To reduce overfitting of the base learner, a weight decay regularization term is added in the learning (Demuth & Beale, 2001). The parameters used in CLUSEN are set as: the number of hidden unit is 8, Ratio is 0.4, Max epoch is 300, Target error is 0.01, and Population of neural network is 20.

Algorithm 2. The CLUSEN algorithm

Input: Training data set Dr, learner L, population size T

Output: Ensemble model N^*

1: **Begin**
2: **for** $t = 1$ to T **do**
3: Dt is bootstrap sampling one third from Dr
4: Train Learner Lt to generate model Nt on Dt
5: **end for**
6: A validation data set V is randomly sampled from Dr
7: **for** $k = 1$ to T **do**
8: Employ clustering algorithm to select subset Mk from all the models **N**
9: Test the ensemble of subset Mk on V and obtain the validation accuracy Rk
10: **end for**
11: Select Mk with the highest Rk and use k as the number of cluster
12: Generate ensemble model N^* on the individual subset of Mk
13: **End**

In the clinical data processing fields, classification accuracy is one of the most important criteria. CLUSEN is used to forecast the degree of malignancy of brain glioma on the D280 data set without any feature selection, results of classification accuracy are listed in Table 3, in which out of bracket is forecast accuracy and inside of bracket is stand deviation. The number of individuals used in CLUSEN in the process of 10-fold cross validation is ranged from 13 to 18 out of 20. From Table 3, it can be seen that classification accuracy of CLUSEN is slightly higher than those of support vector machines, neural networks, and rule induction algorithms (T.-Y. Liu et al., 2006).

Feature Reuse

Computational Methods

In clinical data sets, there are often redundant features, which are weakly relevant to the decision, but may be redundant to other features. These features are removed during the feature selection process, in fact they are still useful, since they really contain information about the disease. To reuse these features, multi-task learning is proposed, which is a form of inductive transfer (Caruana, 1997; Caruana & Sa, 2003). It is applicable to any learning methods that can share some of what is learned between multiple tasks. The basic idea is to use the selected features as the input feature set and to combine the target values with some of the discarded features to form the target output (J. Y. Yang et al., 2008).

There exist several heuristic search methods for multi-task learning (Caruana & Sa, 2003; Li, Yang, Lu, et al., 2004). H-MTL (Heuristic Multi-Task Learning) is a heuristic method with embedded feature selection that is based on the work of Caruana and de Sa (Caruana & Sa, 2003). The embedded model employs the forecast risk criteria (Moody & Utans, 1992; Li, Yang, Liu, & Xue, 2004), which evaluates features by com-

Table 3. Results of forecast accuracy on brain glioma by using CLUSEN and other learning algorithms.

CLUSEN (%)	SVMs (%)	BNN(%)	FMMNN-FRE (%)
87.86(6.02)	85.70 (6.52)	85.62 (7.68)	83.57 (5.10)

puting the change in training accuracy when the features are replaced by their mean values:

$$S_i = R_{acc} - R_{acc}(\overline{\mathbf{x}^i}) \qquad (4)$$

where *Racc* is the training accuracy. $R_{acc}(\overline{\mathbf{x}^i})$ is the test accuracy on the training set with the *i*th feature is replaced by its mean value. The features with zero value are removed, since these features are not useful for learning. Then, the forecast risk criteria is used to rank the remaining features in ascending order; the top quarter of these features are added to the output, and the remaining three quarters are used as the input.

To show the effectiveness of multi-task learning methods, we also implemented a naive feature selection method named GA-FS (Genetic Algorithm based Feature Selection). In GA-FS, we use a binary chromosome with the same length as the feature vector, which equals 1 if the corresponding feature is selected for the input, and 0 if the feature is discarded. The fitness function is defined as

$$fitness = \frac{1}{3} R_{acc} + \frac{2}{3} R_{acc}^v \qquad (5)$$

where *Racc* is the training accuracy of the base learning method, and R_{acc}^v is the forecast accuracy on the validation data set.

In existing heuristic search methods (Caruana & Sa, 2003; Li, Yang, Lu, et al., 2004), the number of features selected for the input and/or the target is decided somewhat arbitrarily. In order to improve performance of feature selection, GA-MTL (Genetic Algorithm based Multi-Task Learning) (Li & Liu, 2006; Li & Yang, 2008), a random method, employs a genetic algorithm (Goldberg, 1998) which simultaneously selects the features for both the input and the target. The number of features for the input and target is automatically determined by the method itself. In both GA-MTL

and GA-FS, the same genetic algorithm is used for the feature selection task. The only difference between GA-MTL and GA-FS is the value of the binary chromosome; in GA-MTL, it equals 0 if the feature is selected to add to the output, whereas in GA-FS, it equals 0 if the feature is removed.

In GA-MTL, the irrelevant features are still present. These may be removed by many feature selection methods (H. Liu & Yu, 2005). Here, we consider using the forecast risk criterion (Moody & Utans, 1992; Li, Yang, Liu, & Xue, 2004) in an embedded method. As shown in Algorithm 3, first the features with a forecast risk value of zero are removed, then GA-MTL is performed on the data set with the selected features. As this method removes the irrelevant features for GA-MTL, it is named GA-MTL-IR (GA-MTL with Irrelevant features Removed) (J. Y. Yang et al., 2008).

GA-MTL-IR removes irrelevant features using an embedded method, but it searches features for MTL using a genetic algorithm. Thus two search algorithms are used in GA-MTL-IR; why not instead use only one genetic algorithm? We propose an enhanced version of GA-MTL (e-GA-MTL) (J. Y. Yang et al., 2008), which is summarized in algorithm 4. It differs from GA-MTL in its binary chromosome; instead of only one bit, two bits are used to represent each feature, where 00 means the corresponding feature is discarded, 10 means it is used as input, 01 means it is added to the output, and 11 means it is used as input and added to the output simultaneously.

In above feature reuse algorithms by using multi-task learning, weight decay based neural networks in a Bayesian framework are used as base learners, which adds a regularization term to the objective function and are to some degree insensitive to the parameter settings (Foresee & Hagan, 1997).

Results on Tumor Classification

On the tumor data sets of microarray, GA-MTL algorithms like GA-MTL, GA-MTL-IR and e-

Algorithm 3. The GA-MTL-IR algorithm

Input: training set Dr, validation set Dv, test set Ds, and the base learner
Output: forecast accuracy on the test set Ds
1: **begin**
2: Train the base learner on training set $Dr \cup Dv$
3: **for** i=from 1 to n, the number of features in $Dr \cup Dv$ **do**
4: Compute the forecast risk value Ri using Equation (4).

5: If Ri is greater than 0, the ith feature is selected, otherwise discarded.
6: **end for**
7: Generate a population of weight vectors
8: Evolve the population where the fitness of a weight vector **w** is measured as in Equation (5)
   on Dr and Dv with the selected features
9: **w*** = the evolved best weight vector
10: Test on Ds with features corresponding to 1's in **w*** as the input and those to 0's be
added to the target
11: **end**

GA-MTL are employed as described in the above subsection. In the experiments, we use the hold out validation procedure. Each data set is used in its entirety, where split data sets are merged, and then the entire data set is randomly split into a training set and a test set Ds; 2/3 of the data is used for training and 1/3 for test. If a validation set is required, the training set is further split so that 2/3 of the original training set is retained for training (forming the set Dr) and 1/3 of the original training set is used for validation (forming the set Dv). Classification results are reported for the test data sets Ds. This process is repeated 50 times. The parameters of the genetic algorithms are set by default as in the MATLAB software, and the parameter of the artificial neural networks is that the number of hidden units is 2.

In order to precisely characterize the performance of different learning methods, BACC (Balanced Accuracy) is defined as

$$\frac{1}{2}\left(\frac{TP}{TP+FN}+\frac{TN}{TN+FP}\right)$$

where TP, TN, FP, and FN, stand for the number of true positive, true negative, false positive, and false negative samples, respectively.,

The following series of experiments using artificial neural networks (ANNs) as classifiers are performed.

- ALL is a baseline method; without any selection, all the genes are input to the ANNs for classification.

Algorithm 4. The e-GA-MTL algorithm

Input: training set Dr, validation set Dv, test set Ds, and the base learner
Output: forecast accuracy on the test set Ds
1: **begin**
2: generate a population of weight vectors
3: evolve the population where the fitness of a weight vector **w** is measured as in Equation (5) on Dr and Dv
4: **w*** = the evolved best weight vector
5: test on Ds with features corresponding to 10's in **w*** to be as the input, those to 01's be added to
  the target, those to 00's be discarded and those to 11's be as the input and output simultaneously
6: **end**

Figure 2. Forecast results on microarray data sets by using multi-task learning algorithms

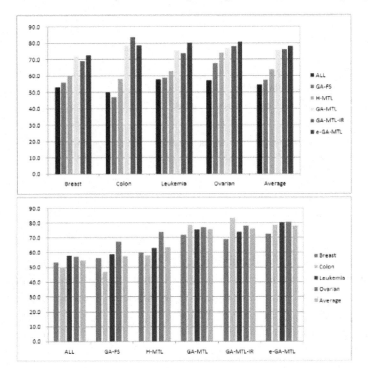

- GA-FS uses a genetic algorithm to select genes and input selected genes to the ANNs.
- H-MTL uses a heuristic embedded feature selection method to search features, where some of the selected features serve as input to the ANNs and some of the features are added to the output.
- GA-MTL uses a genetic algorithm to search features, where some of the selected features are input into ANNs and some of the features are added to the output.
- GA-MTL-IR uses an embedded algorithm to remove irrelevant features and then uses a genetic algorithm to search features, where some of the selected features serve as input to the ANNs and some of the features are added to the output.
- e-GA-MTL also uses a genetic algorithm to search features, and employs two bits to represent one feature; some features

are considered as irrelevant and discarded, some of the selected features serve as input to the ANNs, and some of the features are added to the output.

The average BACC values are shown in Figures 2, where ALL means all the genes are used as input for classification without any gene selection. From Figure 2, we conclude that:

1. On average and for all the data sets, the multi-task learning algorithms H-MTL, GA-MTL, GA-MTL-IR, and e-GA-MTL perform better than the feature selection algorithms GA-FS and ALL.
2. On average and for almost all the data sets, the genetic algorithm based multi-task learning algorithms GA-MTL, GA-MTL-IR and e-GA-MTL perform better than H-MTL, a heuristic algorithm.

Table 4. Statistics values of BACC on the microarray data sets by using GA-MTL series algorithms (%)

DATASET	ALL	GA-FS	H-MTL	GA-MTL	GA-MTL-IR	e-GA-MTL
Breast	53.2(9.2)	56.1(8.6)	59.9(8.5)	71.9(8.4)	69.0(8.3)	72.7(8.4)
Colon	50.0(8.8)	46.9(8.5)	58.1(7.9)	78.6(8.2)	83.7(8.1)	78.6(7.6)
Leukemia	57.7(7.8)	58.8(8.3)	63.1(8.0)	75.5(7.9)	73.8(7.7)	80.2(7.6)
Ovarian	57.2(6.8)	67.6(6.9)	73.9(6.8)	77.1(7.2)	78.2(7.1)	80.6(7.2)
Average	54.5(8.2)	57.4(8.1)	63.8(7.8)	75.8(7.9)	76.2(7.8)	78.0(7.8)

3. On average, e-GA-MTL performs the best among all the learning algorithms.

4. Although GA-FS performs worse than the multi-task learning algorithms, it performs better than those without any gene selection.

Detailed statistical values of BACC are also listed in Table 4, where outside of parentheses represent the mean of BACC values, while Inside of parentheses correspond to the standard deviation across the 50 times of hold out validations. From Table 4 we conclude that:

1. For all the measures, on average, multi-task learning algorithms including H-MTL, GA-MTL, GA-MTL-IR, and e-GA-MTL perform better than GA-FS and ALL, and genetic algorithm based multi-task learning algorithms like GA-MTL, GA-MTL-IR, and e-GA-MTL perform better than H-MTL.

2. Both e-GA-MTL and GA-MTL-IR remove irrelevant genes; both obtain better results than the others.

3. e-GA-MTL performs the best among all the learning algorithms on average. It greatly improves results for the BACC measure.

Discussions

We have demonstrated that genetic algorithm based multi-task learning (GA-MTL) algorithms perform better than the heuristic and feature selection algorithms, and that e-GA-MTL performs

the best of all the methods considered. Several questions come immediately to mind:

Why does multi-task learning succeed? In a previous study, Caruana (1997); Caruana and Sa (2003) gave an explanation of why multi-task learning succeeds. Here we combine their results with the framework presented here. Yu and Liu (2004) proposed to categorize the features into four classes, namely: (1) irrelevant features, (2) weakly relevant and redundant features, (3) weakly relevant but non-redundant features, and (4) strongly relevant features, where (3) and (4) comprise the optimal feature subset and (1) and (2) should be removed using feature selection methods. We have found that II contains useful information. These features should not be discarded, but rather should be used in the learning process. Multi-task learning is a method to use these redundant features to improve the forecast accuracy of the base learning method, which accounts for its improved performance.

Why do genetic algorithms perform better than the heuristic method? Our results demonstrate that genetic algorithm based multi-task learning methods outperform heuristic multi-task learning methods. The chief reason why this is so is that the heuristic method considered here uses the feature ranking technique to select features for the input and the target, which does not consider feature redundancy and/or feature interaction. At the same time, is somewhat arbitrary to use a pre-specified number of features for the input and the target. This is another factor which reduces the performance of the heuristic method. In contrast,

Algorithm 5. The ML-kNN algorithm

1: **Begin**
2: Calculating the conditional probability distribution of each instance associating to each label;
3: for i = 1 to the number of test instances **do**
4: Calculating the distance between the ith test instance and the training instances; then find k instances with the nearest distance in the training data set.
5: According to the labels of k instances and the conditional probability comparing to each label, to forecast the probability of the ith test instance and then produce the forecast results
6: **end for**
7: Output the forecast results of test instances.
8: **End**

---

when the genetic algorithm selects features for the input and the target, it simultaneously considers feature redundancy and/or feature interaction. So it automatically determines the number of features for the input and target. In fact, Kudo and Sklansky proved that genetic algorithms have a higher probability of finding better solutions to naive feature selection problems than other complete, heuristic and random algorithms (Kudo & Sklansky, 2000). Among the genetic algorithm based multi-task learning methods, e-GA-MTL performs better than GA-MTL-IR. The number of features removed by e-GA-MTL is determined automatically by the genetic algorithm, while the number removed by GA-MTL-IR is pre-specified. This is further evidence that genetic algorithm based approaches outperform heuristic approaches.

What effect do irrelevant features have on multi-task learning? The effect of multi-task learning on irrelevant features can be observed by comparing the results obtained by e-GA-MTL, GA-MTL-IR, and GA-MTL; e-GA-MTL and GA-MTL-IR remove irrelevant features, while GA-MTL does not. Here we observed that e-GA-MTL and GA-MTL-IR outperformed GA-MTL, especially for the sensitivity and BACC measures. This shows that irrelevant features degrade the generalization performance of multi-task learning methods, and reduce the robustness of the methods; they should therefore be removed before the learning process.

Multi-Label Learning

Computational Methods

Multi-label learning techniques are used to treat medical data set with multi-labels (Tsoumakas, Katakis, & Vlahavas, 2009). In the clinical practice, there are many cases, which have multi-labels for one sample, e.g. one patient may have a cold and a rhinitis. Single label learners need to model the patient with cold and rhinitis respectively, while multi-label learners are able to model the patient simultaneously. If there is no relation between two labels of cold and rhinitis, single learners are ok. But we know, two diseases exist in one body, these two diseases probably have some relations between each other. In Traditional Chinese Medicine (TCM), one patient often have accompanying symptoms, therefore, modeling symptoms in TCM is a challenge (G.-P. Liu, Li, Wang, & Wang, 2010). Multi-label learning is in great need.

Some multi-label learning algorithms have been proposed (Tsoumakas et al., 2009), of which Multi-label k nearest neighbor (ML-kNN) is a lazy multi-label learning algorithm developed on the basis of k nearest neighbor (kNN) (Zhang & Zhou, 2007). ML-kNN is shown in Algorithm 5, which uses the maximum a posteriori principle in order to determine the label set of the test instance, based on prior and posterior probabilities for the frequency of each label within the k nearest neighbors (Zhang & Zhou, 2007; Tsoumakas et

Figure 3. Forecast results obtained on the 6 labels in syndrome models by using ML-kNN and kNN

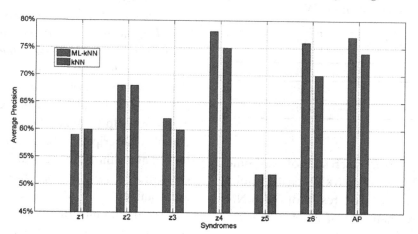

al., 2009). Traditional single kNN learners need to modeling the multi-label data sets one label by one label, which have the possibility of loss information among the labels. While ML-kNN builds models of multi-label data sets one time, which have more precise results.

Results on Coronary Heart Disease

On the data set of coronary heart disease (CHD) in Traditional Chinese Medicine (TCM), the multi-label learning algorithm ML-kNN (Zhang & Zhou, 2007) described in the above subsection is performed. In the CHD data set, 90% of the samples are randomized to be trained and the other 10% are tested. The forecast analysis of models for syndromes of inquiry diagnosis in TCM is performed after re-testing the models for 50 times and taking the mean value.

To evaluate the forecast results of ML-kNN comparing with traditional kNN, the following criteria (Zhang & Zhou, 2007) are used:

- Average precision evaluates the average fraction of labels ranked above a particular label $y \in Y$ which actually are in Y. The performance is perfect when it is 1; the bigger the value of average precision, the better the performance of classifiers.

- Coverage evaluates how far we need, on the average, to go down the list of labels in order to cover all the proper labels of the instance. It is loosely related to precision at the level of perfect recall. The smaller the value of coverage, the better the performance

- Ranking loss evaluates the average fraction of label pairs that are reversely ordered for the instance. The performance is perfect when it is 0; the smaller the value of ranking loss, the better the performance.

On the data set with all symptoms, taken $k = 5$, the models of ML-kNN are employed. The mean accuracy obtained on the 6 labels is shown in Figure 3, and the results of kNN are also shown in the figure as a comparison. In the figure, the horizontal coordinate stands for the label of symptoms forecast, and longitudinal coordinate stands for forecast accuracy with 100% as the highest value. The comparative results of ML-kNN and kNN under three evaluation criteria are listed in Table 5 (G.-P. Liu et al., 2010).

The results in Figure 3 and Table 5 demonstrate that:

Table 5. Results of inquiry diagnosis syndrome models by using ML-kNN and kNN

Evaluation criteria	ML-kNN	kNN
Average Precision	77%	74%
Coverage	3.31	3.44
Ranking Loss	0.28	0.39

1. Comparing the forecast results of syndrome models of ML-kNN with kNN on the whole, the Average Precision result of ML-kNN is 3% more than that of kNN, while the Coverage and Ranking Loss results of ML-kNN are 0.13 and 0.11 lower than kNN, respectively. According to the aforementioned evaluation criteria, the higher Average Precision, the better result obtained, and other indicators are just the opposite. Thus the MK-kNN result is significantly better than kNN;

2. On each label, five out of six syndromes of ML-kNN have better forecast accuracy; the accuracy of ML-kNN is some lower than kNN only in the syndrome of z1;

3. Different labels result in different forecast results, all of them obtain results better than 50%, which means that the inquire model is meaningful.

Clinical Data Sets

The Data Set of Brain Glioma

The brain glioma data set was gathered by neuroradiologists from Hua-Shan Hospital in Shanghai of China. There are more than 20 items in each case, including symptoms on different features, preoperative diagnosis made by some neuroradiologist and, without an exception, a clinical grade (the actual grade of glioma obtained from surgery). With the help of domain experts, we chose fifteen features, *Gender, Age, Shape, Contour, Capsule of*

Tumor, Edema, Mass Effect (Occupation), Post-Contrast Enhancement, Blood Supply, Necrosis/Cyst Degeneration, Calcification, Hemorrhage, Signal Intensity of the T1-weighted Image, Signal Intensity of the T2-weighted Image, and *Clinical Grade*. In some cases, the value of *Post-Contrast enhancement* is unknown. In fact, *Location* and Size also help to make the diagnosis, but their complex descriptions can not be well modeled by our algorithms, so we didn't adopt it. Except *Gender, Age* and *Clinical Grade*, the other items are obtained from MRI of the patient and are described with uncertainty to various extents. In order to forecast the degree of malignancy in brain glioma, descriptions of all features are converted into numerical values.

Originally, four grades are used to mark the degree of malignancy, we merge grade I and II into low-grade and grade III and IV to high-grade. According to the grade, all 280 cases of brain glioma are divided into two classes: low-grade and high-grade, in which 169 are of low-grade glioma and 111 are of high-grade ones. There are 126 cases containing missing values on *Post-Contrast enhancement*, and in the other subset of 154 complete cases, 85 cases are of low-grade gliomas and 69 ones are of high-grade ones. Experiments are performed on D280 and D154, of which D280 is the total data set of 280 cases with missing values in *Post-Contrast enhancement*, while D154 is the the data set of 154 complete cases.

Before the computation, we perform a preprocessing step to normalize the data to the quadrant of [-1, 1] using an affine transformation. More details about this data set, please refer to (Li, Yang, et al., 2006).

The Data Set of Coronary Heart Disease

Coronary heart disease (CHD) is a common cardiovascular disease that is extremely harmful to humans. It would improve the therapeutic effect and decrease mortality to increase the diagnosis rate of CHD. In Traditional Chinese Medicine (TCM), the diagnosis and treatment of coronary heart disease has a long history and ample experience; however, during diagnosis and treatment in TCM, the nonstandard inquiry information influences the treatment effect, which is detrimental to the popularization and application of treating experiences, and hampers the improvement of diagnostic and treatment levels. Here we collect a data set of CHD with inquiry information and syndromes in TCM. This is great significance to the promotion of fundamental and clinical studies for CHD in TCM. In the diagnosis of CHD in TCM, there are several patterns of syndromes. In this chapter, we investigate how to solve this problem by applying novel techniques of multi-label learning.

In this data set, among the 555 patients, 265 patients are male (47.7%, with mean age of 65.15±13.17), and 290 patients are female (52.3%, with mean age of 65.24±13.82). The symptoms collected for inquiry diagnosis included 8 dimensions: cold or warm, sweating, head, body, chest and abdomen, urine and stool, appetite, sleeping, mood, and female gender, a total of 125 symptoms. There are 15 syndromes in differentiation diagnosis, of which 6 commonly-used patterns were selected in our study, including: z1 Deficiency of heart qi syndrome; z2 Deficiency of heart yang syndrome; z3 Deficiency of heart yin syndrome; z4 Qi stagnation syndrome; z5 Turbid phlegm syndrome and z6 blood stasis syndrome.

More details about this data set, please refer to (G.-P. Liu et al., 2010).

Tumor Data Sets in Microarray

The eight microarray data sets used in our study are listed in Table 6.

Breast Cancer: Van't Veer *et al.* (2002) used DNA microarray analysis on primary breast tumors and applied supervised classification methods to identify significant genes for the disease. The data contains 97 patient samples, 46 of which are from

Table 6. Tumor data sets in microarray

Data Sets	Samples	Class Ratio	Features
Breast Cancer	97	46/51	24,481
Colon	62	22/40	2,000
Leukemia	72	25/47	7,129
Ovarian	25	3 91/162	15,154

patients who had developed distance metastases within 5 years (labeled as "relapse"), the remaining 51 samples are from patients who remained free from the disease after their initial diagnosis for an interval of at least 5 years (labeled as "non-relapse"). The number of genes is 24,481 and the missing values of "NaN" are replaced with 100.

Colon: Alon et al. (1999) used Affymetrix oligonucleotide arrays to monitor expression levels of over 6,500 human genes from 40 tumor and 22 normal colon tissue samples. The 2,000 genes with the highest minimal intensity across the 62 tissues were used in the analysis.

Leukemia: The acute leukemia data set, published by Golub et al. (1999b), consists of 72 bone marrow samples with 47 ALL and 25 AML. The gene expression intensities are obtained from Affymetrix high-density oligonucleotide microarrays containing probes for 7,129 genes.

Ovarian: Petricoin et al. (2002) identified proteomic patterns in serum to distinguish ovarian cancer from non-cancer. The proteomic spectral data includes 91 controls (Normal) and 162 ovarian cancers; each sample contains the relative amplitude of the intensity at 15,154 molecular mass/charge (M/Z) identities.

SUMMARY

This chapter reveals some state-of-the-art technologies for clinical data processing in the machine learning field. These techniques include support vector machines, ensemble learning, multi-task learning, multi-label learning, feature selection and feature reuse, all of which have been validated on the real world medical data sets and shown satisfied results. The above works demonstrate how to improve the analysis quality of clinical data processing by using novel machine learning techniques. Though we achieve some improvements, these are just a try to face the great challenges described in the Introduction. Techniques in this chapter only concern the challenges of small sample, high dimension, noise and bias in data sets, multi-labels, etc. More works are needed to improve these techniques and to develop novel techniques to meet the challenges of sparse representation, complex structures, imbalanced classes and interpretation, etc. We believe more people will address the new trend and contribute to the development of clinical data processing. More substantive will appear on this issue.

ACKNOWLEDGMENT

This work was supported by the Natural Science Foundation of China under grant no. 60873129, 30901897, 61005006, the STCSM "Innovation Action Plan" Project of China under grant no. 07DZ19726, the Shanghai Rising-Star Program under grant no. 08QA1403200, the Open Projects Program of National Laboratory of Pattern Recognition.

REFERENCES

Alon, U., Barkai, N., Notterman, D. A., Gish, K., Ybarra, S., Mack, D., et al. (1999). Broad patterns of gene expression revealed by clustering analysis of tumor and normal colon tissues probed by oligonucleotide arrays. In *Proceedings of the National Academy of Sciences of the United States of America*, (pp. 6745-6750).

Bauer, E., & Kohavi, R. (1999). An empirical comparison of voting classification algorithms: Bagging, boosting, and variants. *Machine Learning*, *36*(1-2), 105–139. doi:10.1023/A:1007515423169

Boser, B., Guyon, L., & Vapnik, V. (1992). A training algorithm for optimal margin classifiers. In *Proceedings of the Fifth Annual Workshop on Computational Learning Theory*, (p. 144-152). Pittsburgh: ACM.

Breiman, L. (1996). Bagging predictors. *Machine Learning*, *24*(2), 123–140. doi:10.1007/BF00058655

Caruana, R. (1997). Multitask learning. *Machine Learning*, *28*(1), 41–75. doi:10.1023/A:1007379606734

Caruana, R., & de Sa, V. R. (2003). Benefiting from the variables that variable selection discards. *Journal of Machine Learning Research*, *3*, 1245–1264. doi:10.1162/153244303322753652

Chen, N.-Y., Lu, W.-C., Yang, J., & Li, G.-Z. (2004). *Support vector machines in chemistry*. Singapore: World Scientific Publishing Company. doi:10.1142/9789812794710

Chow, L. K., Gobin, Y. P., Cloughesy, T. F., Sayre, J. W., Villablanca, J. P., & Vinuela, F. (2000). Prognostic factors in recurrent glioblastoma multiforme and anaplastic astrocytoma, treated with selective intra-arterial chemotherapy. *AJNR. American Journal of Neuroradiology*, *21*, 471–478.

Cristianini, N., & Shawe-Taylor, J. (2000). *An introduction to support vector machines*. Cambridge, UK: Cambridge University Press.

Demuth, H., & Beale, M. (2001). *Neural network toolbox user's guide for use with MATLAB* (4th ed.). The Mathworks Inc.

Dudoit, S., Fridlyand, J., & Speed, T. P. (2002). Comparison of discrimination methods for the classification of tumors using gene expression data. *Journal of the American Statistical Association, 97*(457), 77–87. doi:10.1198/016214502753479248

Foresee, F. D., & Hagan, M. T. (1997). Gauss-newton approximation to bayesian regularization. In *Proceedings of the 1997 International Joint Conference on Neural Networks,* (pp. 1930-1935).

Ginsberg, L. E., Fuller, G. N., Hashmi, M., Leeds, N. E., & Schomer, D. F. (1998). The significance of lack of MR contrast enhancement of supratentorial brain tumors in adults: Histopathological evaluation of a series. *Surgical Neurology, 49,* 436–440. doi:10.1016/S0090-3019(97)00360-1

Goldberg, D. E. (1998). *Genetic algorithms in search, optimization, and machine learning.* Boston: Addison Wesley.

Golub, T. R., Slonim, D. K., Tamayo, P., Huard, C., Gaasenbeek, M., & Mesirov, J. P. (1999a). Molecular classification of cancer: Class discovery and class prediction by gene expression. *Bioinformatics &. Computational Biology, 286*(5439), 531–537.

Guyon, I., Gunn, S., Nikravesh, M., & Zadeh, L. (2006). *Feature extraction, foundations and applications. Physica-Verlag.* Springer.

Jain, A., & Zongker, D. (1997). Feature selection: Evaluation, application, and small sample performance. *IEEE Transactions on Pattern Analysis and Machine Intelligence, 19,* 153–158. doi:10.1109/34.574797

Karush, W. (1939). *Minima of functions of several variables with inequalities as side constraints.* Unpublished master's thesis, Department of Mathematics, University of Chicago.

Kohavi, R., & George, J. H. (1997). Wrappers for feature subset selection. *Artificial Intelligence, 97,* 273–324. doi:10.1016/S0004-3702(97)00043-X

Kudo, M., & Sklansky, J. (2000). Comparison of algorithms that select features for pattern classifiers. *Pattern Recognition, 33*(1), 25–41. doi:10.1016/S0031-3203(99)00041-2

Kuhn, H. W., & Tucker, A. W. (1951). Nonlinear programming. In *Proceeding of the 2nd Berkeley Symposium on Mathematical Statistics and Probabilistic,* (p. 481-492). Berkeley, CA: University of California Press.

Lal, T. N., Chapelle, O., Weston, J., & Elisseeff, A. (2006). Embedded methods. In Guyon, I., Gunn, S., & Nikravesh, M. (Eds.), *Feature extraction, foundations and applications. Physica-Verlag.* Springer.

Li, G.-Z., Bu, H.-L., Yang, M. Q., Zeng, X.-Q., & Yang, J. Y. (2008). Selecting subsets of newly extracted features from PCA and PLS in microarray data analysis. *BMC Genomics, 9*(S2), S24. doi:10.1186/1471-2164-9-S2-S24

Li, G.-Z., & Liu, T.-Y. (2006). Improving generalization ability of neural networks ensemble with multi-task learning. *Journal of Computer Information Systems, 2*(4), 1235–1239.

Li, G.-Z., Liu, T.-Y., & Cheng, V. S. (2006). Classification of brain glioma by using SVMs bagging with feature selection. In *BioDM 2006, Lecture Notes in Bioinformatics 3916* (p. 124-130). Springer.

Li, G.-Z., Meng, H.-H., Yang, M., & Yang, J. (2009). Combining support vector regression with feature selection for multivariate calibration. *Neural Computing &. Applications, 18*(7), 813–820.

Li, G.-Z., Yang, J., Kong, A.-S., & Chen, N.-Y. (2004). Clustering algorithm based selective ensemble. *Journal of Fudan University, 2,* 689–691.

Li, G.-Z., Yang, J., Liu, G.-P., & Xue, L. (2004). Feature selection for multi-class problems using support vector machines. In *PRICAI2004, Lecture Notes in Artificial Intelligence 3157,* (p. 292-300). Springer.

Li, G.-Z., Yang, J., Lu, J., Lu, W.-C., & Chen, N.-Y. (2004). *On multivariate calibration problems.* In ISNN2004, (LNCS 3173). (p. 389-394). Springer.

Li, G.-Z., Yang, J., Ye, C.-Z., & Geng, D. (2006). Degree prediction of malignancy in brain glioma using support vector machines. *Computers in Biology and Medicine, 36*(3), 313–325. doi:10.1016/j.compbiomed.2004.11.003

Li, G.-Z., & Yang, J. Y. (2008). Feature selection for ensemble learning and its applications. In *Machine Learning in Bioinformatics.* New York: John Wiley & Sons. doi:10.1002/9780470397428.ch6

Li, G.-Z., & Zeng, X.-Q. (2009). Feature selection for partial least square based dimension reduction. In A. Abraham, A.-E. Hassanien & V. Snasel (Eds.), *Foundations of computational intelligence.* (pp. 3-37). Springer Berlin / Heidelberg.

Liu, G.-P., Li, G.-Z., Wang, Y.-L., & Wang, Y. (2010). Syndrome model of inquiry diagnosis for coronary heart disease in Chinese medicine by using multi-label learning. *BMC Complementary and Alternative Medicine, 10,* 37. doi:10.1186/1472-6882-10-37

Liu, H., & Yu, L. (2005). Toward integrating feature selection algorithms for classification and clustering. *IEEE Transactions on Knowledge and Data Engineering, 17*(3), 1–12.

Liu, T.-Y., Li, G.-Z., & Wu, G.-F. (2006). Degree prediction of malignancy in brain glioma using selective neural networks ensemble. *Journal of Shanghai University, 10*(3), 244–246. doi:10.1007/s11741-006-0123-5

Lopez Gonzalez, M. A., & Sotelo, J. (2000). Brain tumors in Mexico: Characteristics and prognosis of glioblastoma. *Surgical Neurology, 53,* 157–162. doi:10.1016/S0090-3019(99)00177-9

Mitra, P., Murthy, C. A., & Pal, S. K. (2002). Unsupervised feature selection using feature similarity. *IEEE Transactions on Pattern Analysis and Machine Intelligence, 24*(3), 301–312. doi:10.1109/34.990133

Moody, J., & Utans, J. (1992). Principled architecture selection for neural networks: Application to corporate bond rating prediction. In Moody, J. E., Hanson, S. J., & Lippmann, R. P. (Eds.), *Advances in neural information processing systems* (pp. 683–690). Morgan Kaufmann Publishers, Inc.

Petricoin, E. F., Ardekani, A. M., Hitt, B. A., Levine, P. J., Fusaro, V. A., & Steinberg, S. M. (2002). Use of proteomic patterns in serum to identify ovarian cancer. *Lancet, 359*(9306), 572–577. doi:10.1016/S0140-6736(02)07746-2

Pudil, P., Novovicova, J., & Kittler, J. (1994). Floating search methods in feature selection. *Pattern Recognition Letters, 15,* 1119–1125. doi:10.1016/0167-8655(94)90127-9

Tsoumakas, G., Katakis, I., & Vlahavas, I. (2009). Data mining and knowledge discovery handbook. In Maimon, O., & Rokach, L. (Eds.), *Mining multi-label data* (2nd ed.). Springer.

Van't Veer, L. V., Dai, H., Vijver, M. V., He, Y., Hart, A., & Mao, M. (2002). Gene expression profiling predicts clinical outcome of breast cancer. *Nature, 415*(6871), 530–536. doi:10.1038/415530a

Vapnik, V. (1995). *The nature of statistical learning theory.* New York: Springer.

Wang, C., Zhang, J., Liu, A., Sun, B., & Zhao, Y. (2000). Surgical treatment of primary midbrain gliomas. *Surgical Neurology, 53,* 41–51. doi:10.1016/S0090-3019(99)00165-2

Yang, J., & Honavar, V. (1998). Feature subset selection using a genetic algorithm. *IEEE Intelligent Systems, 13,* 44–49. Retrieved from citeseer.ist.psu.edu/yang98feature.html. doi:10.1109/5254.671091

Yang, J. Y., Li, G.-Z., Liu, L.-X., & Yang, M. Q. (2007). Classification of brain glioma by using neural networks ensemble with multi-task learning. In *Proceedings of the 2007 International Conference on Bioinformatics and Computational Biology (BIOCOMP '07),* (p. 515-522). Las Vegas: CSREA Press.

Yang, J. Y., Li, G.-Z., Meng, H.-H., & Yang, M. Q. (2008). Improving prediction accuracy of tumor classification by reusing the discarded genes during gene selection. *BMC Genomics*, *9*(1), S3. doi:10.1186/1471-2164-9-S1-S3

Ye, C.-Z., Yang, J., Geng, D.-Y., Zhou, Y., & Chen, N.-Y. (2002). Fuzzy rules to predict degree of malignancy in brain glioma. *Medical & Biological Engineering & Computing*, *40*, 145–152. doi:10.1007/BF02348118

Yu, L., & Liu, H. (2004). Efficient feature selection via analysis of relevance and redundancy. *Journal of Machine Learning Research*, *5*, 1205–1224.

Zeng, X.-Q., Li, G.-Z., Wu, G.-F., Yang, J., & Yang, M. (2009b). Orthogonal projection weights in dimension reduction based on partial least squares. *International Journal of Computational Intelligence of Bioinformatics & Systematic Biology*, *1*(1), 100–115.

Zeng, X.-Q., Li, G.-Z., Wu, G.-F., Yang, J. Y., & Yang, M. Q. (2009a). Irrelevant gene elimination for partial least squares based dimension reduction by using feature probes. *International Journal of Data Mining & Bioinformatics (Oxford, England)*, *3*(1), 85–103.

Zeng, X.-Q., Li, G.-Z., Yang, J. Y., Yang, M. Q., & Wu, G.-F. (2008). Dimension reduction with redundant genes elimination for tumor classification. *BMC Bioinformatics*, *9*(6), S8. doi:10.1186/1471-2105-9-S6-S8

Zhang, M.-L., & Zhou, Z.-H. (2007). Ml-knn: A lazy learning approach to multi-label learning. *Pattern Recognition*, *40*(7), 2038–2048. doi:10.1016/j.patcog.2006.12.019

Zhou, Z.-H., Wu, J.-X., & Tang, W. (2002). Ensembling neural networks: Many could be better than all. *Artificial Intelligence*, *137*(1-2), 239–263. doi:10.1016/S0004-3702(02)00190-X

KEY TERMS AND DEFINITIONS

Brain Glioma: A type of tumor that starts in the brain, which is a severe disease. If it is of low grade, a surgical operation is needed; otherwise, conservative treatment is needed.

Coronary Heart Disease: Refers to the failure of coronary circulation to supply adequate circulation to cardiac muscle and surrounding tissue. In Traditional Chinese Medicine, there is a systematic therapy.

Ensemble Learning: Uses multiple models to obtain better forecast performance than those which could be obtained from any of the constituent models. It is a popular technique to improve the stability of learners in medical data processing.

Feature Reuse: A technique to reuse the redundant features in the data sets, which might be removed during feature selection. It is useful in medical data processing since all the symptoms contain useful information.

Feature Selection: The technique of selecting a subset of relevant features for building robust learning models, which has three different models like filter, embedded and wrapper. It is a necessary technique to help find the relevant symptoms in clinical data processing.

Multi-Label Learning: A concept in machine learning and its applications, where the examples are associated with a set of labels, e.g. one patient may have a fever and stomach at the same time.

Support Vector Machines: A set of related supervised learning methods used for classification and regression, which are popular techniques to treat small sample problems like most of the medical data sets.

Section 3
Digital Forensics Applications in Dentistry

Chapter 10
Digital Applications in Forensic Odontology

Robert E. Barsley
American Board of Forensic Odontology, Inc.

David R. Senn
American Board of Forensic Odontology, Inc.

Thomas J. David
American Board of Forensic Odontology, Inc.

Franklin D. Wright
American Board of Forensic Odontology, Inc.

Gregory S. Golden
American Board of Forensic Odontology, Inc.

ABSTRACT

Forensic Odontology or forensic dentistry is the use of dental expertise, dental findings, and dental facts in legal proceedings. The principal efforts of dentists in this regard are geared toward establishing the identity of unknown human remains or verifying the identity of visually unrecognizable human remains. The digital revolution has impacted all aspects of forensic odontology. This chapter will discuss the impact on person identification through dental means, dental identification in mass or disaster victim incidents, establishing the age of an unknown individual or human remains through dental examination, digital photography in dentistry and forensic odontology, and the use of digital methods in the analysis and comparison of bite mark evidence.

DENTAL IDENTIFICATION

Dental identification, similar to all forms of identification, involves the comparison of a an unknown object – the dental structures including the teeth and their supporting structures – to a known object – the dental findings recorded during life of the suspected decedent. If a sufficient number of concordant points can be established and no points of difference are observed, the forensic dentist may render the opinion that the two objects derive from a common source – an identification.

DOI: 10.4018/978-1-60960-483-7.ch010

Figure 1. Comparison of antemortem radiographic image (top) to digital postmortem image

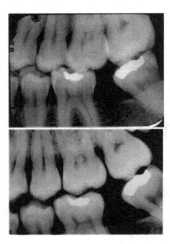

The most commonly used method is a comparison of dental radiographs taken by treating dentists during life with radiographs acquired from the remains in question (Figure 1). The use of digital radiography in clinical situations as well as in the morgue has revolutionized this aspect of forensic odontology (Tabor & Schrader, 2010).

Advances in computer technology coupled with improvement in sensor technology over the past 25 years have resulted in the adoption of digital radiography systems in dental practice. These now include the ability to image orthopanographic, cephalographic, and computed tomographic images for nearly instant delivery to clinical workstations. This stands in marked contrast to film-based dental radiography, particularly in forensic applications, and holds many advantages for the forensic dentist. The dentist-investigator is able to speedily discern whether or not features that might serve to confirm or refute a suspected identification are visible and order re-imaging if needed while the specimen is available. In addition, postmortem and antemortem images can be rapidly transmitted across great distances without any loss of fidelity, questions of orientation (left versus right side), or acquisition date and other provenance issues. In the past,

film-based images were first reproduced or copied onto additional film substrates and then hand-delivered (mail, courier, etc.) for comparison. Loss of detail and possible loss of the original image were not uncommon. Older, film-based images can, by the use of optical scanning hardware and software, be converted to an electronic image (data set) which can be treated similarly to original digital radiographs (transmission, optimization, storage, etc.) (Weems 2010).

Digital radiographic imaging software also allows the investigator to optimize or enhance the image as viewed onscreen, resulting in visualization of greater detail in the captured image – again increasing the likelihood of an identification or exclusion. Many investigators are working to perfect comparative systems (digital image-subtraction, image rectification, point-to-point analysis, etc.) to assist the forensic dentist in analyzing radiographic images.

Although there are many avenues available to authorities to arrive at the identity of unknown human remains, dental identification is rapid, reliable, readily available in most situations, and relatively inexpensive in comparison. For example, DNA requires time-consuming testing and collection of samples. Fingerprinting requires that the unknown remains retain soft tissue suitable for lifting print exemplars as well as the availability of fingerprint records on file. Nowhere is this more evident than in cases involving multiple fatalities. DVI (disaster victim identification) or MFI (multiple fatality incident) situations tax the resources of the medical examiner. In today's fast-paced world, rapid identification is expected, if not demanded, by the next of kin and the press. Digital radiography coupled with computer-aided methods of comparing the postmortem dental information gathered in the morgue to antemortem dental information provided by the families of the missing and law enforcement allows rapid resolution and identification (Molina 2010; Smith & Sweet 2010; Ulhe 2010).

Figure 2. (A) Screen capture of WinID3 odontogram comparison. (B) Screen capture of WinID3 radiographic images. In both images, the antemortem information is displayed in the top half of the image.

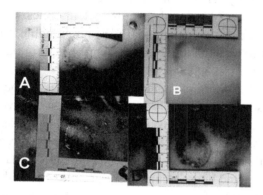

The advent of portable (as opposed to mainframe) computing in the 1980s made possible the adaptation of data bases containing dental information to dental forensics. Algorithms were developed to compare antemortem dental data to postmortem dental data collected in the morgue. Beginning with early DOS-based programs such as CAPMI® (computer aided postmortem identification) and Macintosh-based programs such as ToothPics® among others, there are now several programs vying for supremacy in the international market. These include WinID3® widely used in the U.S.A. (Figure 2), DVI System International® (Plass Data), widely used in Europe, DAVID® (Disaster and Victim Identification) developed in Australia, and UVIS® (developed by the Office of the Chief Medical Examiner in New York City, USA). Differences between these programs include the ability to incorporate and in some cases analyze dental images such as radiographs or whether the comparative data base and search functions are not solely confined to dental information. WinID3® was used during the Hurricane Katrina disaster in the southern United States in 2005 and DVI System International® at the Southeast Asian tsunami disaster in late 2006. DAVID® has not yet been deployed in a large-scale

disaster. UVIS® was designed post 9/11 to better integrate the comparison of data across forensic disciplines such as odontology, anthropology, medical examiner/autopsy, and personal data.

An additional resource useful in dental identification is the OdontoSearch® program operated by the Joint POW-MIA Accounting Command of the U.S. Department of Defense in Hawaii. This program allows a forensic dental investigator to compare the dental data, particularly the pattern of filled and unfilled teeth coupled with missing teeth, of an individual to a large representative sample of the U.S. population. In other words, a frequency value associated with the particular dental configuration at question can be established. Yet another area of growing interest is Ameloglyphics, the analysis of enamel rod end patterns on tooth surfaces. Photomicrographs and interpretation by software originally intended for fingerprint analysis has been recently proposed by some researchers (Gupta 2009; Manjunath 2008; Manjunath 2009).

Dental aging - In some cases the recovered human remains can not be readily linked to a missing person whose antemortem information may confirm identity. In those cases if teeth are present, dental methods can be utilized to estimate the age at death of the remains. Additionally, the age of a living person may be in question. The living person cases include immigration, adoption, and amnesia. Dental aging of the living is commonly relied upon in the United States for immigration matters where the question of whether or not an individual has attained the age of 18 is an important legal question.

In cases where the remains represent an individual under the age of 18, the systematic shedding of the deciduous teeth along with their subsequent replacement by their succedaneous counterparts and permanent molar teeth can be used to estimate developmental age within months – often closely paralleling chronological age. Several researchers over the years have developed graphic depictions of this process (Logan & Kronfeld, 1933; Lunt

& Law, 1974; Schour & Massler, 1940a, Massler 1940b).

For individuals older than approximately 18 other non-developmental dental methods may be used to estimate age within a range of several years. These methods utilize analysis of post formation features such as the attrition or wear of the enamel and dentin of the crowns of teeth, root transparency, cementum apposition, periodontal ligament attachment position, intra-pulpal secondary dentin formation, and analysis of pulp-to-tooth ratios. The anatomical methods have been in use for many years and are more discriminatory for younger individuals. Newer methods developed more recently may allow more discriminatory and more accurate age estimations for adults. The analysis of the ratios of optical isomers of aspartic acid (aspartic acid racemization) and the analysis of the levels of radioactive carbon-14 (^{14}C) included during the formation of dental enamel are the most promising of these techniques. The radioactive ^{14}C levels in enamel result from atmospheric ^{14}C increases following above ground nuclear bomb testing from 1955-1963. The combination of these two techniques can allow accurate age estimations for persons of any age and give estimation of, not only the age at death of an individual, but also his or her date of birth. This is powerful and useful information in criminal investigations (Harris, Mincer, Anderson & Senn, 2010).

Forensic photography has evolved considerably over the last ten years. Film-based forensic photography for documentation of evidence has virtually become non-existent, having now been replaced predominantly with the digital system. This format not only affects the type of cameras used to acquire the image, but also the way those images are viewed, stored, and transmitted.

Digital cameras are now affordable to everyone. The requirements of the photographic task will determine the level of sophistication and the quality of the camera. Members of the general public can purchase very affordable basic consumer "point and push" automatic digital cameras that fulfill most of their requirements for shooting family functions, vacations, etc. For documenting crime scenes, autopsies, and especially bite mark injuries, digital hardware in the "pro-sumer" category is necessary. These higher-end cameras have variable focal lengths, better optics, and software that is manually programmable for whatever situational requirements are appropriate for the task at hand.

With the implementation of numerous computer software programs developed for law enforcement and forensic investigation, odontologists can now paperlessly rectify images, detect and correct certain types of angular distortion and compare suspected biters' dental signatures directly to the bite mark injury.[1] This is all accomplished by computerization of the analysis of bite mark pattern injuries. With the help of programs such as Adobe® Photoshop®, exact stone replicas of the teeth of the suspects are captured on a flat-bed scanner, overlay production, and comparisons to the life-sized image of the injury are done on the computer (Bowers & Johanson, 2000).

Concurrent to the digitization of visible light photography there have been adaptations of several advanced non-visible methods of evidence documentation into the digital domain. Three of the most noteworthy applications for using light at the extreme ends of the spectrum are Infra-Red (IR), Reflective Ultraviolet (UVA), and Alternate Light Imaging (ALI), protocols. Certain digital cameras have been specifically manufactured or can be modified for non-visible techniques (Fugifilm USA, 2010). One major reason these photographic protocols were developed is to track the biochemical changes that occur after an injury takes place. IR and UV photographic techniques are not new, especially to the medical field. They have been in existence for decades. What is new is the fact that they have now been bootstrapped into the digital arena.

Film-based non-visible photography is extremely technique sensitive due to restrictions on handling, exposure, and developing processes of the film emulsion. By removing the film from the process, digital capture has greatly lessened the negative impact. Just as in digital radiography, digital IR, UV, and ALI photography has eliminated the guesswork of capturing images because the immediate results of the exposure are displayed on the camera's LCD. The CCD (sensor chip) of the camera acquires the image and projects it shortly after the camera's software writes it to whatever storage media the camera uses. This gives the photographer the confidence of knowing exactly what the images look like in real time, rather than having to wait for a processing lab to deliver the final results of their efforts. These images can also be sent electronically to any location in the world in a matter of seconds for review and consultation with other experts.

There are many applications of Infra-Red photography to forensic investigation. However in bite mark documentation, the IR image depicts bruising and vascular bleeding at deeper dermal levels in the tissue (Golden & Wright, 2005). Appropriate IR filters and adequate flash must be used to accomplish this. The same advantages hold true for Ultraviolet photography. As with IR techniques, this protocol incorporates specialized camera software and hardware modifications to capture only the ultraviolet range of the light spectrum. With the appropriate filters and illumination, UVA digital images will depict just the surface disruption of damaged tissue that was created from the teeth of the biter. Historically there have been bite mark cases where the UV image proved to be most useful as evidence; more than all other forms of visible and non-visible images collected of the same bite injury. ALI, also referred to as fluorescent photography has numerous applications to forensic investigation. For crime scene documentation, ALI can be used to detect latent prints, fibers, blood spatter, and illicit drugs (Wright & Golden, 2010). This technique is particularly useful in live victims where the bite injury has had time to heal. The technique incorporates using a specialized light

Figure 3. (A) Digital photograph of a bitemark with scale. (B) IR image of same injury. (C) UV image of same injury. (D) ALI image of same injury.

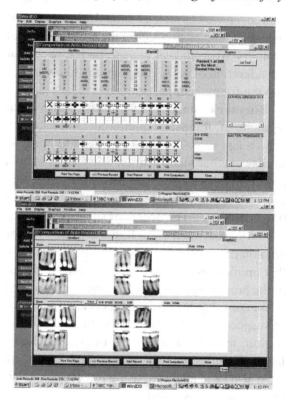

source tuned to a specific wavelength of light, plus blocking filters over the camera lens. The wavelength (color) of light used and blocking filter depends upon what the investigator is trying to photograph. In bite mark documentation the recorded fluorescent image can often delineate normal healthy skin from injured tissues, thereby enhancing the blood distribution pattern of the bruise at levels immediately below the epidermis. What may appear to be a faint or vague injury on the surface of the epidermis may appear more discernable with ALI (Golden, 1994). A typical human bite mark was digitally photographed and is presented for demonstration. (Figure 3)

A great deal of planning should go into the development and acquisition of a digital-based photographic system. Camera considerations should be geared to the level of photographic documentation that is required. Attention must also be given to the size and quality of images desired, as well as storage considerations. Rapid change continues to occur in the world of digital photography from year to year; therefore careful consideration of what equipment is likely to last into the future is important.

Bitemark analysis is the most controversial segment of forensic odontology. Photography plays a key role. The analysis of a bite injury is similar to other identification sciences. A known object (in this case the teeth/dentition of the suspected biter) is compared to an unknown object (the bite injury). The degree of similarity (or dissimilarity) between these forms the basis for the opinion of the forensic odontologist. In forming that opinion the odontologist compares patterns of the properties of the teeth as they are recorded in skin or other inanimate objects to populations of suspected biters. While most bitemarks occur in skin, food substances such as cheese, chocolate and apples, as well as gum and Styrofoam have also been analyzed using bitemark analysis (Wright & Dailey, 2001).

Routine bitemark analysis has been drastically improved with the introduction of digital applications in the methods used for analysis. One of the most commonly used methods in this comparison is referred to as the "overlay" technique. The acceptance and availability of image enhancement software has simplified the production of overlays and other trial aids, has reduced in some respects the degree of "examiner" bias that could be attributed manually produced overlays and trial aids, and easily allows the forensic odontologist to demonstrate to the court the steps taken during the analysis.

The analysis begins with an assessment of the patterned injury to discover if it possesses the class characteristics commonly associated with a bite injury. These include discrete injuries attributable by their size, shape, and position to the location of teeth in the jaw. Are injuries from both the upper and lower jaw (teeth) present? What type of injury was received – abrasion, bruising, puncture, etc.? If the injury is viewed only via photographs, is a scale included in order to determine the dimensions of the injury? Based upon these and other considerations, a forensic dentist can render an opinion as to whether the injury has been caused by a bite and whether the "biter" is human or animal (such as a dog). Animal bites are studied to determine the likely identity of the responsible animal – often a predator of some type. There are numerous recorded cases of cougars, other large felines, dogs, wolves, sharks, and even alligators which have been linked to such an attack.

The patterned injury most often associated with a human bitemark possesses class characteristics of two opposing semi-circular injury patterns with individual tooth marks that would represent injuries from the upper and lower dental arches. If the patterned injury is believed to be a human bitemark, evidence collection of the bitemark will begin using an all-digital format for most forensic dentists. The bitemark injury is digitally photographed, with and without a scale, using color, ultraviolet, infrared and alternate light photography as well as being swabbed for DNA (Wright & Dailey, 2001). The advent of digital photography has had a major impact in this area in the number and quality of photographs available; the ability to "rectify" an image that has not been acquired with the "film" surface, the scale, and the injury pattern all parallel to the same plane; and, the use of image enhancement software to increase the examiner's ability to appreciate fine detail captured in the images. The collection of the evidence from any suspected biters includes digital photographs of the dentition, an intra-occlusal bite registration, DNA swabbing and full arch maxillary and mandibular dental impressions.

Applying digital imaging programs, such as Adobe Photoshop®, the biting edges of the suspected biter's dental stone models are digitized and made nearly life-sized. The photographs of the bitemark are digitized and made nearly life-sized.

Figure 4. Computer generated transparent overlay of maxillary teeth placed over bitemark

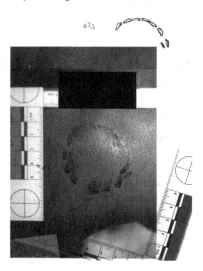

The two digital images are then superimposed to compare the position, size and shape of the suspected biter's teeth to the individual patterns of tooth marks in the bitemark to try to determine if there is a linking between the teeth and the bitemark (Figure 4). The bitemark analysis leads down two separate pathways: inclusion and exclusion. Inclusion pathways are those in which a linking between the uniqueness of the suspected biter's teeth and the resultant patterns in the bitemark is found. More commonly, the exclusion pathway shows no such linking and a determination that the suspected biter's teeth could not have made the bitemark.

Incorporating the results of the digital portion of the bitemark analysis with the other testing done in the analysis, such as a metric analysis of the teeth in the bitemark and the suspected biter's teeth, direct orientation of the suspected biter's teeth onto the bitemark or a nearly life-sized photograph of the bitemark, comparisons of test bites in skin and dental wax leads the forensic dentist to form an opinion regarding a linking between the suspected biter's teeth and the bitemark. The opinion can be expressed with the following American Board of Forensic Odontology bitemark terminology (ABFO, 2010):

Descriptions and terms used to relate a suspected biter to a bitemark (all opinions stated to a reasonable degree of dental certainty):

- The biter
- The probable biter
- Not excluded as the biter
- Excluded as the biter
- Inconclusive

The use of digital photography and digital imaging software has significantly impacted and improved bitemark analysis. Digital images also allow multiple examiners to view the same image across great distance as well as share their results with each other visually across those same distances in real time.

In conclusion, the incorporation of digital methods into the armamentarium of the forensic odontologist has improved the discipline. In addition to the current examples mentioned above, research and development is ongoing in areas such as three-dimensional bitemark analysis and injury reproduction, three-dimensional "overlay" methods, production of bitemark (injury and tooth position) databases that will be subject to query for frequency value determination as in dental comparison for identification. In light of the report on forensic science issued by the National Academy of Sciences in the United States (National Academy Press, 2009), American forensic odontologists are revisiting their methodology and foundations. The authors have no doubt that, as a result of this review, digital methods will play an even greater role in the future.

REFERENCES

American Board of Forensic Odontology. (2010). *Online diplomat's manual.* (p. 116). Retrieved from http://www.abfo.org

Bowers, C. M., & Johanson, R. J. (2000). *Digital analysis of bite mark evidence using Adobe® Photoshop*. Santa Barbara, CA: Forensic Imaging Services.

Fujifilm, U. S. A. (2010). *Finepix camera specifications*. Retrieved from http://www.fujifilmusa.com/products/digital_cameras/is/finepix_ispro/index.html

Golden, G. S. (1994). Use of alternate light source illumination in bite mark photography. *Journal of Forensic Sciences, 39*(3), 815–823.

Golden, G. S., & Wright, F. D. (2005). Photography: Noninvasive analysis. In Dorion, R. B. J. (Ed.), *Bitemark evidence* (pp. 136–139). New York: Marcel Dekker.

Gupta, N., Jadhav, K., & Mujib, B. R. (2009). Is recration of human identity possible using tooth prints? An experimental study to aid in identification. *Forensic Science International, 192*, 67–71. doi:10.1016/j.forsciint.2009.07.017

Harris, E. F., Mincer, H. H., Anderson, K. M., & Senn, D. R. (2010). Age estimation from oral and dental structures. In Senn, D., & Stimson, P. (Eds.), *Forensic dentistry* (2nd ed., pp. 279–293). Boca Raton, FL: Taylor & Francis.

Logan, W., & Kronfeld, R. (1933). Development of the human jaws and surrounding structures from birth to the age of fifteen years. *The Journal of the American Dental Association, 20*(3), 379–427.

Lunt, R. C., & Law, D. B. (1974). A review of the chronology of calcification of deciduous teeth. *The Journal of the American Dental Association, 89*(3), 599–606.

Manjunath, K., Sriram, G., Saraswathi, T. R., & Sivapathasungharam, B. (2008). Enamel rod end patterns: a preliminary study using acetate peel technique adnd automated biometrics. *The Journal of Forensic Odonto-Stomatology, 1*(1), 33–36.

Molina, D. K. (2010). Forensic medicine and human identification. In Senn, D., & Stimson, P. (Eds.), *Forensic dentistry* (2nd ed., pp. 61–78). Boca Raton, FL: Taylor & Francis.

Monjunath, K., Sriram, G., Sarawathi, T., Sivapathasundharam, B., & Porchelvam, S. (2009). Reliability of automated biometrics in the analysis of enamel rod end patterns. *Journal of Forensic Dental Sciences, 1*(1), 32–36. doi:10.4103/0974-2948.50887

National Academies Press. (2009). *Strengthening forensic science in the United States: A path forward*. Retrieved from http://www.nap.edu/catalogue.php?record_id=12589

Schour, I., & Massler, M. (1940a). Studies in tooth development: The growth pattern of human teeth, part 1. *The Journal of the American Dental Association, 27*(11), 1778–1793.

Schour, I., & Massler, M. (1940b). Studies in tooth development: The growth pattern of human teeth, part 2. *The Journal of the American Dental Association, 27*(12), 1918–1931.

Smith, B. C., & Sweet, D. (2010). DNA and DNA evidence. In Senn, D., & Stimson, P. (Eds.), *Forensic dentistry* (2nd ed., pp. 103–136). Boca Raton, FL: Taylor & Francis.

Tabor, M. P., & Schrader, B. A. (2010). Forensic dental identification. In Senn, D., & Stimson, P. (Eds.), *Forensic dentistry* (2nd ed., p. 167). Boca Raton, FL: Taylor & Francis.

Uhle, A. J. (2010). Fingerprints and human identification. In Senn, D., & Stimson, P. (Eds.), *Forensic dentistry* (2nd ed., pp. 79–102). Boca Raton, FL: Taylor & Francis.

Weems, R. A. (2010). Forensic dental radiography. In Senn, D., & Stimson, P. (Eds.), *Forensic dentistry* (2nd ed., pp. 190–191). Boca Raton, FL: Taylor & Francis.

Wright, F. D., & Dailey, J. C. (2001). Human bite marks in forensic dentistry. *Dental Clinics of North America*, *45*(2), 365–397.

Wright, F. D., & Golden, G. S. (2010). Forensic dental photography. In Senn, D., & Stimson, P. (Eds.), *Forensic dentistry* (2nd ed., p. 219). Boca Raton, FL: Taylor & Francis.

KEY TERMS AND DEFINITIONS

Alternate Light Imaging (ALI): Photographic technique utilizing a narrow band of illumination to produce fluorescence which is photographed through a barrier filter that blocks the illumination wavelength.

Bitemark Analysis: The comparison of injury patterns inflicted by teeth to the dental arcade of biters who may be excluded or included as possible biters.

Dental Aging: The use of dental methods to estimate the age of an individual, whether living or dead.

Dental Identification: The use of dental information to link unidentified human remains to a person.

Digital Radiography: A method of radiography in which digital sensors, sensitive to X-rays, are used instead of traditional film-based emulsion to capture images. The image is made viewable on a computer monitor through software.

Non-visible photography: The capture of images, either film-based or digital, using lightwave spectra not visible to the human eye.

Patterned Injury: An injury whose morphology suggests the nature of the injurious item.

Chapter 11
Dental Age Assessment (DAA) of Children and Emerging Adults:
A Practical Guide

Graham J. Roberts
King's College London Dental Institute, UK

Aviva Petrie
UCL Eastman Dental Institute, UK

ABSTRACT

A variety of methods have been used to estimate dental age. Tooth development as a means of estimating age has been used for several centuries. The purpose of the chapter is to describe the method used at the Dental Paediatric Unit of King's College London Dental Institute and the UCL Eastman Dental Institute to carry out Dental Age Assessment (DAA). An important principle is the biological variability of growth of teeth, a factor inappropriately considered in many studies of DAA. This chapter serves to inform colleagues, lawyers, immigration workers, social workers and subjects of unknown date of birth of the way in which DAA is conducted.

INTRODUCTION

General Considerations

Tooth development as a means of estimating age has been used for several centuries. In the early part of the Industrial Revolution in Great Britain children were required to work in underground coal mines on attaining six years of age. Evidence of the attainment of six years was adduced from the presence in the mouth of any of the permanent first molars (Saunders 1837). In general terms this was accepted but was harsh on those children

DOI: 10.4018/978-1-60960-483-7.ch011

whose first permanent molars erupted at under 6 years, sometimes as early as 5 years and 3 months (Ekstrand, Christiansen, & Christiansen 2003). This highlights an important principle, which is the essential biological variability of growth of teeth, a factor inappropriately considered in many studies of Dental Age Assessment (DAA).

Methods of age assessment are used on subjects whose date of birth is unknown either because records are lost or have never existed. The possible techniques are psychological development, height, weight (Demirjian, Buschang, Tenguay, & Patterson, 1985), hand-wrist skeletal development (Tanner, Healy, Goldstein, & Cameron, 2001), sterno-clavicular joint maturation (Kreitner, Schweden, Reipert, Nafe, & Thelen,1998), tooth development (Bolanos, Manrique, Bolanos, & Briones, 2000; Liversidge, Lyons, & Hector, 2003), dental root canal width (Kvaal, Kolltveit, Thomsen, & Solheim, 1995), and/or tooth apical foramen width (Cameriere, Ferrante, & Cingolani, 2006). Occasionally dental age assessment is needed to assist in the identification process of cadaveric remains (Clark, 2008). Studies where different methods of age assessment are compared all indicate that tooth development correlates more closely with chronological age than any of the other techniques (Garn, Lewis, & Kerewsky, 1965; Lewis & Garn, 1960; Demirjian, et al., 1985).

The development of high quality radiographic images, especially the Dental Panoramic Tomograph (DPT), with which the whole of the dentition is viewed on a single image, has provided clinical investigators with a uniquely effective way of assessing dental maturation. This has led to the use of a number of different systems for generating quantitative data from defined stages of tooth development (Liversidge, Chaillet, Mornstad, Nystrom, Rowlings, & Taylor, 2006). The DPT (often referred to as an OPG or OrthoPantomoGraph) is widely used in clinical practice to assess dental disease in otherwise healthy children. This means that very large numbers of DPTs are available which are deemed to be representative of the general population. Occasionally, other radiographic projections which have a limited number of teeth, for example the upper standard occlusal, are used to generate reference data. Thus many studies have been carried out accurately defining the age of attainment of tooth development using clearly defined stages (Demirjian & Goldstein, 1976; Olze, Bilang, Schmidt, Wemecke, Geserick, & Schmeling, 2005).

Careful scrutiny of the literature shows that none of the publications cited explains the detailed method of exactly *how* an individual of

Table 1. Tooth Morphology Types (TMTs) used in the Assessment of Dental Age. [8 Tooth Development Stages] British Dental Journal Nomenclature

Tooth Nomenclature [British Dental Journal Nomenclature]	Anatomical Description of TMTs
UL1	Upper Left Permanent Central Incisor
UL2	Upper Left Permanent Lateral Incisor
UL3	Upper Left Permanent Canine
UL4	Upper Left First Premolar
UL5	Upper Left Second Premolar
UL6	Upper Left Permanent First Molar
UL7	Upper Left Permanent Second Molar
UL8	Upper Left Third Molar
LL8	Lower Left Third Molar
LL7	Lower Left Permanent Second Molar
LL6	Lower Left Permanent First Molar
LL5	Lower Left Second Premolar
LL4	Lower Left First Premolar
LL3	Lower Left Permanent Canine
LL2	Lower Left Permanent Lateral Incisor
LL1	Lower Left Permanent Central Incisor
UR8	Upper Right Third Molar
LR8	Lower Right Third Molar

unknown date of birth is assessed to establish her/his likely age.

A variety of methods have been used to estimate dental age (see Section 6e). The purpose of the present document is to describe the method used at the Dental Paediatric Unit of King's College London Dental Institute and the UCL Eastman Dental Institute to carry out Dental Age Assessment (DAA). This is to inform colleagues, lawyers, immigration workers, social workers and subjects of unknown date of birth of the way in which DAA is conducted.

Nomenclature and Description of TDSs

There are many different shorthand systems used to identify specific teeth (Clark, 2008). In this document the British Dental Journal system (Table 1) is applied to the Demirjian descriptions (Table 2 and Figure 1) of tooth development stages (Demirjian, Goldstein, & Tanner, 1973). The International Dental Federation (FDI) system of nomenclature (Table 3) is applied to the Haavikko descriptions of tooth development stages (Table 4 and Figure 2) (Haavikko, 1970).

Table 2. Descriptions of Tooth Development Stages (TDSs), (Demirjian, 1973; Demirjian & Goldstein, 1976)

Tooth Development Stage (TDS)	Single Rooted Teeth and Multi-Rooted Teeth [Descriptions]
A	In both uniradicular and multiradicular teeth, a beginning of calcification is seen at the superior level of the crypt in the form of an inverted cone or cones. There is no fusion of these calcified points.
B	Fusion of the calcified points forms one or several cusps, which unite to give a regularly outlined occlusal surface.
C	a. Enamel formation is complete at the occlusal surface. Its extension and convergence toward the cervical region is seen. b. The beginning of a dentine deposit is seen. c. The outline of the pulp shape has a curved shape at the occlusal border.
D	a. Crown formation is complete down to the cemento-enamel junction. b. The superior border of the pulp chamber in uniradicular teeth has a definite curved form, being concave towards the cervical region. The projection of the pulp horns, if present, gives an outline like an umbrella top. In molars, the pulp chamber has a trapezoid form. c. Beginning of root formation is seen in the form of a radiopaque spicule.
E	UNIRADICULAR TEETH a. The walls of the pulp chamber now form straight lines, whose continuity is broken by the presence of the pulp horn, which is larger than in the previous stage. b. The root development is still less than the crown. MULTIRADICULAR TEETH a. Initial formation of the radicular bifurcation is seen in the form of either a calcified point or a semilunar shape. b. The root length is still less than the crown height.
F	UNIRADICULAR TEETH a. The walls of the pulp chamber now form a more or less isosceles triangle. The apex ends in a funnel shape. b. root development is equal to or greater than the crown. MULTIRADICULAR TEETH a. The calcified region of the bifurcation has developed further down from its semilunar stage to give the roots a more definite and distinct outline, with funnel shaped endings. b. The root length is equal to or greater than the crown height
G	a. The walls of the root canals are now parallel (distal root of molars) b. The apical ends of the root canals are still partially open.
H	a. The apical end of the root canal is completely closed (distal root in molars) b. The periodontal membrane has a uniform width around the root and apex

Figure 1. Schematic drawings of Demirjian 8 stage system (Demirjian, Goldstein, & Tanner 1973) used in assignment of Tooth Development Stages (A to H)

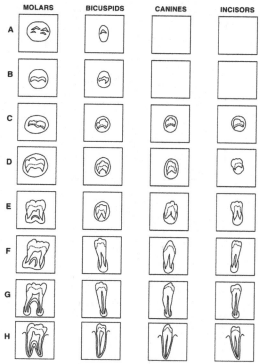

Schematic Representation for Eight Stages of Development

Table 3. Tooth Morphology Types (TMTs) used in the Assessment of Dental Age [12 Tooth Development Stages (Haavikko, 1970)], FDI Nomenclature

Tooth Nomenclature [FDI Notation]	Anatomical Description
21	Upper Left Permanent Central Incisor
22	Upper Left Permanent Lateral Incisor
23	Upper Left Permanent Canine
24	Upper Left First Premolar
25	Upper Left Second Premolar
26	Upper Left Permanent First Molar
27	Upper Left Permanent Second Molar
28	Upper Left Third Molar
31	Lower Left Permanent Central Incisor
32	Lower Left Permanent Lateral Incisor
33	Lower Left Permanent Canine
34	Lower Left First Premolar
35	Lower Left Second Premolar
36	Lower Left Permanent First Molar
37	Lower Left Permanent Second Molar
38	Lower Left Third Molar
18	Upper Right Third Molar
48	Lower Right Third Molar

The application of these two systems is demonstrated in Figure 3 using the same DPT. The remainder of this document only uses the 8 stage system of Demirjian. An exception to this is when Demirjian Stages G and H do not provide sufficiently accurate age assessments, in which case the Haavikko Stage 11 is used (see Section 5.c.iv).

Tooth development is symmetrical thus if a tooth on the left side is missing as a result of early loss (extraction) or hypodontia, the contralateral tooth is usually substituted.

The UR8 and LR8 have been included as a special case because third molars are the moist common teeth for developmental absence.

Each stage is identified by a letter and this is entered into the data proforma (Figure 3) when assessing radiographs that comprise the reference sample.

The identification system for individual TDSs is to combine the Tooth Identification with the Demirjian Stage. For example, LL4G is the Lower Left First Premolar (LL4) Stage G. After Arto Demirjian (Demirjian, Goldstein, & Tanner, 1973). This results in LL4G.

The Tooth Development Stages (TDSs) are those described by Karen Haavikko 1970) and identified as 01 to 12 (Figure 2). This is the 12 stage system of identification. The identification for individual TDSs is to combine the tooth Iden-

Table 4. Definition of Haavikko Stages of Development for Single Rooted and Multi-rooted Teeth (Haavikko, 1970)

Tooth Development Stage (TDS)	Number For Stage	Single Rooted Teeth And Multi Rooted Teeth
0	01	Crypt present, no calcification
C_i	02	Initial calcification
C_{co}	03	Coalescence of cusps
$Cr_{1/2}$	04	Crown ½ complete
$Cr_{3/4}$	05	Crown ¾ complete
Cr_c	06	Crown complete
R_i	07	Initial root formation
$R_{1/4}$	08	Root length ¼
$R_{1/2}$	09	Root length ½
$R_{3/4}$	10	Root length ¾
R_c	11	Root length complete
A_c	12	Apex closed

After Karen Haavikko (1970)

Figure 2. Schematic drawings of Haavikko 12 stage system used to identify Tooth Development Stages (01 to 12)

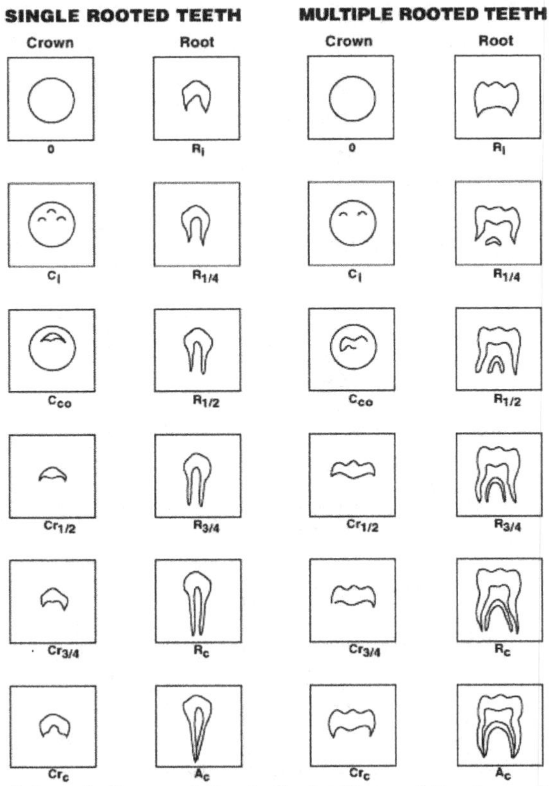

Schematic Representation for Twelve Stages of Development

tification with the Haavikko Stage. For example, 3411 is the Lower Left First Premolar (34) Stage (11) The detailed descriptions of the Haavikko stages are given in Table 4.

Stages of all the teeth discernible on the Left side only are identified. The assessment includes both maxillary and mandibular teeth. Teeth on the right side can be substituted if a tooth on the left side is missing.

The nomenclature for Demirjian (Demirjian, Goldstein, & Tanner, 1973) (8) stages is described in Tables 1 & 2 and Figure 1.

The nomenclature for the Haavikko (1970) (12) stage system is described in Tables 3 & 4 and Figure 2.

Requirements for a Suitable Reference Data

The Scientific reliability of measurements used to determine age is an example of the general problem of assessing Growth and Development and providing referenced data to which individuals are compared

Estimation of age in subjects of unknown date of birth requires that a number of standardised procedures need to be followed. These have been described in a closed document (Sterne 2008) and are listed in Table 5.

"Before a measurement of a child's growth and maturity could have a reliable accuracy attached to it as one which has been scientifically correlated with age, it would be necessary to have been subjected to a series of processes accepted by scientists. For any clinical measurement these are (see Table 5).

Figure 3. Dental Panoramic Tomograph – GW

Right Side   Left Side

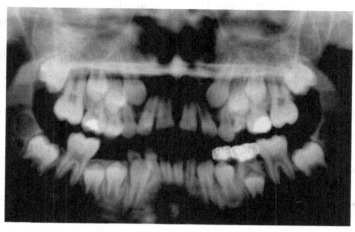

Right Side   Left Side

Stages identified on The DPT shown using the Demirjian 8 stage system	UL1H	UL2G	UL3F	UL4F	UL5E	UL6G	UL7E	-
	LL1H	LL1G	LL3G	LL4F	LL5E	LL6G	LL7E	-

Stages identified on The DPT shown using the Haavikko 12 stage system	2112	2210	2310	2409	2508	2611	2708	-
	3112	3211	3310	3409	3508	3611	3708	3801

Table 5.

1.	...	the measurement must be carried out in a standard way and take into account known genetic patterns
2.	...	many of the same measurements must be carried out on large population
3.	...	these data must be analysed statistically, so as to generate means or medians and standard deviations or standard errors
4.	...	the data and their analyses should be published, in order that they are subjected to peer review. This is a critical step in the confirmation of scientific validity
5.	...	the whole process of measurement should be repeated on a similar population, so as to validate the original data published
6.	...	it would be necessary to repeat the validated measurement on an ethnically different population, in order to establish the presence or absence of ethnic variability
7.	...	in order that any of these clinical measurements might be employed to estimate age, it would be necessary for all these observations to be carried out on populations of children and young people of known age."

ETHICAL ISSUES

Ethical Approval for Research

The research projects from which the data are derived were approved by the ethical committees of University College Hospitals NHS Trust [REC reference 03/E02] (the UCL Eastman Dental Institute) and King's College Hospital NHS Trust [REC reference 06/Q0703/54], and the University of Sydney Research Ethics Committee [REC reference US/23006_1101].

A compelling ethical consideration is that it is *not* permissible to take x-rays solely for research. This means that it is possible only to *re-use* radiographs from patients who have attended for clinical care. This is the only source of x-ray material used to form the sample from which reference data sets are derived. For this reason, studies since 1975 where radiographs have been taken principally for the research will not be quoted in references used to support statements in this document. The radiographs that provide suitable images are Intra-Oral Periapicals (IOPs), Upper Standard Occlusals (USOs), Lower Standard Occlusals (LSOs), Oblique Lateral Jaws (OLJs), and Dental Panoramic Tomographs (DPTs). These radiographs provide high quality images of developing teeth. In essence, any radiograph may be used provided it has a known date of acquisition (dor [date of radiograph]) and a verifiable date of birth (dob) and which provides an image of at least a single tooth (or up to sixteen teeth) that may contribute to the database. The DPT has the enormous advantage of providing images of all teeth present in the mouth – up to the sixteen Tooth Morphology Types (TMTs) of the human permanent dentition.

Ethical Justification for Taking X-Rays for DAA

Radiographs are usually taken for the purpose of diagnosis or monitoring the progress of treatment. That is to say for the net benefit which is usually interpreted as the net benefit for the patient. Regulations also sanction the use of x-rays which may not be for the clinical benefit of the subject (2000). The use of x-rays for non clinical purposes must be of net benefit. That is to say the benefit must be to the subject or society or both.

The British Association of Forensic Odontology supports the use of x-rays for the primary purpose of Dental Age Assessment (British Association of Forensic Odontology). The British Society of Dental and Maxillofacial Radiology support the taking of and x-rays for the primary purpose of assessing age (British Society of Dental and Maxillofacial Radiology 2008). The Royal College of Paediatrics and Child Health do not support the use of x-rays for the purpose of age assessment. An important consideration is the fact that the use of an x-ray is acceptable to the subject who after appropriate explanation provides written consent. This satisfies the ethical requirements.

Informed Consent

All subjects who request Dental Age Assessment have the benefit of independent advice from solicitors working with experience of the UK Border Agency. An individual claiming to be under 18 also has the benefit of a dedicated social worker. The responsibility for explaining the intricacies of informed consent start with the dedicated social worker and/or the legal adviser. The use of interpreters, where needed, is essential. The subjects are provided with an explanation of the procedures to be carried out during the clinical and radiographic examination. The subject provides *written* consent to the procedures, with written endorsement by the interpreter, where appropriate. The issue of consent for subjects under 18 years has been simplified by the ruling of the appeal courts of England which empowers any child to give consent for medical and related procedures provided that s/he understand the implications of the procedures involved. Assessment of capacity for consent requires the three stage test (Hockton, 2002).

The patient must be able to:

1. Comprehend and retain relevant information;
2. Believe it;
3. Weigh it in the balance so as to arrive at a choice.

To assist subjects a short document explaining the issues surrounding Age Assessment is provided to the referring personnel, whether it be the Social Worker, Solicitor, or a relative of the subject (Appendix A).

The law empowers children under the age of 16 to give consent if the child understands the issues of concern. This is known as *Gillick* competence. It is an ongoing matter and will not be lost or acquired on a day to day or week to week basis (Hockton, 2002). The child under 16 years is able to give consent provided the three conditions listed above are met.

In addition, the clinician must be that circumscribed by the fact that the treatment or procedure must be in the child's best interests (Hockton, 2002). This caveat does not apply here as the use of x-rays for age assessment is not a treatment procedure.

In practical terms, patients and/or carers are consenting to providing the following information at the DAA clinic:

- A medical history
- An examination and recording of the condition of oro-dental tissues
- Clinical photographs of teeth
- A facial photograph

- A dental panoramic tomograph (x-ray)
- Occasionally, additional x-rays such as Long Cone Periapicals to show details of wisdom tooth development, or a Hand-Wrist X-Ray and Postero-Anterior Chest views to enable determination beyond reasonable doubt that the subject is older than 18 years (Schmeling et al., 2003). These additional views also give very low radiation exposure to the subject.

ESTABLISHMENT OF A DATABASE

To carry out DAA it is necessary to have access to a suitably large Reference Data Set. This is obtained by establishing a database using demographic data and the information from DPTs from each of a large number of healthy children of known age to provide data on the TDSs described in Section 1 for each tooth for a specific child. Collectively, this gives a range of ages for each of the TDSs which form the database. In practical terms, these TDSs comprise 8 clearly defined stages for each of the 16 Tooth Morphology Types (all the teeth in the

Figure 4. Frequency Distribution of Age for Tooth Development Stage LL8Ef

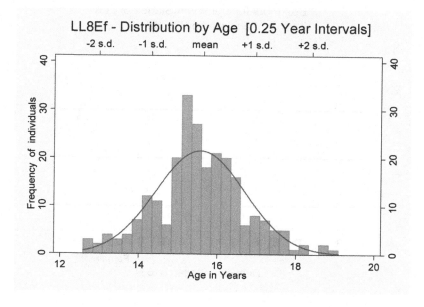

upper and lower jaws on the left side) assessed separately for males and females; this totals 256 TDSs. When the third molars on the right side are included, this increases the total number of TDSs to 288. The actual numbers are less as for some of the TDSs in young patients there are no data available. The distribution of these ages for each TDS, separately for male and female Caucasians, is approximately Normally (symmetrically) distributed. An example for LL8 Stage E for females (LL8Ef) is shown as a histogram in Figure 4, and as a box and whisker plot in Figure 5. All the data for males and females for the LL8 are shown in Figure 6.

This shows the data with the median (50th percentile) as a horizontal bar in the box. The lower and upper limits of the box are the 25th and 75th percentiles, respectively. The whiskers (drawn as bars) extend from the box at both ends and approximately encompass the central 95% of the observations. If the data are approximately normally distributed, the median is near the middle of the box which is in the middle of the whiskers, as shown in the figure.

The 18 year threshold is shown in figure 6. Both males and females have a similar course of development. Note: Some of the age distributions of the early stages for both males and females are skewed, probably a consequence of the relatively small sample sizes for these early stages.

Figure 5. Box plot of LL8Ef 9same data set as in Figure 4.)

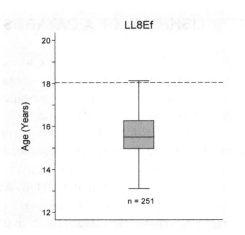

Figure 6. Box plot for whole of data from LL8 comprising the 8 stages partitioned by gender

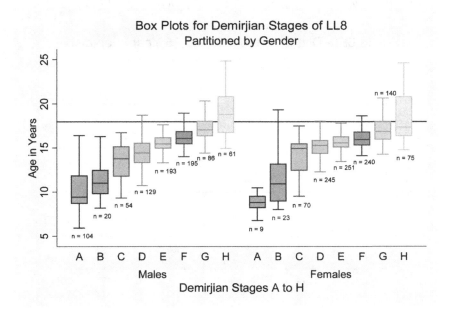

STATISTICAL METHODS

Basic Statistical Theory

The process of Dental Age Assessment is an example of the general biological problem of measuring a variable such as height, weight, or femur length to estimate the age of the individual. This is achieved by taking a sufficiently large and representative sample from the population of interest. From this sample it is possible to create a distribution of ages for a given height, for example, from which the average age for that height can be estimated. This approach has been extended to estimate that age of attainment using Tooth Development Stages (TDS) (Demirjian et al., 1973).

Calculation of Age of Attainment of each Tooth Development Stage

Within the Microsoft Access Database it is possible to raise a query to calculate the age of attainment of each of the TDSs present in an individual subject.

The logical expressions is **LR8Ef: IIf([LR8-E]=0,Null,([dor]-[dob])/365.25).** This gives the ages in years of the lower right third molar Demirjian Stage E for females. By appropriate substitution, the ages of all the Tooth Development Stages (TDSs) of all 16 tooth morphology types (TMTs) on the left side of the mouth for males and females can be calculated. In addition the UR8 and LL8 provide data on third molars on the right side so that substitution can be performed if one of the third molars is developmentally or surgically missing. The complete data set which gives the chronological ages of all the TDSs in all of the subjects is then exported into Excel as a single spreadsheet.

Age Distribution for a Given TDS

Scrutiny of the age data for an individual TDS occasionally shows a value which is impossible; for example, a negative age or an age greater than 30 years. If such an age is noted, the reason for its presence is identified and the age is corrected. Because of the large numbers in the database, it is recognised that it is not possible to always identify these impossible ages, and so a rule has been devised which excludes from any calculations any age less than zero and greater than 30 years.

In addition, in order to exclude outliers that are less clearly defined for a given TDS, any age value which lies beyond 3 standard deviations away from the mean are excluded, i.e. the remaining ages exclude 0.15% of the observations at each end of the age distribution. The remaining 99.7% of the ages are used to calculate the summary statistics for each and every TDS. This ensures a Normal distribution for the summary data for each Tooth Development Stage. The data are periodically checked (once per year) for the effects of outliers and the appropriate assignment for individual teeth

Summary Statistics

From the constrained distribution of ages (the values x_1, x_2, x_3,) for each TDS, the following summary statistics are obtained (Table 6).

Table 6.

• The sample size (*n*)	• The median (i.e. the 50th percentile)
• The arithmetic mean ($\overline{x}$)	• The minimum and maximum ages
• The standard deviation (SD)	• The range (i.e. the difference between the minimum and maximum ages)
• The standard error of the mean (SEM)	• The 0.5th, 5th, 10th, 25th, 50th, 75th, 90th, 95th and 99.5th percentiles.
• The 99% confidence interval for the mean (i.e. the lower and upper limits)	

Calculating the Probability of a Given Age Range

It is possible to use the theory of the Normal (Gaussian) distribution to evaluate the probability that an individual is over or under a specific age from a distribution of ages for a single TDS. This approach utilises an assumed normally distributed data set, the theory of the Normal distribution and the calculated average (mean) and standard deviation (sd) to estimate the probability of interest. This can now be carried out in a straightforward way by using the NORMDIST function (Normal Distribution Function) of Excel [Microsoft Office 2007].

When this function is opened in Microsoft Excel the data are entered as below (a) is the age for which the cumulative probability is sought, (b) is the mean age of the reference data set used – in this case LL8Ef, (c) is the standard deviation from the same reference set, and the word TRUE is entered into the box to give the Cumulative Probability Calculation. A worked example is shown in Table 7.

This calculation can be repeated for each of the ages for cumulative probability is required.

The age at *any* point can be calculated to assist subjects in the support of her/his claimed age. This is the same tooth and stage that provided the data for the boxplot in Figure 5.

The interpretation if this is relatively simple. The cumulative probability is that part of Normal distribution curve below the cut off age chosen.

Calculating an Age from a Given Percentile

If we order the ages from the lowest to the highest values, 50% of the ordered values lie below the 50th percentile and 50% of them lie above the 50th percentile. The 50th percentile is the median of the age distribution. The evaluation of percentiles does not rely on the data being normally distributed. This has the advantage that percentiles can be used with any data set. The 0.5th percentile has 0.5% of the ordered ages below it and 99.5% of the ordered ages above it. It is helpful to use the various percentiles to determine the age below which a specified percentage of the individuals with a given TDS lie (Table 9).

Principles of Meta-Analysis and its Application

When two or more teeth have different TDSs in an individual, it is necessary to combine the

Table 8.

Cumulative probability that subject is under 15 yrs	=	0.32 [32%]
Cumulative probability that subject is under 15.6 yrs	=	**0.50 [50%]**
Cumulative probability that subject is under 16 yrs	=	0.62 [62%]
Cumulative probability that subject is under 17 yrs	=	0.85 [85%]
Cumulative probability that subject is under 18 yrs	=	0.96 [96%]

Table 7. Worked example from the EXCEL NORMDIST function of Cumulative Probability Calculation for LL8Ef with repeated calculations for the 15 yr, 16 yr, 17 yr and 18 yr thresholds. The same cumulative probability as the mean age is also calculated and as is shown this should equal 0.5 (50%) as the mean age of a normally distributed population is exactly at the position of 0.5 cumulative probability

	15	=	A Number – age in years up to which cumulative probability is sought
(a) x	**15.60**	=	Mean age from sample (Reference Data Set)
(c) Standard_dev	**1.31**	=	Standard Deviation from sample (Reference Data Set
(d) Cumulative	**True**	=	Enter TRUE in this box

Table 9. An example is given with the LL8Fm [age in years]

TDS	0.5%-ile	5%-ile	10%-ile	25%-ile	50%-ile	75%-ile	90%-ile	95%-ile	99.5%-ile	TDS
LL8Fm	14.09	14.62	15.02	15.52	16.12	16.97	17.76	18.38	19.18	**LL8Fm**

information from them in order to evaluate the DAA of the individual. We achieve this by using the mathematical techniques of meta-analysis. The main aim of a meta-analysis is to combine the results from individual studies to produce, if appropriate, a weighted estimate of the overall or average effect of interest (e.g. a relative risk or a difference in treatments). In such situations, the direction and magnitude of this average effect, together with a consideration of the associated confidence interval and hypothesis test result, can be used to make decisions about the therapy under investigation and the management of patients (Altman, 1991). In the context of DAA, when we have more than one TDS present in a subject of unknown date of birth (udob) we have used a meta-analysis approach to take advantage of the underlying mathematical techniques to provide a weighted mean of the expected ages of the various TDSs present for that subject. Because the TDSs in a single subject are related in their growth and development, and studies in a meta-analysis should be independent, this approach is likely to lead to an underestimation of the confidence interval for the subject's age. That is to say the confidence interval associated with the meta-analytic calculation for DAA gives a spurious impression of precision. For this reason, we avoid quoting a confidence interval for the estimated Dental Age of an individual subject.

A very simple explanation of the process of meta-analysis is as follows: in principle, in order to obtain the weighted mean age, greater weight is given to those age distributions with larger numbers of observations and smaller variation. The terms 'fixed-effects' and 'random-effects' models arise in the context of meta-analysis. A fixed-effects model in the context of DAA assumes

the mean is the same for every TDS. This is clearly not the case in DAA so we use a random-effects model instead which incorporates the variation between the TDSs into the weight for each TDS. A forest plot is a useful diagrammatic representation of the results: conventionally, it shows the estimated age for each TDS, together with a 99% confidence interval for the mean population age, and an overall estimate of the DAA for that child. Full details of meta-analysis may be found in various texts, for example, Meta-Analysis in Stata (Sterne, 2009).

Assessing Agreement

Kappa Statistic for Comparing TDSs (Intra and Inter-Rater Agreement)

An important consideration in both the development of the database and the assessment of subjects of unknown age is the reliability of the individuals assessing radiographs and the Tooth Development Stage(s) present on a radiograph (Olze et al., 2005). This is a general problem of the consistency of judgement of an anatomical or pathological feature that is undergoing a process of change. This involves assessing intra-rater agreement (often called repeatability) and inter-rater agreement (often referred to as reproducibility) (Altman 1991; Liversidge, 2008). To evaluate agreement, a number of DPTs are chosen randomly and each of the TDSs present on the left side of every DPT are recorded by an observer. For intra-rater agreement, the assessments are made on two occasions, at least a week apart, to ensure that the rater does not remember any of the individual cases used in the assessment. A requirement of the test is that, before the second assessment, a co-worker shuffles the radiographs so that the rater views them in a different order. The index of reliability of intra-rater agreement used is Cohen's Kappa which is also determined to evaluate inter-rater agreement but in this instance each of the TDSs is assessed once by two or more raters. The interpretation of Cohen's Kappa is given in Table 10.

The scaling of the Kappa statistic is 0 when the amount of agreement observed is to be expected from chance and 1 when there is perfect agreement. (Landis & Koch, 1977)

It has been shown that the Demirjian 8 stage system (Demirjian et al., 1973) is slightly more reliable than the Haavikko 12 stage system (Haavikko, 1970) for intra-rater agreement (the same investigator on two occasions) and also for inter-rater agreement (two investigators on separate occasions) [Unpublished data in the DARLInG Archives]. The Kappa values derived from 6 investigators at the Eastman Dental Institute and King's College Dental Hospital show a consistent level of reliability for the Demirjian 8 stage system ranged from 0.8185 to 0.9380 for intra-rater agreement and from 0.6901 to 0.8741 for inter-rater agreement.

Bland and Altman Approach for Comparing Chronological and Dental Age

This approach is commonly used to assess the agreement between two sets of data measured on a numerical variable. In this case, the data relate to chronological and dental age, each measured on a number of individuals, providing a set of paired ages. If the mean difference between the pairs, ($\bar{d}$), is zero (as assessed by the paired *t*-test), there is *no systematic difference* between the pairs of results. Since one set of readings represents the true chronological ages this means that there is no **bias.** Then, *on average*, the chronological and dental ages agree.

In order to draw the Bland and Altman diagram, upper and lower limits of this interval are called the **limits of agreement.** These limits are drawn on the Bland and Altman diagram in which the difference between the pair of ages is plotted on the vertical axis against the mean of the pair of ages on the horizontal axis; together with the **British Standards Institution repeatability coefficient** ($2s_d$) is determined. This coefficient is the maximum difference which is likely to occur between two measurements; from this, it can be judged whether the agreement between pairs of readings in a given situation is acceptable.

It is *inappropriate* to calculate the Pearson correlation coefficient between the *n* pairs of ages (i.e. CA and DA) as a measure of reliability. It is not of interest to decide whether the points in the scatter diagram of the chronological age plotted against the dental age lie on a straight line; it *is* of interest to determine whether they conform to the line of equality (i.e., the 45° line through the origin when the two scales are the same). This will not be established by testing the null hypoth-

Table 10. Values of Cohen's Kappa for assessing intra- and inter-rater agreement

Kappa Value	Level of Agreement	Acceptable?
Below 0.0	Poor	No
0.00 - 0.20	Slight	No
0.21 - 0.40	Fair	No
0.41 - 0.60	Moderate	No
0.61 - 0.80	**Substantial**	**Yes**
0.81 – 1.00	**Almost Perfect**	**Yes**

Figure 7. From Mitchell JC et al. 2009 (Mitchell et al. 2009)

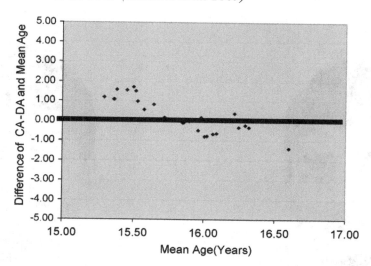

esis that the true Pearson correlation coefficient is zero. It would, in any case, be very surprising if the pairs of CA and DA were not related (Petrie & Sabin, 2009). Instead, Lin's Concordance Correlation Coefficient is calculated as an index of reliability. Lin's coefficient modifies the Pearson correlation coefficient which assesses the closeness of the data about the line of best fit in the scatter plot by taking into account how far the line of best fit is from the 45° line through the origin. The maximum value of Lin's coefficient is 1, achieved when there is perfect concordance, with all the points lying on the 45° line drawn through the origin. The determination of Lin's concordance correlation coefficient may be achieved simply by using Stata (Statacorp, LP 2007).

THE TECHNIQUE OF DAA

General Considerations

History and Examination

Preliminary assessment of an individual presenting for DAA consists of a medical history to exclude conditions which might affect growth and development. In addition, any condition requiring treatment can be brought to the attention of the subject.

A preliminary examination of the individual is made noting the overall physical appearance including stature and facial appearance and any distinguishing features. This overall appraisal is part of the assessment of subjects of all ages. An Oro-Dental Examination is carried out noting the number of Tooth Morphology Types (TMTs). Any signs of disease such as gingival inflammation, periodontal pocketing, and dental caries are recorded as it may be necessary to advise of the possible need for treatment. In addition, the amount of wear on the occlusal surfaces of the 1st, 2nd and 3rd permanent molars is carefully noted as well as wear on other teeth.

Clinical Photographs and X-Rays

A set of clinical photographs is taken with a digital single lens reflex camera (Figures 8 through to 21). An image of the radiograph is also recorded digitally and added to the set of photographs. The whole set of images provides an *aide de memoire* when preparing the written report, a means of

Figure 8. Facial view: Solemn

Figure 9. Facial view: Smiling

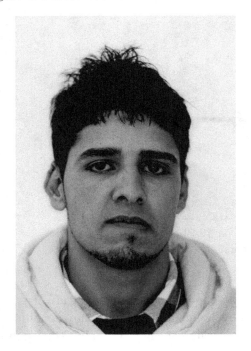

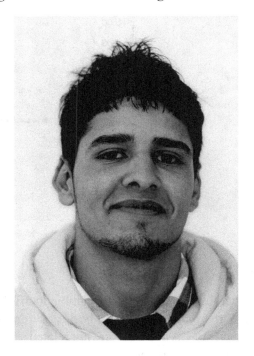

Figure 10. Anterior view

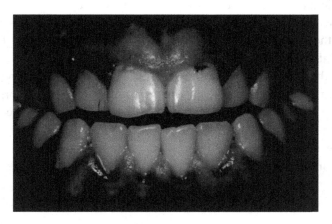

identifying the subject of the report to those that subsequently use the report as part of legal proceedings, and enables the clinician to manipulate the digital image of the xray to improve the assessment of the tooth development stages present. These records allow the clinician to deal with any specific queries that may arise during subsequent proceedings. This occasionally happens when the output clearly looks wrong as occurs when the date of birth and the date of radiograph were entered incorrectly or a tooth development stage is incorrectly assigned.

Note: the facial views are not from the same subject as the intra-oral views and the radiographs. This is to ensure anonymity of the subject. The facial views are from an image library.

Figure 11. Right side in occlusion

Figure 12. Left side in occlusion

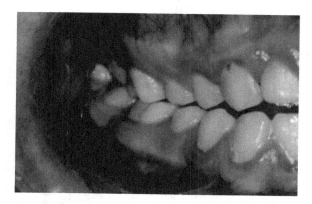

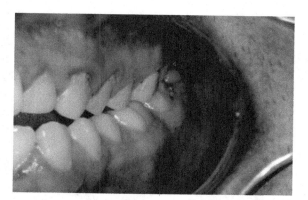

Figure 13. Upper (Maxillary) arch

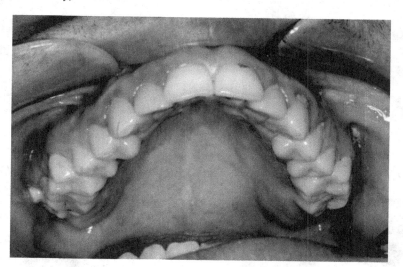

Figure 14. Lower (Mandibular) arch

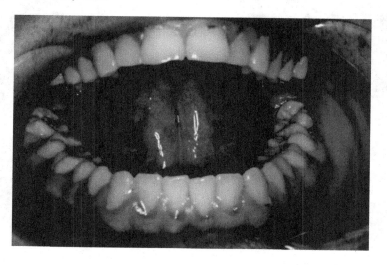

Figure 15. LR6, LR7, LR8 (close up)

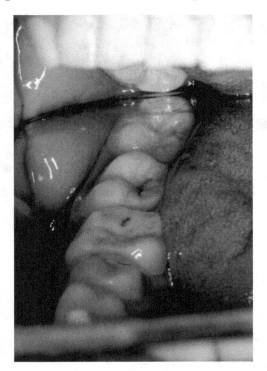

Figure 16. LL6, LL7, LL8 (close up)

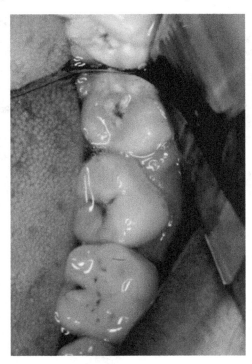

Figure 17. UR6, UR7, UR8 (close up)

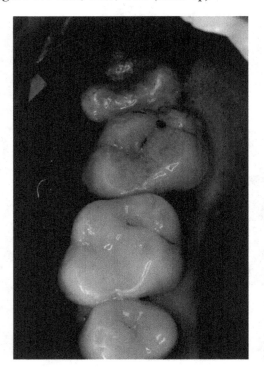

Figure 18. UL6, UL7, UL8 (close up)

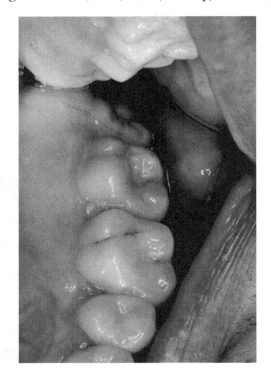

Figure 19.

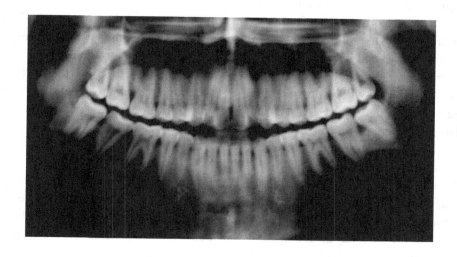

Figure 20.

Figure 21.

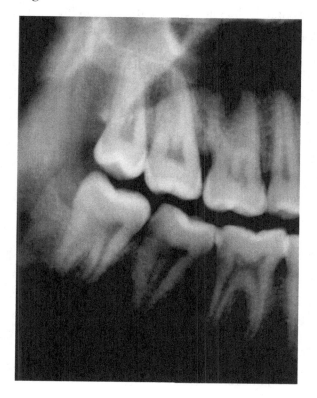

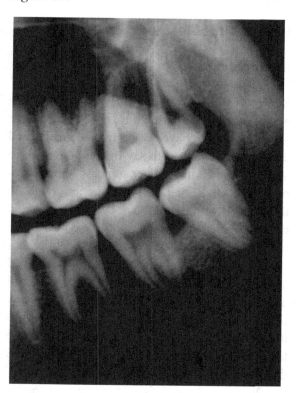

The image of the radiograph is captured in digital format so that it can be viewed on a computer using image manipulation software. This image capture has conventionally been by the production of a silver halide radiation sensitive material on a conventional cellulose acetate base. In the past this image is all that has been available. With modern computer technology it is more convenient to create a digital image of the cellulose acetate specimen. This can be created by a flat bed scanner, a small digital camera, or a single lens reflex camera. Any such camera provides the facility to vary the exposure settings to create the optimum image in terms of contrast and image brightness. [In the near future almost all radiographic images will be derived digitally and will be downloaded to the investigator's computer]. To assist in the handling of large numbers of images it is helpful to name the image with full details of name and ethnicity viz:- [OAK_Gabriel_13245768_1 996_0930_M_2005_0106_nml_Euripoid]. This enables rapid and accurate identification of any radiographic image, should this be required for legal purposes, with the personal details of each subject incorporated into the file name. As with the photographs, the name used is a pseudonym.

Use of Multiple Teeth

Introduction

Subjects of unknown date of birth below the age of 16 Yrs (approximately) are likely to have several teeth that have not completed growth and development. That is to say the teeth may be in stage E, F or G. In younger subjects some stages may be even C, or D. By convention, teeth on the left side of the mouth are used for DAA and this is justified as there is right/left symmetry in tooth development (Haavikko, 1970; Willerhausen, Loffler, & Schulze, 2001). An estimation of age is then performed using only those teeth still developing on the left side of the mouth (i.e. any of the 16 tooth morphology types (TMTs) still developing). This approach involving multiple teeth allows as little as two or as many as 16 developing teeth to be used for the calculation.

The principles of meta-analysis are explained in Section 4b. In the context of DAA, the technique uses the summary statistics derived from the age distributions of the TDSs present on the radiograph of a child of unknown date of birth. These statistics include the sample size, mean, standard deviation and the standard error of the mean of each age

distribution (Table 6). Essentially the mean age for the age distribution of each TDS of the teeth still developing in that child is weighted and they are combined to provide an overall estimate of the mean age for that child; this is then assigned as the estimated dental age of the child of unknown date of birth.

Probabilities

In order to estimate the probability that a child is above (or below) a given age, it is possible to combine the probabilities of being above (or below) this age from all the teeth used for the meta-analysis. A simple approach is to determine the weighted mean of these probabilities: each weight is the number of individuals in the reference data set for a given TDS. If the number of individuals for the ith TDS is n_i and the relevant probability is p_i, the formula for the weighted mean probability is:

$$\frac{\sum n_i p_i}{\sum n_i}$$

For example if there are two TDSs, this formula is:

$$\frac{n_1 p_1 + n_2 p_2}{n_1 + n_2}$$

A specific is example is shown in Table 11. The chance that this child is under 10 years of age is estimated to be 0.05966 which would usually be interpreted to mean that this child has approximately a 6.0% chance of being under 10 years of age.

Example

The DPT shown in Figure 22 is a typical example of a child with multiple developing teeth of known chronological age (12.62 years).

Table 11. Example of calculation for the mean weighted probability that a subject is under a specific age (10 years). This example is based on the stages shown in Table 12

STAGE-male	n_i	SD	MEAN		p_i	%
UL3G	38	1.32	11.87		0.07829	7.83%
UL4G	28	1.46	12.27		0.06000	6.00%
UL5G	28	1.66	12.45		0.06998	6.99%
UL7G	69	1.56	13.34		0.01614	1.16%
UL8D	228	2.01	13.84		0.02804	2.80%
LL3G	36	2.3	11.70		0.22991	22.99%
LL4G	30	1.57	12.10		0.09052	9.05%
LL5F	37	2.96	11.57		0.29792	29.79%
LL7G	113	1.43	13.57		0.00627	0.63%
LL8C	54	2.06	13.43		0.04795	4.70%
		Weighted Probability of subject < 10years			**0.05966**	**5.966%**

The procedure for DAA is as follows:

1. The TDSs for this child using the Demirjian developmental stages (see Section 1b) are entered onto the printed proforma as a permanent record (Figure 23).

2. These stages are entered into a Stata spreadsheet (Acock, 2008) together with the average (mean) age and standard error of the mean (se) for each of these stages derived from the reference data. This information is contained in Table 12. This table has a row of information corresponding to each of the 16 teeth potentially in the left side of the mouth. If a tooth is missing or is at Stage H in the child, the summary statistics are treated as missing values and are marked with a full stop.

Figure 22. Dental Panoramic Tomograph of boy or girl ID No. 04082523, initials DS

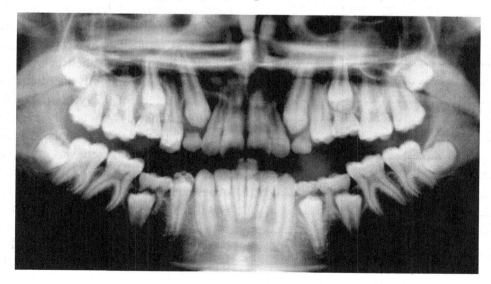

3. Stata calculates the weighted mean age (with 99% confidence interval); this is an estimate of the mean age of children who come from the population from which these reference data are drawn. This estimated mean age is assigned to this child who is of unknown age. However, the precision of the estimate, as indicated by the confidence interval, relates to a population of individuals and not to a single individual. Therefore, it is considered inappropriate to use the confidence interval for the mean determined in this way as an indication of the precision of the estimated age of an individual child. The following

Table 12. Stata spreadsheet for child showing summary statistics (mean age and standard error of the mean) extracted from Table 6 (Morrees & Kent, 1978)

Subject ID	123456789		
Maxillary [L]			
Tooth	Stage	x (Mean age - Yrs)	sem (Standard Error - Yrs)
UL1	H	.	.
UL2	H	.	.
UL3	UL3G	11.87	0.20
UL4	UL4G	12.27	0.22
UL5	UL5G	12.45	0.16
UL6	H	.	.
UL7	UL7G	13.34	0.16
UL8	UL8D	13.84	0.11
Mandibular [L]			
LL1	H	.	.
LL2	H	.	.
LL3	LL3G	11.70	0.68
LL4	LL4G	12.10	0.21
LL5	LL5F	11.57	0.24
LL6	H	.	.
LL7	LL7G	13.57	0.11
LL8	LL8C	13.43	0.26

command provides this information in addition to a forest plot (Figure 23):

meta x se, print level(99) gr(r) cline xlab(5(1)11) id(stage)

The forest plot shows the estimated mean age (the box) and 99% confidence interval of each developing tooth stage. The estimated mean dental age for the population of children with this combination of TDSs is indicated by the dotted line and the 99% confidence interval by the horizontal limits of the diamond. Therefore, the individual child ID No. 123456789 is assigned a dental age of 12.66 years.

The process is simple to carry out. Meta-Analysis software is available free of charge in the Cochrane Collaboration Web site (Review Manager (RevMan) [Computer program]. Version 5.0. Copenhagen: The Nordic Cochrane Centre, The Cochrane Collaboration, 2008.). A tutorial is provided for ease of use. Because it is possible to copy and paste the relevant summary statistics (Table 9) from the Excel spreadsheet directly into Stata (Acock, 2008), it is more convenient to Stata to perform the meta-analysis (Figure 24).

The agreement between CA and the estimated DA was assessed from the test dataset from 50 children using the Bland and Altman method (Section 4c(ii)). All the assessments of the xrays were made with the assessor unaware of the date of the xray or the date of birth of the subject i.e. 'blind'. The differences between CA and the estimated DA were randomly distributed around the mean difference of 0.29years (SD 0.84 years), with the estimated DA generally greater than CA. A paired t-test performed on these data gave p = 0.04, indicating that there was a suggestion of a systematic difference or bias between the pairs of ages. However, Lin's concordance coefficient was 0.95 (95% confidence interval 0.92 to 0.97), which is very close to the upper limit of 1.0 when there is perfect concordance. The British Standards reproducibility coefficient was approximately

Figure 23. Tooth Development Stages from DS (from DPT shown in Figure 22)

Filename:					dob:	dor					
Hospital No:				Ethnicity:							
Mother's origin:					Father's origin:						
Haavikko	21	22	23	24	25	26	27	28		18	28
	31	32	33	34	35	36	37	38		48	38
Demirjian	UL1	UL2	UL3	UL4	UL5	UL6	UL7			UR8	UL8
	H	H	G	G	G	H	G			—	D
	LL1	LL2	LL3	LL4	LL5	LL6	LL7			LR8	LL8
	H	H	G	G	F	H	G			—	C

Figure 24. Results of meta-analysis of child ID No. 123456789, initials DS (generated by Stata Meta – Analysis. Stata version 10.0 California, USA. 2007.)

Subject Research ID No.	Chronological Age (Yrs)	Dental Age (Yrs)	Lower 99%CI (Yrs)	Upper 99%CI (Yrs)
DAA_ST01_25	12.62	12.66	11.96	13.36

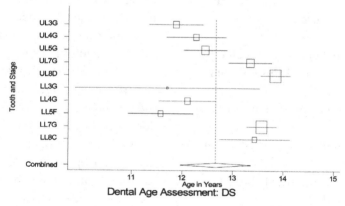

equal to 1.96 x (SD of the differences) = 1.96 x 0.843 = 1.65 years; this indicates that the maximum likely difference between a pair of ages (estimated DA and CA) was approximately 1.7 years. About half of these subjects had a dental age which did not differ from the chronological age by more than three months. (Roberts & Lucas, 1994)

Use of Third Molars

No Third Molar at Stage H

If the third molars have not completed development, the distributions of the age of attainment for the tooth development stages present (C, D, E, F or G) are used to provide an estimate of the DA for the subject.

The possible presentations of the developing third molars are defined below. If more than one third molar is used for the DAA, the technique of meta analysis described in section 5 b iii is applied. The possible presentations are:

a.   All 4 third molars present
    i.   Where there is symmetrical development on the left and right sides, only the third molars on the left side are used for DAA, i.e. UL8 and LL8.
    ii.   Where there is asymmetric development, all four molars are considered.
       •   If either the upper or the lower pairs are asymmetrical but the remaining pair is symmetrical, only the left of the symmetrical pair is used and both of the asymmetrical pair are used.
       •   If there is asymmetry in the development in both the upper and the lower pairs, all four third molars are used

This means that when there is asymmetry, the DAA could be based on 2, 3 or 4 third molars.

b.   Both lower third molars present, upper third molars absent
    i.   If there is symmetry, only the left third molar is used.
    ii.   If they are asymmetrical, both third molars are used

c.   Both upper third molars present, both lower third molars absent
    i.   If there is symmetry, only the left third molar is used.
    ii.   If they are asymmetrical, both third molars are used

d.   One lower third molar and one upper third molar present (other third molars absent), then both teeth are used.

e.   Only one third molar present. The age distribution of the relevant TDS provides an estimated DA for the subject. Note that if age assessment is required on the basis of a single tooth that is not a third molar, this same approach applies.

Example using a Single Third Molar Still Developing (i.e. not at Stage H)

This worked example is that of a female asylum seeker whose claimed age was disputed by the home office. The Dental Panoramic Tomograph revealed the remaining developing teeth were the LR8 and the LL8. There was symmetry in that both these teeth were at the same stage of development which is F. Using the rule (b(i)) defined in section 5c(i), only the LL8Ff summary data are used for DAA.

The summary statistics for the approximately Normally distributed values of age for LL8FfTDS is shown in Table 13.

The approach favoured by the authors is to use the sample mean (16.41 Yrs) from the corresponding TDS in the reference data set to estimate the population mean and to assign this value as the estimated age of the subject of unknown date of birth. This has the advantage of simplicity and, as it is the 'average', it has the benefit of full understanding by non statisticians. The 99% Confidence Interval is not assigned.

Whilst the mean age is, in non statistician terms, an easy concept and comfortable to accept, it does not convey any of the uncertainty that should be associated with an estimate of dental age. One such way of conveying the range of values that might appear reasonable is to calculate the range encompassing one standard deviation above and below the mean. In the case of LL8Ff this would be 15.06 – 17.76 Years [(16.41 – 1.35) = 15.06 years to (16.05 + 1.35) = 17.76 years]. This encompasses 68.27% of the values in the reference data and by inference, we would expect the same percentage of the population from which the sample is drawn to lie in this interval. This is consistent with the usual statement, derived from

Figure 25. The case of the single remaining developing tooth. The LL8Ff

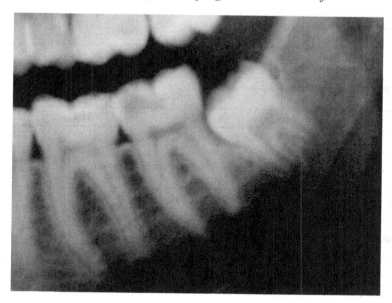

Table 13. Summary data of age (years) for LL8Ff

n	mean	sd	se	med	min	max	range	99%CILL	99%CIUL
240	16.41	1.35	0.09	16.25	11.12	20.51	9.39	16.18	16.63
0.5%ile	**5%ile**	**10%ile**	**25%ile**	**50%ile**	**75%ile**	**90%ile**	**95%ile**	**99.5%ile**	
11.83	14.46	15.03	15.57	16.25	17.13	18.28	18.69	19.85	

Data from EDI-KCL Database (Roberts et al., 2009, unpublished data)

the theory of the Normal distribution, that plus or minus one standard deviation comprises the central 68% of the data in the population.

The Degree of Uncertainty of the Assigned Age using Percentiles

Encompassing 68% of the data in the population (i.e. based on the use of a single sd) is regarded by some as more than is necessary to satisfy the tenet of civil law. That is, a claim is supported and is considered proven if the balance of probability for the claim is greater then 50%. An alternative approach is to provide the range of ages from the 25th percentile (15.57 years) to the 75 percentile (17.13 years). To achieve this it is sufficient to extend the 25th percentile by 0.01 (15.06 − 0.01 = 15.05 years and the 75th percentile by 0.01 (17.13 + 0.01 = 17.14 years) to exceed these limits to satisfy the usual legal requirement that the balance of probability must be greater than 50%. This gives a range of values from 15.05 years to 17.14 years. This is a slightly narrower range than that delimited by plus or minus (+/-) one standard deviation (sd) from the mean (i.e. 15.06 years to 17.76 years).

The Calculated Probability of a Subject being Greater than a Specified Age

Occasionally the query raised is 'how likely is it that Mr / Ms X is over or under 18 years of age?

Table 14.

Value of X for which cumulative Probability is required	*X*	*18.00*
Value of Average (or mean) of the Reference Data Set	*Mean*	*16.41*
Standard Deviation of the (sd) of Reference Data Set	*Standard_dev*	*1.35*
Cumulative Probability	*Cumulative*	*TRUE*

Table 15. Cumulative Probability for LL8Ff at five ages from 15 yrs to 19 yrs

15 yrs cumulative probability is 0.1481; p >15 yrs is estimated as 1 - 0.0148 = 0.9852 = 98.52%.
16 yrs cumulative probability is 0.3807; p > 16 yrs is estimated as 1- 0.3807 = 0.6193 = 61.93%.
17 yrs cumulative probability is 0.6689; p >17 yrs is estimated as 1- 0.6689 = 0.3311 = 33.11%
18 yrs cumulative probability is 0.8805; p > 18 yrs is estimated as 1 - 0.8805 = 0.1195 = 11.95%
19 yrs cumulative probability is 0.9725; p > 19 yrs is estimated as 1- 0.9725 = 0.0275 = 2.75%

It is possible to use the same summary data for the TDS present on the subject's xray to estimate the probability that the subject is under a specified age. The example of the LL8Ff is used with the Normal distribution function (NORMDIST) in Excel [Microsoft Office 2007]. When this statistical function is activated, a small table is opened which requests the user to enter the relevant mean age and standard deviation for this distribution and to indicate that the cumulative probability is required by entering TRUE. These data from LL8Ef are shown in **bold inTable 14**.

Excel outputs the cumulative probability of the individual being of the Reference Data set up to the age of 18.0 Yrs as 0.8806 [88.06%]. To estimate the probability of the subject being 18 Yrs or above it is necessary to subtract the cumulative probability from 1. Thus $1 - 0.8805 = 0.1195$ [11.95%].

Occasionally the request is to indicate the probability of the subject being less than one of several 'pre-determined' ages such as 16 years or 17 years. The same calculation for each of the ages commonly required is shown in Table 15.

Incidentally, a simple check on the veracity of the calculations can be carried out by entering the mean age of the data set as the value for which the cumulative probability is required. The answer should always come to 0.5 or 50% as illustrated below.

16.41 yrs cumulative probability is 0.5 p > 16.41 yrs is estimated as = 0.5 [50%]

One Third Molar at Stage H and One or More Third Molars not at Stage H

The third molar at Stage H is ignored and the age assessment is based on the immature third molar(s). The procedure adopted in this situation is described in Section 5b(i)

All Third Molars at Stage H (Use of a Single Third Molar at Stage H)

If all third molars are present and are at Stage H, only the LL8H (m or f) is used. This is because it is believed that in every individual subject, Stage H is achieved in upper third molars before it is achieved in lower third molars. Sometimes a different third molar will be used for age assessment if the LL8 is missing.

An important belief is that a tooth with completed growth (Stage H) for any Tooth Morphology Type (TMT) should not be used for DAA (Liversidge, 2008). This is based on the premise that it is impossible, when viewing different TMTs to identify precisely when all subjects in a reference sample have achieved Stage H (Kullman, 1995). However, most investigators use Stage H but in various ways. Usually these investigators cap the age for such a subject at some defined value (i.e. any subject whose age is above this cap is excluded from the data set), although these values for capping vary from one investigator to another. For example Levesque and Demirjian caps it at 19.0 years (Levesque, Demirjian, & Tanguay, 1981), Bolanos caps it at 20.0 years (Bolanos, Moussa, Manrique, & Bolanos, 2008), Nortje (1983) caps it at 21.0 years, Willerhausen at 24.0 years (Willerhausen, Loffler & Schulze, 2001), Mincer caps it at 24 years (Mincer, Harris & Berryman, 1993), Liversidge (2008) at 24 years, and Olze caps it at 26.0 years (Olze et al., 2004). Altogether these cover a time interval of 7 years. The corresponding mean age of attainment of Stage H are 19.0 years (Nortje, 1983), 19.2 years (Levesque, Demirjian, & Tanguay, 1981), 19.26 years (Liversidge, 2008), 19.45 years (Bolanos, Moussa, Manrique, & Bolanos, 2008), 20.2 years (Mincer et al., 1993), 21.3 years (Willerhausen et al., 2001), and 22.5 years (Olze et al. 2004), a range of just over 3.5 years. This wide range of age of attainment for stage H is ostensibly for male caucasians. This is clearly questionable and is a consequence of these investigators failing to indicate how they identified the appropriate age at which to cap or censor the data. For future reference, we refer to the use of a data set which has been capped in this way as an '*arbitrarily censored*' data set.

Recent work has shown that the age at which 100% of the population have achieved completion

of root development in lower 3rd molars (Stage H) can be identified in the following way [Roberts, Parekh, Petrie, Lucas 2008]. Initially, the age data for each third molar tooth attaining stages G and H were arranged in ascending order. All cases were Stage G at the younger ages, then cases were a mixture of Stages G and H, and at the older ages only Stage H was present. This enabled the identification of the youngest age beyond which there were only cases of Stage H (i.e. no more cases of stage G) for the single third molar. All cases older than this age were excluded from the data set. The remaining data are referred to as the '*appropriately censored*' data as opposed to the 'arbitrarily censored' data which has an 'arbitrary' cut-off point.

The different estimates of the mean age obtained using the arbitrarily censored (at age 26 years) data set and the appropriately censored data set are shown in Table 16.

The use of Stage H of 3rd molars needs to be interpreted cautiously. It is important to qualify the uncertainty surrounding this by indicating that the subject is *at least* this age and *could be* older. It is hoped that the use of sterno-clavicular joint maturation may be of use in improving the accuracy of DAA in the emerging adult. This is currently 'work in progress'. Other factors that may provide an indication of an age older than 19.81 Yrs are the root canal widths of the 3rd molar and / or the relative width of root canals in the 1st, 2nd, and 3rd lower permanent molars.

Example of a Single Third Molar at Stage H

A common presentation for age assessments is to determine whether an individual is above or below 18 years of age. The clinical presentation may or may not show the presence of 3rd molars erupted in the mouth. It is always advisable to obtain a radiograph to show the degree of root development (Figure 26). As can be seen, the root of the LL8 is at Stage H

Table 16. Comparison between summary data of Stage H using the arbitrarily (at age 26 years) censored data set and the appropriately censored data set for males and Females

Tooth Br Den J	Stage H - Males			Stage H - Females		
	Statistic	Arbitrarily censored (at 26yrs)	Appropriately Censored	Arbitrarily censored (at 26yrs)	Appropriately Censored	Statistic
UR8	**n**	74	72	101	93	**n**
	Mean	19.57	19.42	20.08	19.81	**Mean**
	99% CI	19.07 to 20.1	18.96 to 19.88	19.70 to 20.45	19.47 to 20.15	**99% CI**
UL8	**n**	70	68	101	91	**n**
	Mean	19.53	19.38	20.13	19.70	**Mean**
	99% CI	18.67 to 19.66	18.91 to 19.85	19.74 to 20.49	19.43 to 20.09	**99% CI**
LL8	**n**	50	45	59	51	**n**
	Mean	19.91	19.46	20.78	20.34	**Mean**
	99% CI	19.25 to 20.57	18.87 to 20.05	20.32 to 21.24	19.94 to 20.74	**99% CI**
LR8	**n**	49	47	60	58	**n**
	Mean	20.02	19.81	20.70	19.71	**Mean**
	99% CI	19.35 to 20.68	19.18 to 20.45	20.24 to 21.17	20.27 to 21.16	**99% CI**

Using the data set which provided the summary information in Table 8 above, the esimated age of this subject would be 19.46 years (sd = 2.42 yrs). From the distribution of ages for LL8Hm, the estimated probability of a subject being at or below a given age can be calculated. These probabilities are 7.63% (16yrs) and 27.31%.

The data set is continually being updated and we provide the analagous results for March 31st 2009. The estimated age of this subject would be 19.04 years (sd = 2.36 years). From the distribution of ages for LL8Hm, the estimated probability of a subject being at or below a given age can be calculated. These probabilities are 9.88% (16yrs), 19.4% (17.0) and 32.9% (18 years). Table 17. shows the full summary statistics for this data set for LL8Hm.

Age summary statistics for the updated data set for all third molars at Stage H for males and females are provided in Table 17.

PROBLEMS WITH DAA DIFFICULTIES WITH THE TECHNIQUE(S) OF DAA

There are a number of problems associated with the techniques of DAA which require elaboration so that commissioners of DAA reports have a reference document to answer frequently asked questions and further questions that, perhaps, commissioners should, but have not asked.

Ethnic and Global Differences

In general terms, it is not difficult to identify different major racial groups (Black, White, Asian and other) by visual inspection. However, within these major racial groupings are many subgroups which are difficult to define precisely in a way which can be properly related to physical growth and development. These difficulties become manifest when attempting to obtain suitable reference samples. Despite differences claimed, recent extensive work has shown that racial and ethnic differences are minimal as regards the age

Figure 26. Lower Left 3ʳᵈ Molar Stage H [complete apex] - LL8Hm

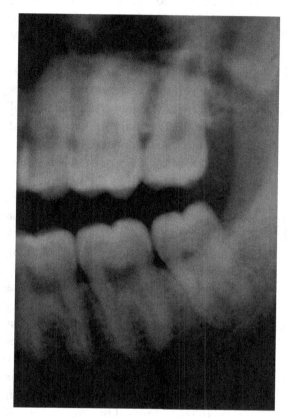

of the later stages of tooth development(Olze, van Nierkerk, Ishikawa, Zhu, Schulz, Maeda, & Schmeling, 2007; Liversidge, 2008).

The problem that needs to be addressed is the appropriateness of using data from U.K. Caucasians for subjects from, for example, Afghanistan, West Africa, South America and the Far East. From the above work (Olze et al., 2007; Liversidge, 2008) it is deemed acceptable, in the absence of

reference data from specific racial/ethnic groups, to assign the ages from the U.K. Caucasian data base with the proviso that there are small statistically significant differences which are unlikely to be clinically significant. Notwithstanding this, it is recognised that the acquisition of racial specific data is likely to be the preferred approach to dental age assessment.

Nutritional Influences

The effect of food intake in terms of its calorific, mineral and vitamin content is only discernable with extreme deprivation such as occurs with severe Vitamin D deficiency (Garn et al., 1965) Most of the data comes from animal experimentation. However, in humans, even severe nutritional deprivation in children, as occurs in children with Dystrophic Epidermolysis Bullosa, has minimal affect on dental development and maturity (Kostara, Roberts, & Gelbier, 2000; Liversidge et al. 2005). A further example of the minimal effect of metabolic disturbance occurs in children who have undergone renal transplantation and who are on immune suppressant therapy (Jaffe, Roberts, Chantler, & Carter, 1990). These children have only a slight delay in dental development.

Syndromal Conditions Affecting Growth of Teeth

A variety of syndromes such as familial short stature (Vallejo-Bollanos & Espana-Lopez, 1997), genetic anomalies (Garn, Lewis, & Bonne, 1962), and growth hormone deficiency (Garn, Lewis, &

Table 17. This is the format of the table of results for LL8Hm

n	mean	sd	se	med	min	max	range	99%CILL	99%CIUL
61	19.08	2.38	0.31	19.28	14.94	23.62	8.68	18.29	19.97
0.5%ile	**5%ile**	**10%ile**	**25%ile**	**50%ile**	**75%ile**	**90%ile**	**95%ile**	**99.5%ile**	
15.10	15.55	15.88	17.01	19.28	21.13	22.26	23.02	23.57	

Blizzard, 1965). It is usually clearly apparent that there is a systemic genetic disorder that is likely to have affected tooth growth and development. In such circumstances the process of DAA cannot be used.

Radiology

Radiological Techniques

Historically, the imaging techniques used for assessing dental development have comprised intra-oral periapical (IOP) radiographs, oblique lateral jaw views (bimolars), dental panoramic tomographs (DPT) and, more recently, cone beam tomography (CBT).

- *Intra-oral periapical (IOP) radiographs:* This is the most commonly used radiological view in dental clinical practice. It is not used much for DAA because it only provides images of only two or possibly three teeth. This compares unfavourably with the DPT which provides an image of all 16 tooth morphology types on one film. However, the IOP is often used to supplement images of individual teeth of insufficient clarity on the DPT. The IOP is particularly useful in post-mortem work as mortuaries as a rule do not have x-ray machines capable of taking DPTs. In general terms, the high quality images from IOPs are comparable with images of individual teeth on DPTs.

- *Oblique lateral jaw views (bimolars.* This view was used for many decades before the introduction in 1968 of DPTs. It provides a view of the buccal segment of the lower jaw comprising the first and second premolars and the first and second permanent molars (four teeth). A skilled radiographer can usually provide an image of all the teeth from the permanent central incisor to the second permanent molar. The upper teeth are rarely clearly discernable because of superimposition of teeth from one jaw on to the other. This limitation explains the use of only four or seven teeth in the early publications (Demirjian et al. 1976)

- *Dental panoramic tomographs (DPT)*: This view is the most commonly used because it provides a high quality image of the 16 TMTs. The main limitation is that it is currently recommended that this view is not taken below the age of seven years, unless there is benefit to the patient. This means that the reference data on the younger age group is dependent on bimolars or periapical views. This means that not all of the 16 Tooth Morphology Types and their Developmental Stages are available in sufficient numbers to provide an adequate Reference Data Set. Occasionally, artifacts are present because of incorrect position of the patient in the DPT apparatus, movement of the subject or anatomical features which may lead a poor image. The clear advantage of having images of upper teeth is sometimes attenuated by one or more of these teeth providing an unusable image.

- *Cone beam tomography*: This relatively new technique provides images of high quality. Its great advantage is that the investigator has the ability to reformat the image in any plane. This overcomes the occasional problems of superimposition, common with IOPs, or loss of part of the image because it is outside the focal plane of DPTs. Currently the amount of radiation associated with this technique is too great to justify its routine use.

Radiation Protection

All radiographs have to be ordered by a clinician following examination of the patient. Under the IR(MER) regulations, the exposure of the subject to radiation has to be justified. The use of radiographs for DAA is legally permitted. A requirement is to ensure that the dosage used is as low as reasonably achievable. In terms of obtaining consent from the patient, it is not necessary to indicate that, for example, the taking of a DPT has a one in two million chance of causing a lifetime fatal cancer, as this is considered too remote a possibility to draw to the patient's attention. The estimates of risks from radiation are available from the Health Protection Agency on www.hpa.org.uk (see National Patient Dose Database (NPDD).

Methods of Assessment

Investigators have used a variety of techniques to assess maturity and from that estimate age. These include the maturity index from Arto Demirjian (Demirjian et al., 1973), age of attained stages described by Karen Haavikko (1970), linear regression (Cameriere et al., 2007), measurement of tooth length (Liversidge, Dean, & Molleson, 1993), measurement of the width of the opening at the apex of developing teeth (Cameriere et al., 2007) and occlusal wear (Akpata, 1975). All of these approaches have their merits, but the general applicability is limited by the need for specialised measuring equipment, such as a computer digitizer, or statistical manipulation beyond the ability of most dental surgeons. The methods described in this document have the advantage of general applicability because of the use of easily obtainable reference data (Roberts et al., 2008) by using DPTs obtained for clinical purposes. The DPTs taken for DAA can be easily assessed in a reliable way (Maber, Liversidge, & Hector, 2006) and the manipulation of the data is carried out using software which is widely used.

MEDICO LEGAL STATUS OF THE DAA PROCESS

The law in relation to the Dental Age Assessment relates to two sets of circumstances.

- *Civil Cases*: The usual approach is to use the estimated mean value of the population from which the subject is believed to belong as the estimated dental age of the subject of unknown date of birth. If the lawyers and social workers require further information, it is possible to estimate the probability that the subject is below (or above) a specified age. In civil cases, the legal burden of proof of being above or below a certain age is on the balance of probability, i.e. the probability must be greater than 0.50 (50%). If DAA is based on a single tooth (e.g., third molar), simple probability theory associated with the Normal distribution provides an estimate of the required probability (see Section 4 a iv). If multiple teeth are used for DAA, a simple approach to estimate the relevant probability is to calculate the weighted mean of the probabilities associated with each of the teeth used in the age assessment (see Section 5 b ii).
- *Criminal Cases*: The same approach is used in criminal cases as in civil cases, ie. providing an estimated mean age and, often, the probability that the subject is above (or below) a specified age. The essential difference between the two scenarios is that in criminal cases, legal burden of proof of being above or below a certain age is not on the "balance of probabilities" but is "beyond reasonable doubt". This is a considerably more demanding requirement but it is really up to the judicial authorities to decide exactly what this means.

CLOSING REMARKS

This document describes a simple approach to assessing dental age. We are interested in developing this further by giving consideration to other statistical methods, such as use of the sensitivity and the specificity of the technique of assigning a subject above or below a given age and logistic regression analysis for estimating the probability that the subject is above or below that age. In addition, once sufficient data is accumulated, we will be looking at the effect of ethnicity on dental age assessment.

The acquisition of Reference Data Sets for specific populations or Identifiable Human Groups (IHG) is an important aspect of Dental Age Assessment that is currently an active process.

ACKNOWLEDGMENT

We wish to acknowledge Professor Tim Cole of the Institute of Child Health, University College London for advice during the preparation of this manuscript. Teelana Boonpitaksathit, from the Department of Orthodontics, UCL Eastman Dental Institute, Susan Parekh, from the Department of Paediatric Dentistry, UCL Eastman Dental Institute, Tricia Percival, from the Department of Paediatric Dentistry, University of the West Indies, Port of Spain, Trinidad, Julie Mitchell, Monica Yadava, Kevin Moze and Victoria S Lucas, from the Department of Paediatric Dentistry, King's College Dental Institute, Bessemer Road, London, SE5 9RS, UK, Norah Donaldson, from the Department of Biostatistics, King's College Dental Institute, Bessemer Road, London SE5 9RS, UK are acknowledged for their contribution to this chapter.

REFERENCES

Acock, A. (2008). *A gentle introduction to Stata* (2nd ed.). Texas: Stata Press.

Akpata, E. S. (1975). Molar tooth attrition in a selected group of Nigerians. *Community Dentistry and Oral Epidemiology*, *3*, 132–135. doi:10.1111/j.1600-0528.1975.tb00294.x

Altman, D. (1991). *Practical statistics for medical research*. London: Chapman & Hall.

Bolanos, M. V., Manrique, M. C., Bolanos, M. J., & Briones, M. T. (2000). Approaches to chronological age assessment based on dental calcification. *Forensic Science International*, *110*, 97–106. doi:10.1016/S0379-0738(00)00154-7

Bolanos, M. V., Moussa, H., Manrique, M. C., & Bolanos, M. J. (2008). Radiographic evaluation of third molar development in Spanish children and young people. *Forensic Science International*, *133*, 212–219. doi:10.1016/S0379-0738(03)00037-9

Cameriere, R., Brkic, H., Ermenc, B., Ferrante, L., Ovsenik, M., & Cingolani, M. (2007a). The measurement of open apices of teeth to test chronological age over 14-year olds in living subjects. *Forensic Science International*, *174*, 217–221. doi:10.1016/j.forsciint.2007.04.220

Cameriere, R., Ferrante, L., Belcastro, M. G., Bonfiglioli, B., Rastelli, E., & Cingolani, M. (2007b). Age estimation by pulp/tooth ratio in canines by peri-apical x-rays. *Journal of Forensic Sciences*, *52*, 166–170. doi:10.1111/j.1556-4029.2006.00336.x

Cameriere, R., Ferrante, L., & Cingolani, M. (2006). Age estimation in children by measurement of open apices in teeth. *International Journal of Legal Medicine*, *120*, 49–52. doi:10.1007/s00414-005-0047-9

Clark, H. C. (2008). *Practical forensic odontology*. Oxford: Wright.

Demirjian, A., Buschang, P. H., Tenguay, T., & Patterson, D. K. (1985). Interrelationships among measures of somatic, skeletal, dental, and sexual maturity. *American Journal of Orthodontics, 88,* 433–438. doi:10.1016/0002-9416(85)90070-3

Demirjian, A., & Goldstein, H. (1976). New systems for dental maturity based on seven and four teeth. *Annals of Human Biology, 3,* 411–421. doi:10.1080/03014467600001671

Demirjian, A., Goldstein, H., & Tanner, J. M. (1973). A new system of dental age assessment. *Human Biology, 45,* 211–227.

Dept. of Health. (2000). The ionising radiation (medical exposure) regulations 2000. Retrieved from www.opsi.gov.uk/si/si2000/20001059.htm

Ekstrand, K. R., Christiansen, J., & Christiansen, M. E. C. (2003). Time and duration of eruption of first and second permanent molars: A longitudinal investigation. *Community Dentistry and Oral Epidemiology, 31,* 344–350. doi:10.1034/j.1600-0528.2003.00016.x

Garn, S., Lewis, A. B., & Bonne, B. (1962). Third molar formation and its development course. *The Angle Orthodontist, 32,* 270–279.

Garn, S., Lewis, A. B., & Kerewsky, R. S. (1965). Genetic, nutritional, and maturational correlates of dental development. *Journal of Dental Research, 44*(1), 228–242. doi:10.1177/00220345 650440011901

Garn, S. M., Lewis, A. B., & Blizzard, R. M. (1965). Endocrine factors in tooth development. *Journal of Dental Research, 44*(1), 243–257. doi:10.1177/00220345650440012001

Haavikko, K. (1970). The formation and the alveolar and clinical eruption of the permanent teeth. *Suom Hammaslaken Toimen, 66,* 103–170.

Hockton, A. (2002). *The law of consent to medical treatment.* London: Sweet & Maxwell.

Jaffe, E. C., Roberts, G. J., Chantler, C., & Carter, J. E. (1990). Dental maturity in children with chronic renal failure assessed ITom dental panoramic tomographs. *Journal of the International Association of Dentistry for Children, 20,* 54–58.

Kostara, A., Roberts, G. J., & Gelbier, M. (2000). Dental maturity in children with Dystrophic Epidermolysis Bullosa. *Pediatric Dentistry, 22,* 385–388.

Kreitner, K. F., Schweden, F. J., Reipert, T., Nafe, B., & Thelen, M. (1998). Bone age determination based on the study of the medial extremity of the clavicle. *European Radiology, 8,* 1116–1122. doi:10.1007/s003300050518

Kullman, L. (1995). Accuracy of two dental and one skeletal age estimation method in Swedish adolescents. *Forensic Science International, 75,* 225–226. doi:10.1016/0379-0738(95)01792-5

Kvaal, S., Kolltveit, K. M., Thomsen, O., & Solheim, T. (1995). Age estimation of adults from dental radiographs. *Forensic Science International, 74,* 175–185. doi:10.1016/0379-0738(95)01760-G

Landis, J. R., & Koch, G. G. (1977). The measurement of observer agreement for categorical data. *Biometrics, 33,* 159–174. doi:10.2307/2529310

Levesque, G. Y., Demirjian, A., & Tanguay, R. (1981). Sexual dimorphism in the development, emergence, and agenesis of the mandibular third molar. *Journal of Dental Research, 60,* 1735–1741. doi:10.1177/00220345810600100201

Lewis, A. B., & Gam, S. M. (1960). The relationship between tooth formation and other maturational factors. *The Angle Orthodontist, 30,* 70–77.

Liversidge, H. M. (2008). Timing of human mandibular third molar formation. *Annals of Human Biology, 35,* 294–321. doi:10.1080/03014460801971445

Liversidge, H. M., Chaillet, N., Mornstad, H., Nystrom, M., Rowlings, K., & Taylor, J. (2006). Timing of Demirjian's tooth formation stages. *Annals of Human Biology*, *33*, 454–470. doi:10.1080/03014460600802387

Liversidge, H. M., Dean, M. C., & Molleson, T. (1993). Increasing human tooth length between birth and 5.4 years. *American Journal of Physical Anthropology*, *90*, 307–313. doi:10.1002/ajpa.1330900305

Liversidge, H. M., Kosmidou, A., Hector, M. P., & Roberts, G. J. (2005). Epidermolysis bullo'sa and dental development age. *International Journal of Paediatric Dentistry*, *15*, 335–341. doi:10.1111/j.1365-263X.2005.00649.x

Liversidge, H. M., Lyons, M., & Hector, M. P. (2003). The accuracy of three methods of age estimation using radiographic measurements of developing teeth. *Forensic Science International*, *131*, 22–29. doi:10.1016/S0379-0738(02)00373-0

Maber, M., Liversidge, H. M., & Hector, M. P. (2006). Accuracy of age estimation of radiographic methods using developing teeth. *Forensic Science International*, *159S*, S68–S73. doi:10.1016/j.forsciint.2006.02.019

Mincer, H. H., Hams, E. F., & Berryman, H. E. (1993). The ABFO study of third molar development. *Journal of Forensic Sciences*, *38*, 379–390.

Mitchell, J. C., Roberts, G., Donaldson, A. N., & Lucas, V. S. (2009). Dental Age Asessment (DAA): Reference data for British caucasians at the 16 year threshold. *Forensic Science International*, *189*, 19–23. doi:10.1016/j.forsciint.2009.04.002

Morrees, C. F. A., & Kent, R. L. (1978). A step function model using tooth counts to assess the developmental timing of dentititon. *Annals of Human Biology*, *5*, 55–68. doi:10.1080/03014467800002641

Nortje, C. J. (1983). The permanent mandibular third molar. It's value in age determination. *The Journal of Forensic Odonto-Stomatology*, *1*, 27–31.

Olze, A., Bilang, D., Schmidt, S., Wemecke, K. D., Geserick, G., & Schmeling, A. (2005). Validation of common classification systems for assessing mineralization of third molars. *Internal Journal of Legal Medicine*, *119*, 22–26. doi:10.1007/s00414-004-0489-5

Olze, A., Schmeling, A., Taniguchi, M., Van Niekerk, P., Wemecke, K. D., & Geserick, G. (2004). Forensic age estimation in living subjects: The ethnic factor in wisdom teeth mineralization. *International Journal of Legal Medicine*, *118*, 170–173. doi:10.1007/s00414-004-0434-7

Olze, A., van Nierkerk, P., Ishikawa, T., Zhu, B. L., Schulz, R., & Maeda, H. (2007). Comparative study on the effect of ethnicity on wisdom tooth eruption. *International Journal of Legal Medicine*, *121*, 445–448. doi:10.1007/s00414-007-0171-9

Petrie, A., & Sabin, C. (2009). *Medical statistics at a glance* (3rd ed.). Oxford: Wiley Blackwell.

Roberts, G. L., & Lucas, V. S. (1994). Growth of the nasal septum of in the Snell strain of hypopituitary dwarf mouse. *European Journal of Orthodontics*, *16*, 138–148.

Roberts, G. L., Parekh, S., Petrie, A., & Lucas, V. S. (2008). Dental age assessment (DAA): A simple method for children and emerging adults. *British Dental Journal*, *204*, E7–E9. doi:10.1038/bdj.2008.21

Saunders, E. (1837). *The teeth a test of age, considered with reference to the factory children: Addressed to both Houses of Parliament, Westminster, London UK*. London: H. Renshaw.

Schmeling, A., Olze, A., Reisinger, W., Rosing, F. W., Muhler, M., & Wemecke, K. D. (2003). Forensic age diagnostics of living individuals in criminal proceedings. *Homo, 54*, 162–169. doi:10.1078/0018-442X-00066

Statacorp, L. P. (2007). *Stata reference manual* (10th ed.).

Sterne, C.M.M. (2008). *Age assessment in young people: Witness statement to the courts.*

Sterne, J. A. C. (2009). *Meta-analysis in stata.* College Station, TX: Stata Corp LP.

Tanner, J. M., Healy, M. J. R., Goldstein, H., & Cameron, N. (2001). *Assessment of skeletal maturity* (3rd ed.). London: W.B. Saunders.

Vallejo-Bollanos, E., & Espana-Lopez, A. J. (1997). The relationship between dental age, bone age and chronological age in 54 children with short familial stature. *International Journal of Paediatric Dentistry, 7*, 15–17. doi:10.1111/j.1365-263X.1997.tb00267.x

Willerhausen, B., Loffler, N., & Schulze, R. (2001). Analysis of 1202 orthopantomograms to evaluate the potential of forensic age determination based on third molar developmental stages. *European Journal of Medical Research, 6*, 377–384.

KEY TERMS AND DEFINITIONS

Dental Age: An indication of the maturity of the developing dentition, i.e. how far along the course of development the dentition of an individual has progressed. It is expressed in decimal years.

Meta-Analysis: The statistical technique where data from a number of different studies of similar design are integrated to provide a weighted average. In the context of DAA the age

of attainment of different TDSs from a single person is averaged to provide an estimate of the Dental Age. The averaging process is weighted by the distribution and number of individuals in the Tooth Development Stages of the Reference Data Set. The process of DAA is *not* meta-analysis but uses the same mathematical techniques of meta-analysis.

Radiological Techniques: The creation of a latent image of the jaws by passing ionising radiation through the jaw. The image is captured on a suitable sensor. In recent times this has been a photographic emulsion on an acetate sheet. Increasingly the images are created and stored in digital format

Reference Data Set [RDS]: The numerical data comprising the n-tds, mean, standard deviation, maximum, minimum, range, and 0.5^{th}, 5th, 10th, 25th, 50th, 75th, 90th, 95th, and 99.5^{th} percentiles. There is s full RDS for each Tooth Development Stage for each gender. This comprises a total of 256 TDSs for the 8 stage Demirjian system and 384 TDSs for the 12 stage Haavikko system

Tooth Development Stages [TDSs]: This is the core of any system of Age Assessment. Each TMT is divided into discrete stages. The systems used in this communication are the 8 Stage Definitions (Demirjian - Table 2 and Figure1) and the 12 Stage Definitions (Haavikko – Table 4 and Figure 2.)

Tooth Morphology Types (TMTs): The human dentition comprises 32 teeth. The teeth on one side are mirror images of the teeth on the other and *vice versa*. The 16 teeth on one side consist of 8 upper teeth and 8 lower teeth. Each of these 16 teeth is a unique Tooth Morphology Type. The significance of this is that each TMT has a unique developmental tempo.

Tooth Nomenclature: Each of the 32 teeth in the human dentition can be referred to by a form of shorthand. There are over 10 styles of notation available. In this text notation that lends itself to computer input has been used. These details are described in Table 1 – the British Dental Journal [BDJ] system of nomenclature combined with the 8 stage system of Demirjian and Table 3 – the

Fedaire Dentaire Internationale [FDI] system of nomenclature combined with the 12 stage system of Haavikko

APPENDIX A

DENTAL AGE ASSESSMENT (DAA): at King's College Hospital Information sheet for Clients, Lawyers, Interpreters and Social Workers

Introduction

Many of the subjects attending the DAA clinic have concerns about the processes involved. This document is to explain the procedures that will be carried out and the risks associated with the taking of a Dental Panoramic X-ray.

Practical Procedure

The process of DAA is straight forward and comprises four parts

1. An overall appraisal of the subject.
2. An Oral and Dental Examination.
3. An X-ray usually a Dental Panoramic Tomograph.
4. Clinical photographs.

None of these procedures cause any pain although the plastic lip and cheek retractors used for the photographs may cause some discomfort.

Risks Associated with the Procedure

There are no risks associated with the clinical procedures.
There is a 1 in 2 million adult life-time risk of developing a cancer from the x-ray.
To put this in perspective, that is a 1 in 50 million chance of developing a cancer in any one year.
This is a vanishingly small risk.

Consent

This is an ongoing process which starts with the social worker, or legal advisor, suggesting that the subject undergoes a Dental Age Assessment. The implications of this are that an 'age' will be assigned to the subject. The DAA is not the sole method of assessment, there are several methods used to help children, adolescents and emerging adults. The important outcome is the age assigned. This is, on the balance of probability, of benefit to the subject and the community.

Documentation

The subject and/or the person acting *in loco parentis* will be asked to sign the consent at the bottom of the sheet comprising the clinical findings.
The words used are:

I give my consent (permission) for a Dental Examination, a Dental Panoramic Radiograph (X-ray of the teeth) and photographs of my teeth and face to enable an assessment of my age.

Print Name:..

Signed:...Date:...............................

Witness:...Title:.........................Date:.....................

Please contact Christine Bell: christine.bell@kcl.ac.uk Tel: 020 3299 3375 or

Fax: 020 3299 4074 for any more information, queries etc.

APPENDIX B

Summary Data for all Demirjian Tooth Development Stages for males and females.

DENTAL AGE ASSESSMENT - Demirjian 8 stage Summary Data

Table 18. Summary Data for Females and Males for All tooth Development Stages for UR8 f & m Caucasians from the UK [London and its environs].

TDS	n	mean	sd	se	med	min	max	range	99%CIL	99%CIU	0.5%ile	5%ile	10%ile	25%ile	50%ile	75%ile	90%ile	95%ile	99.5%ile	TDS
UR8Af	21	9.48	1.29	0.28	9.22	7.33	13.68	6.35	8.76	10.21	7.39	7.92	8.46	9.13	9.22	9.71	10.18	11.67	13.47	UR8Af
UR8Am	57	9.71	0.74	0.10	9.92	7.78	11.03	3.25	9.46	9.97	7.90	8.46	8.77	9.22	9.92	10.37	10.41	10.53	10.98	UR8Am
UR8Bf	36	10.14	1.63	0.27	9.20	8.56	14.88	6.32	9.43	10.84	8.65	9.09	9.09	9.10	9.20	10.97	12.76	13.63	14.71	UR8Bf
UR8Bm	48	9.92	1.22	0.18	9.83	5.95	12.45	6.51	9.47	10.38	6.48	8.22	8.54	9.26	9.83	10.59	11.70	11.79	12.35	UR8Bm
UR8Cf	92	11.66	2.51	0.26	10.61	7.86	16.65	8.80	10.98	12.33	8.02	9.03	9.13	9.85	10.61	13.65	15.71	16.04	16.51	UR8Cf
UR8Cm	91	11.50	2.32	0.24	10.55	8.99	17.15	8.80	10.87	12.13	9.01	9.20	9.37	9.83	10.55	12.92	15.47	15.93	17.13	UR8Cm
UR8Df	296	14.23	1.90	0.11	14.70	10.00	18.28	8.28	13.95	14.51	10.26	10.81	11.51	12.81	14.70	15.56	16.38	16.89	18.05	UR8Df
UR8Dm	228	13.67	2.01	0.13	13.72	9.77	18.71	8.94	13.33	14.02	9.83	10.43	10.67	12.35	13.72	15.38	16.32	16.81	18.24	UR8Dm
UR8Ef	240	15.09	1.20	0.08	15.22	11.48	18.61	7.12	14.89	15.29	12.11	12.94	13.41	14.27	15.22	15.92	16.54	16.76	18.08	UR8Ef
UR8Em	166	15.41	0.88	0.07	15.44	13.67	17.71	4.04	15.23	15.59	13.68	13.92	14.19	14.91	15.44	16.00	16.59	16.89	17.40	UR8Em
UR8Ff	191	16.56	0.82	0.06	16.47	15.37	19.15	3.78	16.41	16.71	15.39	15.51	15.62	15.92	16.47	17.04	17.70	18.09	18.77	UR8Ff
UR8Fm	149	15.59	0.69	0.06	15.66	13.62	16.69	3.08	15.45	15.74	13.92	14.36	14.61	15.18	15.66	16.10	16.47	16.61	16.67	UR8Fm
UR8Gf	155	17.33	1.21	0.10	17.47	15.01	20.64	5.64	17.08	17.58	15.11	15.48	15.62	16.33	17.47	18.19	18.82	19.05	20.32	UR8Gf
UR8Gm	105	16.97	0.97	0.09	17.18	15.22	19.26	4.04	16.72	17.21	15.28	15.49	15.72	16.40	17.18	17.82	18.32	18.79	19.16	UR8Gm
UR8Hf	120	18.71	2.08	0.19	18.84	14.76	22.28	7.52	18.22	19.20	15.01	15.61	15.97	16.75	18.84	20.52	21.60	22.06	22.27	UR8Hf
UR8Hm	90	18.88	2.15	0.23	18.76	14.94	23.62	8.68	18.30	19.47	15.17	15.93	15.93	17.02	18.76	20.34	21.63	22.58	23.55	UR8Hm
TDS	n	mean	sd	se	med	min	max	range	99%CIL	99%CIU	0.5%ile	5%ile	10%ile	25%ile	50%ile	75%ile	90%ile	95%ile	99.5%ile	TDS

Table 19. Summary Data for Females and Males for All tooth Development Stages for LL8 f & m Caucasians from the UK [London and its environs]

TDS	n	mean	sd	se	med	min	max	range	99%CIL	99%CIU	0.5%ile	5%ile	10%ile	25%ile	50%ile	75%ile	90%ile	95%ile	99.5%ile	TDS
LL8Af	9	10.85	3.04	1.01	8.92	6.98	15.30	8.32	8.24	13.47	7.03	7.50	8.01	8.83	8.92	13.60	14.00	14.65	15.24	LL8Af
LL8Am	104	10.04	1.48	0.15	10.04	5.95	16.41	10.46	9.67	9.67	7.12	8.25	8.77	9.13	10.04	10.37	11.34	13.00	16.05	
LL88A																				
m																				
LL8Bf	23	12.28	2.00	0.42	12.34	8.83	15.49	6.66	11.21	13.36	8.93	9.77	9.99	10.57	12.34	13.97	14.84	15.27	15.47	LL8Bf
LL8Bm	20	11.78	2.16	0.48	11.43	9.03	16.74	7.72	10.53	13.03	9.03	9.04	9.25	10.55	11.43	12.89	14.13	16.31	16.70	LL8Bm
LL8Cf	70	14.23	1.91	0.23	14.67	9.22	18.28	9.06	13.64	13.64	14.82	11.12	11.86	12.96	14.67	15.46	16.38	16.83	18.19	LL8Cf
LL8Cm	54	13.66	2.06	0.28	14.08	5.95	16.76	10.80	12.93	14.38	6.85	9.99	11.75	12.51	14.08	15.22	15.86	16.22	16.71	LL8Cm
LL8Df	245	14.75	1.52	0.10	15.02	10.26	18.61	8.35	14.50	15.00	10.74	12.24	13.75	15.02	15.02	15.76	16.53	16.88	18.25	LL8Df
LL8Dm	129	14.47	1.44	0.13	14.56	10.75	18.71	7.96	14.14	14.79	11.21	12.12	12.66	13.43	14.56	15.59	16.04	16.48	17.82	LL8Dm
LL8Ef	251	15.60	1.31	0.08	15.53	12.08	21.37	9.28	15.38	15.81	12.28	13.46	14.02	15.01	15.53	16.29	17.11	17.62	20.01	LL8Ef
LL8Em	193	15.41	1.05	0.08	15.42	12.40	18.20	5.80	15.21	15.60	12.67	13.59	14.06	14.88	15.42	16.13	16.68	16.96	17.95	LL8Em
LL8Ff	240	16.41	1.35	0.09	16.25	11.12	20.51	9.39	16.18	16.63	11.83	14.46	15.03	15.57	16.25	17.13	18.28	18.69	19.85	LL8Ff
LL8Fm	195	16.29	1.11	0.08	16.12	14.02	19.36	5.34	16.09	16.50	14.09	14.62	15.02	15.52	16.12	16.97	17.76	18.38	19.18	LL8Fm
LL8Gf	140	17.42	1.33	0.11	17.27	14.96	20.96	6.00	17.13	17.71	15.11	15.60	15.81	16.34	17.27	18.39	19.06	19.79	20.89	LL8Gf
LL8Gm	86	17.28	1.15	0.12	17.41	14.41	19.86	5.45	16.96	17.60	14.75	15.44	15.75	16.44	17.41	18.10	18.70	19.10	19.66	LL8Gm
LL8Hf	75	18.89	2.31	0.27	19.16	14.76	22.52	7.76	18.20	19.57	14.93	15.55	15.91	16.66	19.16	20.88	21.89	22.15	22.52	LL8Hf
LL8Hm	61	19.04	2.36	0.30	19.28	14.94	23.62	8.68	18.26	19.82	15.10	15.55	15.88	16.98	19.28	21.13	21.65	22.81	23.57	LL8Hm
TDS	n	mean	sd	se	med	min	max	range	99%CIL	99%CIU	0.5%ile	5%ile	10%ile	25%ile	50%ile	75%ile	90%ile	95%ile	99.5%ile	TDS

Table 20. Summary Data for Females and Males for All tooth Development Stages for LR8 f & m Caucasians from the UK [London and its environs].

TDS	n	mean	sd	se	med	min	max	range	99%CIL	99%CIU	0.5%ile	5%ile	10%ile	25%ile	50%ile	75%ile	90%ile	95%ile	99.5%ile	TDS
LR8Af	9	10.87	2.69	0.90	10.86	6.98	14.83	7.84	8.56	13.19	7.06	7.72	8.46	8.92	10.86	13.60	13.91	14.37	14.78	LR8Af
LR8Am	17	10.96	2.71	0.66	9.85	8.00	16.41	8.41	9.27	12.66	8.06	8.61	8.79	9.00	9.85	12.00	15.79	16.29	16.40	LR8Am
LR8Bf	20	12.43	2.00	0.45	12.87	8.83	15.32	6.49	11.27	13.58	8.92	9.71	9.89	10.60	12.87	13.93	14.87	15.31	15.31	LR8Bf
LR8Bm	19	11.74	1.78	0.41	11.43	8.77	14.29	5.52	10.68	12.79	8.79	9.02	9.23	10.75	11.43	13.31	13.93	14.12	14.27	LR8Bm
LR8Cf	71	14.18	1.84	0.22	14.66	9.22	18.01	8.79	13.62	14.75	9.35	11.13	11.90	12.93	14.66	15.51	16.21	16.44	17.83	LR8Cf
LR8Cm	43	13.60	1.85	0.28	13.95	9.34	16.29	6.95	12.87	14.33	9.38	10.24	11.73	12.45	13.95	15.22	15.87	16.17	16.28	LR8Cm
LR8Df	240	14.77	1.55	0.10	15.00	10.26	19.35	9.09	14.51	15.02	10.73	12.23	12.66	13.75	15.00	15.83	16.58	16.89	18.77	LR8Df
LR8Dm	131	14.43	1.47	0.13	14.56	10.52	17.28	6.75	14.10	14.76	10.67	12.06	12.43	13.44	14.56	15.58	16.08	16.63	17.03	LR8Dm
LR8Ef	244	15.66	1.37	0.09	15.54	12.08	21.37	9.28	15.44	15.89	12.28	13.48	14.11	15.02	15.54	16.35	17.28	17.92	20.02	LR8Ef
LR8Em	207	15.52	1.15	0.08	15.51	12.03	18.71	6.68	15.31	15.73	12.81	13.52	14.07	14.91	15.51	16.31	16.96	17.36	18.32	LR8Em
LR8Ff	193	15.87	0.77	0.06	15.92	13.83	17.18	3.35	15.73	16.01	14.02	14.43	14.93	15.31	15.92	16.54	16.86	16.95	17.14	LR8Ff
LR8Fm	195	16.23	1.09	0.08	16.11	14.02	19.36	5.34	16.03	16.43	14.09	14.60	14.99	15.48	16.11	16.83	17.74	18.34	19.18	LR8Fm
LR8Gf	140	17.60	1.37	0.12	17.53	15.18	20.96	5.78	17.30	17.90	15.20	15.64	15.87	16.57	17.53	18.49	19.50	20.23	20.92	LR8Gf
LR8Gm	84	17.42	1.21	0.13	17.45	15.20	20.33	5.13	17.08	17.76	15.21	15.49	15.93	16.45	17.45	18.23	18.99	19.34	20.33	LR8Gm
LR8Hf	79	19.35	2.48	0.28	19.59	14.76	23.92	9.16	18.63	20.07	14.94	15.58	15.99	17.02	19.59	21.53	22.33	23.20	23.79	LR8Hf
LR8Hm	61	19.08	2.38	0.31	19.28	14.94	23.62	8.68	18.29	19.87	15.10	15.55	15.88	17.01	19.28	21.13	22.26	23.02	23.57	LR8Hm
TDS	n	mean	sd	se	med	min	max	range	99%CIL	99%CIU	0.5%ile	5%ile	10%ile	25%ile	50%ile	75%ile	90%ile	95%ile	99.5%ile	TDS

Table 21. Summary Data for Females and Males for All tooth Development Stages UL1 f & m Caucasians from the UK [London and its environs].

TDS	n	mean	sd	se	med	min	max	range	99%CIL	99%CIU	0.5%ile	5%ile	10%ile	25%ile	50%ile	75%ile	90%ile	95%ile	99.5%ile	TDS
UL1Af	no data																			UL1Af
UL1Am	no.data																			UL1Am
UL1Bf	no data																			UL1Bf
UL1Bm	no data																			UL1Bm
UL1Cf	no data																			UL1Cf
UL1Cm	no data																			UL1Cm
UL1Df	12	4.90	1.02	0.29	5.00	3.04	6.37	3.33	4.14	5.66	3.08	3.43	3.78	4.11	5.00	5.71	6.02	6.18	6.35	UL1Df
UL1Dm	14	4.70	0.72	0.19	4.84	3.56	5.58	2.02	4.20	5.20	3.57	3.65	3.73	4.08	4.84	5.35	5.52	5.55	5.58	UL1Dm
UL1Ef	12	5.95	1.00	0.29	5.74	4.44	8.07	3.64	5.21	6.69	4.46	4.70	4.96	5.50	5.74	6.27	7.24	7.66	8.03	UL1Ef
UL1Em	24	5.85	1.06	0.22	5.67	4.21	8.79	4.58	5.30	6.41	4.25	4.53	4.66	5.28	5.67	6.29	6.83	7.81	8.70	UL1Em
UL1Ff	14	7.03	1.10	0.29	7.10	4.19	8.48	4.29	6.27	7.79	4.31	5.39	6.07	6.74	7.10	7.69	8.22	8.34	8.47	UL1Ff
UL1Fm	21	7.21	1.15	0.25	7.19	5.44	9.48	4.04	6.56	7.85	5.45	5.52	5.82	6.50	7.19	7.92	8.81	8.84	9.41	UL1Fm
UL1Gf	34	8.41	1.26	0.22	8.51	6.43	11.11	4.68	7.99	8.84	6.45	6.76	6.97	7.31	8.51	8.93	9.92	11.01	11.10	UL1Gf
UL1Gm	27	8.94	1.73	0.33	8.79	6.31	12.87	6.56	8.08	9.79	6.31	6.53	7.07	7.82	8.79	9.79	11.55	11.92	12.75	UL1Gm
UL1Hf	20	10.00	0.76	0.17	10.23	8.29	11.12	2.83	9.56	10.45	8.34	8.84	8.87	9.56	10.23	10.61	10.76	10.87	11.09	UL1Hf
UL1Hm	56	11.41	1.34	0.18	11.98	7.58	12.80	5.23	10.95	11.87	7.90	8.97	9.23	10.56	11.98	12.43	12.69	12.79	12.80	UL1Hm
TDS	n	mean	sd	se	med	min	max	range	99%CIL	99%CIU	0.5%ile	5%ile	10%ile	25%ile	50%ile	75%ile	90%ile	95%ile	99.5%ile	TDS

Table 22. Summary Data for Females and Males for All tooth Development Stages UL2 f & m Caucasians from the UK [London and its environs].

TDS	n	mean	sd	se	med	min	max	range	99%CIL	99%CIU	0.5%ile	5%ile	10%ile	25%ile	50%ile	75%ile	90%ile	95%ile	99.5%ile	TDS
UL2Af	No data																			UL2Af
UL2Am	no data																			UL2Am
UL2Bf	no data																			UL2Bf
UL2Bm	no data																			UL2Bm
UL2Cf	3	3.32	0.55	0.32	3.04	2.97	3.95	0.98	2.50	4.14	2.97	2.98	2.99	3.00	3.04	3.49	3.77	3.86	3.94	UL2Cf
UL2Cm	12	4.99	0.95	0.28	5.28	3.56	6.70	3.14	4.28	5.70	3.58	3.70	3.83	4.05	5.28	5.57	5.75	6.19	6.65	UL2Cm
UL2Df	13	5.75	1.05	0.29	5.69	4.16	8.07	3.91	5.00	6.49	4.20	4.53	4.82	5.02	5.69	6.03	7.08	7.62	8.03	UL2Df
UL2Dm	23	5.59	1.31	0.27	5.52	3.70	8.90	5.20	4.89	6.30	3.73	3.98	4.26	4.78	5.52	6.06	7.20	8.24	8.84	UL2Dm
UL2Ef	13	6.33	1.19	0.33	6.15	4.44	8.21	3.77	5.47	7.18	4.47	4.72	5.02	5.52	6.15	7.32	7.99	8.14	8.20	UL2Ef
UL2Em	18	6.36	1.09	0.26	6.17	4.62	8.84	4.22	5.69	7.02	4.68	5.26	5.44	5.58	6.17	6.79	7.60	8.80	8.84	UL2Em
UL2Ff	30	7.72	1.18	0.22	7.82	4.19	9.66	5.47	7.16	8.27	4.46	6.21	6.71	6.97	7.82	8.77	8.96	9.28	9.62	UL2Ff
UL2Fm	96	8.82	1.23	0.13	9.11	5.44	10.97	5.53	8.50	9.15	5.46	6.49	7.17	7.95	9.11	9.89	10.15	10.38	10.75	UL2Fm
UL2Gf	18	9.06	1.34	0.31	8.70	6.98	11.24	4.25	8.25	9.87	7.01	7.24	7.57	8.08	8.70	9.93	11.01	11.05	11.22	UL2Gf
UL2Gm	22	9.67	1.63	0.35	9.23	7.08	12.87	5.79	8.77	10.56	7.10	7.31	7.86	8.77	9.23	11.20	11.81	11.99	12.77	UL2Gm
UL2Hf	25	10.52	0.74	0.15	10.65	8.87	11.46	2.60	10.14	10.90	8.91	9.28	9.54	10.12	10.65	11.14	11.33	11.34	11.45	UL2Hf
UL2Hm	33	11.25	1.17	0.20	11.88	7.58	12.40	4.82	10.72	11.78	7.81	9.22	9.59	10.66	11.88	12.08	12.23	12.34	12.40	UL2Hm
TDS	n	mean	sd	se	med	min	max	range	99%CIL	99%CIU	0.5%ile	5%ile	10%ile	25%ile	50%ile	75%ile	90%ile	95%ile	99.5%ile	TDS

Table 23. Summary Data for Females and Males for All tooth Development Stages UL3 f & m Caucasians from the UK [London and its environs].

TDS	n	mean	sd	se	med	min	max	range	99%CIL	99%CIU	0.5%ile	5%ile	10%ile	25%ile	50%ile	75%ile	90%ile	95%ile	99.5%ile	TDS
UL3Af	No data																			UL3Af
UL3Am	No data																			UL3Am
UL3Bf	No data																			UL3Bf
UL3Bm	No data																			UL3Bm
UL3Cf	6	4.30	0.87	0.36	4.46	2.97	5.12	2.15	3.38	5.22	2.99	3.17	3.36	3.81	4.46	5.01	5.07	5.10	5.12	UL3Cf
UL3Cm	14	4.88	1.02	0.27	5.08	3.40	6.50	3.10	4.17	5.58	3.41	3.51	3.61	4.01	5.08	5.51	6.18	6.42	6.49	UL3Cm
UL3Df	15	5.86	1.21	0.31	5.95	3.63	8.07	4.44	5.06	6.67	3.67	4.00	4.27	5.27	5.95	6.40	7.32	7.54	8.02	UL3Df
UL3Dm	18	5.40	0.97	0.23	5.46	3.81	7.19	3.38	4.81	5.99	3.82	3.93	4.31	4.71	5.46	5.71	6.84	7.14	7.18	UL3Dm
UL3Ef	30	7.01	1.20	0.22	6.98	4.19	9.34	5.15	6.45	7.58	4.34	5.31	5.54	6.16	6.98	7.86	8.52	8.93	9.28	UL3Ef
UL3Em	41	7.51	1.70	0.26	7.30	5.47	15.52	10.05	6.83	8.19	5.47	5.56	5.82	6.48	7.30	8.16	8.80	8.96	14.31	UL3Em
UL3Ff	28	8.53	0.85	0.16	8.58	6.98	10.21	3.23	8.12	8.95	7.01	7.22	7.34	7.97	8.58	8.92	9.71	9.91	10.17	UL3Ff
UL3Fm	26	9.23	1.61	0.32	9.08	5.95	11.99	6.04	8.42	10.05	5.97	6.39	7.17	8.48	9.08	10.28	11.43	11.46	11.92	UL3Fm
UL3Gf	41	11.56	1.55	0.24	11.14	9.23	15.30	6.08	10.94	12.18	9.28	9.62	9.90	10.49	11.14	12.46	13.60	15.21	15.30	UL3Gf
UL3Gm	38	11.98	1.32	0.21	12.12	9.04	14.22	5.18	11.43	12.53	9.09	9.43	9.68	11.50	12.12	12.82	13.55	13.68	14.14	UL3Gm
UL3Hf	104	12.93	0.63	0.06	13.01	11.12	13.80	2.68	12.77	13.09	11.22	11.76	12.04	12.58	13.01	13.43	13.69	13.74	13.80	UL3Hf
UL3Hm	93	13.39	0.74	0.08	13.55	10.75	14.23	3.47	13.19	13.58	10.79	12.14	12.62	12.96	13.55	13.97	14.18	14.21	14.22	UL3Hm
TDS	n	mean	sd	se	med	min	max	range	99%CIL	99%CIU	0.5%ile	5%ile	10%ile	25%ile	50%ile	75%ile	90%ile	95%ile	99.5%ile	TDS

Table 24. Summary Data for Females and Males for All tooth Development Stages UL4 f & m Caucasians from the UK [London and its environs].

TDS	n	mean	sd	se	med	min	max	range	99%CIL	99%CIU	0.5%ile	5%ile	10%ile	25%ile	50%ile	75%ile	90%ile	95%ile	99.5%ile	TDS
UL4Af	No data																			UL4Af
UL4Am																				UL4Am
UL4Bf	3	4.50	1.21	0.70	5.02	3.12	5.36	2.24	2.70	6.30	3.14	3.31	3.50	4.07	5.02	5.19	5.29	5.32	5.35	UL4Bf
UL4Bm	6	4.44	0.96	0.39	4.26	3.40	5.70	2.30	3.43	5.46	3.40	3.44	3.48	3.69	4.26	5.22	5.59	5.64	5.69	UL4Bm
UL4Cf	15	4.91	0.84	0.22	5.02	3.63	6.15	2.52	4.35	5.47	3.64	3.72	3.84	4.17	5.02	5.61	5.93	6.07	6.14	UL4Cf
UL4Cm	21	4.82	0.66	0.15	5.02	3.70	5.58	1.88	4.45	5.19	3.71	3.81	3.93	4.21	5.02	5.43	5.54	5.56	5.58	UL4Cm
UL4Df	31	7.24	1.08	0.19	7.16	5.44	10.21	4.77	6.74	7.74	5.46	5.59	5.91	6.58	7.16	7.96	8.21	8.84	10.06	UL4Df
UL4Dm	34	7.07	1.08	0.19	6.84	5.44	9.48	4.04	6.59	7.55	5.44	5.51	5.78	6.29	6.84	7.88	8.83	8.89	9.39	UL4Dm
UL4Ef	19	8.08	1.35	0.31	8.29	4.19	9.96	5.77	6.98	8.88	5.67	5.93	6.85	7.27	8.29	8.85	9.63	9.84	9.95	UL4Ef
UL4Em	24	7.89	1.35	0.28	7.79	5.58	10.28	4.70	7.18	8.60	5.62	5.95	6.06	7.08	7.79	8.79	9.33	10.16	10.28	UL4Em
UL4Ff	21	10.03	1.48	0.32	9.90	7.29	12.54	5.25	9.19	10.86	7.35	7.92	8.09	8.92	9.90	11.11	12.27	12.34	12.52	UL4Ff
UL4Fm	18	10.51	1.66	0.39	10.38	8.01	13.59	5.57	9.50	11.52	8.03	8.14	8.78	9.12	10.38	11.65	12.46	13.55	13.58	UL4Fm
UL4Gf	22	12.04	1.60	0.34	11.48	9.62	15.31	5.69	11.37	12.70	9.69	10.26	10.42	11.01	11.48	13.35	13.83	15.23	15.31	UL4Gf
UL4Gm	28	12.05	1.46	0.28	12.24	8.38	14.29	5.91	11.34	12.76	8.50	9.29	9.97	11.43	12.24	12.85	13.83	14.12	14.28	UL4Gm
UL4Hf	89	12.78	0.76	0.08	12.94	10.49	13.85	3.36	12.57	12.99	10.56	10.56	11.86	12.34	12.94	13.30	13.67	13.77	13.84	UL4Hf
UL4Hm	80	13.25	0.89	0.10	13.48	9.52	14.25	4.72	13.00	13.51	10.01	11.98	12.15	12.81	13.48	13.91	14.19	14.22	14.24	UL4Hm
TDS	n	mean	sd	se	med	min	max	range	99%CIL	99%CIU	0.5%ile	5%ile	10%ile	25%ile	50%ile	75%ile	90%ile	95%ile	99.5%ile	TDS

Table 25. Summary Data for Females and Males for All tooth Development Stages UL5 f & m Caucasians from the UK [London and its environs].

TDS	n	mean	sd	se	med	min	max	range	99%CIL	99%CIU	0.5%ile	5%ile	10%ile	25%ile	50%ile	75%ile	90%ile	95%ile	99.5%ile	TDS
UL5Af	4	3.60	0.48	0.24	3.61	3.04	4.17	1.13	2.99	4.22	3.04	3.10	3.16	3.35	3.61	3.86	4.04	4.11	4.16	UL5Af
UL5Am	4	4.16	1.05	0.53	3.78	3.40	5.70	2.30	2.80	5.52	3.40	3.43	3.45	3.52	3.78	4.42	5.19	5.44	5.67	UL5Am
UL5Bf	7	4.72	1.40	0.53	5.02	2.28	6.15	3.87	3.35	6.09	2.32	2.68	3.09	4.04	5.02	5.75	6.15	6.15	6.15	UL5Bf
UL5Bm	7	4.69	0.80	0.30	4.46	3.70	5.58	1.88	3.91	5.47	3.71	3.77	3.84	4.07	4.46	5.47	5.54	5.56	5.58	UL5Bm
UL5Cf	14	6.00	1.47	0.39	5.62	3.95	10.21	6.25	4.99	7.02	4.02	4.65	4.65	5.05	5.62	6.03	7.27	8.33	10.02	UL5Cf
UL5Cm	19	5.17	0.69	0.16	5.37	3.81	6.48	2.67	4.76	5.58	3.82	3.94	4.36	4.73	5.37	5.50	5.72	6.39	6.47	UL5Cm
UL5Df	29	7.40	0.89	0.17	7.32	5.63	9.22	3.59	6.97	7.82	5.67	5.93	6.34	6.92	7.32	8.02	8.51	8.74	9.16	UL5Df
UL5Dm	37	7.23	1.11	0.18	7.09	5.44	9.48	4.04	6.76	7.70	5.45	5.57	5.90	6.31	7.09	7.92	8.81	8.87	9.38	UL5Dm
UL5Ef	20	8.61	2.12	0.47	8.38	4.19	15.06	10.87	7.38	9.83	4.43	6.62	6.86	7.61	8.38	9.02	10.11	11.67	14.72	UL5Ef
UL5Em	23	8.71	1.36	0.28	8.77	5.95	11.97	6.02	7.98	9.44	6.07	7.07	7.15	7.87	8.77	9.12	10.28	10.95	11.87	UL5Em
UL5Ff	24	10.70	1.58	0.32	10.39	8.09	13.55	5.46	9.87	11.53	8.15	8.62	8.92	9.61	10.39	12.27	12.82	13.28	13.53	UL5Ff
UL5Fm	21	11.10	1.79	0.39	11.43	6.81	13.94	7.13	10.10	12.11	6.97	8.38	9.10	9.85	11.43	12.40	12.40	13.00	13.59	13.91
UL5Gf	37	12.58	1.53	0.25	12.61	10.26	15.79	5.53	11.94	13.23	10.28	10.60	10.71	11.14	12.61	13.68	14.91	15.30	15.70	UL5Gf
UL5Gm	28	12.60	1.66	0.31	12.57	9.27	16.91	7.64	11.79	13.40	9.30	9.77	10.53	12.02	12.57	12.99	14.54	15.20	16.68	UL5Gm
UL5Hf	306	14.26	0.98	0.06	14.56	10.49	15.30	4.81	14.12	14.40	11.33	12.35	12.89	13.64	14.56	14.56	15.07	15.26	15.29	UL5Hf
UL5Hm	179	14.11	0.94	0.07	14.25	10.75	15.24	4.48	13.93	14.29	10.97	12.20	12.81	13.54	14.25	14.98	15.11	15.16	15.23	UL5Hm
TDS	n	mean	sd	se	med	min	max	range	99%CIL	99%CIU	0.5%ile	5%ile	10%ile	25%ile	50%ile	75%ile	90%ile	95%ile	99.5%ile	TDS

Table 26. Summary Data for Females and Males for All tooth Development Stages UL6f & m Caucasians from the UK [London and its environs].

	n	mean	sd	se	med	min	max	range	99%CIL	99%CIU	0.5%ile	5%ile	10%ile	25%ile	50%ile	75%ile	90%ile	95%ile	99.5%ile	
UL6Af	No data																			UL6Af
UL6Am	No data																			UL6Am
UL6Bf	No data																			UL6Bf
UL6Bm	No data																			UL6Bm
UL6Cf	No data																			UL6Cf
UL6Cm	No data																			UL6Cm
UL6Df	9	3.80	0.71	0.24	3.76	2.97	5.02	2.05	3.20	4.41	2.98	3.00	3.02	3.12	3.76	4.17	4.65	4.83	5.00	UL6Df
UL6Dm	12	4.12	0.58	0.17	3.97	3.40	5.43	2.03	3.69	4.55	3.41	3.49	3.58	3.70	3.97	4.46	4.75	5.07	5.39	UL6Dm
UL6Ef	11	5.28	0.65	0.20	5.21	4.16	6.37	2.20	4.77	5.79	4.18	4.30	4.44	5.00	5.21	5.71	6.03	6.20	6.35	UL6Ef
UL6Em	20	5.59	1.07	0.24	5.53	3.81	8.80	4.99	4.98	6.21	3.85	4.19	4.58	5.02	5.53	5.88	6.52	6.98	8.62	UL6Em
UL6Ff	16	6.72	0.92	0.23	6.94	5.44	8.07	2.63	6.13	7.31	5.45	5.50	5.54	5.85	6.94	7.35	7.96	8.03	8.07	UL6Ff
UL6Fm	14	6.17	0.75	0.20	6.17	5.37	7.78	2.41	5.65	6.69	5.37	5.41	5.45	5.49	6.17	6.62	7.12	7.46	7.74	UL6Fm
UL6Gf	42	7.93	1.22	0.19	8.05	4.19	10.44	6.25	7.44	8.41	4.55	6.05	6.57	7.17	8.05	8.86	9.19	9.93	10.37	UL6Gf
UL6Gm	46	8.19	1.59	0.23	7.98	5.52	12.79	7.27	7.59	8.79	5.59	6.04	6.43	7.10	7.98	8.84	9.47	11.43	12.72	UL6Gm
UL6Hf	15	9.51	0.81	0.21	9.66	7.69	10.40	2.71	8.97	10.06	7.71	7.85	8.28	9.36	9.66	10.05	10.30	10.35	10.40	UL6Hf
UL6Hm	68	9.32	0.78	0.09	9.46	5.95	10.09	4.15	9.08	9.56	5.99	8.22	8.36	9.18	9.46	9.84	9.96	10.03	10.08	UL6Hm
TDS	n	mean	sd	se	med	min	max	range	99%CIL	99%CIU	0.5%ile	5%ile	10%ile	25%ile	50%ile	75%ile	90%ile	95%ile	99.5%ile	TDS

Table 27. Summary Data for Females and Males for All tooth Development Stages UL7 f & m Caucasians from the UK [London and its environs].

TDS	n	mean	sd	se	med	min	max	range	99%CIL	99%CIU	0.5%ile	5%ile	10%ile	25%ile	50%ile	75%ile	90%ile	95%ile	99.5%ile	TDS
UL7Af	2	3.79																		UL7Af
UL7Am	2	5.08	0.88	0.62	5.08	4.46	5.70	1.24	3.48	6.68	4.46	4.52	4.58	4.77	5.08	5.39	5.58	5.64	5.69	UL7Am
UL7Bf	10	4.19	0.85	0.27	4.30	2.28	5.12	2.84	3.49	4.89	2.34	2.89	3.50	3.81	4.30	4.86	5.03	5.08	5.12	UL7Bf
UL7Bm	16	4.87	0.83	0.21	4.90	3.70	6.48	2.78	4.33	5.40	3.72	3.88	3.94	4.05	4.90	5.46	5.67	5.94	6.43	UL7Bm
UL7Cf	13	6.01	1.21	0.34	5.69	5.02	9.83	4.81	5.14	6.87	5.03	5.13	5.24	5.44	5.69	6.03	6.32	7.75	9.62	UL7Cf
UL7Cm	20	5.94	1.26	0.28	5.53	3.81	8.80	4.99	5.21	6.67	3.87	4.42	4.66	5.39	5.53	6.60	7.83	8.05	8.72	UL7Cm
UL7Df	50	7.87	1.57	0.22	7.90	4.19	15.26	11.07	7.30	8.45	4.52	5.93	6.54	7.00	7.90	8.47	9.35	9.82	14.02	UL7Df
UL7Dm	41	7.65	1.20	0.19	7.43	5.37	10.28	4.91	7.17	8.13	5.46	5.95	6.25	6.72	7.43	8.77	8.96	9.48	10.28	UL7Dm
UL7Ef	15	9.27	1.19	0.31	8.93	6.98	11.14	4.16	8.48	10.06	7.00	7.20	7.81	8.85	8.93	10.01	10.77	10.94	11.12	UL7Ef
UL7Em	21	9.45	1.68	0.37	9.27	5.95	12.00	6.05	8.50	10.40	5.98	6.25	7.06	9.00	9.27	10.97	11.43	11.73	11.97	UL7Em
UL7Ff	15	11.42	1.70	0.44	11.11	9.59	15.66	6.07	10.29	12.56	9.59	9.61	9.68	10.37	11.11	12.50	13.27	14.18	15.51	UL7Ff
UL7Fm	18	11.48	1.33	0.31	11.89	8.38	13.59	5.21	10.67	12.29	8.47	9.30	9.51	10.99	11.89	12.33	12.63	12.96	13.53	UL7Fm
UL7Gf	86	13.93	1.81	0.19	14.15	10.26	19.87	9.61	13.43	14.44	10.40	11.01	11.42	12.63	14.15	15.25	15.91	16.24	18.95	UL7Gf
UL7Gm	69	14.31	1.56	0.19	14.44	10.52	17.53	7.01	13.82	14.79	10.57	11.98	12.38	13.00	14.44	15.39	16.12	16.66	17.40	UL7Gm
UL7Hf	398	14.45	0.99	0.05	14.86	11.58	15.52	3.93	14.32	14.58	11.58	12.29	12.96	13.95	14.86	15.21	15.38	15.47	15.51	UL7Hf
UL7Hm	321	14.70	0.90	0.05	15.02	11.99	15.72	3.73	14.57	14.82	12.03	12.89	13.31	14.20	15.02	15.42	15.59	15.64	15.71	UL7Hm
TDS	n	mean	sd	se	med	min	max	range	99%CIL	99%CIU	0.5%ile	5%ile	10%ile	25%ile	50%ile	75%ile	90%ile	95%ile	99.5%ile	TDS

Table 28. Summary Data for Females and Males for All tooth Development Stages LL7 f & m Caucasians from the UK [London and its environs].

TDS	n	mean	sd	se	med	min	max	range	99%CIL	99%CIU	0.5%ile	5%ile	10%ile	25%ile	50%ile	75%ile	90%ile	95%ile	99.5%ile	TDS
LL7Af	No data																			LL7Af
LL7Am	No data																			L7L7Am
LL7Bf	No data																			LL7Bf
LL7Bm	No data																			LL7Bm
LL7Cf	18	5.54	1.09	0.26	5.67	2.28	7.45	5.17	4.88	6.20	2.44	3.88	4.76	5.14	5.67	6.12	6.44	6.73	7.38	LL7Cf
LL7Cm	28	6.04	1.01	0.19	5.57	3.81	8.01	4.21	5.55	6.53	3.93	4.80	5.07	5.46	5.57	6.83	7.34	7.67	7.97	LL7Cm
LL7Df	42	7.72	1.09	0.17	7.79	4.19	10.21	6.02	7.29	8.16	4.55	6.44	6.74	7.07	7.79	8.27	8.93	9.33	10.16	LL7Df
LL7Dm	32	7.44	1.19	0.21	7.35	3.40	9.48	6.08	6.90	7.98	3.78	6.01	6.26	6.84	7.35	8.28	8.79	8.82	9.38	LL7Dm
LL7Ef	13	9.06	0.93	0.26	8.92	6.98	10.65	3.67	8.39	9.72	7.06	7.75	8.33	8.58	8.92	9.66	10.07	10.33	10.62	LL7Ef
LL7Em	26	8.97	2.29	0.45	9.08	0.27	11.73	11.45	7.81	10.13	0.98	6.04	6.87	8.82	9.08	10.27	11.23	11.43	11.69	LL7Em
LL7Ff	98	10.42	1.41	0.14	10.15	7.86	15.30	7.45	10.06	10.79	8.34	9.10	9.10	9.38	10.15	11.08	11.78	13.33	15.19	LL7Ff
LL7Fm	28	11.75	2.04	0.39	11.97	5.95	15.39	9.43	10.76	12.75	6.28	8.69	9.32	10.80	11.97	12.80	13.88	14.82	15.35	LL7Fm
LL7Gf	140	14.24	1.55	0.13	14.26	10.66	19.87	9.21	13.90	14.58	10.72	11.89	12.27	13.00	14.26	15.30	15.94	16.29	18.34	LL7Gf
LL7Gm	113	14.31	1.43	0.13	14.48	10.24	17.53	7.29	13.96	14.65	10.40	12.07	12.32	13.25	14.48	15.35	15.91	16.20	17.32	LL7Gm
LL7Hf	464	14.91	0.86	0.04	15.16	12.08	15.92	3.84	14.81	15.01	12.25	13.10	13.65	14.46	15.16	15.55	15.78	15.85	15.92	LL7Hf
LL7Hm	321	14.70	0.90	0.05	15.02	11.99	15.72	3.73	14.57	14.82	12.03	12.89	13.31	14.20	15.02	15.42	15.59	15.64	15.71	LL7Hm
TDS	n	mean	sd	se	med	min	max	range	99%CIL	99%CIU	0.5%ile	5%ile	10%ile	25%ile	50%ile	75%ile	90%ile	95%ile	99.5%ile	TDS

Table 29. Summary Data for Females and Males for All tooth Development Stages LL6 f & m Caucasians from the UK [London and its environs].

TDS	n	mean	sd	se	med	min	max	range	99%CIL	99%CIU	0.5%ile	5%ile	10%ile	25%ile	50%ile	75%ile	90%ile	95%ile	99.5%ile	TDS
LL6Af	No data																			LL6Af
LL6Am	No data																			LL6Am
LL6Bf	No data																			LL6Bf
LL6Bm	No data																			LL6Bm
LL6Cf	No data																			LL6Cf
LL6Cm	No data																			LL6Cm
LL6Df	7	3.25	0.57	0.22	3.12	2.28	3.95	1.68	2.69	3.81	2.30	2.49	2.70	3.00	3.12	3.69	3.84	3.89	3.95	LL6Df
LL6Dm	7	4.70	1.00	0.38	4.46	3.56	5.95	2.39	3.73	5.68	3.57	3.60	3.64	3.87	4.46	5.60	5.85	5.90	5.95	LL6Dm
LL6Ef	10	4.96	0.64	0.20	4.99	4.16	6.03	1.86	4.44	5.49	4.16	4.17	4.17	4.47	4.47	5.30	5.81	5.92	6.018029	LL6Ef
LL6Em	23	5.07	0.90	0.19	5.14	3.70	6.89	3.19	4.59	5.56	3.71	3.82	3.94	4.33	5.14	5.58	6.26	6.47	6.84	LL6Em
LL6Ff	17	6.37	0.88	0.21	6.37	5.02	8.02	2.99	5.82	6.92	5.04	5.17	5.35	5.63	6.37	6.98	7.37	7.56	7.97	LL6Ff
LL6Fm	18	6.39	1.20	0.28	6.21	5.02	9.48	4.45	5.67	7.12	5.05	5.32	5.42	5.49	6.21	6.79	7.75	8.90	9.42	LL6Fm
LL6Gf	45	8.00	1.60	0.24	8.02	4.19	15.30	11.11	7.39	8.62	4.58	6.05	6.48	7.16	8.02	8.83	9.10	9.83	14.16	LL6Gf
LL6Gm	42	8.05	1.62	0.25	7.91	5.52	14.25	8.73	7.40	8.69	5.52	5.96	6.33	7.08	7.91	8.79	9.09	11.32	13.67	6.02
LL6Hf	199	10.43	1.09	0.08	10.26	7.69	12.36	4.67	10.23	10.63	7.86	9.00	9.11	9.57	10.26	11.46	12.02	12.24	12.35	LL6Hf
LL6Hm	170	10.30	0.83	0.06	10.24	7.39	11.91	4.52	10.14	10.46	8.14	9.03	9.24	9.83	10.24	10.75	11.56	11.73	11.91	LL6Hm
TDS	n	mean	sd	se	med	min	max	range	99%CIL	99%CIU	0.5%ile	5%ile	10%ile	25%ile	50%ile	75%ile	90%ile	95%ile	99.5%ile	TDS

Table 30. Summary Data for Females and Males for All tooth Development Stages LL5 f & m Caucasians from the UK [London and its environs].

TDS	n	mean	sd	se	med	min	max	range	99%CIL	99%CIU	0.5%ile	5%ile	10%ile	25%ile	50%ile	75%ile	90%ile	95%ile	99.5%ile	TDS
LL5Af	6	9.58	4.82	1.97	9.07	3.63	14.83	11.19	4.50	14.65	3.70	4.26	4.89	6.21	9.07	13.97	14.77	14.80	14.82	LL5Af
LL5Am	10	5.70	3.88	1.23	4.20	3.40	16.27	12.87	2.53	8.86	3.41	3.47	3.55	3.69	4.20	5.63	7.76	12.02	15.85	LL5Am
LL5Bf	5	4.85	1.59	0.71	5.36	2.28	6.15	3.87	3.01	6.69	2.32	2.71	3.14	4.44	5.36	6.03	6.10	6.13	6.15	LL5Bf
LL5Bm	3	4.55	0.90	0.52	4.06	3.99	5.58	1.59	3.21	5.88	3.99	4.00	4.01	4.03	4.06	4.82	5.28	5.43	5.57	LL5Bm
LL5Cf	15	5.57	1.47	0.38	5.44	3.95	10.21	6.25	4.58	6.55	3.97	4.10	4.17	5.02	5.44	5.74	6.38	7.69	9.95	LL5Cf
LL5Cm	23	5.34	1.03	0.21	5.42	3.81	8.80	4.79	4.79	5.89	3.82	3.98	4.26	4.73	5.42	5.53	6.36	6.47	8.54	LL5Cm
LL5Df	63	8.20	1.32	0.17	8.10	5.63	10.33	4.70	7.77	8.63	5.64	5.98	6.57	7.12	8.10	9.21	10.21	10.32	10.33	LL5Df
LL5Dm	29	7.18	1.46	0.27	6.89	5.52	12.47	6.95	6.48	7.88	5.52	5.52	5.57	6.31	6.89	7.81	8.80	9.22	12.05	LL5Dm
LL5Ef	25	8.76	2.33	0.47	8.48	4.19	16.96	12.76	7.56	9.96	4.50	6.74	6.80	7.40	8.48	9.49	9.93	12.27	16.46	LL5Ef
LL5Em	27	8.51	1.42	0.27	8.77	5.95	11.97	6.02	7.81	9.22	5.95	6.16	6.90	7.49	8.77	9.05	10.28	10.80	11.85	LL5Em
LL5Ff	128	10.44	1.55	0.14	9.98	7.69	16.76	9.07	10.08	10.79	7.80	8.89	9.10	9.44	9.98	10.96	12.66	13.63	15.99	LL5Ff
LL5Fm	37	12.10	2.96	0.49	12.00	0.27	17.11	16.84	10.85	13.36	1.73	8.91	9.24	10.66	12.00	14.06	15.24	15.52	16.93	LL5Fm
LL5Gf	61	12.92	1.41	0.18	12.83	10.26	16.07	5.81	12.45	13.39	10.36	10.66	11.01	12.02	12.83	13.85	14.95	15.14	15.84	LL5Gf
LL5Gm	50	13.22	1.64	0.23	12.91	9.27	16.79	7.52	12.62	13.82	9.33	10.51	11.78	12.21	12.91	14.34	15.43	15.95	16.62	LL5Gm
LL5Hf	531	14.84	1.08	0.05	15.21	9.83	16.01	6.18	14.72	14.97	10.03	12.76	13.25	14.38	15.21	15.60	15.85	15.94	16.00	LL5Hf
LL5Hm	542	15.43	1.17	0.05	15.59	10.75	17.19	6.44	15.30	15.56	11.64	13.10	13.69	14.91	15.59	16.34	16.76	16.97	17.16	LL5Hm
TDS	n	mean	sd	se	med	min	max	range	99%CIL	99%CIU	0.5%ile	5%ile	10%ile	25%ile	50%ile	75%ile	90%ile	95%ile	99.5%ile	TDS

Table 31. Summary Data for Females and Males for All tooth Development Stages LL4 f & m Caucasians from the UK [London and its environs].

TDS	n	mean	sd	se	med	min	max	range	99%CIL	99%CIU	0.5%ile	5%ile	10%ile	25%ile	50%ile	75%ile	90%ile	95%ile	99.5%ile	TDS
LL4Af	No data																			LL4Af
LL4Am	No data																			LL4Am
LL4Bf	4	3.76	0.85	0.43	3.55	2.97	4.97	1.99	2.66	4.86	2.98	3.05	3.12	3.34	3.55	3.97	4.57	4.77	4.95	LL4Bf
LL4Bm	5	3.88	0.42	0.19	3.93	3.40	4.46	1.06	3.40	4.37	3.40	3.43	3.47	3.56	3.93	4.06	4.30	4.38	4.45	LL4Bm
LL4Cf	13	5.00	1.21	0.34	5.36	2.28	6.37	4.09	4.13	5.87	2.37	3.16	3.80	4.16	5.36	6.03	6.15	6.24	6.36	LL4Cf
LL4Cm	22	4.91	0.75	0.16	5.08	3.69	6.25	2.57	4.50	5.32	3.69	3.71	3.82	4.27	5.08	5.47	5.58	5.69	6.20	LL4Cm
LL4Df	25	6.58	1.30	0.26	6.55	4.17	10.21	6.04	5.91	7.25	4.27	5.04	5.16	5.63	6.55	7.36	7.97	8.06	9.95	LL4Df
LL4Dm	24	6.53	1.03	0.21	6.49	4.78	8.84	4.06	5.98	7.07	4.85	5.44	5.49	5.55	6.49	6.95	7.77	8.67	8.84	LL4Dm
LL4Ef	31	8.21	1.16	0.21	8.29	4.19	9.96	5.77	7.67	8.75	4.57	6.80	6.98	7.65	8.29	8.90	9.49	9.71	9.94	LL4Ef
LL4Em	36	7.77	1.17	0.20	7.82	5.58	10.24	4.66	7.27	8.28	5.62	5.92	6.13	7.08	7.82	8.77	9.02	9.47	10.11	LL4Em
LL4Ff	27	10.27	2.64	0.51	9.90	6.75	16.96	10.20	8.96	11.58	6.78	7.03	7.25	8.58	9.90	11.26	13.66	15.77	16.82	LL4Ff
LL4Fm	24	10.50	2.89	0.59	10.40	0.27	15.39	15.11	8.98	12.03	1.18	8.26	8.88	9.16	10.40	11.98	13.23	15.00	15.37	LL4Fm
LL4Gf	24	11.88	1.39	0.28	11.40	9.76	15.04	5.28	11.15	12.61	9.82	10.28	10.43	10.92	11.40	12.86	13.58	14.01	14.93	LL4Gf
LL4Gm	30	12.00	1.57	0.29	12.04	8.38	14.56	6.18	11.26	12.74	8.51	9.38	9.72	11.43	12.04	12.96	14.08	14.26	14.52	LL4Gm
LL4Hf	154	12.99	0.98	0.08	13.17	10.14	14.27	4.14	12.78	13.19	10.20	11.03	11.58	12.31	13.17	13.82	14.09	14.09	14.26	14.26
LL4Hm	102	13.20	0.81	0.08	13.42	10.75	14.22	3.47	12.99	13.40	10.75	11.72	12.17	12.67	13.42	13.83	14.11	14.19	14.22	LL4Hm
TDS	n	mean	sd	se	med	min	max	range	99%CIL	99%CIU	0.5%ile	5%ile	10%ile	25%ile	50%ile	75%ile	90%ile	95%ile	99.5%ile	TDS

Table 32. Summary Data for Females and Males for All tooth Development Stages LL3 f & m Caucasians from the UK [London and its environs].

TDS	n	mean	sd	se	med	min	max	range	99%CIL	99%CIU	0.5%ile	5%ile	10%ile	25%ile	50%ile	75%ile	90%ile	95%ile	99.5%ile	TDS
LL3AF	No data																			LL3AF
LL3Am	No data																			LL3Am
LL3Bf	2	3.08	0.06	0.04	3.08	3.04	3.12	0.08	2.97	3.18	3.04	3.04	3.04	3.06	3.08	3.10	3.11	3.11	3.12	LL3Bf
LL3Bm	3	5.31	0.25	0.14	5.43	5.02	5.47	0.45	4.94	5.68	5.03	5.10	5.23	5.23	5.43	5.45	5.46	5.47	5.47	LL3Bm
LL3Cf	6	4.72	1.56	0.64	4.59	2.97	7.32	4.34	3.07	6.36	2.99	3.09	3.22	3.63	4.59	5.27	6.34	6.83	7.27	LL3Cf
LL3Cm	7	4.40	0.80	0.30	4.21	3.40	5.42	2.02	3.63	3.41	3.45	3.50	3.81	3.81	4.21	5.08	5.25	5.33	5.41	LL3Cm
LL3Df	12	5.27	1.27	0.37	5.16	3.63	8.02	4.38	4.33	6.21	3.64	3.70	3.78	4.32	5.16	6.00	6.35	7.11	7.93	LL3Df
LL3Dm	18	5.13	1.10	0.26	5.50 *	3.69	7.19	3.50	4.46	5.80	3.69	3.70	3.78	4.11	5.50	5.67	6.52	7.14	7.18	LL3Dm
LL3Ef	31	6.91	1.32	0.24	6.92	4.19	9.96	5.77	6.30	7.53	4.31	5.20	5.52	5.97	6.92	7.74	8.57	9.14	9.86	LL3Ef
LL3Em	40	6.75	1.18	0.19	6.60	4.62	9.48	4.86	6.38	7.12	4.65	5.34	5.48	5.92	6.60	7.53	8.63	8.80	9.35	LL3Em
LL3Ff	32	8.36	0.92	0.16	8.38	10.21	10.21	3.47	7.94	8.78	6.74	6.88	7.16	7.79	8.38	8.92	9.58	9.74	10.15	LL3Ff
LL3Fm	34	9.22	1.49	0.26	8.98	7.06	13.59	6.53	8.56	9.87	7.10	7.29	7.45	8.22	8.98	10.14	11.22	11.91	13.32	LL3Fm
LL3Gf	29	11.13	1.44	0.27	11.01	7.69	14.09	6.40	10.44	11.82	7.91	9.38	9.73	10.33	11.01	12.25	13.06	13.75	14.05	LL3Gf
LL3Gm	36	11.52	2.30	0.38	11.98	0.27	14.22	13.95	10.53	12.50	1.81	9.21	9.63	11.33	11.98	12.53	13.21	13.76	14.19	LL3Gm
LL3Hf	157	12.96	0.83	0.07	13.10	10.64	14.05	3.41	12.79	13.13	10.66	11.30	11.77	12.44	13.10	13.66	13.87	13.97	14.05	LL3Hf
LL3Hm	71	12.83	0.69	0.08	12.96	10.75	13.66	2.90	12.62	13.05	10.75	11.40	12.03	12.55	12.96	13.38	13.54	13.60	13.64	LL3Hm
TDS	n	mean	sd	se	med	min	max	range	99%CIL	99%CIU	0.5%ile	5%ile	10%ile	25%ile	50%ile	75%ile	90%ile	95%ile	99.5%ile	TDS

Table 33. Summary Data for Females and Males for All tooth Development Stages LL2 f & m Caucasians from the UK [London and its environs].

TDS	n	mean	sd	se	med	min	max	range	99%CIL	99%CIU	0.5%ile	5%ile	10%ile	25%ile	50%ile	75%ile	90%ile	95%ile	99.5%ile	TDS
LL2Af	No data																			LL2Af
LL2Am	No data																			LL2Am
LL2Bf	No data																			LL2Bf
LL2Bm	No data																			LL2Bm
LL2Cf	3	3.32	0.55	0.32	3.04	2.97	3.95	0.98	2.50	4.14	2.97	2.98	2.99	3.00	3.04	3.49	3.77	3.86	3.94	LL2Cf
LL2Cm	2	5.31	FALSE	0.17	5.31	5.14	5.48	0.34	4.87	5.74	5.74	5.14	5.17	5.22	5.31	5.39	5.44	5.46	5.47	LL2Cm
LL2Df	10	4.65	1.19	0.38	4.59	3.12	6.61	3.49	3.68	5.62	3.13	3.27	3.42	3.66	4.59	5.50	6.02	6.31	6.58	LL2Df
LL2Dm	16	4.77	0.96	0.24	4.85	3.56	6.38	2.82	4.15	5.38	3.57	3.66	3.69	3.92	4.85	5.47	5.98	6.29	6.37	LL2Dm
LL2Ef	11	6.12	1.59	0.48	5.69	4.44	9.34	4.90	4.88	7.35	4.46	4.70	4.97	5.11	5.69	6.15	8.93	9.14	9.32	LL2Ef
LL2Em	18	5.36	0.62	0.15	5.52	4.21	6.48	2.27	4.98	5.74	4.23	4.42	4.46	4.94	5.52	5.57	6.02	6.21	6.45	LL2Em
LL2Ff	18	7.06	1.11	0.26	7.10	5.44	9.49	4.05	6.38	0.00	5.45	5.51	5.54	6.12	7.10	7.87	8.13	8.40	9.38	LL2Ff
LL2Fm	20	7.15	1.19	0.27	6.96	5.37	9.48	4.11	6.46	7.84	5.39	5.53	5.79	6.45	6.96	7.90	8.86	9.06	9.43	LL2Fm
LL2Gf	33	8.04	1.44	0.25	7.92	4.19	11.01	6.82	7.39	8.68	4.49	6.27	6.59	7.16	7.92	8.83	9.90	10.76	11.01	LL2Gf
LL2Gm	31	8.56	1.45	0.26	8.38	6.31	12.18	5.87	7.89	9.24	6.34	6.81	7.13	7.68	8.38	8.98	10.52	11.77	12.12	LL2Gm
LL2Hf	44	9.43	0.81	0.12	9.65	7.18	10.49	3.31	9.12	9.75	7.36	8.11	8.47	8.77	9.65	10.02	10.34	10.43	10.49	LL2Hf
LL2Hm	61	10.22	0.96	0.12	10.28	7.43	11.70	4.27	9.91	10.54	7.67	8.53	9.06	9.59	10.28	10.97	11.43	11.52	11.70	LL2Hm
TDS	n	mean	sd	se	med	min	max	range	99%CIL	99%CIU	0.5%ile	5%ile	10%ile	25%ile	50%ile	75%ile	90%ile	95%ile	99.5%ile	TDS

Table 34. Summary Data for Females and Males for All tooth Development Stages LL1 f & m Caucasians from the UK [London and its environs].

TDS	n	mean	sd	se	med	min	max	range	99%CIL	99%CIU	0.5%ile	5%ile	10%ile	25%ile	50%ile	75%ile	90%ile	95%ile	99.5%ile	TDS
LL1Af	No data																			LL1Af
LL1Am	No data																			LL1Am
	no data																			
LL1Bf	no data																			LL1Bf
LL1Bm	no data																			LL1Bm
LL1Cf	no data																			LL1Cf
LL1Cm	no data																			LL1Cm
LL1Df	4	3.84	0.83	0.42	3.61	3.12	5.02	1.91	2.77	4.91	3.12	3.17	3.22	3.37	3.61	4.07	4.64	4.83	5.00	LL1Df
LL1Dm	11	4.67	0.81	0.24	5.02	3.56	5.58	2.02	4.04	5.29	3.57	3.62	3.69	3.97	5.02	5.42	5.48	5.53	5.58	LL1Dm
LL1Ef	8	5.06	0.84	0.30	5.07	3.63	6.03	2.40	4.30	5.83	3.65	3.82	4.00	4.77	5.07	5.71	5.98	6.00	6.03	LL1Ef
LL1Em	11	5.33	0.62	0.19	5.48	4.46	6.48	2.02	4.85	5.81	4.46	4.46	4.46	4.85	5.48	5.64	5.76	6.12	6.44	LL1Em
LL1Ff	14	5.88	0.75	0.20	5.74	4.44	7.16	2.72	5.36	6.40	4.49	4.94	5.25	5.46	5.74	6.15	6.99	7.08	7.15	LL1Ff
LL1Fm	17	5.95	1.18	0.29	5.54	4.21	9.48	5.26	5.21	6.69	4.24	4.53	4.71	5.44	5.54	6.50	6.77	7.39	9.27	LL1Fm
LL1Gf	34	7.85	1.18	0.20	7.96	4.19	9.96	5.77	7.33	8.37	4.49	6.29	6.74	7.19	7.96	8.84	9.30	9.55	9.91	LL1Gf
LL1Gm	22	7.65	1.09	0.23	7.55	5.82	10.52	4.70	7.05	8.26	5.87	6.31	6.33	7.07	7.55	8.29	8.84	8.96	10.36	LL1Gm
LL1Hf	44	8.57	0.77	0.12	8.59	6.55	9.63	3.07	8.27	8.87	6.63	7.02	7.75	8.16	8.59	9.11	9.57	9.62	9.63	LL1Hf
LL1Hm	73	9.03	1.03	0.12	9.10	5.95	10.44	4.50	8.72	9.34	5.99	7.32	7.60	8.31	9.10	9.85	10.24	10.30	10.44	LL1Hm
TDS	n	mean	sd	se	med	min	max	range	99%CIL	99%CIU	0.5%ile	5%ile	10%ile	25%ile	50%ile	75%ile	90%ile	95%ile	99.5%ile	TDS
3811f	135	17.65	1.58	0.14	17.48	14.96	22.78	7.82	17.30	18.00	15.10	15.62	15.82	16.54	17.48	18.49	19.55	20.89	22.44	3811f
3811m	85	17.40	1.18	0.13	17.43	15.22	20.33	5.11	17.07	17.74	15.27	15.45	15.95	16.47	17.43	18.22	18.81	19.33	20.33	3811m

Chapter 12
Automating Human Identification Using Dental X–Ray Radiographs

Omaima Nomir
Univeristy of Mansoura, Egypt

Mohamed Abdel Mottaleb
University of Miami, USA

ABSTRACT

The goal of forensic dentistry is to identify individuals based on their dental characteristics. This chapter presents a system for automating that process by identifying people from dental X-ray images. Given a dental image of a postmortem (PM), the proposed system retrieves the best matches from an antemortem (AM) database. The system automatically segments dental X-ray images into individual teeth and extracts representative feature vectors for each tooth, which are later used for retrieval. This chapter details a new method for teeth segmentation, and three different methods for representing and matching teeth. Each method has a different technique for representing the tooth shape and has its advantages and disadvantages compared with the other methods. The first method represents each tooth contour by signature vectors obtained at salient points on the contour of the tooth. The second method uses Hierarchical Chamfer distance for matching AM and PM teeth. In the third method, each tooth is described using a feature vector extracted using the force field energy function and Fourier descriptors. During retrieval, according to a matching distance between the AM and PM teeth, AM radiographs that are most similar to a given PM image, are found and presented to the user. To increase the accuracy of the identification process, the three matching techniques are fused together. The fusion of information is an integral part of any identification system to improve the overall performance. This chapter introduces some scenarios for fusing the three matchers at the score level as well as at the fusion level.

DOI: 10.4018/978-1-60960-483-7.ch012

INTRODUCTION

Human identification is a fundamental activity at the heart of our society and culture. For many applications, ensuring the identity and authenticity of people is a prerequisite. Biometrics identification refers to identifying an individual based on his or her distinguishing characteristics. It is being accepted by government and industry alike that automated biometric identification will become a necessary fact of life.

Forensic identification is typically defined as the use of science or technology in identifying human beings in the court of law. It has a wide area of applications in criminal investigations, court evidences and security applications.

Forensic identification may take place prior to death and is referred to as ante mortem (AM) identification. Identification may as well be carried out after death and is called postmortem (PM) identification. While behavioral characteristics (e.g. speech) are not suitable for PM identification, most of the physiological characteristics are not appropriate for PM identification as well, especially under severe circumstances encountered in mass disasters (e.g. airplane crashers) or when identification is being attempted more than a couple of weeks postmortem, because of the decay of soft tissues of the body. Therefore, a postmortem biometric identifier has to survive such severe conditions and resist early decay that affects body tissues. Because of their survivability, the best candidates for postmortem biometric identification are the dental features and now the importance of using dental records for human identification is well recognized (Jain, & Ross, 2002).

Forensic odontology (Brogdon, 1998) is the branch of forensics concerned with identifying humans based on their dental features. Dental identification is a comparative technique, where the PM dental records are analyzed and compared against AM records to confirm identity and establish the degree of certainty that the dental records

obtained from the remains of a decedent and the AM dental records of a missing person are for the same individual. Currently the identification is carried out manually by comparing extracted features from a postmortem (PM) dental record to extracted fractures from a database of ante mortem (AM) records. According to forensic experts (Brogdon, 1998), dental characteristics preserve their shape after death for a long period of time. Several individual teeth may get missed or filled after its AM record is taken, hence dental features need to be recorded based on the contour/shape of individual teeth rather than the contour of the whole jaw. This would require reliable automatic segmentation techniques that can extract the contour of each individual tooth for latter retrieval purposes to allow for retrieval based on teeth shapes.

The objective of our research is to automate the process of forensic odontology using image processing and pattern recognition techniques. There are several advantages for automating this procedure. An automatic system can perform identification on a large scale database while a manual or semi-automatic system is useful for verification on a small data set. Also, automating this process will come up with an ordered list of closest matches that we may refer to in order to decide the best match. Accordingly, this will facilitate for forensic odontologists to only manually verify through this best match short list instead of manually searching a large number of AM records. In order to achieve this goal, we need to automate the process of segmenting the dental radiographs and to separate each individual tooth. For the automated identification, the dental records are usually available as radiographs. An automated dental identification system consists of two main stages: feature extraction and feature matching. During feature extraction, certain salient information of the teeth such as contours, artificial prosthesis, number of cuspids, etc. is extracted from the radiographs.

Figure 1. Dental identification system logical diagram

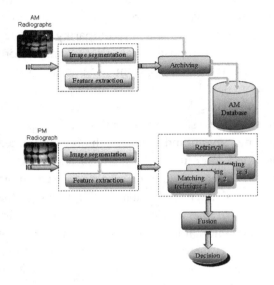

In this Chapter, we present a fully automated dental biometrics system (Nomir, 2006). A block diagram of the proposed dental identification system is shown in Figure 1. This dental identification system can be used by both law enforcement and security agencies in both forensic and biometric identification. The system archives AM dental images in a database, and searches the database for the best matches to a given PM image. The AM images are archived by segmenting and separating the individual teeth in bite-wing images and then extracting a set of features for each individual tooth.

The goal of the segmentation is to separate the teeth from the rest of the radiograph. Then, the individual teeth are separated by first separating the upper jaw from the lower jaw and then separating each tooth, this step is achieved using integral projection. After separating each tooth, we use and compare between three different methods to search the database for a given PM subject. In the first method, a set of salient points on the contour of each tooth is identified and signatures for these points are extracted. These signatures are vectors that are extracted for each salient point. During searching, matching scores are generated

based on the distances between the signature vectors of AM and PM teeth. In the second method, we use a hierarchical edge matching algorithm at different resolution levels. The technique is based on matching teeth contours using Hierarchical Chamfer distance. Using this hierarchical structure; the search space is reduced significantly as well as the computational load. In the third method, instead of using only the contour points as the features, we combine region and boundary information to overcome the inherent limitations of using either representation alone. The process of matching is carried out based on two sets of features, where the first set is extracted using a force field transformation to represent the appearance of the tooth and the second set consists of the Fourier descriptors of the contour of the tooth to represent the shape.

Finally, to increase the accuracy of the overall identification process, we fuse the three matching techniques. The fusion of information is an integral part of any identification systems. We analyze some scenarios for fusing the introduced matchers. Some scenarios are boolean while the others are statistical and accordingly the results are recorded using the different fusion scenarios.

Currently we are building an Automated Dental Identification System (ADIS) (Fahmy, Nassar, Said, Chen, Nomir, Zhou, Howell, Ammar, Abdel-Mottaleb, & Jain, 2004a, 2004b, 2004c, 2005) and (Nomir, & Abdel-Mottaleb, 2005, 2006) for identifying individuals using their dental X-ray records. ADIS is a process automation tool, for postmortem identification, that is being designed to achieve accurate and timely identification results with minimum amount of human intervention. To this end, ADIS automates and facilitates some of the steps taken by forensic experts to examine missing and unidentified persons (MUP) cases.

The rest of this chapter is organized as follows: first Section presents the automatic dental image segmentation technique, second Section presents the matching techniques, third Section presents the fusion of the three matching techniques using different scenarios to increase the accuracy of the overall identification process, fourth Section concludes the Chapter.

AUTOMATIC DENTAL IMAGE SEGMENTATION

Dental X-ray images are classified according to the view they are captured from, and their coverage (Brogdon, 1998). The most commonly used images are panoramic, periapical, and bite-wing. A panoramic image is taken to give a complete view of the upper and lower jaws; it does not show fine details as bite-wing and periapical images. A periapical image is captured to obtain a view of the entire teeth area including the tip of the root and the surrounding tissues. A bite-wing image is captured to view back teeth, only the crowns and parts of the roots for two to four adjacent teeth in both upper and lower jaws are captured. The bite-wing images hold more information about the curvature, and the roots, and these images are the most common views made by dentists, therefore, we used them in our system.

This Section introduces our automatic dental segmentation technique (Nomir, & Abdel-Mottaleb, 2005) and (Abdel-Mottaleb, Nomir, Nassar, Fahmy, & Ammar, 2003). Our segmentation method consists of two stages. The first stage separates the teeth from the background using a two-step thresholding technique; this stage is detailed in the first Subsection. The second stage separates the upper jaw from the lower jaw and then separates each tooth using integral projection; this stage is detailed in the second Subsection. Figure 2 shows a block diagram of the main steps of the

segmentation algorithm. In the third Subsection the experimental results for the segmentation algorithm are presented.

Radiograph Segmentation

Dental X-ray images have three different regions: the background or air, which has the lowest intensity, corresponds to soft tissues. The bone areas have average intensity and the teeth have highest intensity. In some cases the intensity of the bone areas is close to the intensity of the teeth, which makes it difficult to use a single threshold for segmenting the whole image.

The first stage of the radiograph segmentation, is to separate the teeth from the background using a two-step thresholding technique. It starts by iterative thresholding followed by adaptive thresholding (Gonzalez & Wood, 2003) to segment the teeth from both the background and the bone areas. In the next two Subsections, we present the iterative thresholding step, and the adaptive thresholding step respectively.

Iterative Thresholding

In this technique, the initial thresholding is estimated by first detecting the edges in the original image using Canny edge detection (Jain, Kasturi, & Schnck, 1995). Then, it applies a morphological dilation to the binary edge image to obtain pixels around the edge locations. The reason for applying this step is to select the pixels around areas of high contrast in the original image. Usually about half of the pixels in the resulting image will belong to the teeth areas and the other half will belong to the background and the bones. Figure

Figure 2. The segmentation algorithm

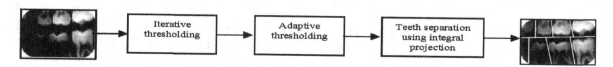

Figure 3. (a) The original image; (b) The binary edge image; (c) The dilated edge image

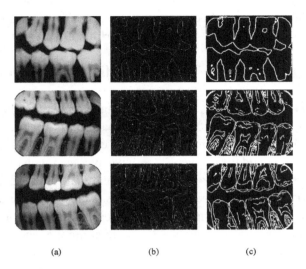

(a)   (b)   (c)

3(b), and Figure 3(c) show the binary edge images and the results of the dilation respectively for the images in Figure 3(a). After obtaining the dilated image, we use the average gray value of the corresponding pixels, from the original image, as an initial threshold. Then, the iterative thresholding is done as follows:

Let $f(i, j)$ be the gray scale value at pixel (i, j), and T_i be the segmentation threshold at step i. To obtain a new threshold, we threshold the original image using T_i to separate the image into teeth areas and non-teeth areas, and obtain μ^i_0 and μ^i_B, which are the mean gray values for the two areas respectively.

$$\mu^i_0 = \frac{\sum_{(i,j)\varepsilon dental} f(i, j)}{\# dental\_pixels} \qquad (1)$$

$$\mu^i_B = \frac{\sum_{(i,j)\varepsilon background} f(i, j)}{\# background\_pixels} \qquad (2)$$

The threshold for step $i + 1$ is then obtained as

$$T_{i+1} = \frac{\mu^i_0 + \mu^i_B}{2} \qquad (3)$$

The iterative threshold updating step is repeated until there is no change in the threshold, i.e. $T_i = T_{i+1}$. The final threshold segments the image into teeth areas, (pixels with values higher than the threshold) and background areas, (pixels with values lower than the threshold). Four to ten iterations were found to be sufficient for convergence. Figure 4(b) shows the resulting binary images for the images in Figure 4(a). It also shows the result of masking the original images with the binary images (Figure 4(c)), i.e., the ones in the binary image have been replaced with the original image gray values, and the zeros are kept. This is the image to which adaptive thresholding is applied.

Adaptive Thresholding

From the experimental results, applying the iterative thresholding technique to segment the teeth from the background sometimes did not lead to good results. Applying adaptive thresholding to the result of masking the original images in 4(c) always produces more accurate results. The reason is that using adaptive thresholding after the iterative thresholding makes the valleys between the teeth clearer because it gets rid of some of the remaining background bones from the first step

Figure 4. (a) The original image; (b) Result of iterative thresholding; (c) The original image after masking by the binary image

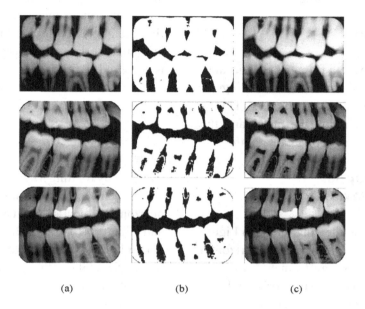

(a)   (b)   (c)

thresholding. This results in locating the separating lines between teeth more easily. We can notice that in Figure 5 the teeth are separated better than in Figure 4(b), and that leads to correctly locate the separation lines between the teeth, as will be explained in the second Subsection.

The idea of the adaptive thresholding is to threshold the pixel at the center of a window according to the average gray value of the non-zero pixels inside this window. Using a window of size $I \times J$ pixels, the following is applied to each pixel of the image that results from masking the original image with the binary image obtained from the iterative thresholding.

$$T(i,j) = \frac{\sum_{S=-I/2}^{I/2} \sum_{t=-J/2}^{J/2} f(i+s, j+t)}{\# \, non - zero \_ pixels} \qquad (4)$$

If the center pixel value of the window is $C(i, j)$, then

$$C'(i,j) = \begin{cases} 1 & C(i,j) \geq T'(i,j) \\ 0 & otherwise \end{cases} \qquad (5)$$

By randomly selecting 30 images from the database as our training set (these images were

Figure 5. Result of adaptive thresholding

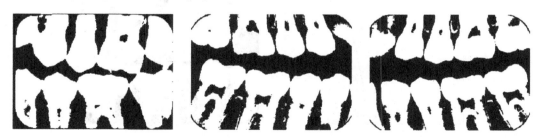

not used in testing), $T'(i, j) = 0.9 \times T(i, j)$ was found to be a suitable threshold value.

Teeth Separation

After segmenting the teeth from the background, each tooth is separated from its surroundings in order to prepare for feature extraction. This is achieved by first separating the upper and the lower jaws, and then separating each tooth.

Separating the Upper and the Lower Jaws

If we consider the first bitewing image in Figure 5, it is clear that a horizontal or a near horizontal line can separate the upper jaw from the lower jaw.

This can be achieved by using horizontal projection as follows: Let $f(i, j)$ be the *mxn* binary image obtained from the segmentation stage, the horizontal integral projection is

$$H(i) = \sum_{j=1}^{n} f(i, j) \qquad (6)$$

Assuming that it is possible to separate the upper jaw from the lower jaw by a straight line, the integral projection along that line will be minimal.

Since it is not always the case that this line is horizontal, we need to rotate the image in a small range of angles. To estimate that range of angles, we randomly selected 40 images from the database as a training set and found that the range [-20:20] is a suitable range of angles. We iteratively rotate the image in that range, and find the angle at which a line that produces the minimum horizontal projection is obtained. This is achieved as follows:

$$\theta, i = \arg \min_{\theta,i} H_{\theta,i}(i) \qquad (7)$$

where $H_{\theta}(i)$ is the horizontal integral projection obtained by rotating $f(i, j)$ with an angle θ. Figure 6 shows an example, in Figure 6(a) the minimum horizontal projection point is marked with a circle, and Figure 6(b) shows the corresponding horizontal line in the image. It is clear that this is the best horizontal line that can separate the two jaws without cutting through the teeth.

In many cases, there is no single straight line that can separate the upper and the lower jaws. Therefore, the initial straight line obtained from the horizontal projection is incrementally modified by reapplying the projection process in adjacent vertical strips in order to find the piece-wise linear separation of the two jaws. The stripes are $h \times w$ pixels around the line, where h is the height of the strip and w is the width of the strip, in our experiments we used $h = 40$, and $w = 20$. Figure 7 shows an example of separating the two jaws using this method. Figure 7(a) shows a case where there is no single line that can separate the two jaws. Figure 7(b), and Figure 7(c) show the result of using the piecewise separation method and

Figure 6. (a) Horizontal integral projection; (b) The initial line segmenting the two jaws

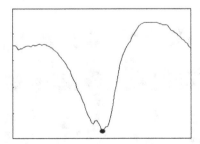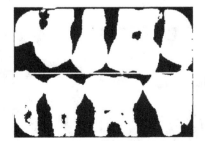

Figure 7. (a) The original image; (b) The binary image with the exact locations for separating the two jaws; (c) The upper and the lower jaws after separation

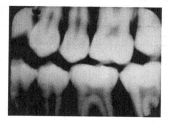 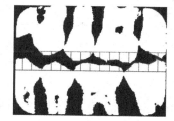 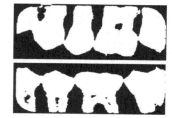

show the upper and lower jaws after the separation.

Separating Each Individual Tooth

To separate each individual tooth we use a technique similar to the one used for separating the two jaws. The goal is to find the lines that separate the adjacent teeth. This can be achieved by using the integral projection method in the vertical direction. If $f(i, j)$ is the mxn binary image obtained from the segmentation stage, the vertical projection is

$$V(i) = \sum_{i=1}^{m} f(i, j) \qquad (8)$$

The separating lines are located by finding valleys in the result of the vertical projection. Due to different teeth alignment, the lines are always neither vertical nor parallel. Therefore, we rotate the image in a small range of angles, e.g. [-20:20] (we used a set of training data to estimate this range), and calculate the vertical projection for each angle in this range. For each projection, we use a threshold value to obtain the valleys that identify locations of vertical lines between adjacent teeth. In the experiments, we used a threshold value equal to 0.35 of the maximum number of ones in the result of the projection. We then select the separating lines and the corresponding angles which produce the minimum vertical projection among all the rotation angles. Figure 8 shows

the detected separating lines overlaid over the original image.

Experiments and Results

Our database was provided by the FBI's Criminal Justice Information Service (CJIS) division, which includes records of different dental radiographs types of AM as well as PM records.

The proposed segmentation technique was applied to 187 bite-wing images. It always correctly segments the upper jaw from the lower jaw for all the images.

Summary of the results for segmenting individual teeth are shown in Table 1. A few teeth segmentation/separation results are shown in Figure 9.

Figure 8. Result of teeth separation

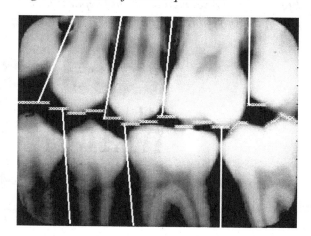

Table 1. The segmentation results

	Upper Jaw	Lower Jaw
Total # of teeth in the 187 images	627	569
# of correctly separated teeth	519	456
Ratio of correctly separated teeth	83%	80%

The cases where teeth were incorrectly separated are due to the images' poor quality. This is especially true for teeth at the borders of the images. In these cases the method can not correctly locate the separation lines, sometimes bones were considered as part of the tooth because of failure of the segmentation stage.

DENTAL MATCHING TACHNIQUES

This Section introduces our dental radiograph matching techniques. Each technique extracts a set of features from the previously segmented X-ray images.

The first Subsection introduces a dental X-ray teeth matching technique that uses signature vectors. The second Subsection introduces the hierarchal contour matching technique. The third Subsection introduces the matching technique based on teeth shapes and appearances. And finally, the fourth Subsection gives a comparison between the three techniques.

Dental X-Ray Teeth Matching using Signature Vectors

This method relies on selecting a set of salient points from the object's contour and generating a signature vector for each salient point (Nomir & Abdel-Mottaleb, 2005) and (Abdel-Mottaleb, et al., 2003). The signature vectors capture the curvature information for each salient point (Yamany & Farag, 2003). Each element in the vector is the distance between the salient point and a point on the contour. Teeth matching is then performed by minimizing the Euclidean distance between the signature vectors of the PM and the AM teeth. Salient points are identified as the points of high curvature on the contour.

Figure 9. Teeth segmentation and separation results (a) The original images; (b) The images after applying adaptive thresholding; (c) The detected separating lines overlaid over the original image

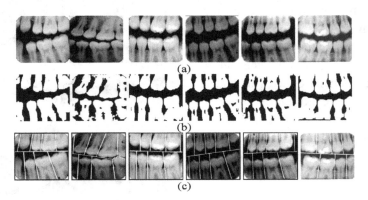

Contour Extraction and Teeth Numbering

To extract the contour points from the binary image that results from the segmentation a connected component analysis using 8-connectivity (Gonzalez & Wood, 2003) is applied.

For all the teeth in the database as well as for the PM query teeth, each tooth contour is represented by equal number of points by applying equal points sampling technique on the extracted tooth contour pixels. To increase the accuracy of our matching and reduce the search space when matching, we only consider corresponding teeth (i.e., teeth that have the same number). Each tooth is numbered according to the universal teeth numbering system (Figure 10) using our algorithm described in (Mahoor & Abdel-Mottaleb, 2005).

Figure 10. Upper and lower jaws with teeth numbered according to the universal system

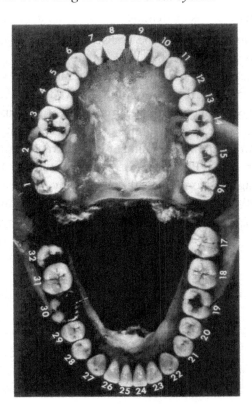

Generating the Signature Vectors and Matching

We developed a method for shape description and matching. The method relies on selecting a set of salient points from the object's contour and generating a signature vector for each salient point (Yamany & Farag, 2003). The algorithm calculates the curvature for every point on the contour. Then, selects the N points with the highest curvature as the salient points. A test is performed to eliminate spike points that have considerable higher curvature than their neighbors.

These points are considered as noise. Figure 11 shows an example, where the contour of the tooth is marked with black. For each salient point, p, defined by its *2D* coordinates, each point p_i on the contour can be related to p by the distance

$$d_i = \left\| p - p_i \right\| \tag{9}$$

and the signature vector V_p of the point p is defined as

$$V_p = [d_1, d_2, \ldots, d_M] \tag{10}$$

where M is the number of points on the tooth contour. This is done for all the N salient points, in the experiments we chose $N = 20$.

Figure 11. Generating the signature vector Vp for point p

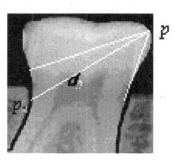

Before matching, the contour of each tooth in a PM image has to be aligned with the contour of a corresponding tooth (i.e. have the same universal tooth number) in an AM image. There may be variations between the AM and PM teeth, regarding scale, rotation, and translation. To solve this problem, we apply a transformation T for aligning both teeth, which results in the minimum matching distance between both teeth. The alignment step assumes that the image of the PM tooth, P, is transformed with respect to the image of the AM tooth, P', by an affine transformation as follows

$$T(p) = A \ X \ P + \tau \qquad (11)$$

where $P = (x, y)^T$ represents a point in the query contour, $T(P)$ is the result of applying the affine transformation to the query tooth P. A is a transformation matrix that includes both rotation and scaling, and τ is a translation vector. The parameters A and τ can be represented as

$$A = \begin{bmatrix} \cos\theta & \sin\theta \\ -\sin\theta & \cos\theta \end{bmatrix} X \begin{bmatrix} S_x & 0 \\ 0 & S_y \end{bmatrix} \qquad (12)$$

$$\tau = \begin{bmatrix} \tau_x \\ \tau_y \end{bmatrix} \qquad (13)$$

where θ is the rotation angle, S_x and S_y are vertical and horizontal scale factors, and τ_x and τ_y are vertical and horizontal translations. The five parameters, (i.e., $\theta, S_x, S_y, \tau_x, \tau_y$), are optimized to obtain the minimum matching distance between the transformed contour of the query AM tooth and the contour of the AM database tooth. Suppose we have a query tooth contour, q, and a database tooth contour, k, their signature vectors Q_i and K_i are defined as follows:

$$Q_{i,j} = \left\| qc_i - q_j \right\|, i = 1...N, j = 1....M \qquad (14)$$

where qc_i is a high curvature point, q_j is a point on the contour, N is the number of high curvature points, and M is the number of points on the contour,

$$K_{i,j} = \left\| kc_i - k_j \right\|, i = 1...N, j = 1....M \qquad (15)$$

where kc_i is a high curvature point, and k_j is a point on the contour of the AM database tooth. After aligning the contour of a PM tooth with the contour of a corresponding tooth in an AM image, the matching distance is calculated by

$$D(T(q), K) = \sqrt{\sum_{i=1}^{N} \frac{1}{k_i'} \sum_{j=1}^{M} (Q_{i,j}' - K_{i,j})^2} \qquad (16)$$

where $Q_{i,j}'$ is the feature j in the signature vector Q_i after applying the transformation T to the query PM tooth q. By ranking the values of D in an ascending order, the best matching AM tooth corresponds to the minimum D. In order to obtain the best matching image, majority voting is used so that the best matching AM image is the image with the maximum number of teeth ranked first. For a given PM image, we order the matched AM images according to the maximum number of teeth that ranked first, then to the maximum number of teeth that ranked second and so on. The best AM match is the first image in the list. If there is a tie, the one that has the minimum average matching distance for the whole AM image is chosen.

Experiments and Results

The AM database contains 187 AM images. Figure 12 shows a sample of the X-ray images in the AM database. The matching method was evaluated using 50 PM query images, which contain 217 teeth. Among the 217 queries, 172 correct matches were ranked first. Based on the majority voting, the correct matches were always retrieved for the 50 PM query images, 40 were ranked first, three were ranked second, two were ranked third, four were ranked fifth, and one was ranked seventh. The matching performance curve is shown in Figure 13. Figure 14 shows the retrieval results for one of the query PM images, the left column shows the PM query tooth, the middle column shows the retrieved AM tooth without applying the numbering technique and the right column shows the retrieved AM tooth when applying the numbering technique before matching. The

matching distance D is listed under each retrieved tooth. The PM image in Figure 14(a) contains six teeth, Figure 14(b) shows four out of the six teeth are correctly matched to an AM image of the same person. Figure 14(c) shows five out of the six teeth are correctly matched to the same person.

By studying the misclassified teeth, we found that there are different reasons for misclassification. In some cases the contour of the tooth is not correctly extracted during the segmentation step because of the poor quality of the image. In other cases, the teeth at the corners of the image have poor quality and sometimes parts of the teeth do not appear in the image. Because the X-ray image is a *2D* projection of a *3D* object, and it is not a unique representation. In some cases, the

Figure 12. Sample of X-ray AM images from the database

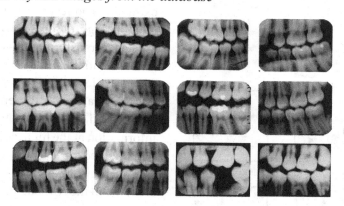

Figure 13. Performance curve of the signature vectors matching technique when using the Euclidean distance

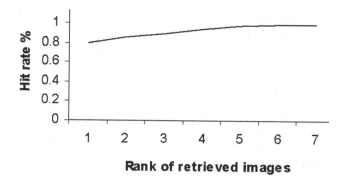

Figure 14. Example of the retrieval results using the signature vectors matching (a) Query tooth marked with black; (b) Best matched tooth in the database (1, 2, 5, and 6 are correct matches); (c) Best matched tooth in the database when using numbering technique (1, 2, 4, 5, and 6 are correct matches)

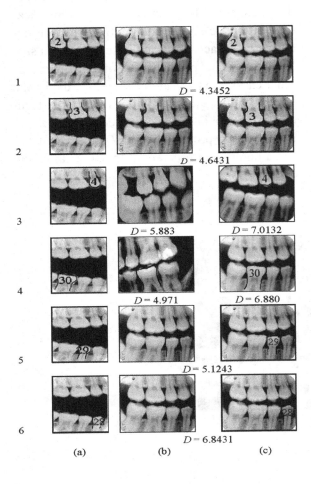

(a)   (b)   (c)

results by about 10%, but also eliminates the possibility of matching teeth that have different numbers as we may notice from the third row of Figure 14.

Hierarchal Contour Matching of Dental X-Ray Radiographs

In this section we introduce the second technique for dental X-ray matching (Nomir & Abdel-Mottaleb, 2006, 2008a). This technique is based upon edge matching using the Hierarchical Chamfer Matching algorithm (Borgefors, 1998). The algorithm finds the best match for a given image by minimizing a predefined matching criterion in terms of the distance between the contour points of the two images. The matching is performed in a hierarchical fashion using multi-resolution levels. The algorithm has two main stages: feature extraction and teeth matching. At the feature extraction stage, the contour pixels are extracted and a distance transformation (DT) image (Borgefors, 1998) is built for all the AM teeth in the database. Then, a hierarchical structure, which contains the DT images at different resolution levels, is constructed for each tooth from the AM tooth information at the higher resolution level, as will be explained in the feature extraction section. The DTs at all resolution levels for each AM tooth are archived in the AM database. At the teeth matching stage, given a PM query image, the teeth are first segmented, and numbered.

At any resolution level, the matching scores are generated based on the distance between the contours of the PM tooth and each AM tooth that have the same tooth number. This is achieved by superimposing the contour pixels of the PM tooth on the DT of each AM tooth, and then, calculating the distance between the PM and the AM contours. The contour of the PM tooth at any resolution level is constructed from the contour of the PM tooth at the higher resolution level, as will be explained in the feature extraction section.

2D shapes of the contours were similar, which leads to wrong matches. It is also important to note that, if the PM images are captured long after the AM images were captured, the shapes of the teeth can change because of artificial prosthesis, teeth growth, and teeth extraction.

We also noticed that, applying the teeth numbering step before the matching step, not only decreases the search space and enhances the final

The AM teeth are ranked according to the matching distance in an ascending order, i.e., the first ranked AM tooth is the one with the minimum matching distance and so on. Then, majority voting is used, as explained in the previous Subsection, dental X-ray teeth matching using signature vectors.

The distance transformation can be computed by two methods as it will be detailed later. Our goal is to reduce the retrieval time of the identification procedure.

Using the multi-resolution hierarchy; the search space is significantly reduced and consequently the computational load. Accordingly, the retrieval time is improved. The details of the feature extraction step are presented in the first next Subsection, and the details of the matching step are presented in the second next Subsection. Also the experimental results are presented in the third next Subsection.

Feature Extraction

The technique starts by extracting the contour pixels for all the AM teeth in the database. A DT (Barrow, Tenenbuam, Bolles, & Wolf, 1977). is created and archived for each AM tooth. For each AM tooth contour, the DT is computed iteratively by setting each contour point to zero and non-contour points to infinity, each pixel obtains a new value $v_{i,j}^k$ equal to

$$v_{i,j}^k = \min \begin{cases} v_{i,j}^{k-1} \\ v_{i,p}^{k-1} + 3 & p = j-1, j+1 \\ v_{m,j}^{k-1} + 3 & m = i-1, i+1 \\ v_{m,p}^{k-1} + 4 & m = i-1, i+1; p = j-1, j+1 \end{cases} \tag{17}$$

where $v_{i,j}^k$ is the value of the pixel at position i,j at iteration k. This iterative procedure continues till no changes occur in the values. We can notice that the global distances in the DT image are approximated by propagating local distances, i.e., distances between neighboring pixels over the image, which is the main idea of building the DT. This computation is only applied for an area around the contour points rather than the whole image, which further reduces the number of computations. From our experimental results, 10 to 15 iterations were sufficient for convergence. Figure 15 shows an example of a DT.

The distance transformation can be computed by two methods. In the first method, given the contour of the AM tooth, at a certain resolution level, the contour of the AM tooth is constructed from its contour information at the higher resolution level. Then, the DT (Barrow et al., 1977) is computed from the AM tooth contour information at that resolution level (Nomir & Abdel-Mottaleb, 2006). In the second method, given the contour of the AM tooth, the DT, is computed first for the highest resolution level (Nomir & Abdel-Mottaleb, 2008a). For the following, lower resolution,

Figure 15. Example of the distance transformation: the zero entries represent the pixels' positions of an AM tooth contour. The dark-edge entries represent the pixels' positions of a given PM tooth contour

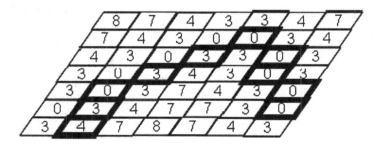

levels the DT, is computed using the DT information from the higher resolution level without creating the pyramid of the AM contours. This method requires less computation than the first method.

Using the first method, the tooth contour image at a given resolution level in the hierarchical pyramid is constructed from the contour image at the higher resolution level by replacing each block of four pixels by one pixel. This new pixel is the result of the "OR" of the four parent pixels. In (Borgefors, 1998), this process is repeated till only one pixel is left, but from our experimental results, we found that it is sufficient to use six levels. This is due to the fact that there is no much details in the lower resolution levels. This previous procedure is applied to the contour of all the AM teeth in the database. Using the second method, the DT at a given resolution level in the hierarchical pyramid is constructed from the DT at the higher resolution level by replacing each block of four pixel values by one pixel. This new pixel value is the result of averaging the four parent pixel values.

For the PM tooth, we need to construct the contour images at the different resolutions to perform matching. The contour image at a given resolution level in the hierarchical pyramid is constructed from the contour image at the higher resolution level by replacing each block of four pixels by one pixel. This new pixel is the result of the "OR" of the four parent pixels.

For a given resolution level, l, if the coordinates of a point at the original image are x and y, then the corresponding pixel coordinates at resolution level l will be

$$x_l = 2^{-l}(x + 2^l - 1) \qquad (18)$$

$$y_l = 2^{-l}(y + 2^l - 1) \qquad (19)$$

Teeth Matching

The idea of our matching technique is to perform matching using different resolution levels. Starting at a low resolution level, the search space is large, i.e. contains all the images, while the matching between two teeth is fast. At each resolution level, the distance between the AM and the PM teeth contours is calculated. Then, the AM teeth are arranged in an ascending order based upon the calculated distance. Half of the AM teeth with the largest distances are removed from the search space and the remaining AM teeth are marked as the possible candidates for further match. As a result, the search space is decreased while moving to higher resolution levels. Before calculating the matching distance between a PM image and an AM image, the contour of each tooth in the PM image has to be aligned with the contour of the corresponding tooth (i.e., tooth that has the same number) in the AM image using the same transformation previously mentioned in previous Subsection, dental X-ray teeth matching using signature vectors. The matching distance is

$$D(T(q), k) = \sqrt{\frac{1}{M} \sum_{i=1}^{M} v_i^2} \qquad (20)$$

where q in the query tooth, $T(q)$ is the query tooth after applying the transformation T, k is the AM database tooth, v_i is the value of the DT at position i after superimposing the transformed contour of the PM tooth, where position i lies on the transformed contour of the PM tooth, and M is the number of contour points. D will be zero if we have a perfect match between the contours of the AM and the PM teeth.

Our goal is to search for the best match between a given PM and the AM teeth in the database. This is one of the important advantages of using hierarchal algorithm, i.e., to speed up the search. In order to obtain the best matched image, majority voting is used, as explained in the previous

Subsection, dental X-ray teeth matching using signature vectors, so that the best matched AM image is the image with the maximum number of teeth ranked first.

Experiments and Results

We tested the Hierarchical teeth matching algorithm using the same set of bitewing dental images that was used in the previous matching technique.

The matching technique was evaluated using 50 PM query images, the correct matches were always retrieved for the 50 PM query images, 42 were ranked first, three were ranked second, two were ranked fourth, and three were ranked fifth. The matching performance curve is shown in Figure 16.

Figure 17 shows the retrieval results for one query PM image. Each row contains the query PM tooth and the best matched AM tooth from the database, in columns *a,* and *b,* respectively. Column *c* shows the corresponding AM tooth for the same person when it is not ranked first. The matching distance *D* is shown under each retrieved tooth. The PM image in Figure 17 contains six teeth; four out of the six teeth were correctly matched to an AM image of the same person, while for the other two incorrectly matched teeth, their correct matches were ranked fourth and third.

By studying the misclassified teeth, we found that the reasons for misclassification are the same as mentioned in the previous Subsection, dental X-ray teeth matching using signature vectors. We also applied the same matching technique to our testing set using only the original images without applying the hierarchical technique. Comparing the retrieval time of both methods, the hierarchical method reduces the retrieval time by 31%, on average.

Matching X-Ray Dental Radiographs Using Teeth Shapes and Appearances

The contour is one of the important features that can discriminate between teeth. However, because of the poor quality of some images, the resulting contours can have poor quality and this strongly affects the final matching results (Nomir & Abdel-Mottaleb, 2005, 2006, 2008a) and (Abdel-Mottaleb et al., 2003). In this Section, we introduce a teeth matching technique which uses two sets of features (Nomir & Abdel-Mottaleb, 2007a), which overcomes the drawback of using only the contour of the tooth in matching. It uses features that represent the contour as well as features which describe the appearance of the tooth.

The contour is represented using Fourier descriptors, and the appearance is described using force field energy function. Fourier descriptors are calculated for the contour of the tooth, hence they represent the shape of the contour. On the

Figure 16. Performance curve of the hierarchical matching technique

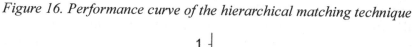

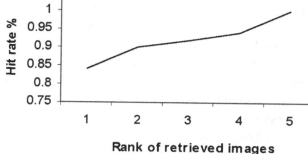

Figure 17. Retrieval results using the Hierarchical Matching algorithm (a) Query PM tooth marked with black; (b) the AM tooth for the correct person marked with black; (c) The ranked 1st tooth, when matched with a wrong person, marked with black (rows 3, and 6)

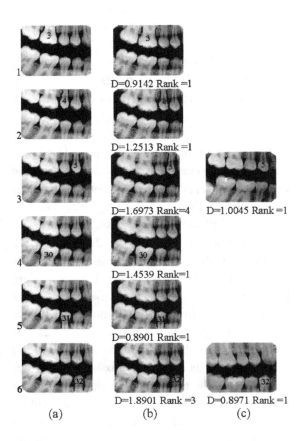

The details of the feature extraction step are presented in the first Subsection, and the details of the matching step are presented in the second Subsection. Also the experimental results are presented in the third Subsection.

Feature Extraction

Feature Extraction using Fourier Descriptors Considering the *2D N* points of the tooth's contour as a discrete function $u(n) = (x(n), y(n))$ (Arbter, Snyder, Burhardt, & Hirzinge, 2002), we can define a discrete complex function, *f(n)*, to represent the contour of the tooth as

$$f(n) = x(n) + jy(n) \tag{21}$$

By assuming that *f(n)* is a periodic signal with period *N* (Arbter et al., 2002), and applying Discrete Fourier transformation (DFT) to the complex function, we obtain

$$F(s) = \frac{1}{N} \sum_{i=0}^{N-1} f(i)e^{\frac{-2\pi si}{N}}, \; s = 0,1,\ldots N-1 \tag{22}$$

The coefficients $F(s)$ are called Fourier descriptors. By setting the first Fourier descriptor $F(0)$ to zero, which moves the centroid of the contour to 0, dividing the remaining coefficients by $F(1)$, and taking only the absolute values of the *F's* we can achieve translation invariance, scale invariance, and rotation invariance, respectively (Costa, & Cesar, 2000). We use the feature vector that corresponds to the low frequency components as follows:

$$V = \left[\frac{|F(2)|}{|F(1)|}, \frac{|F(3)|}{|F(1)|}, \ldots\ldots, \frac{|F(21)|}{|F(1)|} \right] \tag{23}$$

other hand, the calculation of the force field function uses the pixels within the tooth area, hence it emphasizes the texture. The overall feature vector is the concatenation of the features extracted by the two methods.

The extracted features for the AM images are archived in a database. During searching, matching scores are generated based on the Euclidean distance between the features extracted from the AM and the PM teeth. The result of this search will be a set of AM candidates that best match the PM query image.

Using a set of training images, we found that the first 20 Fourier descriptors were sufficient to characterize each individual tooth.

Teeth Analysis and Feature Extraction Using Force Field Transformation

A set of features are extracted to represent each individual tooth. First, the tooth is preprocessed by applying an energy transformation method called force field transformation. This transformation was used in (Hurley, Nixon, & Carter, 2000, 2002) for ear recognition, it smoothes the original grayscale image while preserving the important features. In this approach, the *2D* intensity image *f(x, y)* is treated as a surface. The surface is defined as *w = f(x, y)*, where *w* is the image intensity at pixel *(x, y)*. Under this representation, the most distinctive features are surface feature points. The algorithm starts by converting a tooth image into a force field by pretending that each pixel exerts an isotropic force on all the other pixels. Following the gradient direction of the potential energy associated with that force field forms energy channels along the way. Eventually, these channels become trapped in a small number of energy wells. These wells are the peaks of the potential energy surface and they are used to describe the appearance of each individual tooth. Assume that each tooth image has *N* pixels. A pixel at position r_i with intensity $p(r_i)$ is considered to exert a spherically symmetric force field $F_i(r_j)$ on a pixel of unit intensity at the pixel location r_i defined as follows:

$$F_i(r_j) = p(r_i) * d_{ji} \tag{24}$$

$$d_{ji} = \frac{(r_i - r_j)}{|r_i - r_j|^3} = \frac{1}{((x_i - x_j)^2 + (y_i - y_j)^2)} \angle\theta \tag{25}$$

where $r_i = [x_i, y_i]$, and $r_j = [x_j, y_j]$, d_{ji} is represented by an absolute, and an angle values, $\theta = \tan^{-1}\dfrac{(y_i - y_j)}{(x_i - x_j)}$ the angle gives the direction of the force field.

This force field is associated with potential energy field $E_i(r_j)$ which is given by

$$E_i(r_j) = \frac{p(r_i)}{|r_i - r_j|} \tag{26}$$

To calculate the total potential energy at a given pixel *j*, the sum of the potential energy functions from all the pixels within the region is taken into account and is given by

$$E(r_j) = \sum_{i=0, i \neq j}^{N-1} E_i(r_j) \tag{27}$$

Figure 18(b) is the energy potential surface for the tooth image in Figure 18(a).

To extract the potential wells, an initialization procedure takes place. The initialization procedure starts by arranging a set of 100 test pixels (see Figure 19(a)) in an ellipse around each tooth and is allowed to iteratively follow the gradient of the potential energy, which captures the general flow of the force field.

Figure 18. The potential energy surface (a) The original tooth; (b) The potential energy surface for the tooth in (a)

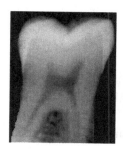 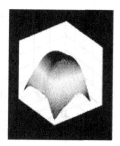

Figure 19. Extraction of potential wells and channels (a) 100 pixels for initialization; (b) field lines are terminating into five wells; (c) wells positions

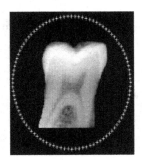 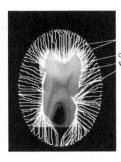 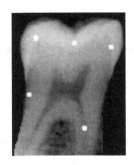

By following the field lines, each field line will continue moving until it reaches a maximum in the potential energy surface. The field lines flow into a small number of channels. The channel is modulating the natural flow of the field lines towards a single well at the center of the field. The field lines flow eventually terminate in wells, the maximum in the potential energy surface where no force is exerted and no further movement is possible, joining up with other channels on the way. These locations for the image in Figure 19(a) are shown on Figure 19(c). Using a set of training data, we found that initializing the procedure with 100 pixels is enough for extracting all the wells. We apply this procedure to all the images of the AM teeth in the database. Also, the same procedure is applied for the teeth of a given PM image, to obtain the corresponding feature vector. Suppose that a tooth has W wells, we define the feature vector as,

$$V^t = [d_{1,2}, d_{1,3}, \ldots\ldots, d_{w-1,w}], \qquad (28)$$

$$d_{j,k} = \frac{1}{d'} \left\| w_j - w_k \right\| \qquad (29)$$

where $d_{j,k}$ is the normalized distance between well j, w_j and well k, w_k; W is the total number of wells; $j = 1,\ldots, W-1$; $k = j+1,\ldots, W$; $j \neq k$, and d' is the mean value of the components of the tooth's

feature vector V. d' is used to normalize the distance between each pair of wells, e.g., j and k, to be independent of the scale.

We found from the experimental results, using a set of training images, that each tooth has around four to seven wells on average. We store the positions of all the extracted wells for each tooth in our database. During matching, when we match two teeth with different number of wells, the matching is based on the smallest number of wells as will be explained later in the next matching Subsection.

The computational cost for extracting the wells is high since the force field calculation uses all the pixels within the tooth area. Converting the tooth image into force field requires that each pixel exerts an isotropic force on all other pixels, which is time consuming.

In order to reduce the computations, we examined the locations of the extracted wells for a set of training images, we found that the wells are usually located in an area around the contour of the tooth. Based on this observation, we only apply the force field energy function for a subset of pixels around the tooth's contour, which tremendously reduces the number of computations compared with the number of computations when we use all the pixels. After locating the wells positions, the feature vector is calculated by computing the normalized distances between all extracted wells.

Teeth Matching

Matching is performed by minimizing the matching distance between the feature vector of the PM tooth and the feature vector of an AM tooth. There may be variations in scale, rotation, and translation between the AM and the PM teeth. During matching, the image of a PM tooth is aligned with that of a corresponding AM tooth (they should also have the same universal tooth number). We use the same transformation mentioned in the matching technique introduced in the previous Subsection, dental X-ray teeth matching using signature vectors. Suppose we have a query tooth with feature vector Q, and a database tooth with feature vector K, which are defined as,

$$Q = [q_i], i = 1, \ldots, ((W-1) * W / 2) + 20 \tag{30}$$

$$K = [k_j], j = 1, \ldots, ((W-1) * W / 2) + 20 \tag{31}$$

where q_i is the ith feature in the Q vector, k_j is the jth feature in the K vector, W is the number of wells, and $(W-1) * W/2$ is the number of features corresponding to the well positions and the remaining 20 features are the Fourier descriptors.

As the number of extracted wells in both the query and the database teeth may be different, so if the number of wells in the query and the database teeth are W_i and W_j respectively, we only need to compare the corresponding W wells in the AM and the PM teeth, where,

$$W = min(W_i, W_j) \tag{32}$$

This is achieved by choosing the W wells from the AM and the PM teeth, which result in the minimum distance between AM and PM teeth. This technique has the advantage of representing each tooth by a small set of features that represent both shape and appearance, in order

to avoid the drawbacks of using only incorrect contours obtained in case of poor quality images. The best matches are obtained by minimizing the distance, $D_{q,k}$, between the PM query tooth, q, and the AM tooth, k, considering the transformation T as follows

$$D_{T(q),k} = \sqrt{\sum_{i=1}^{((W-1)*W/w)+20} (q_i' - k_i)^2} \tag{33}$$

where $T(q)$ is the transformed query tooth, and q_i' is the ith feature of the query tooth after applying the transformation T. The best matched AM tooth, with distance D, corresponds to the minimum $D_{T(q),k}$,

$$D = \arg \min_k D_{T(q),k} \tag{34}$$

In order to obtain the best matched image, majority voting is used as explained in the previous Subsection, dental X-ray teeth matching using signature vectors, so that the best matching AM image is the image with the maximum number of teeth ranked first.

Experiments and Results

We tested the algorithm using the same set of bitewing dental images that was used in the previous matching techniques. The matching method was evaluated using 50 PM query images. For the 50 PM query images, the correct matches were always retrieved for the 50 PM query images, 43 were ranked first, four were ranked second, two were ranked third, and one was ranked fifth.

We applied the same matching technique to our testing set, but using only the force field features. The correct matches were also retrieved for the 50 PM query images, 37 were ranked first, four were ranked second, one was ranked third, three were ranked fourth, four were ranked sixth, and one was ranked seventh. We also applied the same

Figure 20. Matching using force field and Fourier descriptors: the matching performance curves for the three cases

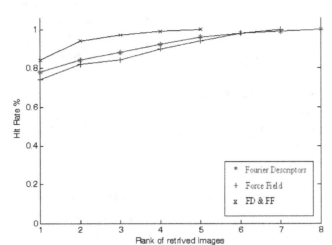

matching technique to our test set, but using only the Fourier descriptors as features. The correct matches were also retrieved for the 50 PM query images, 39 were ranked first, three were ranked second, two were ranked third, two were ranked fourth, two were ranked fifth, two were ranked sixth, and one was ranked eighth. We notice that using the two sets of features results in better performance. The matching performance curves for the three cases are shown in Figure 20. Table 2 shows the summary of the results.

Figure 21, shows the retrieval results for one of the query PM images. The left column shows the well positions superimposed on each PM query tooth. The second column shows the corresponding AM teeth for the same subject with the well positions marked. The third and fourth columns show the AM teeth that best match the query teeth along with the complete AM image if the correct AM tooth was not ranked first. The matching distance D is listed under each retrieved tooth. The PM image in Figure 21 contains seven teeth, where five out of the seven teeth were correctly matched to an AM image of the same person while the correct match for the two mismatched teeth were ranked second. Majority voting is then used to find the best matched AM image. In our example, since five out of seven teeth were ranked first and retrieved from the same person, it is considered the best match.

By studying the misclassified teeth, we found that the reasons for misclassification are the same as mentioned in the previous Subsection, dental X-ray teeth matching using signature vectors.

Table 2. Matching using force field and Fourier descriptors: the experimental results for the three cases

Method	The number of retrieved images							
	Rank1	Rank2	Rank3	Rank4	Rank5	Rank6	Rank7	Rank8
FF	37	4	1	3		4	1	
FD	39	3	2	2	1	2		1
FF & FD	43	4	2		1			

Figure 21. Retrieval results (a) The wells positions in a query PM tooth; (b) The wells positions in the matching tooth in the corresponding AM image and its rank; (c) The ranked first AM tooth if the correct AM tooth was not ranked first; (d) The complete AM image for the tooth in (c), marked with black if the correct AM tooth was not ranked first

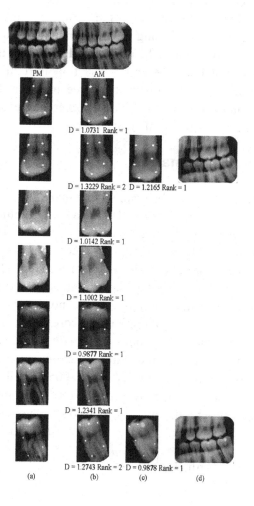

Comparison between the Introduced Matching Techniques

In this Chapter, we introduced three techniques for teeth matching. Table 3 shows the summary of the experimental results using the three matching techniques. To compare between the performance of the three matching techniques, we use the ML-One-Err and the ML-coverage measures, which are commonly used in multi-label environments (Provost, & Fawcett, 2001) to compare between the performance of more than one classifier. These two measures are defined as follows,

$$ML - One - Err = \frac{\bigcup \{x \varepsilon X : r_x \neq 1\}}{|X|} \quad (35)$$

where x is a query image, X is the set of all query images, r_x is the rank of image x, U is the number of images with $r_x \neq 1$, and |X| is the total number of query images.

$$LM - \text{cov} erage = \frac{\sum_{x \varepsilon X} (r_x - 1)}{|X|} \quad (36)$$

where x is a query image, X is the set of all query images, r_x is the rank of image x, and |X| is the total number of query images. Small values of these measures indicate better performance. The range for the ML-One-Err is from zero to one, while for the ML-Coverage measure it is zero

Table 3. Summary of the experimental results of the three matching methods

Method	The number of retrieved images						
	Rank 1	Rank 2	Rank 3	Rank 4	Rank 5	Rank 6	Rank 7
Signature vectors	40	3	2		4		1
Hierarchical	42	3		2	3		
FF & FD	43	4	2		1		

for perfect performance and increases with lower performance.

Table 4 shows the results when using the Euclidean and the Huasdorff distances for matching. We can notice that Hierarchical matching outperforms the matching using signature vectors. Matching using force field and Fourier descriptors outperforms the matching using signature vectors and the Hierarchical matching.

FUSION OF MATCHING TECHNIQUES

In this Section, we fuse the matching techniques introduced in the second Section using three approaches, fusion at the matching level, which is detailed in the first Subsection, and fusion at the decision level, which is detailed in the second Subsection. Also, we use another approach to fuse the three matchers using a Bayesian framework based on given constraints (error costs), the third Subsection. The goal is to improve the performance of the fused matchers i.e., the three matchers that were introduced in the third Section (Nomir & Abdel-Mottaleb, 2007b, 2007c, 2008b).

Fusion at the Matching Level

In this approach, the scores or decisions of an individual matcher are available for fusion while the features used by one matcher are not accessible to the others. As mentioned in the second Section, our final result from the matching step is an ordered list. This representation may not be ap-

propriate for fusion at the matching level, because fusion at the matching level requires fusing the scores of these matchers. Therefore, for a given PM image we have to assign a score to each AM image proportional to the distance between the given PM image and that AM image.

In the following two Subsections, we discuss some scenarios for fusing the three matchers at the matching level. The first Subsection introduces the scenario for fusing the three matchers using the average sum of the normalized scores for the three matchers. Second Subsection introduces the scenarios for fusing the three matchers by estimating a weight for each matcher that results in the minimum total error.

Score Summation

The easiest way for fusion at the matching level is by score summation. The idea is to calculate the average of the matching scores, produced by the three different matchers. According to the average scores, a decision of reject or accept takes place. Before applying this method, the generated scores are first normalized. The normalization typically involves mapping the scores from multiple domains into a common domain. We use the Tanh to normalize the matching scores (Snelick, Uludag, Mink, Indovina, & Jain, 2005). The Tanh technique maps the raw scores to the (0, 1) range, and computes the new normalized score value as,

$$S = \frac{1}{2}\left[\tanh(0.01\frac{(S_b - mean_{S_b})}{std_{S_b}} + 1\right] \qquad (37)$$

where S_b, and S are the score values before and after the normalization, while $mean_{Sb}$ and std_{Sb} represent the mean and standard deviation of all possible values of S_b that will be observed, respectively.

Table 4. Performance evaluation for the three methods

Method	ML-One-Err	ML-Coverage
Signature vectors	0.20	0.58
Hierarchical	0.16	0.42
FF & FD	0.14	0.24

Weight Estimation

Weights are used to indicate the importance of each individual matcher for the fusion. In this section, we introduce three scenarios to estimate a weight for each individual matcher. These calculated weights are used to fuse the three matchers together. The fusion of the three matchers' scores will be the weighted sum of the individual matchers' normalized scores. The first scenario uses exhaustive search to estimate the weights, which result in the minimum total error using a set of training data (Jain, & Ross, 2002). The second scenario uses a defined function of the normalized scores, of each individual matcher, for a set of training data to estimate the weight for that matcher (Cheung, Mak, & Kung, 2005). The third scenario uses each matchers' performance on a set of training data to obtain the weights.

- Calculating weights using exhaustive search

A different weight is initially assigned for each individual matcher. The method exhaustively searches the space of weights (w_1, w_2, *and* w_3) for the three matchers, such that the total error rate for a training set is minimized. The weights are considered to be multiples of 0.01 over the range [0, 1]. The fused score is computed under the constraints

$$w_1 + w_2 + w_3 = 1,$$ (38)

$$w_i \geq 0, i = 1, 2, 3$$ (39)

and, it is equal to

$$S_j = \sum_{i=1}^{3} w_i S_{i,j}$$ (40)

where $S_{i,j}$ is the normalized score of matcher i for subject j, and S_j is the fused score for subject j.

The search for the optimum weights is achieved by iteratively changing the value of each weight by 0.01 while applying the constraints in Equations 38, and 39, then calculating the total error each iteration. Applying all possible weight combinations, then choosing the set of weights that minimizes the total error, which is in the form of costs associated with the two types of errors, over the training data set

$$E = C_{FA} F_{AR} + C_{FR} F_{RR}$$ (41)

where C_{FA} is the cost of accepting a false match, F_{AR} is the false acceptance rate, C_{FR} is the cost of falsely rejecting a true match, and F_{RR} is the false rejection rate. For simplicity, we assign equal costs ($C_{FA} = C_{FR} = 1$), i.e., the risk is equivalent to the total error.

This scenario needs many iterations to choose the final weights, since all possible combinations of the weight values need to be considered.

- Deriving the Weights from the Scores

Each matcher is assigned a weight, which is a function of the matcher's normalized scores derived using a set of training data. In this case each matcher weight is inversely proportional to the error rate, and it is in the form

$$w_{i,j} = \frac{\exp((s_{i,j} - \mu_i / 2\sigma_i^2)}{\sum_{j=1}^{m} \exp((s_{i,j} - \mu_i)^2 / 2\sigma_i^2)}$$ (42)

where $w_{i,j}$ is the weight of matcher i for subject j, $s_{i,j}$ is the normalized score of matcher i for subject j, μ_i is the mean score for matcher i, σ_i is the standard deviation for matcher i's scores, and m is the number of the training subjects.

$$\mu_i = \frac{\sum_{j=1}^{m} s_{i,j}}{m} \quad (43)$$

$$\sigma_i^2 = \frac{1}{m} \sum_{j=1}^{m} (s_{i,j} - \mu_i)^2 \quad (44)$$

After calculating the weights for the three matchers, the weights are normalized so that $w_{1,j} + w_{2,j} + w_{3,j} = 1$. Then, the set of weights that results in the minimum total error is selected.

- Assigning weights based on the performance

Different weights may be assigned to each matcher based on their individual performance (Ross, Nandakumar, & Jain, 2006). In this scenario, we assign for each matcher a weight, which is a function of the matcher's performance derived using a set of training data. The weights are calculated as follows

$$w_i = \frac{1 - (F_{AR_i} + F_{RR_i})}{3 - \sum_{j=1}^{3} (F_{AR_j} + F_{RR_j})} \quad (45)$$

where w_i is the weight for matcher i, F_{ARi}, and F_{RRi} are the false acceptance rate and the false rejection rate for matcher i respectively, and $i = 1, 2, 3$.

The values for F_{ARi}, and F_{RRi} are threshold dependent, i.e., when the value of the operation point (F_{ARi}, and F_{RRi}) for each matcher is changed, the weights assigned to the individual matcher will be suitably modified.

Fusion at the Decision Level

In this approach, a separate decision is made for each matcher. These decisions are then combined into a final vote. This approach has become in-creasingly popular in multi-biometric systems. Many different strategies are available to combine the distinct decisions into a final decision. They range from majority votes to sophisticated statistical methods (Ross, & Jain, 2003). In practice, however, developers seem to prefer the easiest method: boolean conjunctions. In the following two Subsections, we discuss some scenarios for fusing our introduced matchers at the decision level, some are boolean while the others are statistical.

Boolean Scenarios

The most prevalent rules for fusing multiple matchers are the AND and the OR rules. Given the decisions from the three matching techniques, D_{M1}, D_{M2}, and D_{M3}, we fuse the three matchers using the boolean functions.

- **AND rule (D_{M1}.AND. D_{M2}.AND. D_{M3}):** this requires a positive decision from the three matchers, otherwise it fails to identify.

If F_{ARi} is the false acceptance rate, and F_{RRi} is the false rejection rate for matcher i, where $i = 1, 2, 3$. Using the AND rule, a false accept can only occur for the fused matchers, if the three matchers outcomes are falsely accepted.

A false reject occurs if at least one matcher outcome is falsely rejected.

- **OR rule (D_{M1}.OR. D_{M2}.OR. D_{M3}):** this scenario requires positive decision from at least one matcher in order to accept. For the OR rule, a false accept can occur if at least one matcher outcome is falsely accepted. On the other hand, a false reject can only occur if the three matchers, outcomes are falsely rejected.
- **AND-OR rule ((D_{M1}.AND. D_{M2}).OR. (D_{M1}.AND. D_{M3}).OR. (D_{M2}.AND. D_{M3})):** this scenario is more reliable than the AND

rule because it requires positive decision from only two matchers at a time.

Statistical Scenario

Let X_i, for $i = 1,...,N$ be a set of independent random variables that represent the decisions of N matchers. $p(X_i/w_j)$ is the conditional probability function for X_1, where $j = T/F$ (True/False), w_T represents a true match, and w_F represents a false match.

For a given matcher, the class-conditional probability density functions ($p(X_i/w_T)$, and $p(X_i/w_F)$) are usually unknown. A critical issue in this decision fusion scheme is to estimate the class conditional probability density functions from a set of training data. Assuming that X_i, $i = 1, 2, 3$ are independent decisions from the three matchers, and using a set of training data, the probability density functions for the three matchers are shown in Figure 22, and the joint probability density function has the following form

$$p(X_1,......X_N / w_j) = \prod_{i=1}^{3} p(X_i / w_j) \qquad (46)$$

A given observation $X^0 = (X_1^0, X_2^0, X_3^0)$ is classified as

$$(X_1^0, X_2^0, X_3^0)\varepsilon \begin{cases} w_T & if\ \dfrac{p(X_1^0, X_2^0, X_3^0 / w_T)}{p(X_1^0, X_2^0, X_3^0 / w_F)} > \lambda \\ w_F & otherwise \end{cases}$$

$$(47)$$

where λ depends on the performance requirements of the fusion result. It is usually specified in terms of C_{FA} (cost of accepting a false match), and C_{FR} (cost of rejecting a true match) for the result of fusion. By assigning a value for λ, the decision for any given observation can be obtained using Equation 47.

Figure 22. The probability density functions for the three matchers

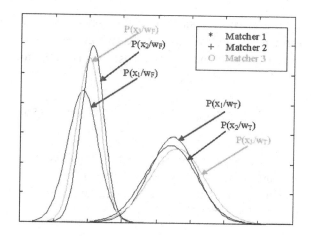

Bayesian Framework for Building the System

In biometrics systems, the performance requirement is usually specified in terms of F_{AR}, and F_{RR}, therefore, the fusion scheme should establish a decision boundary which satisfies the requirements on F_{AR} and F_{RR} (Jain, Bolle, & Pankanti, 1999). A Bayesian framework can be automatically adapted by selecting the C_{FA} and C_{FR} costs to reflect the security level and uniqueness of the biometrics, i.e., high C_{FA} is typically required for a high security system, and high C_{FR} is required for biometric systems. The idea is to minimize a weighted sum of the probabilities of the two types of error (Bayesian cost), where the weights are the costs associated with the two types of errors, which is in the form,

$$E = C_{FA}F_{AR} + C_{FR}F_{RR} \qquad (48)$$

where C_{FA} is the cost of accepting a false match, F_{AR} is the false acceptance rate, C_{FR} is the cost of falsely rejecting a true match, and F_{RR} is the false rejection rate. This error rate can be rewritten in terms of a single cost,

$$C_{FR} = 2 - C_{FA} \qquad (49)$$

Equation 49 results from the fact that global error is simply the sum of the two error rates if cost is ignored, thus the two costs are assumed to equal 1, accordingly,

$$E = C_{FA}F_{AR} + (2 - C_{FA})F_{RR} \qquad (50)$$

The optimum Bayesian fusion rule (Veeramachaneni, Osadciw, & Varshney, 2005), which minimizes the Bayesian cost in equation 50, for fusing N matchers is,

$$\sum_{i=1}^{N} \left\{ X_i \log(\frac{1 - F_{RR_i}}{F_{AR_i}}) + (1 - X_i) \right.$$
$$\left. \log(\frac{F_{RR_i}}{1 - F_{AR_i}}) \right\} \begin{array}{c} X_g = 1 > \\ X_g = 0 < \end{array} \log(\frac{C_{FA}}{C_{FR}}) \qquad (51)$$

where X_i is the individual matcher decision (1 for accept and 0 for reject), X_g is the decision resulting from the fusion, and N is the number of matchers, which is three in our case. This rule in Equation 51 assumes an equal a priori probabilities of a true match and a false match.

In this scenario, the False Acceptance Rate, F_{AR_i} (type II error), and False Rejection Rate, F_{RR_i} (type *I* error) are calculated separately for each matcher using a set of training data.

There are a total of 2^{2^N} (256, where $N = 3$) possible fusion rules considering all possible combinations of the matcher decisions, Table 5 shows the fusion rules for the three matchers. By selecting a set of C_{FA}, and C_{FR} error costs, we look for the fusion rule that achieves the best identification performance by minimizing the total cost. This is achieved by selecting the rule, out of the 256 rules, that combines the individual biometric decisions.

The matchers' decisions are assumed to be independent. Costs have been included in Equation 51 to allow relative changes in the cost weights for F_{AR}, and F_{RR} depending upon the application. Higher cost for false acceptance is typically required for a high security system. Higher cost for false rejection is, however, required for forensic applications in which the system might accept everyone who has even a slightest match. Varying these costs affects the fusion rule selection. To study the system performance, a set of error costs are selected under a chosen operating point (F_{RR}, and F_{AR} for each individual matcher). Based on these selections, the optimum fusion rule is obtained.

Experiments and Results

The matching techniques were fused using the scenarios previously introduced. The following three Subsections show the results of the fusion

Table 5. Fusion rules for the three matchers

X_1	X_2	X_3	f_1	f_2	f_3	....	f_{254}	f_{255}	f_{256}
0	0	0	0	0	0	....	1	1	1
0	0	1	0	0	0	....	1	1	1
0	1	0	0	0	0	....	1	1	1
0	1	1	0	0	0	....	1	1	1
1	0	0	0	0	0	....	1	1	1
1	0	1	0	0	0	....	1	1	1
1	1	0	0	0	1	....	0	1	1
1	1	1	0	1	0	....	1	0	1

of the three matchers at the matching level, at the decision level, and using the Bayesian framework.

Fusion at the Matching Level

Using the score summation scenario, Figure 23 shows the performance of the sum rule compared to the performance of the three individual matchers, where each matcher is assigned an equal weight (1/3). From the Receiver operating characteristic (ROC) curves, we can notice that the overall performance of the sum is better than the performance of each individual matcher.

Using the weight estimation scenario, based on the exhaustive search, we found that the weights for the matchers that results in the minimum error are $w_1 = 0.29$, $w_2 = 0.32$, and $w_3 = 0.39$, respectively. Figure 24 shows the performance of the exhaustive search scenario. Using the scenario for deriving the weights from the scores, we found

Figure 23. ROC curves showing an improvement in performance when scores are combined using the sum rule with equal weights

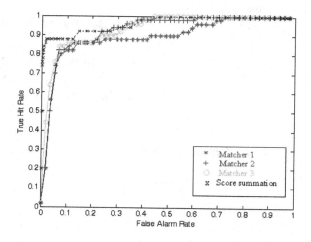

Figure 24. ROC curves showing the performance when matchers' weights are derived using exhaustive search

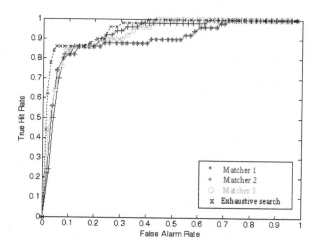

that the weights for the matchers that results in the minimum error are $W_1 = 0.22$, $W_2 = 0.27$, and $W_3 = 0.51$, respectively. Figure 25 shows the performance curve for this fusion scenario.

Using the scenario which assigns weights based on the performance, Table 6 shows the calculated weights corresponding to given operating points (F_{AR}, and F_{RR}) for each matcher, and Figure 26 shows the performance of this fusion scenario.

From the ROC curves, we can notice that the overall performance of the fused matchers, when calculating the weights based on the matcher's performance (using a certain operating point), is better than the overall performance of the fused matchers when calculating the weights using exhaustive search or deriving the weights from the normalized scores.

Fusion at the Decision Level

Figures 27, 28, and 29 show the performance of fusing the three matchers using the AND, OR, and AND − OR rules respectively.

Comparing the ROC curves of the three scenarios for fusing the matchers using boolean functions, we can notice that, when we use the AND rule, the F_{RR} (false rejection rate) for the fused matchers is higher than it is for any individual matcher. Also, we can notice that, when we use the OR rule, the F_{AR} (false acceptance rate) for the fused matchers is higher than the F_{AR} for any individual matcher.

The Bayesian Framework for Fusion

By selecting a set of error costs under a chosen operating point (F_{RR}, and F_{AR} for each individual matcher), the Bayesian framework obtains the

Figure 25. ROC curve showing the performance when matchers' weights are derived from the scores

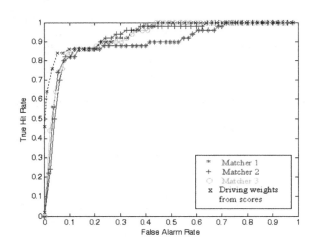

Table 6. The calculated weights based on the matchers performance

	F_{RR}	F_{AR}	Weight
Matcher 1	18%	6.5%	0.31
Matcher 2	15%	6.0%	0.34
Matcher 3	13%	4.5%	0.35

optimum fusion rule for building the system. Some experimental results are shown in Table 7. We analyzed the 256 fusion rules using two sets of operating points.

First set, uses the same operating points for the three matchers. If the F_{AR} is more costly (C_{FA} = 1.0000 to 1.9685), the AND rule, (f_2), is the optimal rule (Equation 51). If the F_{RR} is more costly (C_{FA} = 0.0035 to 1.0000), the OR rule, (f_{128}), becomes the optimal rule. There is a very small range of costs (C_{FA} = 0 to 0.0035) in which the

fused result is to accept regardless of the decisions from the three matchers, rule (f_{256}), i.e., whatever the decisions from the three matchers, the fused matcher decision is to accept, as shown in Table 5. Another small cost range (C_{FA} = 1.9685 to 2.0000) corresponds to reject regardless of the decisions from the three matchers, rule (f_1), as shown in Table 5.

In the second set, the third matcher has the smallest F_{AR}, but has the largest F_{RR}. On the other hand, the first matcher has the smallest F_{RR}, and

Figure 26. ROC curve showing the performance when weights are derived from the individual matcher performance

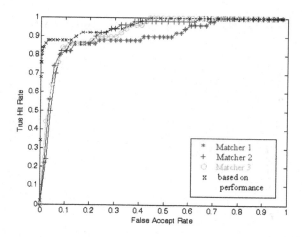

Figure 27. ROC curve showing the performance of the three matchers fused using AND rule

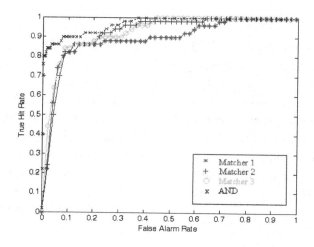

Figure 28. ROC curve showing the performance of fusing the three matchers using OR rule

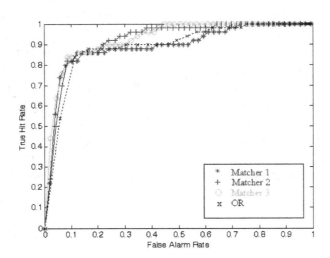

Figure 29. ROC curve showing the performance of fusing the matchers using AND-OR rule

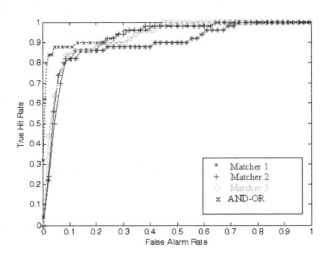

has the largest F_{AR} value. Table 7 shows that the AND rule, (f_2), remains optimal for C_{FA} ranges from 1.2064 to 1.9643. Conversely, the OR rule, (f_{128}), becomes optimal for C_{FA} ranges from 0.000861 to 0.6891. It is important to note that the optimal fusion rule for C_{FA} ranges from 0.6891 to 0.8745 relies only on the third matcher, (f_{85}). Also, the optimal fusion rule for C_{FA} ranges from 0.8745 to 1.2064 relies on the AND–OR, (f_{23}), rule of the three matchers.

CONCLUSION

With the advancements in information technology and the huge volume of cases that need to be investigated by forensic specialists, automation of forensic identification became inevitable. In this Chapter, we have introduced an automated dental identification system. The system archives AM dental images in a database, and searches the database for the best matches to a given PM image.

Table 7. Example of optimal fusion rules for the same and different operating points

Operating points	Optimal fusion rule	Range of C_{FA} cost
$F_{AR1} = 10\%$ $F_{RR1} = 10\%$ $F_{AR2} = 10\%$ $F_{RR2} = 10\%$ $F_{AR3} = 10\%$ $F_{RR3} = 10\%$	$f_{256}(11111111)$	
	$f_{128}(11111111)$	
	$f_2(00000001)$	
	$f_1(00000000)$	
$F_{AR1} = 8\%$ $F_{RR1} = 3\%$ $F_{AR2} = 5\%$ $F_{RR2} = 4\%$ $F_{AR3} = 1\%$ $F_{RR3} = 8\%$	$f_{256}(11111111)$	
	$f_{128}(11111111)$	
	$f_{85}(01010101)$	
	$f_{23}(00010111)$	
	$f_2(00000001)$	
	$f_1(00000000)$	

The system can be used by both law enforcement and security agencies in both forensic and biometric identification. The goal of our research is to automate the process of extracting a representation from the dental radiographs and to automate the process of matching PM and AM records. An automatic system can perform identification on a large scale database while a manual or semiautomatic system is useful for verification on a small data set. Also, automating this process will come up with an ordered list of closest matches that we may refer to in order to decide the best match. Accordingly, this will facilitate for forensic odontologists to only manually verify a short list instead of manually searching a large number of AM records.

We presented a new technique for dental X-ray image segmentation as well as three techniques for teeth matching. These techniques address the issues of representing each individual tooth by a set of features and calculating the similarity between teeth based on these features. Then, finding the best matching teeth from the AM database, and finding the best matched individuals using majority voting. To improve the overall system performance, we fuse the three matchers. We introduced some scenarios to fuse the matchers at the matching level as well as at the decision level. Also, using the Bayesian framework gives the flexibility to design a robust system with different operating points (F_{AR}, and F_{RR}) for the fused matchers under given error costs.

REFERENCES

Abdel-Mottaleb, M., Nomir, O., Nassar, D., Fahmy, G., & Ammar, H. (2003). Challenges of developing an automated dental identification system. *IEEE Mid-West Symposium for Circuits and Systems,* (pp. 411–414). Cairo, Egypt.

Arbter, K., Snyder, W. E., Burhardt, H., & Hirzinge, G. (2002). Content-based image retrieval using Fourier descriptors on a logo database. *Journal of Pattern Recognition, 3,* 521–524.

Barrow, H. G., Tenenbuam, J. M., Bolles, R. C., & Wolf, H. C. (1977). Parametric Correspondence and Chamfer matching: Two new techniques for image matching. In *Proceedings of the 5th International Joint Conference on Artificial Intelligence,* (pp. 659–663). Cambridge, MA, USA.

Borgefors, G. (1998). Hierarchical Chamfer matching: A parametric edge matching algorithm. *IEEE Transactions on Pattern Analysis and Machine Intelligence, 10*(6), 849–865. doi:10.1109/34.9107

Brogdon, B.G. (1998). *Forensic radiology.* Boca Raton, FL: CRC Press. doi:10.1201/9781420048339

Cheung, M., Mak, M., & Kung, S. (2005). A two-level fusion approach to multimodal biometric verification. *International Conference on Acoustics, Speech, and Signal Processing, 5,* 485–488. Philadelphia, PA, USA.

Costa, L. F., & Cesar, R. M. (2000). *Shape analysis and classification: Theory and practice.* Boca Raton, FL: CRC Press.

Fahmy, G., Nassar, D., Said, E., Chen, H., Nomir, O., Zhou, J., et al. (2004a). Towards an automated dental identification system. *IEEE International Conference of Biometric Authenticity,* (pp. 789–796). Hong Kong.

Fahmy, G., Nassar, D., Said, E., Chen, H., Nomir, O., Zhou, J., et al. (2004b). A Web based tool for an Automated Dental Identification System (ADIS). *Proceedings of National Conference on Digital Government Research,* (pp. 1–2). Seattle, WA, USA.

Gonzalez, R., & Wood, R. (2003). *Digital image processing.* Addison Wesley.

Hurley, D., Nixon, M., & Carter, J. (2000). *Automatic ear recognition by force field transformation* (pp. 789–796). London, UK: IEEE Colloquium on Visual Biometrics.

Hurley, D., Nixon, M., & Carter, J. (2002). Force field energy function for image feature extraction. *Image and Vision Computing,* 311–317. doi:10.1016/S0262-8856(02)00003-3

Jain, A. K., Bolle, R. M., & Pankanti, S. (1999). *Biometrics: Personal identification in networked society.* Boston: Kluwer Academic Publishers.

Jain, A. K., & Ross, A. (2002). Learning user-specific parameters in a multibiometric System. [Rochester, New York, USA.]. *Proceedings of the International Conference on Image Processing, 1,* 57–60. doi:10.1109/ICIP.2002.1037958

Jain, A. K., Ross, A., & Prabhakar, S. (2004). An introduction to biometric recognition. *IEEE Transactions on Circuits and Systems for Video Technology. Special Issue on Image and Video-Based Biometrics, 14*(1), 4–20.

Jain, R., Kasturi, R., & Schnck, B. G. (1995). *Machine vision.* McGraw-Hill Inc.

Mahoor, M., & Abdel-Mottaleb, M. (2005). Classification and numbering of teeth in Bitewing dental images. *Journal of Pattern Recognition, 38,* 577–586. doi:10.1016/j.patcog.2004.08.012

Nassar, D., Said, E. H., Abaza, A., Chekuri, S., Zhou, J., Mahoor, M., et al. (2005). Automated Dental Identification System (ADIS). *Proceedings of National Conference on Digital Government Research,* (pp. 165–166). Atlanta, GA, USA.

Nomir, O. (2006). *A framework for automating human identification using dental X-ray radiograph.* Unpublished doctoral dissertation, University of Miami, 2006.

Nomir, O., & Abdel-Mottaleb, M. (2005). A system for human identification from X-ray dental radiographs. *Journal of Pattern Recognition, 38*(8), 1295–1305. doi:10.1016/j.patcog.2004.12.010

Nomir, O., & Abdel-Mottaleb, M. (2006). Hierarchical dental X-ray radiographs matching. *International Conference on Image Processing ICIP,* (pp. 2677–2680). Atlanta, GA, USA.

Nomir, O., & Abdel-Mottaleb, M. (2007a). Dental biometrics: Matching X-ray dental images using teeth shapes and appearances. *IEEE Transactions on Information Forensics and Security, 2*(2), 188–197. doi:10.1109/TIFS.2007.897245

Nomir, O., & Abdel-Mottaleb, M. (2007b). Combining matching algorithms for human identification using dental X-ray radiographs. *International Conference on Image Processing ICIP,* (pp. 409–412). San Antonio, Texas, USA.

Nomir, O., & Abdel-Mottaleb, M. (2007c). Human identification based on fusing matching algorithms using dental X-ray radiographs. *International Conference on Computer Theory and Applications,* (pp. 85–88). Alexandria, Egypt.

Nomir, O., & Abdel-Mottaleb, M. (2008a). Hierarchical contour matching for dental X-ray radiographs. *Journal of Pattern Recognition, 41*(1), 130–138. doi:10.1016/j.patcog.2007.05.015

Nomir, O., & Abdel-Mottaleb, M. (2008b). Fusion of matching algorithms for human identification using dental X-ray radiographs. *IEEE Transactions on Information Forensics and Security, 3*(2), 223–233. doi:10.1109/TIFS.2008.919343

Provost, F. J., & Fawcett, T. (2001). Robust classification for imprecise environments. *Machine Learning, 42*(3), 203–231. doi:10.1023/A:1007601015854

Ross, A., & Jain, A. K. (2003). Information fusion in biometrics. *Pattern Recognition Letters, 24,* 2115–2125. doi:10.1016/S0167-8655(03)00079-5

Ross, A., Nandakumar, K., & Jain, A. K. (2006). *Handbook of biometrics.* Springer-Verlag.

Snelick, R., Uludag, U., Mink, A., Indovina, M., & Jain, A. K. (2005). Large-scale evaluation of multimodal biometric authentication using state-of-the-art systems. *IEEE Transactions on Pattern Analysis and Machine Intelligence, 27*(3). doi:10.1109/TPAMI.2005.57

Veeramachaneni, K., Osadciw, L., & Varshney, P. K. (2005). An adaptive multimodal biometric management algorithm. *IEEE Transactions on Systems, Man, and Cybernetics, 35*(3).

Yamany, S., & Farag, A. (2003). Adaptive object identification and recognition using neural networks and surface signatures. *IEEE Conference on Advanced Video and Signal Based Surveillance,* (pp. 137–142). Miami, FL, USA.

KEY TERMS AND DEFINITIONS

Antemortem (AM) Identification: Is identification prior to death, is usually possible through comparison of many biometric identifiers.

Biometrics: Identification refers to identifying an individual based on his or her distinguishing characteristics. Biometrics is the science of identifying, or verifying the identity of a person based on physiological or behavioral characteristics. Physiological characteristics, include measures obtained from fingerprints, facial features, DNA, or hand geometry. Behavioral characteristics, like signature or voice, on the other hand, represent the way some action is carried over time.

Database: A database is a collection of X-ray dental radiographs. It includes records of different dental radiographs types of AM as well as PM records. It also includes the extracted features for all AM included radiographs. It is provided by the FBI's Criminal Justice Information Service (CJIS) division.

Dental Image Segmentation: Is to separate the teeth areas from the rest of the radiograph. Then, the individual teeth are separated by first separating the upper jaw from the lower jaw (in case of bitewing and panoramic radiographs), and then separating each tooth.

Dental Radiograph: Commonly referred to as X-ray films, or informally, X-rays, are pictures of the teeth, bones, and surrounding soft tissues to screen for and help identify problems with the teeth, mouth, and jaw. X-ray pictures can show cavities, cancerous or benign masses, hidden dental structures (such as wisdom teeth) and bone loss that cannot be seen during a visual examination. Dental X-rays may also be done as follow-up after dental treatments.

Force Field: Transformation smoothes the original grayscale image while preserving the important features. It uses to extract a set of features that uniquely represent each tooth. There is a potential energy surface associated with this force field. The directional property of the force field is exploited to automatically locate a small number of potential energy wells that are used to describe each individual tooth.

Forensic Odontology: The branch of forensics that deals with human identification based on dental features.

Fourier descriptors: Method is a powerful method for shape description. FDs can be used for representing the boundary of a two-dimensional shape. FDs have useful properties including simplicity of implementation and concentration of the contour information in the first few coefficients. The Fourier descriptors represent each tooth's contour by the first few Fourier descriptors.

Fusion: Is to integrate information form different sources using the strategies for information fusion. There are fusion, at the feature extraction level (tightly coupled integration), fusion at the matching level, and fusion at the decision level (loosely coupled integration).

Hierarchical Matching: Is performed at different resolution levels for the AM and PM teeth. Using the Hierarchical matching technique reduces the computational load which improves the retrieval time significantly.

Postmortem (PM) Identification: Is identification after death. From the definition, PM identification is impossible using behavioral biometrics (e.g. speech, gait).

Chapter 13
Left–Right Asymmetries and other Common Anatomical Variants of Temporomandibular Articular Surfaces

Aldo Scafoglieri
Vrije Universiteit Brussel, Belgium

Peter Van Roy
Vrije Universiteit Brussel, Belgium

Steven Provyn
Vrije Universiteit Brussel, Belgium & Haute École Paul Henri Spaak, Belgium

Jonathan Tresignie
Vrije Universiteit Brussel, Belgium

Jan Pieter Clarys
Vrije Universiteit Brussel, Belgium

ABSTRACT

In this chapter, the authors describe systematically left-right asymmetries and other common anatomical variants of the temporomandibular articular surfaces as they can appear in daily clinical practice. Digital photography and macroscopic observation were used to evaluate morphologic features of TMJ surfaces of elderly subjects at 100 glenoid fossae and articular eminences of dried skull bases, and at 100 dried mandibles. Mandibular condyle shape in the horizontal plane and in the frontal plane were evaluated using a standardized classification devised by Öberg et al. (1971). Degenerative form and surface changes of the TMJ were assessed using a scale devised by Wedel et al. (1978). The antero-posterior and medio-lateral diameter of the temporomandibular articular surfaces were measured using a digital caliper. The orientation was determined using a clinical goniometer. Morphologic left-right asymmetries of the temporomandibular articular surfaces were frequently present in mandibular condyles and in glenoid fossae. In general, mandibular condyles showed more often morphologic left-right

DOI: 10.4018/978-1-60960-483-7.ch013

asymmetries than glenoid fossae. Anatomical variants of the articular surfaces of the left and right mandibular condyles resulted from differences in shape. The majority of the articular surfaces had an oblong horizontal outline and a rounded frontal outline. One fifth of the mandibular condyles showed pear-shaped horizontal outlines and flat or ridge-shaped frontal outlines. An important incidence of left-right asymmetries and other common anatomical variants of the temporomandibular articular joint surfaces must be considered at observation and therapy of the temporomandibular joint; arthrokinematic functional consequences may result.

INTRODUCTION

Development of the Temporomandibular Joint

Formation of the TMJ starts during embryologic development but completion normally stops before the age of 30 years (Björk, 1955; Ingervall et al., 1976; Morimoto et al., 1987; Mérida-Velasco et al., 1999; Katsavrias, 2002). The inferior joint cavity is formed in the ninth week of embryologic development. The glenoid fossa and the superior joint cavity are formed two weeks afterwards (Mérida-Velasco et al., 1999). The articular eminence of the TMJ develops after birth and enchondral calcification of the mandibular condyle periphery begins during the teen-age period (Figure 1) (Ingervall et al., 1976; Katsavrias, 2002).

The morphology of the temporomandibular articular surfaces changes constantly during life time. Changes after the age of 30 are considered adaptations to altered functions. Consequently,

the function of the TMJ is assumed to show up anatomical variants and specifically asymmetries (Katsavrias, 2002).

Asymmetries of the Mandibular Condyle

In literature only a few publications about left-right asymmetries and anatomical variants of the TMJ are available. There is a lack of systematic investigations concerning asymmetries of the temporomandibular articular surfaces in recent dried skulls. Available information relates to morphologic differences of mandibular condyles.

In a western population of 286 patients, Sheppard (1982) found mandibular condyle asymmetry in 40% of the cases. In a study conducted by Capurso and Bonazza (1990), macroscopic observation of 100 dry Sardinian skulls revealed asymmetry of mandibular condyles in 30% of the cases. Evaluation of 26 X-rays of patients with temporomandibular joint dysfunction by

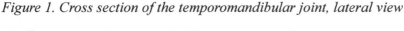

Figure 1. Cross section of the temporomandibular joint, lateral view

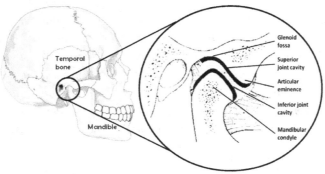

Cros et al. (1977) showed a systematic asymmetry in the orientation of medio-lateral condylar axis. Pirttiniemi and Kantomaa (1992) ascribed asymmetry of the TMJ to reciprocal interaction between developmental aspects of the skull base and impaired directional function.

Variants of the Mandibular Condyle

Variants of mandibular condyle shape in the horizontal plane and in the frontal plane were described previously (Öberg et al., 1971; Solberg et al., 1985; Wedel et al., 1978; Wittaker et al., 1985). Wedel et al. (1978) and Whittaker et al. (1985) used the classification devised by Öberg et al. (1971) to describe these variants. Solberg et al. (1985) devised another classification to describe variants of the mandibular condyles in the horizontal, frontal and sagittal plane. In this chapter, the classification devised by Öberg et al. (1971) was used (see below). Only Whittaker et al. (1985) provided data of left-right differences of mandibular condyles, resulting from the study of a Romano-British collection of 204 dry skulls. In all studies the majority of the articular surfaces had oblong horizontal outlines and rounded frontal outlines. On the basis of macroscopic observation of 115 dissected TMJ's Öberg et al. (1971) found that one third of the articular surfaces revealed round to oval horizontal outlines and one fifth presented flat frontal outlines. Observing 48 medieval skulls, Wedel et al. (1978) reported that more than 10% of the articular surfaces had pear-shaped horizontal outlines and ridge-shaped frontal outlines. From a series of 92 disarticulated TMJ's at autopsy, Solberg et al. (1985) documented the association of specific shapes of the articular eminence and the mandibular condyles. A slightly rounded mandibular condyle in the frontal plane was related to an elliptical condyle in the horizontal plane and a curved articular eminence in the frontal plane. Mandibular condyles with deviations in form were more often gable-shaped, cylindrical and irregular in appearance.

Since the knowledge of TMJ kinematics is essentially based on mandible movement and the latter is determined by TMJ morphology, the following paragraphs will compare systematically the morphology of the left and right temporomandibular articular surfaces in relation to possible asymmetries and previously described variants.

EVALUATION OF TEMPOROMANDIBULAR ARTICULAR SURFACE MORPHOLOGY

Hundred articular eminences and glenoid fossae of dried skull bases and 100 dried mandibles were selected at random from the scientific collection of macerated bones of the Vrije Universiteit Brussel. Sixty-three mandibles were edentate, 23 partially dentate and 14 were fully dentate. No paired relationship between the selected temporal and mandibular articular surfaces was available. Morphology of the skull material was studied by digital photography and macroscopic observation. Shape, size, orientation and degree of degeneration of the TMJ surfaces were evaluated. Superior and posterior views of the mandibular condyles were made. Glenoid fossae were photographed from below and articular eminences from the side.

Evaluation of Mandibular Condyle Shape

Concerning the shape of the mandibular condyles a classification devised by Öberg et al. (1971) was used:

Horizontal mandibular condyle outline was encoded as follows (Figure 2):

1. oblong (antero-posterior diameter < ½ medio-lateral diameter)
2. rounded to oval (antero-posterior diameter ≥ ½ medio-lateral diameter)
3. tapering laterally, pear-shaped

Figure 2. Mandibular condyle shape in the horizontal plane

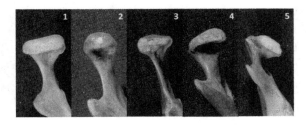

4.   tapering medially, pear-shaped
5.   other shapes

In order to increase the discernment of the classification the notion "pear-shaped" was further defined: pear-shape was considered to be present if the anterior and posterior tangent lines to the mandibular condyles revealed an angle larger than 10°.

Frontal mandibular condyle outline was encoded as follows (Figure 3):

1.   rounded or slightly convex
2.   largely plane (straight)
3.   ridge-shaped (inverted V-shaped)
4.   other shapes

Mandibular condyles were considered asymmetric in the horizontal and/or frontal plane concerning their shape if left and right joint surfaces were encoded differently.

Figure 3. Mandibular condyle shape in the frontal plane

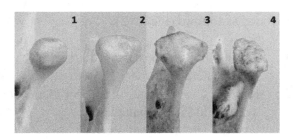

Measurement of Temporomandibular Articular Surface Size

Concerning the size of the mandibular condyles and glenoid fossae, the antero-posterior and medio-lateral diameters were read out using a digital caliper with an accuracy to 1/10 of a millimetre. The following definitions were used to evaluate the diameter:

1.   The antero-posterior mandibular condyle diameter is the shortest distance between the most prominent anterior and posterior aspect of the articular surface measured at right angles to the oblique connection line between the medial and lateral end of the mandibular condyle.
2.   The antero-posterior glenoid fossa diameter is the shortest distance between the most prominent anterior aspect of the articular eminence and the postglenoid process measured at right angles to the oblique connection line between the medial and lateral end of the glenoid fossa.
3.   The medio-lateral mandibular condyle diameter is the shortest distance between the most prominent medial and lateral aspects of the articular surface measured at right angles to the antero-posterior diameter of the mandibular condyle.
4.   The medio-lateral glenoid fossa diameter is the shortest distance between the points of intersection of the sphenotemporal suture with the squamotympanical fissure medially and the most posterior aspect of the articular tubercle measured at right angles to the antero-posterior diameter of the glenoid fossa.

Left-right differences in antero-posterior and/or medio-lateral diameters larger than 10% were considered to be asymmetric.

Figure 4. Construction of the orientation angle (α) of the mandibular condyle

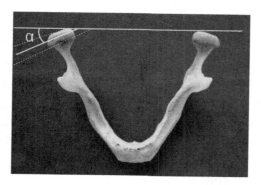

Measurement of Temporomandibular Articular Surface Orientation

The orientation of the mandibular condyles, glenoid fossae and articular eminences in the transverse plane was determined using a clinical goniometer read out to 1 degree.

The following definitions were used to evaluate the orientation of the articular surfaces:

1. The mandibular condyle orientation angle in the horizontal plane is the angle measured between the tangent line connecting the two condyles posteriorly and the bisector of the parallels to the anterior and posterior condylar outline (Figure 4).
2. The glenoid fossa orientation angle in the horizontal plane is the angle measured between the frontal axis and a straight line connecting the point of intersection of the sphenotemporal suture and the squamo-tympanical fissure medially and the most posterior aspect of the articular tubercle laterally (Figure 5).
3. The articular eminence orientation angle in the sagittal plane is the angle measured between the Frankfurter-horizontal and the tangent line to the lateral border of the articular eminence (Figure 6).

Figure 5. Construction of the orientation angle (α) of the glenoid fossa in the horizontal plane

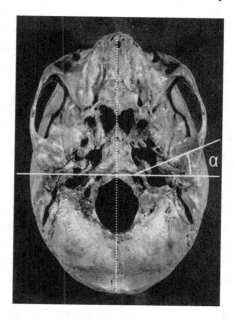

Mandibular condyles, glenoid fossae and articular eminences were considered asymmetric concerning their orientation if a left-right difference of at least 10° existed.

Test-retest reliability of the orientation measurements. The reliability of the orientation measurements studied by digital photography is presented in Table 1. No significant differences between test and retest measurements ($p > 0.05$)

Figure 6. Construction of the orientation angle (α) of the articular eminence in the sagittal plane

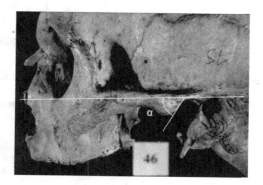

Table 1. Test-retest reliability of orientation measurements of the temporomandibular articular surfaces (n=20)

Articular surface	p	r
Left mandibular condyle	.263	.97
Right mandibular condyle	.517	.95
Left glenoid fossa	.587	.76
Right glenoid fossa	.306	.70
Left articular eminence	.109	.98
Right articular eminence	.321	.97

were found. Very high reliability coefficients (r>0.95) were found for the orientation measurements of the mandibular condyles and the articular eminences. The reliability of glenoid fossae orientation measurements proved to be high (r>0.70).

Evaluation of Temporomandibular Articular Surface Degeneration

In relation to the degeneration of the mandibular condyles and glenoid fossae a scale devised by Wedel et al. (1978) was used:

Form changes of the TMJ were encoded as follows (Figure 7):

1. normal
2. slight remodelling/flattening
3. marked remodelling
4. deforming change

Surface changes of the TMJ were evaluated as follows (Figure 8):

1. normal
2. uneven surface, unbroken compact layer
3. marked irregular surface/local perforation of the compact bone layer
4. compact layer broken up in areas >3mm^2/ largely distributed small perforations

Mandibular condyles and glenoid fossae were considered asymmetric concerning their degeneration if left and right joint surfaces were encoded differently.

Statistical analysis was conducted using an SPSS/PC package. Paired t-tests (p<0.05) were

Figure 7. Degree of degeneration of temporomandibular articular form

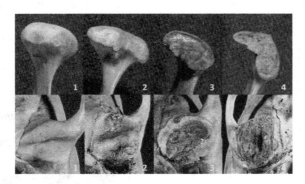

Figure 8. Degree of degeneration of mandibular condyle surface

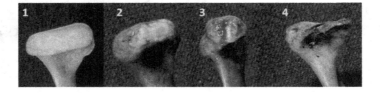

used to compare size and orientation of left and right TMJ surfaces. Pearson correlation coefficients were calculated to assess the reliability of the orientation measurements.

INCIDENCE OF LEFT-RIGHT ASYMMETRIES AND ANATOMICAL VARIANTS OF THE TEMPORMANDIBULAR ARTICULAR SURFACES

Incidences for left-right asymmetries of TMJ surfaces are shown in Table 2. Morphologic left-right asymmetries of the temporomandibular articular surfaces were frequently present in mandibular condyles and in glenoid fossae. In general mandibular condyles showed more frequently morphologic left-right asymmetries than glenoid fossae.

Left-Right Asymmetries of the Mandibular Condyle

Thirty percent of the articular surfaces of the mandibular condyles showed left-right asymmetries in 7 studied features. Intra-individual differences in shape and in antero-posterior diameter resulted the highest incidence (42%) for left-right asymmetries. Form and surface changes as a result of

degeneration of the mandibular articular surfaces were present in 24% to 39%. Whereas differences in the medio-lateral diameter and in the orientation resulted in lower incidences, respectively 10 and 16 percent.

Left-Right Asymmetries of the Glenoid Fossae

The articular surfaces of the glenoid fossae showed left-right asymmetries in 13% of the 6 investigated features. Form changes and surface changes as a result of degeneration of the articular surfaces resulted in high incidences, respectively 18 and 27%, for left-right asymmetries. In 24% of the dried skulls, differences in the orientation angle of the articular eminence resulted in left-right asymmetries. Low incidences for left-right asymmetries were found as a result of differences in antero-posterior (4%) and medio-lateral diameter (4%) and in orientation of the glenoid fossae in the horizontal plane (1%).

Variants of the Mandibular Condyle

The incidence of variants in shape of the mandibular condyles in the horizontal and in the frontal plane was calculated and is showed in Figures 9 and 10. Two thirds of the mandibular condyles had an oblong outline in the horizontal plane.

Table 2. Incidence of left-right asymmetries of the temporomandibular articular surfaces in percentage

Feature	Mandibular condyle	Glenoid fossa	Articular eminence
Shape in the horizontal plane	42	-	-
Shape in the frontal plane	37	-	-
Antero-posterior diameter	42	4	-
Medio-lateral diameter	10	4	-
Orientation	16	1	24
Degenerative form changes	39	18	-
Degenerative surface changes	24	27	-

Figure 9. Incidence of left and right mandibular condyle variants in the horizontal plane

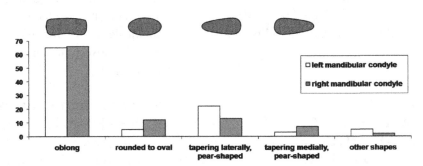

Figure 10. Incidence of left and right mandibular condyle variants in the frontal plane

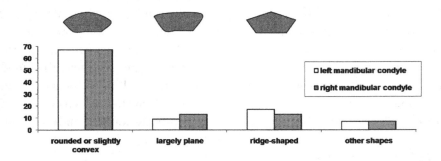

Rounded or tapered outlines were found in 31% of the cases. The left mandibular condyles were more often medially tapered (22%) than the right ones (13%). Right mandibular condyles were more often rounded to oval (12%) than the left ones (5%). Left and right condyles were laterally tapered in 3% and 7% of the cases respectively.

Sixty-seven percent of the mandibular condyles had a rounded or slightly convex outline in the frontal plane. Left and right mandibular condyles were plane shaped in 9% and 13% of the cases respectively. Ridge-shaped condyles occurred in 17% for left mandibular articular surfaces and in 13% for the right mandibular articular surfaces. The incidences for variants in shape were similar for left and the right mandibular articular surfaces.

MORPHOLOGICAL AND FUNCTIONAL ASPECTS RELATED TO LEFT-RIGHT ASYMMETRIES OF THE TEMPOROMANDIBULAR ARTICULAR SURFACES

In this chapter osteometric and descriptive data concerning left-right asymmetries and variants of TMJ surfaces are provided. Additional results were provided concerning size and orientation of the articular surfaces. Data were provided from skull material of elderly subjects after maceration. This may raise the question whether these can be considered as representative of a larger population. As mentioned in the introduction, formation of TMJ surface is completed after the age of 20. In literature, by the knowledge of the authors, no data concerning asymmetries of the TMJ surfaces in young and in elder individuals are available. Thus the results provided in this chapter can't be extrapolated immediately to a large population. Elder patients represent an important group in daily clinical practice so left-right asymmetries caused by degenerative changes can therefore be significant. On the other hand Solberg et al. (1985) showed that form and surface changes in TMJ caused by degeneration frequently occurred in young adults and that the incidence barely increased in older age groups.

Morphological Aspects Related to Left-Right Asymmetries of the Temporomandibular Articular Surfaces

In this chapter incidences for left-right asymmetries were higher in mandibular condyles than in glenoid fossae. Herewith form and surfaces changes caused by degeneration are more important and extensive in mandibular condyles. It is supposed that the chance of finding left-right asymmetries is bigger in mandibular condyles than in glenoid fossae because developmental failures of the TMJ reveal themselves as form changes of the mandibular condyle and because the structural adaptability of the mandibular condyle after the third decade is bigger. This is the result of an unequal left-right TMJ loading due to asymmetric dentition and muscle function (Luder, 2002). As far as the mandible is concerned high incidences of left-right asymmetries were also reported previously (Sheppard, 1982; Capurso & Bonazza, 1990). Left-right asymmetries of the temporal articular surfaces were also frequently found at the level of the articular eminence. The existence of left-right asymmetries in the TMJ can only be explained partially by developmental failure and degenerative changes. Therefore it is proposed that morphologic left-right asymmetries do not always imply pathology of the temporomandibular joint but confirm the adaptability of the masticatory system to changing circumstances. Solberg et al. (1985) studied mandibular condyle shape in the frontal, horizontal and sagittal plane. A convex mandibular condyle in the frontal plane often was associated to an elliptical condyle in the horizontal plane. On the contrary a rounded or slightly convex condyle often was associated to an oblong condyle. This can possibly be explained by the use of a different terminology and population of investigation.

It must be pointed out that concerning the shape of glenoid fossae, by knowledge of the authors, no classification in the horizontal plane and only one in the frontal plane is available. To compare the incidences of mandibular condyle and glenoid fossa asymmetries a classification should be devised. Although glenoid fossa asymmetries were observed, they were not systematically investigated by lack of a classification.

Functional Aspects Related to Left-Right Asymmetries of the Temporomandibular Articular Surfaces

The TMJ is a synovial junction with a saddle-shaped articulating disc. The disc separates the joint into two separate pressure-bearing compounds and compensates the lack of congruence between the mandibular condyle and the glenoid fossa and articular eminence during roll-glide mechanism. Knowledge of TMJ kinematics is essentially based on mandible movement. Mandible movement is determined also by TMJ morphology. Since the two TMJ's form a bilateral lever system for mandible movement, left-right asymmetries could be structural factors causing arthrokinematic changes observed in practice. In the light of the findings presented in this chapter the basic assumption of symmetrical mandible motion made in clinical practice must be questioned.

Several arthrokinematic studies proved that the mandible moves asymmetrically. Bushang et al. (2000) showed that during laterotrusion the contralateral and ipsilateral condyles move in opposite directions. According to Gallo et al. (1997, 2000) finite helical axis pathways of the mandibular condyles do not coincide during mastication. The mandible shifts laterally toward the working side during opening. During closing the working condyle essentially only rotates while the balancing condyle moves dorsally and cranially. It is self-evident that knowledge of temporomandibular articular surface morphology is necessary in understanding movement disorders of the TMJ. At this moment, by knowledge of the authors in this chapter, only Palla et al. (2003) assessed mandibular motion taking into account TMJ bony anatomy. Since left-right asymmetries frequently occur in normal population and since it isn't clear yet whether these asymmetries can influence TMJ arthrokinematics, biomechanical studies in combination with three-dimensional reconstructions of the bony anatomy of the TMJ are likely to be the most appropriate method to understand normal mandible motion at this moment.

CONCLUSION

Left-right asymmetries of mandibular condyles and glenoid fossae are frequently found in an elder population. Further investigations should clarify which relationships can be found between the morphological characteristics of the temporomandibular articular surfaces considering left-right asymmetries on the one hand and kinematical or functional anatomic differences on the other hand.

REFERENCES

Björk, A. (1995). Cranial base development. A follow-up X-ray study of the individual variation in growth occurring between the ages of 12 and 20 years and its relation to brain case and face development. *American Journal of Orthodontics*, *41*, 198–225. doi:10.1016/0002-9416(55)90005-1

Buschang, P. H., Hayasaki, H., & Throckmorton, G. S. (2000). Quantification of human chewing-cycle kinematics. *Archives of Oral Biology*, *45*, 461–474. doi:10.1016/S0003-9969(00)00015-7

Capurso, U., & Bonazza, M. (1990). Le variazioni morfologiche dell' articolazione temporomandibolare. *Minerva Stomatologica*, *39*, 629–636.

Cros, P., Chollat, L., & Dumas, P. (1977). Dissymétrie des axes des condyles mandibulaires sur le plan horizontal. *Revue de Stomatologie et de Chirurgie Maxillo-Faciale*, *78*, 429–432.

Gallo, L. M., Airoldi, G. B., Airoldi, R. L., & Palla, S. (1997). Description of mandibular finite helical axis pathways in asymptomatic subjects. *Journal of Dental Research*, *76*, 704–713. doi:10.1177/00220345970760021201

Gallo, L. M., Fushima, K., & Palla, S. (2000). Mandibular helical axis pathways during mastication. *Journal of Dental Research*, *79*, 1566–1572. doi:10.1177/00220345000790080701

Ingervall, B., Carlsson, G. E., & Thilander, B. (1976). Postnatal development of the human temporomandibular joint. A microradiographic study. *Acta Odontologica Scandinavica*, *34*, 133–139. doi:10.3109/00016357609002560

Katsavrias, E. G. (2002). Changes in articular eminence inclination during the craniofacial growth period. *The Angle Orthodontist*, *72*, 258–263.

Luder, H.-U. (2002). Factors affecting degeneration in human temporomandibular joints as assessed histologically. *European Journal of Oral Sciences*, *110*, 106–113. doi:10.1034/j.1600-0722.2002.11212.x

Mérida-Velasco, J. R., Rodriguez-Vazquez, J. F., Mérida-Velasco, J. A., Sanchez-Montesinos, I., Espin-Ferra, J., & Jimenez-Collado, J. (1999). Development of the human temporomandibular joint. *The Anatomical Record*, *255*, 20–33. doi:10.1002/(SICI)1097-0185(19990501)255:1<20::AID-AR4>3.0.CO;2-N

Morimoto, K., Hashimoto, N., & Suetsugu, T. (1987). Prenatal developmental process of human temporomandibular joint. *The Journal of Prosthetic Dentistry, 57,* 723–729. doi:10.1016/0022-3913(87)90372-6

Öberg, T., Carlsson, G. E., & Fajers, C.-M. (1971). The temporomandibular joint. A morphologic study on a human autopsy material. *Acta Odontologica Scandinavica, 29,* 349–389. doi:10.3109/00016357109026526

Palla, S., Gallo, L. M., & Gossi, D. (2003). Dynamic stereometry of the temporomandibular joint. *Orthodontics & Craniofacial Research, 1,* 37–47. doi:10.1034/j.1600-0544.2003.233.x

Pirttiniemi, P., & Kantomaa, T. (1992). Relation of glenoid fossa morphology to mandibulofacial asymmetry, studied in dry human Lapp skulls. *Acta Odontologica Scandinavica, 50,* 235–243. doi:10.3109/00016359209012768

Sheppard, S. M. (1982). Asymptomatic morphologic variations in the mandibular condyle-ramus region. *The Journal of Prosthetic Dentistry, 47,* 539–544. doi:10.1016/0022-3913(82)90306-7

Solberg, W. K., Hansson, T. L., & Nordtrom, B. (1985). The temporomandibular joint in young adults at autopsy: A morphologic classification and evaluation. *Journal of Oral Rehabilitation, 12,* 303–321. doi:10.1111/j.1365-2842.1985.tb01285.x

Wedel, A., Carlsson, G. E., & Sagne, S. (1978). Temporomandibular joint morphology in a medieval skull material. *Swedish Dental Journal, 2,* 177–187.

Whittaker, D. K., Davies, G., & Brown, M. (1985). Tooth loss, attrition and temporomandibular joint changes in a Romano-British population. *Journal of Oral Rehabilitation, 12,* 407–419. doi:10.1111/j.1365-2842.1985.tb01546.x

KEY TERMS AND DEFINITIONS

Anatomical Variants: These are structures of living things that display a morphology that is a little different from other structures of the same type.

Asymmetry: This is the absence of symmetry.

Enchondral Calcification: This is an essential process during fetal development of the mammalian skeletal system resulting in the creation of bone tissue, also known as *enchondral ossification.*

Frankfurter Horizontal: This is the horizontal plane represented in profile by a line between the lowest point on the margin of the orbit and the highest point on the margin of the auditory meatus, also called *Frankfort horizontal plane.*

Glenoid Fossa: This is a concave depression in the temporal bone, also frequently referred to as *fossa mandibularis,* which articulates with the convex mandibular condyle.

Maceration: This is a bone preparation technique whereby parts of a vertebrate corpse are left to rot inside a closed container at near-constant temperature, to get a clean skeleton.

Osteometric Data: These are numerical data obtained by measurement of the human skeleton.

Sphenotemporal Suture: This is a fairly rigid joint between the sphenoid bone and the temporal bone of the cranium, also known as *sutura sphenotemporale.*

Squamotympanical Fissure: this is the groove on the temporal bone of the skull situated behind the glenoid fossa, also called *fissura tympanosquamosa.*

Temporomandibular Joint: This is the synovial joint of the jaw that allows the mouth to open and to close, and is frequently referred to as *TMJ.*

Chapter 14
Forensic Statistics in Health Sciences

Amit Chattopadhyay
National Institutes of Health, USA

ABSTRACT

This chapter reviews the application of forensic statistical methods related issues such as: methods of deciphering evidence, DNA profile matching, searching a database of DNA profiles, scientific reliability, discrimination in presentation of statistical evidence in legal settings, assumptions in underlying statistical analysis when evidence is presented, precision & accuracy, role of using extreme values in evidence, and decision analysis in forensic science. The emphasis of the chapter is on concepts from statistical application, nature, and use of evidences in everyday clinical practice and in the court of law. Another goal of the chapter is to serve as a central reference to access of information about resources related to this topic.

INTRODUCTION

Forensic statistics may be defined as the application of statistics to forensic science and the law to seek the truth in a way that truth is identified with high degree of confidence from among a variety of possible solutions to the problem at hand. Forensic statisticians help to quantify evidence in criminal cases (The Royal Statistical Society, 2005). Statistics is a scientific system that analyzes data collected from a pool of observations by collection, and interprets the data to provide explanation(s) for the observed event or phenomenon. Usually, an appropriate evaluation of evidence and a comparison of probabilities of the evidence under two different propositions are required while making a decision. This evidence generated by forensic statistics may be used subsequently to either implicate or exonerate a person suspected of committing that crime, or just

DOI: 10.4018/978-1-60960-483-7.ch014

to gain further insight into the incident. Over the years, with increasing technological advancement, forensic science has become a key part of criminal investigations worldwide (The Royal Statistical Society, 2005).

The Logical Basis of Forensic Statistics

Statistics, like all scientific systems runs on logical reasoning, especially when investigating causation. Logical reasoning involves an argument consists of one or more premises (statement that is either true or false that is offered in support of a claim) and one conclusion (a sentence that is true or false). The conclusion should follow from the premises based on the claims (Chattopadhyay, 2010). Errors in logical reasoning leading to fallacious conclusions occur in health research, and are a major threat to concluding causal association. Logic may be defined as the science of those principles, laws, and methods that guides correct and proper reasoning.

Critical thinking involves knowledge of the science of logic; including the skills of logical analysis, correct reasoning, and understanding statistical methods. Critical thinking, however, involves more than just an understanding of logical procedures. A good critical thinker must also understand the sources of knowledge, the nature of knowledge, and the nature of truth. Logic is not intended merely to inform or instruct. It is also a directive and aims at assisting us in the proper use of our power of reasoning (Dolhenty, 2010). An argument is simply a set of statements, one of which is designated as a conclusion and the remaining statements, called premises, are asserted as being true and are offered as evidence that supports or implies the conclusion. The first step in recognizing an argument for the purposes of understanding and evaluating the argument is to identify the premises and the conclusion which make up the argument.

Scientific methodology uses synthesis and analysis to determine evidence in factor of truth about a question employing the two parts of logic: inductive reasoning and deductive reasoning. Fallacies arise from a discontinuity in logical chain of reasoning. Although there are several important errors in logical arguments that occur, important ones in science are: inductive argument fallacy, deductive fallacy, inductive fallacy, and factual error.

DECIPHERING EVIDENCE

Evidence is the information that supports a certain conclusion. In the courts, usually, the existence of means, motive and opportunity drives the conclusions towards commitment of crime, and loads the dice towards potentially biasing a decision against the suspect, whether the crime was committed on not. Technicalities towards admission of evidence may also play a role. Thus there always exists the possibility that the weight of evidence in court may at times deviate from the truth. Therefore Types I and II error rates may indicate efficiency of the justice process.

Scientific Reliability

It is common in courts to see most associations be interpreted as causal associations. Even if no such direct claims are made, several studies interpret the associations as causal in the discussion of the articles. However, inferring causal association is a tedious and rigorous proposition and requires quality insight, sound judgment and careful assessment of evidence. In making such inferences, design of the study must be considered as the limiting framework within which conclusions may be drawn. Errors in study designs may lead to incorrect conclusions and may color expert opinion about evidence in question in courts.

The Duhem-Quine thesis (or the Duhem-Quine problem) states that it is impossible to test a scientific hypothesis in isolation of its environment because background assumptions about associated issues form the basis of empirical tests (Gillies, 1998). Therefore, when a study is conducted under assumptions, the study results are also a statement on those assumptions themselves because all assumptions are proved to be valid prior to the study. Therefore, the mere demonstration of an observed association cannot be taken as evidence for causality at face value.

Usually, scientific evidence is stated in terms of probabilities that the jury/judge must assess by itself or in light of other corroboration/ conflicting evidences. However, in some situations, such as paternity testing, DNA evidence is generally considered to be clinching evidence about the case. However, even such scientifically advanced technology is subject to the same statistical assumptions about the probability of the DNA matches between the suspect and the available databases. These issues are discussed in DNA profiling section.

Decision Analysis in Forensic Science

Although formal decision analysis protocols and algorithms are being developed for use in forensic sciences (for example, Taroni et al, 2005), clear guidelines are not yet available. Such guidelines may be suitable for certain types of crimes, but because of the dynamic nature of the human mind and its creativity, a cook-book approach may not be the best way to deal with evidence. To deal with the uncertainties and potentially confecting evidence, a formal approach may be useful though.

One of the key philosophical issues dealing with statistical evidence is the heavy reliance on p-value of a test for statistical conclusions. It is already well-known that given whatever "significance" threshold, any point can be proven with a sufficiently large sample size. P-value is the most used statistic sin scientific literature, and has become the most controversial statistic in social

and epidemiologic research. Correct interpretation of the p-value must emphasize the last part of the definition - the assumption for p-value i.e. that the null hypothesis is true. Therefore, the p-value does not provide evidence that the alternate hypothesis under study is true/ false. The logical fallacy of mistaking the null P-value for the probability that the null hypothesis is true is common (Chattopadhyay, 2009).

"Routine statistical testing does not answer questions such as: How often is the null hypothesis true when we fail to reject it? When we do reject the null hypothesis, how often is the alternative hypothesis true? These are the probabilities of ultimate concern in significance testing - the predictive values of significant/ non-significant statistical tests. It has been suggested that we should avoid exact interpretation of p-values in observational research where they may lack theoretical basis; stop interpreting P-values as if they measure probability of alternative hypotheses (which should be done using Bayesian methods); and we should get serious about precision of effect estimates and look for narrow confidence intervals instead of low P-values to identify results that are least influenced by random error (Poole 2001). However, for most statistical tests that are conducted under assumptions, "healthy looking" p-value continues to be the most sought after statistic" (Chattopadhyaya, 2009).

Precision, Accuracy and Meaningfulness

Precision is the degree to which a variable has nearly the same value when measured several times. Normally the estimate provided by different studies varies from each other. If the range of the estimate from different studies is close by then the estimates are generally considered to be precise and vice-versa. Accuracy, on the other hand, assesses the degree to which a variable actually represents what it is supposed to represent. It is possible to obtain very precise, but inaccurate results. Even if results are statistically precise and accurate, their meaningfulness in context of the situation under examination (such as a specific trial) may be in question. For example a positive or negative DNA matches against a convenience (and biased) database that does not correctly population prevalence of all possible genotypes may lead to inappropriate results and bias the jury. That statistical significance does not necessarily coincide with contextual meaningfulness of the information needs to be kept in mind all the time.

Sample Size in Statistical Evidence

Another role of a forensic statistician relates to sampling problems and determination of sample size. In some cases, it is necessary to examine a consignment of similar-looking items, and it is often not practical to examine every item. This may be purely on financial grounds but may be on health grounds also. The question then arises as to how many items should be examined on a sampling basis. For example, the consignment to be examined may be a set of CDs, some of which are thought to contain pornographic material. Then it is desirable for the examining officers to examine as few CDs as is commensurate with a good description of the proportion of the CDs which are illicit. The sample size determination is really just a quality control problem; there are UN Guidelines where the problem concerns drugs (The Royal Statistical Society, 2005).

Increasing the sample size in a study increases its power and precision of estimates derived from it. "If an association between exposure and outcome exists in reality, and it is also detected by the study; or if an association does not exist in reality and study correctly detects absence of an association, then a correct decision has been made. However, if there is no real association, but the study detects an association, then the situation is similar to a false-positive test, and such errors are called Type I errors or alpha errors (finding

a difference that does not exist). Alternately, if a study fails to detect a true association, then the situation is similar to false negative test and such errors are called Type-II errors or beta errors (not finding difference which exists). Studies need to guard against and minimize both these types of errors" (Chattopadhyay, 2009).

ASSUMPTIONS IN UNDERLYING STATISTICAL ANALYSIS WHEN EVIDENCE IS PRESENTED

In general, statistical methods rely on a variety of assumptions about the nature of the underlying data on which tests are run and from which conclusions are drawn. When the data do not meet those assumptions, the results often are not valid. Furthermore, unless the sampling is done in specific way (and analyses done in ways suitable for the sampling scheme) the results may not be generalizable to the rest of the population. Therefore, it is important for courts assessing the evidentiary relevance of statistical studies to check that those assumptions are satisfied, at least, approximately.

The validity of a hypothesis test is partly determined by whether the assumptions underlying the test are satisfied. In the past, a preliminary analysis of the data has been suggested prior to the use of the statistical test. In this article, the authors describe several limitations of preliminary tests (e.g., influence on significance levels). Another strategy that uses theoretical knowledge in conjunction with prior empirical evidence and reason, prior to data collection, is described (Wells & Hintze, 2007). Determining the appropriate statistical test for the specific involves the consideration of several factors such as: the study's research questions, type of independent variable(s) and dependent variable(s), and design are useful in identifying a set of possible statistical techniques. One of the last limiting factors that is helpful in deciding which statistical test is appropriate is determining which assumptions will be satisfied:

Hypothesis testing is a powerful technique for testing theories and answering research questions primarily due to the use of probability to control the likelihood of making an incorrect conclusion. Two types of errors may be committed when performing a hypothesis test: Type I or II. A Type I error occurs when a true null hypothesis (H0) is rejected, whereas a Type II error occurs when a false H0 is not rejected. Because we can control the Type I error rate strictly, the null and alternative hypotheses are typically constructed so the worse mistake is associated with a Type I error. As a result, the Type I error is considered the more severe of the two errors and the one that must be controlled first and foremost. The Type II error rate is often conceptualized as power, that is, the probability of rejecting a false H0. The ultimate goal of any hypothesis test is to control the Type I error rate at the nominal alpha level (e.g.,.05) while exhibiting a reasonable amount of power (e.g., at least.80) to detect a meaningful effect. Anything that impedes the control of these two error rates must be avoided for hypothesis testing to remain valid and useful.

The ultimate goal of any hypothesis test is to answer a research question, whether explicitly or implicitly stated, which is done by testing whether a specific parameter, which is associated with the research question, differs from a specific value or range of values. The general procedure for performing a hypothesis test is, first, to compute a statistic that summarizes the data (e.g., sample mean). Then the summary statistic is converted to a test statistic by comparing the sample statistic to the parameter value specified under H0. The test statistic is then compared to a reference distribution, known as the null distribution. (Wells & Hintze, 2007)

PATTERN RECOGNITION, VOICE RECOGNITION, AND FACIAL RECOGNITION

Pattern Recognition

Statistical pattern recognition covers all stages of an investigation including formulation of the problem, data collection by employing discrimination and classification assessment of results and interpretation. Computerized pattern recognition has been defined as: automatic (machine) recognition, description, classification, and grouping of patterns are important problems in a variety of engineering and scientific disciplines such as biology, psychology, medicine, marketing, computer vision, artificial intelligence, and remote sensing (Jain et al, 2000)

More recently, neural network techniques and methods imported from statistical learning theory have been receiving increasing attention. The design of a recognition system requires careful attention to the following issues: definition of pattern classes, sensing environment, pattern representation, feature extraction and selection, cluster analysis, classifier design and learning, selection of training and test samples, and performance evaluation. In spite of almost 50 years of research and development in this field, the general problem of recognizing complex patterns with arbitrary orientation, location, and scale remains unsolved. New and emerging applications, such as data mining, web searching, retrieval of multimedia data, face recognition, and cursive handwriting recognition, require robust and efficient pattern recognition techniques. The objective of this review paper is to summarize and compare some of the well-known methods used in various stages of a pattern recognition system and identify research topics and applications which are at the forefront of this exciting and challenging field. (Jain et al, 2000)

Pattern recognition problems go through eight distinct steps as described by Fukunaga (1990), outlined below.

1. **Formulation of the problem:** gaining a clear understanding of the aims of the investigation and planning the remaining stages.
2. Data collection: making measurements on appropriate variables and recording details of the data collection procedure (ground truth).
3. **Initial examination of the data:** checking the data, calculating summary statistics and producing plots in order to get a feel for the structure.
4. **Feature selection or feature extraction:** selecting variables from the measured set that are appropriate for the task. These new variables may be obtained by a linear or nonlinear transformation of the original set (feature extraction). To some extent, the division of feature extraction and classification is artificial.
5. **Unsupervised pattern classification or clustering:** this may be viewed as exploratory data analysis and it may provide a successful conclusion to a study. On the other hand, it may be a means of preprocessing the data for a supervised classification procedure.
6. **Apply discrimination or regression procedures as appropriate:** the classifier is designed using a training set of exemplar patterns.
7. **Assessment of results:** this may involve applying the trained classifier to an independent test set of labeled patterns.
8. **Interpretation.**

In the statistical approach, each pattern is represented in terms of d features or measurements and is viewed as a point in a d-dimensional space. The goal is to choose those features that allow pattern vectors belonging to different categories to occupy compact and disjoint regions in a d-dimensional feature space. The effectiveness of the representation space (feature set) is determined by how well patterns from different classes can be separated. Given a set of training patterns from each class, the objective is to establish decision boundaries in the feature space which separate patterns belonging to different classes. In the statistical decision theoretic approach, the decision boundaries are determined by the probability distributions of the patterns belonging to each class, which must either be specified or learned.

One can also take a discriminant analysis-based approach to classification: First a parametric form of the decision boundary (e.g., linear or quadratic) secified; then the 'best' decision boundary of the specified form is found based on the classification of training patterns. Such boundaries can be constructed using, for example, a mean squared error criterion. The direct boundary construction approaches are supported by Vapnik's philosophy If you possess a restricted amount of information for solving some problem, try to solve the problem directly and never solve a more general problem as an intermediate step. It is possible that the available information is sufficient for a direct solution but is insufficient for solving a more general intermediate problem. (Jain et al, 2000)

Voice Recognition

Automatic speaker recognition technology appears to have reached a sufficient level of maturity for realistic application in the field of forensic science. Forensic speaker recognition is the process of determining if a specific individual (suspected speaker) is the source of a questioned voice recording (trace). Forensic automatic speaker recognition (FASR) methods now may provide a coherent way of quantifying and presenting recorded voice as biometric evidence. In such methods, the biometric evidence consists of the quantified degree of similarity between speaker-dependent features extracted from the trace and speaker-dependent features extracted from recorded speech of a suspect. The interpretation of recorded voice as evidence in the forensic context presents particular challenges, including within-speaker (within-source) variability and between-speakers (between-sources) variability. Consequently, FASR methods must provide a statistical evaluation which gives the court an indication of the strength of the evidence given the estimated within-source and between-sources variabilities.

To assess the state of the technology, the Federal Bureau of Investigation (FBI) built a speech corpus that included multiple levels of increasing difficulty based on text-independence, channel-independence, speaking mode, and speech duration. An evaluation of multiple automatic speaker recognition programs indicated that a large GMM model-based recognition algorithm operating with features that are robust with respect to channel variations had the best performance. (Nakasone & Beck, 2000)

Drygajlo et al. (2003) described a Bayesian double statistical approach for interpreting recorded speech data. "The means proposed for dealing with them is through Bayesian inference and corpus based methodology. A probabilistic model – the odds form of Bayes' theorem and likelihood ratio – seems to be an adequate tool for assisting forensic experts in the speaker recognition domain to interpret this evidence. In forensic speaker recognition, statistical modelling techniques are based on the distribution of various features pertaining to the suspect's speech and its comparison to the distribution of the same features in a reference population with respect to the questioned recording. In this paper, the state-of-the-art automatic, text-independent speaker recognition system, using Gaussian mixture model (GMM), is adapted to the Bayesian interpretation (BI) framework to estimate the within-source variability of the suspected speaker and the between-sources variability, given the questioned recording. This double statistical approach (BI-GMM) gives an adequate solution for the interpretation of the recorded speech as evidence in the judicial process" (Drygajlo et al., 2003).

Facial Recognition

Forensic facial reconstruction is the reproduction of the lost or unknown facial features of an individual, for the purposes of recognition and identification. "It is generally accepted that facial reconstruction can be divided into four categories: (1) replacing and repositioning damaged or distorted soft tissues onto a skull; (2) the use of photographic transparencies and drawings in an identikit-type system; (3) the technique of graphic, photographic or video superimposition; (4) plastic or three-dimensional reconstruction of a face over a skull, using modeling clay" (Aulsebrook et al., 1995). Facial reconstruction has become a complementary technique in forensic anthropology, in addition to showing the relation between soft tissues and craniofacial bone structure and has major role in identification and biometrics in future.. In a recent forensic paleopathology case study, Gaytán et al., (2009) described using findings obtained from images of a skull with leontiasis ossea. This unique specimen is on display in the National Museum of Anthropology and History in Mexico. They found the skull to show "tissue overgrowth, periosteal bone proliferation, which produced a cortical and diploid thickening involving the entire bone matrix. Furthermore, the study of images, X-rays, and helical computed tomography "revealed generalized hyperostosis obliterating the maxillary and sphenoid sinuses, and two exuberant bony masses arising from the maxilla with encroachment of the anterior nasal opening." They suggested that "in order to reconstruct an image of the external appearance in life", they obtained a copy of the image using a stereolithography machine followed by application of a three dimensional (3-D) facial reconstruction technique to create an approximation of the external appearance of the specimen (Gaytán et al., 2009).

This study comes in early stages of the facial reconstruction and imaging technology. Gaytán et al., (2009) identified a series of problems when interpreting the cortical topography, the position of eyes and oral cavity. "In this sense, facial reconstruction allows only for a moderate investigation due to the limited information that can be obtained from the skull and the significant alterations observed (Gaytán et al., 2009). These problems included: (A) Choosing the facial thickness markers to be used. The location of the craniofacial points was a major problem, in particular the location of medial landmarks, specifically the nasion, supranasal, infranasal, and prosthion. (B) Recognition of the location of muscular and fibrous areas, as the marked deformities and tissue proliferation had significantly altered the places where muscles attached. (C) Exact location of the eyes - the eyeball must keep a relation based on the tangent that crosses the orbit longitudinally, with the center in the orbit (Gaytán et al., 2009).

Statistical assessment of facial structure and potential standardization of identifying data-point inputs for developing a reference database are yet to start in this area. Such standardization will require statistical assessment of the interaction between different image methods is helpful in developing a visual idea of an unknown face.

Surface scanning of the face of a suspect is presented as a way to better match the facial features with those of a perpetrator from CCTV footage. We performed a simple pilot study where we obtained facial surface scans of volunteers and then in blind trials tried to match these scans with 2D photographs of the faces of the volunteers. Fifteen male volunteers were surface scanned using a Polhemus FastSCAN Cobra Handheld Laser Scanner. Three photographs were taken of each volunteer's face in full frontal, profile and from above at an angle of 45° and also 45° laterally. Via special software (MIMICS© and Photoshop©) the surface scans were matched

with the photographs in blind trials. The matches were graded as: a good fit; possible fit; and no fit. All the surface scans and photos were matched correctly, although one surface scan could be matched with two angled photographs, meaning that the discriminatory value was 86.7%. We also tested the surface scanner in terms of reliability in establishing point measures on skulls, and compared with physical measurements performed by calipers. The variation was on average 1 mm for five cranial measures. We suggest how surface scanning might be applied in forensic facial identification (Lynnerup, 2009).

DNA PROFILING

Office of Justice Programs of the US Federal Government provides funding, training and assistance to ensure that forensic DNA reaches its full potential to solve crimes, protect the innocent and identify missing persons. Their web site can be accessed for online training and up-to-date information on DNA forensics (www.dna.gov). DNA analysis is a powerful tool because each person's DNA is unique (with the exception of identical twins). Therefore, DNA evidence collected from a crime scene can implicate or eliminate a suspect, similar to the use of fingerprints. It also can analyze unidentified remains through comparisons with DNA from relatives (DNAGov, 2010).

DNA-based human identification was instituted in 1985. "Since the development of the technology, experts called for setting of standards and use of proficiency tests for quality assurance measures. The response of the National Institute of Standards and Technology to DNA forensic standards needs was catalyzed by the Technical Working Group on DNA Analysis Methods, sponsored by the Federal Bureau of Investigation with funding provided by the National Institute of Justice. Standard reference materials were developed for the original technologies used in DNA identification and for the newer polymerase chain reaction-based technologies. Adoption of recommended standards developed through the Federal Bureau of Investigation-commissioned DNA Advisory Board show the acceptance of National Institute of Standards and Technology standards for calibration of laboratory protocols. New technologies will require a process of validation and continued testing through the use of proficiency tests, such as those provided through the College of American Pathologists. Robotics and parallel processing of samples will lead to increased efficiency in DNA testing. The use of DNA data banks of convicted felons will increase dramatically with the Federal Bureau of Investigation's national implementation of a computerized identification system known as the Combined DNA Index System. Finally, sample collection and training are of major concern for those who look at the long-term impact of DNA testing in forensic laboratories" (Reeder, 1999).

"The DNA Identification Act of 1994 was designed to improve the capability and quality control in state and local crime laboratories. This legislation also authorized the FBI director to establish a national DNA identification index and provides penalties for the disclosure of DNA data held by data banks that participate in the Combined DNA Index System (CODIS). The database CODIS facilitates the exchange of information in DNA data banks in different states. CODIS coordinates a data bank that will store digital information from DNA samples from thousands of convicted criminals across the country" (Reeder, 1999).

The advent of DNA profiling a big change occurred in the way the legal system viewed quantitative data. Now a quantitative approach is being requested in many areas, far removed from the original area of DNA profiling. The earlier research and development work is being applied and further work is being done to tackle the increasingly more complex cases which arise in bringing a sound statistical approach to the assessment of evidence (The Royal Statistical Society, 2005).

One example of casework that a forensic statistician may be involved with is DNA profiling, which is a powerful method of identification using genetics. Often, the evidence to be evaluated involves human (or sometimes animal) biological material such as blood, semen or vaginal fluid. Considerable work has been done in statistical and population genetics in assessing the importance of such evidence. Applications, however, are often not restricted to simple cases with one sample of DNA left at the scene of a crime and one suspect. Complications very often arise, for example because relatives may be involved, or the suspect may have been identified by a search through a DNA profile database, or the sample found at the crime scene may be a mixture of body fluids from more than one person. More advanced statistical methods are required in such situations (The Royal Statistical Society, 2005).

DNA-based lab tests are crucial evidence in many cases and are assuming more importance. A non-match results in exclusion of the suspect. However, decisions may ne definitive with a match or inconclusive. These results are based on estimation of frequencies of the alleles in the population. The question may be framed as:

1. Does the sample match the suspect (complete match/ partial match)?
2. Does the sample uniquely match the suspect (no others could match the profile)?

Such questions may be answered by measuring the frequency of alleles in populations to make a quantitative statement that expresses the rarity or common occurrence of DNA profile in the population (Planz, 2008) by assessing frequency at each locus and frequency across all loci and by examining polymorphisms and mutations. More than 99% of human DNA sequences are the same across the population. In general, mutations create variability in gene pool and are responsible for the intra-species variation, and are also an important contributor to evolution. The National Human

Figure 1. Why complicated statistical tests are needed in forensic sciences (adapted from Planz, 2008)

- Estimation of frequencies are needed for biological identification and DNA databases are needed for placing statistical weight on DNA profiles
- Specific genotypes are rare - about 99.5% of the genome is common between people. Variations that are unique to individuals are very rare
- Several of the genotypes in questions may not be easily seen in some populations
- Hardy Weinberg Equilibrium
- Linkage equilibrium (condition where genomes are composed of a random association of gametes. Linkage disequilibrium between two loci means that knowledge of a genotype at one locus gives at least a statistical clue as to the genotype at the other locus. It can exist either because of population substructure or because of physical linkage.
- Joint probability of unique features in the genome of an individual makes the features still rarer.

Genome Research Institute of NIH estimates that there are more sites that are polymorphic in the entire human population, "than the number of sites that differ between any particular pair of chromosomes. Altogether, there may be anywhere from 6 million to 30 million nucleotide positions in the genome at which variation can occur in the human population" (NHGRI, 2008). It also says that approximately one in every 100 to 500 bases in human DNA may be polymorphic.

Statistical tests form the basis for genetic analysis (Figure 1). Types of genetic analyses often used to establish identity include:

- **Genetic risk studies:** Risk studies establish the occurrence of greater risk of a trait/disease in persons with a certain genotype.
- **Segregation analyses:** The next step, after establishing the genetic basis is to establish the inheritance pattern of the trait in question.
- **Linkage studies:** Linkage implies cosegragation of loci (and not cosegragation of alleles) within families i.e. joint inheritance of genetic loci or alleles.
- **Association studies:** Association, resulting from direct gene involvement or linkage disequilibrium with the trait/ disease gene, is studied at the population level and allows fine mapping.

Tests results may be assessed and communicated in many ways such as by making a qualitative statement without any quantitative results, by stating the probability of exclusion; likelihood ratio estimates; presumptive genotype assignment based on peak heights

Several problems may impact decision making based on genetic tests. these include: appropriate control selection; avoiding selection bias resulting from definition of source and target population; genotyping errors; lack of quality control in molecular methods; inappropriate choice of marker/ allele/genotype frequency (for comparisons); failure to evaluate the mode of inheritance in a genetic disease; failure to account for the linkage disequilibrium (LD) structure of the gene (only haplotype-tagging markers will show the association, other markers within the same gene may fail to show an association); likelihood that the gene studied account for a small proportion of the variability in risk; True variability among different populations in allele frequencies, information bias, disease and exposure misclassification, and potential confounding from a variety of variables (measured and unmeasured) (Chattopadhyay, 2009).

According to the Hardy-Weinberg principle, allele and genotype frequencies in a population remain constant and are in equilibrium (the Hardy-Weinberg Equilibrium - HWE). This equilibrium is maintained through generations unless some specific disturbances occur. Such disturbances may include: non-random mating, mutations, selection, limited population size, random genetic drift and gene flow (HWP, 2009). In nature, however, HWE is rarely achieved.

It is important to remember that static allelic frequencies are used assuming that: the population size is large; allele pairs are independent, mating occurs randomly; no mutation occur, no migration (no exchange of alleles between populations), and no natural selection occurs. However, nature usually violates all these assumptions. This necessitates a test for departure from HWE. (usually performed employing using Pearson's chi-squared test, using the observed genotype frequencies obtained from the data and the expected genotype frequencies obtained under HWE (see potential sources of variations and errors above). If HWE is violated then the assumptions are violated and no allelic association test may be used. Lack of HWE in controls is usually an indication of problems with typing rather than selection, admixture, nonrandom mating or other reasons for violation of HWE (HWP, 2009).

Presence of systematic differences in allele frequencies between subpopulations in a population is called population stratification. Furthermore, pooling of data from two countries, might lead to population stratification (Wacholder et al., 2000; Millikan, 2001). Migration of individuals between populations is the main cause of population stratification. This phenomenon can pose serious problems in association studies using case control designs because associations could be found essentially due to the structure of the population resulting from population stratification and not due to loci associated with disease giving rise to spurious associations (Wacholder et al., 2000).

Forensic evidentiary samples routinely contain DNA from multiple contributors. The interpretation of these mixtures can be a challenging. The process of mixture interpretation can be straightforward or quite complex, involving laboratory and statistical considerations. While many of the technical challenges are routine features of forensic laboratory analysis and therefore cannot be eliminated, use of conservative statistical methods should obviate court objections and reduce the difficulties in mixture genotype assignment (Ladd et al, 2001).

In human identification, the victim's toothbrush is an invaluable personal item as the deposited cellular material contains DNA from which a reference profile can be produced. We also tested two commonly used DNA extraction methods: QIAamp1 DNA Mini Kit and Chelex1 100 to explore the efficiency of these protocols in recovering DNA from toothbrushes. In this experiment, volunteers brushed their teeth for 1, 7, 14, or 30 days. It was also found that, with a suitable method of recovery, DNA samples from five bundles of bristles from all of the toothbrushes generated complete profiles. Based on the experimental results, a general guideline concerning the appropriate extraction method and the quantity of the starting material for the analysis of DNA from toothbrushes could be suggested (Bandhaya and Panvisavas, 2008).

DNA Assessment

Steps in processing forensic DNA samples with Single Tandem Repeats (STR) markers are outlined in Figure 2. A brief description of statistical concepts used in DNA analysis is provided in Figure 3. The specific methods used for DNA typing are validated by individual laboratories to ensure that reliable results are obtained and before new technologies are implemented. DNA databases to match Montaret Davis to his crime scene are valuable tools and will continue to play an important role in law enforcement efforts (DNA.Gov, 2010).

The resulting DNA profile for a sample, which is a combination of individual STR genotypes, is compared to other samples. In the case of a forensic investigation, these other samples would include known reference samples such as the

Figure 2. Outline of processing forensic DNA samples with Single Tandem Repeats (STR) markers (Adapted from DNA.Gov) and identification if "unique profiles"

Steps in DNA Testing
- DNA extraction from sample
- Measurement of DNA quantity
- DNA isolation
- DNA copying using PCR
- Separation of PCR products to assess STR regions. Separation is usually carried out by: slab gel and capillary electrophoresis. Fluorescence detection methods have greatly aided the sensitivity and ease of measuring PCR-amplified STR alleles.
- Genotyping - determination of number of repeats in a DNA sequence
- The resulting DNA profile for a sample, is compared to other samples
- Reporting of DNA testing

Types of Samples Suitable for DNA Testing
- Questioned or Unknown Samples
- Samples From Unidentified Bodies
- Reference Samples From Known Individuals
- Samples to Use When No Conventional Reference Samples Are Available
- Reference Samples From Individuals Who Have Been Transfused
- Use of Samples From Relatives for Testing
- Determination of Paternity or Maternity of a Child or Fetus

Possible Results From DNA Tests
- Inclusions
- Exclusions
- Inconclusive Results

Commonly Conducted Analysis
- PCR
- STR
- Y-chromosome analysis (Y-STR)
- Mitochondrial analysis

Unique Profile Identification
- Identify genotype of suspect and demarcate identifying alleles
- Check for zygosity (homozygous/ heterozygous)
- Assess population prevalence of genotype
- Calculate genotype frequency at each loci
- Calculate overall genotype frequency for the suspect

Worked example: If the frequency of allele "A" is 0.4; then the frequency of genotype AA is: 0.4 x 0.4 = 0.16 (16%). If the allele frequency of "B" is 0.6 and "C" is 0.3, the frequency of genotype BC is: 0.6 x 0.3 = 0.18 (18%). The overall genotype frequency for someone with alleles: AA and BC is: 0.16 x 0.18 = 0.0288 (2.88%). Identification of individuals with "unique" genotypes is based on such identification of characteristics that era so rare so that the genotype frequency is very low imparting a "unique" profile for the individual.

Potential Sources of Errors in DNA Profiling
Contamination during collection, mixed samples, amplification errors, degradation, peak height imbalance during primer building, dye pull up, spikes, DNA mutation

Figure 3. Outline of important genetic and statistical concepts in DNA evidence assessment

- Chromosomes: Bundles of DNA material that carry biological characteristics across generations. There are two sets of 23 different chromosomes, each set being contributed by one parent.
- Sex chromosomes: One set is "sex chromosomes" (they determine the biological sex of the child): contribution from Mother: "X chromosome"; contribution from father: "Y chromosome". The "Sex chromosome" in men: XY; in women: XX.
- Allele is a DNA sequence for a gene that is located at a specific position on a specific chromosome. Alleles determine distinct traits that can be passed on from parents to the child. Each parent contributes one allele to the child. Allele also serves as a genetic marker variant. Alleles are usually represented by letters and numbers to represent their characteristic and contribution from parent. For example $A_1 A_1$ indicates allele of type "A_1" was contributed by each parent; whereas $A_1 A_2$ indicates that one parent contributed "A_1" and the other contributed "A_2". Allele frequency is the proportion of the allele found in the population.
- Homozygous: Both alleles for a train are the same: For example: $A_1 A_1$.
- Heterozygous: Two different alleles contribute to a single trait: for example: $A_1 A_2$.
- Probability: Quantitative term calculated by dividing the number of events that occur (outcomes) by the number of possible outcomes. In case of tossing a coin, the possible outcomes are 2 ("heads"/ "tails"). Therefore in any one toss, the probability of getting "heads" [P(h)] is ½ = 0.5 or 50% (i.e. one heads divided by two possible outcomes). The probability of getting tails [P(t)] is also 50%.
- Joint probability: Probability of two or more events occurring together.
- Product rule (rule of multiplication): The probability that independent events will occur simultaneously is the product of their individual probabilities. Therefore the probability that two events A and B will occur together is: P(A and B): P(A) x P(B).
- Sum rule (addition rule): The probability of an event that can occur in two or more independent ways is the sum of the separate probabilities of the different ways. Therefore the probability that two events A and B will occur together is: P(A or B): P(A) + P(B).
- Locus: Location of allele on the chromosome.
- Linkage equilibrium: State where the haplotype proportion in the population have the same value even if the alleles at each locus were to combine at random. It is defined in terms if disequilibrium i.e. linkage equilibrium occurs when there is no linkage disequilibrium. Linkage disequilibrium is defined as the non-random association of alleles at two or more loci which may/ may not be on the same chromosome.
- Haplotype: A combination of alleles at one or different locus/loci on the chromosome that are transmitted together.
- Genotype: Profile of genes (DNA) in an individual. Groups of individuals may share common DNA profile, but small sections may differ, giving rise to the possibility of identifying "unique" profile for each individual.
- Hardy-Weinberg Principle (Theory): Allele and genotype proportions in a population generally remain constant across generations (i.e. they remain in equilibrium) unless specific influences are introduced in the populations that may disturb the equilibrium.
Genotype frequency: Proportion of a certain genotype found in the population. For example, if the frequency of allele "A" is 0.4; then the frequency of genotype AA is: 0.4 x 0.4 = 0.16 (16%).

tion between the groups, African-Americans and Caucasians have different population databases for comparison purposes.

Finally a case report or paternity test result is generated. This report typically includes the random match probability for the match in question. This random match probability is the chance that a randomly selected individual from a population will have an identical STR profile or combination of genotypes at the DNA markers tested (DNAGov, 2010).

Searching a Database of DNA Profiles

When evidence from one crime scene is compared with evidence from another scene using CODIS,

victim or suspects that are compared to the crime scene evidence. With paternity investigations, a child's genotype would be compared to his or her mother's and the alleged father(s) under investigation. If there is not a match between the questioned sample and the known sample, then the samples may be considered to have originated from different sources. The term used for failure to match between two DNA profiles is 'exclusion'.

If a match or 'inclusion' results, then a comparison of the DNA profile is made to a population database, which is a collection of DNA profiles obtained from unrelated individuals of a particular ethnic group. For example, due to genetic varia-

those crime scenes can be linked to the same perpetrator locally, statewide, and nationally. DNA is also a powerful tool because when biological evidence from crime scenes is collected and stored properly, forensically valuable DNA can be found on evidence that may be decades old. Therefore, old cases that were previously thought unsolvable may contain valuable DNA evidence capable of identifying the perpetrator. DNA collection and analysis gives the criminal justice field a powerful tool for convicting the guilty and exonerating the innocent" (DNAGov, 2010).

In 1986, Paul Hildwin was convicted of murdering Vronzettie Cox, a 42-year-old woman whose body was found in the trunk of her car 25 years ago (the case of Paul C. Hildin vs. State of Florida (http://www.law.fsu.edu/library/flsupct/89658/89658b2.pdf), In 2003, the DNA test results proved that Hildwin was not the man whose semen and saliva were found on key items of evidence in the vehicle of the woman he was convicted of murdering in 1986. On June 9th, 2010, a petition has been filed asking the Florida Supreme Court to order a DNA database search (CODIS and Florida's state database system) that could prove beyond any doubt whether a Hernando County man on death row, Paul Hildwin, was wrongfully convicted.

Controversy over DNA profile evidence was generated in 1999 stemming from a 1996 report on DNA profile evidence issued by the U.S. National Research Council (NRC). The issue concerns the evidential weight of a DNA profile match when the match results from a search through a profile database (Balding, 2002). The differing viewpoints of the statisticians involved in the NRC report and authors raising the issue (Stockmarr, 1999) lead to dramatically different assessments of evidence. Meester and Sjerps (2003) raised the question: Does the evidential strength of a DNA match depend on whether the suspect was identified through database search or through other evidence ("probable cause")? They suggested that "by concentrating on the posterior odds", the

problems could be eliminated. The central cause of the conflict stems from Bayesian use of posterior probabilities in assessing additional evidence over a single match. At the heart of the matter is the manner in which the statistics are calculated (the authors cited above used likelihood ratios). The two quantities differ substantially and have given rise to the DNA database search controversy. Recently, Storvik and Egeland (2007) have suggested that "a P-value in a frequentist hypothesis setting is approximately equal to the result of the np rule. We argue, however, that a more reasonable procedure in this case is to use conditional testing, in which case a P-value directly related to posterior probabilities and the likelihood ratio is obtained. This way of viewing the problem bridges the gap between the Bayesian and frequentist approaches. At the same time it indicates that the np rule should not be used to quantify evidence" (Storvik & Egeland, 2007).

What is "Uniqueness"?

Generally, "uniqueness" implies existence of a set of characteristics in a person that are not present in any one else. In forensic DNA analysis, this means that genotype frequency of the suspect should be extremely low (See Figure 3 for common terms and Figure 2 for calculating genotype frequency). In general, we need to be able to distinguish between two individuals with certainty, which characterizes the power of discrimination to the analyses (power of discrimination is the ability of individualizing the suspect). Power of exclusion, on the hand implies the ability to exclude a genotype. Power of exclusion and calculation of probabilities for exclusion has been controversial. It is calculated as: 1 − sum of squares of all the expected phenotype/genotypes (Planz, 2008).

Random match probability is defined as the probability that two randomly selected persons will have the same genotype just by chance alone (i.e. the sum of the squares of the observed genotype (or phenotype) frequencies in a database). Therefore, this weighs heavily the fact that the database is a true representation of the genotype frequencies of the population. This probability should be as low as possible to make a call for unique match for a suspect against a database.

To generate frequency estimates that may be as rare as one in a billion, or even one in a trillion, from a data base of several hundred individuals, forensic laboratories typically follow a three-step procedure. First, they estimate the frequency of each allele in the DNA profile by simply counting to determine the proportion of people in the data base who have it. If two percent of the alleles (of a particular locus) are type A and three percent are type B, their frequencies would be stated as .02 and .03 respectively.

Second, they estimate the frequency of each genotype by using the formula 2pq, where p and q are the frequencies of the two alleles in the genotype. Suppose, for example, that a genotype consisted of alleles A and B. The frequency of genotype AB would be estimated to be $2 \times .02 \times .03 = .0012$ (approximately 1 in 833).[29] This formula assumes that the frequencies of the two alleles in a genotype are statistically independent and may significantly underestimate the frequency of genotypes if the allele frequencies are not independent.

Third, they estimate the frequency of the overall DNA profile by multiplying the frequencies of each genotype. For example, suppose that there is a three-locus match between the suspect and the evidentiary sample. At the first locus, both have genotype AB, which has an estimated frequency of 0.0012; at the second locus, both have genotype CD, which has an estimated frequency of 0.005; at the third locus both have genotype EF, which has an estimated frequency of 0.01. An analyst would typically report that the frequency of the overall profile, across the three loci, is .0012 x .005 x .01 = .00000006, or one in 16.7 million. This formula, sometimes called the product rule, assumes that the frequencies of the genotypes are statistically independent and may significantly underestimate

the frequency of the multilocus genotype if the frequencies are not independent. (Krane, 2003)

One of the major criticisms has been that the reference database, which is a "convenience sample" from compilation of names of criminals, blood donors and paternity case litigants, is a convenience database, and therefore does not represent population frequencies of genotypes which lead to statistical validity issues related to the results. Forensic laboratories generally provide estimates of the frequency of a matching DNA profiles among members of three broad racial groups in North America. In parentage testing using DNA markers, the formulae for calculating the probability of exclusion generally overstate the power of a test battery by considering its ability to exclude a random person. It is know that in many cases, in particular immigration applications, the false father is more likely to be a relative, e.g. brother, of the true father than an unrelated man (Fung et al., 2002).

There may occur situations when alleles are not represented in the population database (or are extremely rare in the database itself). However, although ideally, frequencies of all genotypes should be known and represented in the reference database, that is not the case.

Recent discussions on a forensic discussion group highlighted the prevalence of a practice in the application of inclusion probabilities when dropout is possible that is of significant concern. "In such cases, there appears to be an unpublished practice of calculation of an inclusion probability only for those loci at which the profile of interest (hereafter the suspect) is fully included among the alleles present in the crime scene sample and to omit those loci at which the suspect has alleles that are not fully represented among the alleles in the mixture. The danger is that this approach may produce apparently strong evidence against a surprisingly large fraction of non-contributors. In this paper, the risk associated with the approach of ignoring loci with discordant alleles is assessed by simulation" (Curran & Buckleton,

2010). However, there are a series of potential errors that may lead to problems with identification using DNA profiles, such as: Contamination during collection, mixed samples, amplification errors, degradation, peak height imbalance during primer building, dye pull up, spikes, DNA mutation related errors (tri-allelic patterns; off ladder alleles), data: signal/noise ratio, allelic imbalance, examiner bias.

Computer Programs for Statistical Genetics

Genetic analyses leading to population genetics estimates, linkage analyses, genome analyses, comparative genomics, genotype assessment, individual identification, genetic diversity in populations and cross-matching against large databases are possible only because of the substantial computer analytical power that are available today.

Table 1 provides a working list of commonly available statistical; programs and their websites. A comprehensive list of genetic analysis programs is available at: http://www.nslij-genetics.org/soft/.

The analysis of genetic diversity within species is vital for understanding evolutionary processes at the population level and at the genomic level. A large quantity of data can now be produced at an unprecedented rate, requiring the use of dedicated computer programs to extract all embedded information. Several statistical packages have been recently developed, which offer a panel of standard and more sophisticated analyses (Excoffier & Heckel, 2006). For a thorough description of functionalities, special features and assumptions of commonly used programs, how those programs can interoperate, and discussion of new directions that could lead to improved software and analyses the reader is referred to an excellent review of these programs provided by Excoffier and Heckel (2006).

PRESENTATION OF STATISTICAL EVIDENCE IN LEGAL SETTINGS

One of the key criteria of presenting forensic evidence is to be able to establish causation between the charges and the charged i.e. to establish whether the offence was committed as charged or not. The information, analyses and opinion of the Statistician should also be communicated to others in clear and unambiguous terms to those concerned, who may/ may not have statistical technical understanding. Forensic statisticians are often required to attend court cases as "expert witnesses". This involves reporting calculated probabilities, or other statistical measures, to the jury, and explaining to them how the calculations were performed. This is a challenge in itself, as the jury will typically consist of people who have little knowledge of statistical methods, and is further complicated by the need to choose careful wording (so as not to "lead" the jury into a decision on guilt or innocence of a defendant). (The Royal Statistical Society, 2005).

"Confusion may occasionally arise through wrong usage of the terms allele, gene, or marker in an association study. Some investigators state that they compare allele or haplotype frequencies, but only count each individual once. They, therefore, refer to what used to be phenotype frequencies in serological HLA studies, or in the case of genotyping studies, to marker frequencies (MF), which correspond to inferred phenotype frequencies if it is an expressed genotype. Allele (AF) or haplotype frequency (HF) is analogous to gene frequency (GF) in that they are always calculated in terms of the total number of chromosomes not individuals" (Dorak, 2007). Other common statistical issues that impact genetic epidemiology studies include: lack of power, excessive sub-group analyses and post-hoc analyses being treated as a-priori instead of exploratory analyses, possible one-tailed tests, ignoring multiple comparison; ignoring correlated data (e.g. using chi-square test where McNemar's

Table 1. Programs dealing with population genetics and statistics

Program	Website
Individual purpose programs	
BayesAss+	http://www.rannala.org/labpages/software.html
BAPS	http://www.rni.helsinki.fi/~jic/bapspage.html
GeneClass	http://www.montpellier.inra.fr/URLB/index.html
Geneland	http://www.inapg.inra.fr/ens_rech/mathinfo/personnel/guillot/Geneland.html
NewHybrids	http://ib.berkeley.edu/labs/slatkin/eriq/software/software.htm
Structure	http://pritch.bsd.uchicago.edu/software/structure2_1.html
Multipurpose programs	
Arlequin	http://cmpg.unibe.ch/software/arlequin3/
DnaSP	http://www.ub.es/dnasp/
FSTAT	http://www2.unil.ch/popgen/softwares/fstat.htm
GDA	http://hydrodictyon.eeb.uconn.edu/people/plewis/software.php
Genepop	http://ftp.cefe.cnrs.fr/PC/MSDOS/GENEPOP
Genetix	http://www.univ-montp2.fr/~genetix/genetix/genetix.htm
MEGA	http://www.megasoftware.net/
MSA	http://i122server.vu-wien.ac.at/MSA/MSA_download.html
SPAGeDi	http://www.ulb.ac.be/sciences/ecoevol/spagedi.html
Specialized programs	
BATWING	http://www.mas.ncl.ac.uk/~nijw/
COLONISE	http://www-leca.ujf-grenoble.fr/logiciels.htm
FDIST2	http://www.rubic.rdg.ac.uk/~mab/software.html
Hickory	http://darwin.eeb.uconn.edu/hickory/hickory.html
IM	http://lifesci.rutgers.edu/~heylab/HeylabSoftware.htm#IM
LAMARC	http://evolution.gs.washington.edu/lamarc/lamarc_prog.html
Migrate	http://popgen.csit.fsu.edu/
MSVAR	http://www.rubic.rdg.ac.uk/~mab/software.html
Conversion programs	
Convert	http://www.agriculture.purdue.edu/fnr/html/faculty/Rhodes/Students%20and%20Staff/glaubitz/software.htm
Formatomatic	http://taylor0.biology.ucla.edu/~manoukis/Pub_programs/Formatomatic/

A comprehensive list of genetic analysis software is available at: http://www.nslij-genetics.org/soft/ (last update: June 5, 2010; last accessed June 9, 2010).

test should be used); and non-consideration of alternative genetic models (Chattopadhyay, 2009).

Referring to the DNA database search controversy mentioned above, Balding (2002) pointed out the need to use better communication strategies by Statisticians: "One noticeable feature of the controversy under discussion is that Stockmarr and the statisticians behind the NRC report had little practical experience of DNA profile evidence in the courtroom prior to making their contributions to the debate. The criminal legal setting has some customs and requirements that appear to conflict with established statistical conventions. For example, the notion that evidence that has led to the identification of the suspect should not subsequently be used as evidence in court is analogous with some modes of statistical reasoning. But it is inconsistent with legal practice and would, I believe, be regarded as absurd by legal commentators. A statistician may in some instances reasonably take the view that it is the legal practice that is flawed, not the statistical conventions" (Balding, 2002).

ACKNOWLEDGMENT

The views expressed in this chapter are those of the author and do not represent the position of NIH/ NIDCR/ United States Government

REFERENCES

Aulsebrook, W. A., Iscan, M. Y., Slabbert, J. H., & Becker, P. (1995). Superimposition and reconstruction in forensic facial identification: A survey. *Forensic Science International, 75*(2-3), 101–120. doi:10.1016/0379-0738(95)01770-4

Balding, D. J. (2002). The DNA database search controversy. *Biometrics, 58*(1), 241–244. doi:10.1111/j.0006-341X.2002.00241.x

Bandhaya, A., & Panvisavas, N. (2008). Optimization of DNA recovery from toothbrushes. *Forensic Science International. Genetics Supplement Series, 1*, 9–10. doi:10.1016/j.fsigss.2007.10.053

Chattopadhyay, A. (2010). *Oral health epidemiology: Principles and practice*. Sudbury, MA: Jones & Bartlett publishers.

Curran, J.M. & Buckleton, J. (2010). Inclusion probabilities and dropout. *Journal of Forensic Science*.

DNA.gov. (2010). DNA *initiative: Advancing criminal justice through DNA technology*. Retrieved June 9, 2010, from www page: http://www.dna.gov/more/contactus/

Dolhenty, J. (2010). *Logic and critical thinking*. The Jonathan Dolhenty Archive.

Dorak, M. T. (2007). Statistical analysis in HLA and disease association studies. Retrieved from www.dorak.info/hla/stat.html

Drygajlo, A., Meuwly, D., & Alexander, A. (2003). Statistical methods and Bayesian interpretation of evidence in forensic automatic speaker recognition. In [Geneva, Switzerland.]. *Proceedings of Eurospeech, 2003*, 689–692.

Excoffier, L., & Heckel, G. (2006). Computer programs for population genetics data analysis: A survival guide. *Nature Reviews. Genetics, 7*(10), 745–758. doi:10.1038/nrg1904

Fukunaga, K. (1990). *Introduction to Statistical pattern recognition* (2nd ed.). Academic Press.

Fung, W. K., Chung, Y. K., & Wong, D. M. (2002). Power of exclusion revisited: Probability of excluding relatives of the true father from paternity. *International Journal of Legal Medicine, 116*(2), 64–67. doi:10.1007/s004140100210

Gaytán, E., Mansilla-Lory, J., Leboreiro, I., & Pineda, S. C. (2009). Facial reconstruction of a pathological case. *Forensic Science, Medicine, and Pathology, 5*(2), 95–99. doi:10.1007/s12024-009-9088-6

Gillies, D. (1998). The Duhem thesis and the Quine thesis. In M. Curd & J.A. (Eds.), *Philosophy of science: The central issues*. (pp. 302-319). New York: Norton

Jain, A. K., Duin, R. P. W., & Mao, J. (2000). Statistical pattern recognition: A review. *IEEE Transactions on Pattern Analysis and Machine Intelligence, 22*, 4–37. doi:10.1109/34.824819

Krane, D. (2003). Random match probability. In *Proceedings of Forensic Bioinformatics 2nd Annual Conference on Statistics and DNA Profiling*. August 29-30, 2003. Retrieved on June 9, 2010, from http://www.bioforensics.com/conference/RMP/index.html

Ladd, C., Lee, H. C., Yang, N., & Bieber, F. R. (2001). Interpretation of complex forensic DNA mixtures. *Croatian Medical Journal, 42*(3), 244–246.

Lynnerup, N., Clausen, M. L., Kristoffersen, A. M., & Steglich-Arnholm, H. (2009). Facial recognition and laser surface scan: A pilot study. *Forensic Science, Medicine, and Pathology, 5*(3), 167–173. doi:10.1007/s12024-009-9094-8

Meester, R., & Sjerps, M. (2003). The evidential value in the DNA database search controversy and the two-stain problem. *Biometrics, 59*(3), 727–732. doi:10.1111/1541-0420.00084

Millikan, R. C. (2001). Re: Population stratification in epidemiologic studies of common genetic variants and cancer: Quantification of bias. *Journal of the National Cancer Institute, 93,* 156. doi:10.1093/jnci/93.2.156

Nakasone, H., & Beck, S. D. (2001). Forensic automatic speaker recognition. *2001: A Speaker Odyssey - The Speaker Recognition Workshop.* June 18-22, 2001, Crete, Greece.

NHGRI. (2008). National Human Genome Research Institute methods for discovering and scoring single nucleotide polymorphisms. Retrieved from www.genome.gov/10001029

Planz, J. V. (2008). *Validation theory and its effect on the interpretation of DNA mixtures.* 19th International Symposium on Human Identification, October 15, 2008. Hollywood, CA.

Poole, C. (2001). Low p-values or narrow confidence intervals: Which are more durable? *Epidemiology (Cambridge, Mass.), 12,* 291–294. doi:10.1097/00001648-200105000-00005

Reeder, D. J. (1999). Impact of DNA typing on standards and practice in the forensic community. *Archives of Pathology & Laboratory Medicine, 123*(11), 1063–1065.

Stockmarr, A. (1999). Likelihood ratios for evaluating DNA evidence when the suspect is found through a database search. *Biometrics, 55,* 671–677. doi:10.1111/j.0006-341X.1999.00671.x

Storvik, G., & Egeland, T. (2007). The DNA database search controversy revisited: Bridging the Bayesian-frequentist gap. *Biometrics, 63*(3), 922–925. doi:10.1111/j.1541-0420.2007.00751.x

Taroni, F., Bozza, S., & Aitken, C. (2005). Decision analysis in forensic science. *Journal of Forensic Sciences, 50*(4), 894–905. doi:10.1520/JFS2004443

The Royal Statistical Society. (2005). *A career as a forensic statistician.* Retrieved June 9, 2010, from http://www.rss.org.uk/pdf/Careers_forensic4.pdf

Wacholder, S. (2000). Population stratification in Epidemiologic studies of common genetic variants and cancer: Quantification of bias. *Journal of the National Cancer Institute, 92,* 1151–1158. doi:10.1093/jnci/92.14.1151

Wells, C. G., & Hintze, J. M. (2007). Dealing with assumptions underlying statistical tests. *Psychology in the Schools, 44,* 495–502. doi:10.1002/pits.20241

KEY TERMS AND DEFINTIONS

Accuracy: Accuracy, on the other hand, assesses the degree to which a variable actually represents what it is supposed to represent.

Duhem-Quine Thesis: The Duhem-Quine thesis states that it is impossible to test a scientific hypothesis in isolation of its environment because background assumptions about associated issues form the basis of empirical tests.

Hardy-Weinberg Principle: The Hardy-Weinberg principle states that allele and genotype frequencies in a population remain constant and are in equilibrium; and this equilibrium is maintained through generations unless some specific disturbances occur.

Precision: Precision is the degree to which a variable has nearly the same value when measured several times.

Statistical Pattern Recognition: Statistical pattern recognition covers all stages of an investigation including formulation of the problem, data collection by employing discrimination and classification assessment of results and interpretation.

Compilation of References

Abdel-Mottaleb, M., Nomir, O., Nassar, D., Fahmy, G., & Ammar, H. (2003). Challenges of developing an automated dental identification system. *IEEE Mid-West Symposium for Circuits and Systems*, (pp. 411–414). Cairo, Egypt.

Acock, A. (2008). *A gentle introduction to Stata* (2nd ed.). Texas: Stata Press.

(1968). Reduction of dimensionality in biological diffusion processes. In Adam, G., & Delbruck, M. (Eds.), *Structural chemistry and molecular biology*. San Francisco: W.H. Freeman and Company.

Adams, M. D., Dubnick, M., Kerlavage, A. R., Moreno, R., Kelley, J. M., & Utterback, T. R. (1992). Sequence identification of 2,375 human brain genes. *Nature*, *355*(6361), 632–634. doi:10.1038/355632a0

Adams, M. D., Kelley, J. M., Gocayne, J. D., Dubnick, M., Polymeropoulos, M. H., & Xiao, H. (1991). Complementary DNA sequencing: Expressed sequence tags and human genome project. *Science*, *252*(5013), 1651–1656. doi:10.1126/science.2047873

Adams, J. E. (1997). Single and dual energy X-ray absorptiometry. In Guglielmi, G., Passariello, R., & Genant, H. K. (Eds.), *Bone densitometry: An update. European Radiology, 7(2), S20–S31*.

Aghayev, E., Yen, K., Sonnenschein, M., Jackowski, C., Thali, M., & Vock, P. (2005). Pneumomediastinum and soft tissue emphysema of the neck in post-mortem CT and MRI: A new vital sign in hanging? *Forensic Science International*, *153*, 181–188. doi:10.1016/j.forsciint.2004.09.124

Aguda, B., Kim, Y., Piper-Hunter, M., Friedman, A., & Marsh, C. (2008). MicroRNA regulation of a cancer network: Consequences of the feedback loops involving miR-17-92, E2F, and Myc. [PNAS]. *Proceedings of the National Academy of Sciences of the United States of America*, *105*(50), 19678–19683. doi:10.1073/pnas.0811166106

Akiba, N., Saitoh, N., & Kuroki, K. (2007). Fluorescence spectra and images of latent fingerprints excited with a tunable laser in the ultraviolet region. *Journal of Forensic Sciences*, *52*(5), 1103–1107. doi:10.1111/j.1556-4029.2007.00532.x

Akpata, E. S. (1975). Molar tooth attrition in a selected group of Nigerians. *Community Dentistry and Oral Epidemiology*, *3*, 132–135. doi:10.1111/j.1600-0528.1975.tb00294.x

Alberty, R. A. (1959). The rate equation for an enzymatic reaction. In Boyer, P. (Eds.), *Kinetics, thermodynamics, mechanisms and basic properties. The enzymes* (pp. 143–155). New York: Academic Press.

Alon, U., Barkai, N., Notterman, D. A., Gish, K., Ybarra, S., Mack, D., et al. (1999). Broad patterns of gene expression revealed by clustering analysis of tumor and normal colon tissues probed by oligonucleotide arrays. In *Proceedings of the National Academy of Sciences of the United States of America*, (pp. 6745-6750).

Altman, N. S., & Hua, J. (2006). Extending the loop design for two-channel microarray experiments. *Genetical Research*, *88*(3), 153–163. doi:10.1017/S0016672307008476

Altman, D. (1991). *Practical statistics for medical research*. London: Chapman & Hall.

Alvarez-Garcia, I., & Miska, E. A. (2006). MicroRNA functions in animal development and human disease. *Development*, *132*, 4653–4662. doi:10.1242/dev.02073

Ambros, V. (2004). The functions of animal microRNAs. *Nature*, *431*, 350–355. doi:10.1038/nature02871

American Board of Forensic Odontology. (2010). *Online diplomat's manual.* (p. 116). Retrieved from http://www.abfo.org

Andenmatten, M. A., Thali, M. J., Kneubuehl, B. P., Oesterhelweg, L., Ross, S., & Spendlove, D. (2008). Gunshot injuries detected by post-mortem multislice computed tomography (MSCT): A feasibility study. *Legal Medicine*, *10*, 287–292. doi:10.1016/j.legalmed.2008.03.005

Andersen, S. T., & Bertelsen, F. (1972). Scanning electron microscope studies of pollen of cereals and other grasses. *Grana*, *12*, 79–86. doi:10.1080/00173137209428830

Arbter, K., Snyder, W. E., Burhardt, H., & Hirzinge, G. (2002). Content-based image retrieval using Fourier descriptors on a logo database. *Journal of Pattern Recognition*, *3*, 521–524.

Aronson, D. G., & Weinberger, H. F. (1975). *Nonlinear diffusion in population genetics, combustion, and nerve pulse propagation.* New York: Springer–Verlag.

Audic, S., & Claverie, J. M. (1997). The significance of digital gene expression profiles. *Genome Research*, *7*(10), 986–995.

Aulehla, A., & Pourquie, O. (2006). On periodicity and directionality of somitogenesis. *Anatomy and Embryology*, *211*(7), 3–8. doi:10.1007/s00429-006-0124-y

Aulsebrook, W. A., Iscan, M. Y., Slabbert, J. H., & Becker, P. (1995). Superimposition and reconstruction in forensic facial identification: A survey. *Forensic Science International*, *75*(2-3), 101–120. doi:10.1016/0379-0738(95)01770-4

Axelrod, D., & Wang, M. D. (1994). Reduction-of-dimensionality kinetics at reaction-limited cell surface receptors. *Biophysical Journal*, *66*(3 Pt 1), 588–600. doi:10.1016/S0006-3495(94)80834-3

Baccino, E., Ubelaker, D. H., Hayek, L. C., & Zerilli, A. (1999). Evaluation of seven methods of estimating age at death from mature human skeletal remains. *Journal of Forensic Sciences*, *44*(5), 931–936.

Bailey, L. C. Jr, Searls, D. B., & Overton, G. C. (1998). Analysis of EST-driven gene annotation in human genomic sequence. *Genome Research*, *8*(4), 362–376.

Bailly, G., Bérar, M., Elisei, F., & Odisio, M. (2003). Audio-visual speech synthesis. *International Journal of Speech Technology*, *6*(4), 331–346. doi:10.1023/A:1025700715107

Bainbridge, M. N., Warren, R. L., Hirst, M., Romanuik, T., Zeng, T., & Go, A. (2006). Analysis of the prostate cancer cell line LNCaP transcriptome using a sequencing-by-synthesis approach. *BMC Genomics*, *7*, 246. doi:10.1186/1471-2164-7-246

Baker, L. (2009). Biomolecular applications. In Blau, S., & Ubelaker, D. H. (Eds.), *Handbook of forensic anthropology and archaeology* (pp. 322–334). Walnut Creek, CA: Left Coast Press, Inc.

Balding, D. J. (2003). Likelihood-based inference for genetic correlation coefficients. *Theoretical Population Biology*, *63*(3), 221–230. doi:10.1016/S0040-5809(03)00007-8

Balding, D. J., & Nichols, R. A. (1994). DNA profile match probability calculation: How to allow for population stratification, relatedness, database selection, and single bands. *Forensic Science International*, *64*(2-3), 125–140. doi:10.1016/0379-0738(94)90222-4

Balding, D. J. (2002). The DNA database search controversy. *Biometrics*, *58*(1), 241–244. doi:10.1111/j.0006-341X.2002.00241.x

Bandhaya, A., & Panvisavas, N. (2008). Optimization of DNA recovery from toothbrushes. *Forensic Science International. Genetics Supplement Series*, *1*, 9–10. doi:10.1016/j.fsigss.2007.10.053

Banks, L. M., van Juijk, C., & Genant, H. K. (1995). Radiographic technique for assessing osteoporotic vertebral fracture. In Genant, H. K., Jergas, M., & van Juijk, C. (Eds.), *Vertebral fracture in osteoporosis* (pp. 131–147). San Francisco: University of California Osteoporosis Research Group.

Bar-Even, A., Paulsson, J., Maheshri, N., Carmi, M., O'Shea, E., & Pilpel, Y. (2006). Noise in protein expression scales with natural protein abundance. *Nature Genetics*, *38*(6), 636–643. doi:10.1038/ng1807

Barnett, E., & Nordin, B. E. C. (1960). Radiographic diagnosis of osteoporosis: New approach. *Clinical Radiology, 11*, 166–174. doi:10.1016/S0009-9260(60)80012-8

Barrett, P. J. (1980). The shape of rock particles, a critical review. *Sedimentology, 27*, 291–303. doi:10.1111/j.1365-3091.1980.tb01179.x

Barrett, J. C., & Kawasaki, E. S. (2003). Microarrays: The use of oligonucleotides and cDNA for the analysis of gene expression. *Drug Discovery Today, 8*(3), 134–141. doi:10.1016/S1359-6446(02)02578-3

Barrett, T., Troup, D. B., Wilhite, S. E., Ledoux, P., Rudnev, D., & Evangelista, C. (2009). NCBI GEO: Archive for high-throughput functional genomic data. *Nucleic Acids Research, 37*(Database issue), D5–D15. doi:10.1093/nar/gkn764

Barrow, H. G., Tenenbuam, J. M., Bolles, R. C., & Wolf, H. C. (1977). Parametric Correspondence and Chamfer matching: Two new techniques for image matching. In *Proceedings of the 5th International Joint Conference on Artificial Intelligence,* (pp. 659–663). Cambridge, MA, USA.

Bartel, D. (2004). MicroRNAs: Genomics, biogenesis, mechanism and function. *Cell, 116*, 281–297. doi:10.1016/S0092-8674(04)00045-5

Basso, C., & Vetter, T. (2005). Statistically motivated 3D faces reconstruction. In Buzug, T. M., Sigl, K.-M., Bongartz, J., & Prüfer, K. (Eds.), *Facial reconstruction* (pp. 450–469). München: Wolters/Kluwer.

Bauer, E., & Kohavi, R. (1999). An empirical comparison of voting classification algorithms: Bagging, boosting, and variants. *Machine Learning, 36*(1-2), 105–139. doi:10.1023/A:1007515423169

Bautin, N. N. (1984). *Povedenie dinamichnih sistem v blizi granits oblasti ustoichivisti.* Nauka, Moskva.

Beesley, K. M., Damaskinos, S., & Dixon, A. E. (1995). Fingerprint imaging with a confocal scanning laser macroscope. *Journal of Forensic Sciences, 40*(1), 10–17.

Beissbarth, T., Fellenberg, K., Brors, B., Arribas-Prat, R., Boer, J., & Hauser, N. C. (2000). Processing and quality control of DNA array hybridization data. *Bioinformatics (Oxford, England), 16*(11), 1014–1022. doi:10.1093/bioinformatics/16.11.1014

Belintsev, B. N., Beloussov, L. V., & Zarayski, A. G. (1985). Model of epithelial morphogenesis basing on the elastic forces and contact polarization of cells. *Ontogenesis, 16*(1), 5–13.

Belintsev, B. N., Beloussov, L. V., & Zarayski, A. G. (1987). Model of pattern formation in epithelial morphogenesis. *Journal of Theoretical Biology, 129*, 369–394. doi:10.1016/S0022-5193(87)80019-X

Beloussov, L. V. (2001). Somitogenesis in vertebrate embryos as a robust macromorphological process. In Sanders, E. J. (Ed.), *The origin and fate of somites.* IOS Press.

Berar, M., Desvignes, M., & Bailly, G. (2006). 3D semi-landmarks-based statistical face reconstruction. *Journal of Computing and Information Technology, 14*(1), 31–43. doi:10.2498/cit.2006.01.04

Bérar, M., Desvignes, M., Bailly, G., & Payan, Y. (2004). *3D meshes registration: Application to statistical skull model* (pp. 100–107). Berlin, Heidelberg: Springer.

Berg, H. C., & Purcell, E. M. (1977). Physics of chemoreception. *Biophysical Journal, 20*(2), 193–219. doi:10.1016/S0006-3495(77)85544-6

Bevan, B. (1996). Geophysical exploration of the U. S. national parks. *Northeast Historical Archaeology, 25*, 69–84.

Bevan, B. W. (1983). Electromagnetics for mapping buried earth features. *Journal of Field Archaeology, 10*(1), 47–54. doi:10.2307/529747

Bilban, M., Buehler, L. K., Head, S., Desoye, G., & Quaranta, V. (2002). Defining signal thresholds in DNA microarrays: Exemplary application for invasive cancer. *BMC Genomics, 3*(1), 19. doi:10.1186/1471-2164-3-19

Bilder, D. (2004). Epithelial polarity and proliferation control: Links from the Drosophila neoplastic tumor suppressors. *Genes & Development, 18*, 1909–1925. doi:10.1101/gad.1211604

Björk, A. (1995). Cranial base development. A follow-up X-ray study of the individual variation in growth occurring between the ages of 12 and 20 years and its relation to brain case and face development. *American Journal of Orthodontics, 41*, 198–225. doi:10.1016/0002-9416(55)90005-1

Blake, G. M., Rea, J. A., & Fogelman, I. (1997). Vertebral morphometry studies using dual-energy X-ray absorptiometry. *Seminars in Nuclear Medicine*, 27, 276–290. doi:10.1016/S0001-2998(97)80029-3

Blake, J. M., Jagathesan, T., Herd, R. J. M., & Fogelman, I. (1994). Dual X-ray absorptiometry of the lumbar spine: The precision of paired anteroposterior/lateral studies. *The British Journal of Radiology*, 67, 624–630. doi:10.1259/0007-1285-67-799-624

Blanchard, A. P., Kaiser, R. J., & Hood, L. E. (1996). High density oligonucleotide arrays. *Biosensors & Bioelectronics*, 11(6/7), 687–690. doi:10.1016/0956-5663(96)83302-1

Bock, J. H., & Norris, D. O. (1997). Forensic botany: An under-utilized resource. *Journal of Forensic Sciences*, 42(3), 364–367.

Boguski, M. S., Lowe, T. M., & Tolstoshev, C. M. (1993). dbEST-database for expressed sequence tags. *Nature Genetics*, 4(4), 332–333. doi:10.1038/ng0893-332

Boguski, M. S., & Schuler, G. D. (1995). Establishing a human transcript map. *Nature Genetics*, 10(4), 369–371. doi:10.1038/ng0895-369

Boguski, M. S., Tolstoshev, C. M., & Bassett, D. E. Jr. (1994). Gene discovery in dbEST. *Science*, 265(5181), 1993–1994. doi:10.1126/science.8091218

Bolanos, M. V., Manrique, M. C., Bolanos, M. J., & Briones, M. T. (2000). Approaches to chronological age assessment based on dental calcification. *Forensic Science International*, 110, 97–106. doi:10.1016/S0379-0738(00)00154-7

Bolanos, M. V., Moussa, H., Manrique, M. C., & Bolanos, M. J. (2008). Radiographic evaluation of third molar development in Spanish children and young people. *Forensic Science International*, 133, 212–219. doi:10.1016/S0379-0738(03)00037-9

Boldsen, J. L., Milner, G. R., Konigsberg, L. W., & Wood, J. W. (2002). Transition analysis: A new method for estimating age from skeletons. In Hoppa, R. D., & Vaupel, J. W. (Eds.), *Paleodemography: Age distributions from skeletal samples* (pp. 73–106). Cambridge, UK: Cambridge University Press.

Boles, T. C., Snow, C. C., & Stover, E. (1995). Forensic DNA testing on skeletal remains from mass graves: A pilot project in Guatemala. *Journal of Forensic Sciences*, 40(3), 349–355.

Bolstad, B. M., Irizarry, R. A., Astrand, M., & Speed, T. P. (2003). A comparison of normalization methods for high density oligonucleotide array data based on bias and variance. *Bioinformatics (Oxford, England)*, 19(2), 185–193. doi:10.1093/bioinformatics/19.2.185

Bonaldo, M. F., Lennon, G., & Soares, M. B. (1996). Normalization and subtraction: Two approaches to facilitate gene discovery. *Genome Research*, 6(9), 791–806. doi:10.1101/gr.6.9.791

Bookstein, F. L. (1997). Landmark methods for forms without landmarks: Morphometrics of group difference in outline shape. *Medical Image Analysis*, 1, 225–243. doi:10.1016/S1361-8415(97)85012-8

Borgefors, G. (1998). Hierarchical Chamfer matching: A parametric edge matching algorithm. *IEEE Transactions on Pattern Analysis and Machine Intelligence*, 10(6), 849–865. doi:10.1109/34.9107

Boser, B., Guyon, L., & Vapnik, V. (1992). A training algorithm for optimal margin classifiers. In *Proceedings of the Fifth Annual Workshop on Computational Learning Theory*, (p. 144-152). Pittsburgh: ACM.

Bouvier, M., & Ubelaker, D. H. (1977). A comparison of two methods for the microscopic determination of age at death. *American Journal of Physical Anthropology*, 46(3), 391–394. doi:10.1002/ajpa.1330460303

Bowers, C. M., & Johanson, R. J. (2000). *Digital analysis of bite mark evidence using Adobe® Photoshop*. Santa Barbara, CA: Forensic Imaging Services.

Braun, R., Rowe, W., Schaefer, C., Zhang, J., & Buetow, K. (2009). Needles in the haystack: Identifying individuals present in pooled genomic data. *PLOS Genetics*, 5(10), e1000668. doi:10.1371/journal.pgen.1000668

Braz, V. S. (2009). Anthropological estimation of sex. In Blau, S., & Ubelaker, D. H. (Eds.), *Handbook of forensic anthropology and archaeology* (pp. 201–207). Walnut Creek, CA: Left Coast Press, Inc.

Breiman, L. (1996). Bagging predictors. *Machine Learning*, 24(2), 123–140. doi:10.1007/BF00058655

Brenner, S., Johnson, M., Bridgham, J., Golda, G., Lloyd, D. H., & Johnson, D. (2000a). Gene expression analysis by massively parallel signature sequencing (MPSS) on microbead arrays. *Nature Biotechnology, 18*(6), 630–634. doi:10.1038/76469

Brenner, S., Williams, S. R., Vermaas, E. H., Storck, T., Moon, K., & McCollum, C. (2000b). In vitro cloning of complex mixtures of DNA on microbeads: Physical separation of differentially expressed cDNAs. *Proceedings of the National Academy of Sciences of the United States of America, 97*(4), 1665–1670. doi:10.1073/pnas.97.4.1665

Brogdon, B. G. (1998). *Forensic radiology.* Boca Raton, FL: CRC Press. doi:10.1201/9781420048339

Brown, P. O., & Botstein, D. (1999). Exploring the new world of the genome with DNA microarrays. *Nature Genetics, 21*(Suppl. 1), 33–37. doi:10.1038/4462

Bruewer, M., Hopkins, A. M., & Nusrat, A. (2003). Proinflammatory cytokines disrupt epithelial barrier function by apoptosis-independent mechanisms. *Journal of Immunology (Baltimore, MD.: 1950), 171*, 6164–6172.

Bruschweiler, W., Braun, M., Dirnhofer, R., & Thali, M. J. (2003). Analysis of patterned injuries and injury-causing instruments with forensic 3D/CAD supported photogrammetry (FPHG): An instruction manual for the documentation process. *Forensic Science International, 132*, 130–138. doi:10.1016/S0379-0738(03)00006-9

Buck, M. J., & Lieb, J. D. (2004). ChIP-chip: Considerations for the design, analysis, and application of genome-wide chromatin immunoprecipitation experiments. *Genomics, 83*(3), 349–360. doi:10.1016/j.ygeno.2003.11.004

Budowle, B., Adamowicz, M., Aranda, X. G., Barna, C., Chakraborty, R., & Cheswick, D. (2005). Twelve short tandem repeat loci Y chromosome haplotypes: Genetic analysis on populations residing in North America. *Forensic Science International, 150*(1), 1–15. doi:10.1016/j.forsciint.2005.01.010

Budowle, B., Giusti, A. M., Waye, J. S., Baechtel, F. S., Fourney, R. M., & Adams, D. E. (1991). Fixed-bin analysis for statistical evaluation of continuous distributions of allelic data from VNTR loci, for use in forensic comparisons. *American Journal of Human Genetics, 48*(5), 841–855.

Budowle, B., Schutzer, S. E., Ascher, M. S., Atlas, R. M., Burans, J. P., & Chakraborty, R. (2005). Toward a system of microbial forensics: From sample collection to interpretation of evidence. *Applied and Environmental Microbiology, 71*(5), 2209–2213. doi:10.1128/AEM.71.5.2209-2213.2005

Budowle, B., Schutzer, S. E., Einseln, A., Kelley, L. C., Walsh, A. C., & Smith, J. A. (2003). Public health. Building microbial forensics as a response to bioterrorism. *Science, 301*(5641), 1852–1853. doi:10.1126/science.1090083

Budowle, B., & van Daal, A. (2008). Forensically relevant SNP classes. *BioTechniques, 44*(5), 603–608, 610. doi:10.2144/000112806

Budowle, B., & van Daal, A. (2009). Extracting evidence from forensic DNA analyses: Future molecular biology directions. *BioTechniques, 46*(5), 339–340, 342–350. doi:10.2144/000113136

Burke, J., Davison, D., & Hide, W. (1999). d2_cluster: A validated method for clustering EST and full-length cDNA sequences. *Genome Research, 9*(11), 1135–1142. doi:10.1101/gr.9.11.1135

Buschang, P. H., Hayasaki, H., & Throckmorton, G. S. (2000). Quantification of human chewing-cycle kinematics. *Archives of Oral Biology, 45*, 461–474. doi:10.1016/S0003-9969(00)00015-7

Butler, J. M., Schoske, R., Vallone, P. M., Redman, J. W., & Kline, M. C. (2003). Allele frequencies for 15 autosomal STR loci on U.S. Caucasian, African American, and Hispanic populations. *Journal of Forensic Sciences, 48*(4), 908–911.

Butte, A. (2002). The use and analysis of microarray data. *Nature Reviews. Drug Discovery, 1*(12), 951–960. doi:10.1038/nrd961

Buzug, T. (2006). Special issue on computer assisted craniofacial reconstruction and modelling [Editorial]. *Journal of Computing and Information Technology, 14*(1), 1–6. doi:10.2498/cit.2006.01.01

Cai, X., Hagedorn, C., & Cullen, B. (2004). Human microRNAs are processed from capped, polyadenylated transcripts that can also function as mRNAs. *RNA (New York, N.Y.), 10*, 1957–1966. doi:10.1261/rna.7135204

Calin, G., & Croce, C. (2006). MicroRNA signatures in human cancer. *Nature Reviews. Cancer, 6*, 259–269. doi:10.1038/nrc1997

Cameriere, R., Brkic, H., Ermenc, B., Ferrante, L., Ovsenik, M., & Cingolani, M. (2007a). The measurement of open apices of teeth to test chronological age over 14-year olds in living subjects. *Forensic Science International, 174*, 217–221. doi:10.1016/j.forsciint.2007.04.220

Cameriere, R., Ferrante, L., Belcastro, M. G., Bonfiglioli, B., Rastelli, E., & Cingolani, M. (2007b). Age estimation by pulp/tooth ratio in canines by peri-apical x-rays. *Journal of Forensic Sciences, 52*, 166–170. doi:10.1111/j.1556-4029.2006.00336.x

Cameriere, R., Ferrante, L., & Cingolani, M. (2006). Age estimation in children by measurement of open apices in teeth. *International Journal of Legal Medicine, 120*, 49–52. doi:10.1007/s00414-005-0047-9

Capurso, U., & Bonazza, M. (1990). Le variazioni morfologiche dell' articolazione temporomandibolare. *Minerva Stomatologica, 39*, 629–636.

Carthew, R. (2006). Gene regulation by microRNAs. *Current Opinion in Genetics & Development, 16*(2), 203–208. doi:10.1016/j.gde.2006.02.012

Caruana, R. (1997). Multitask learning. *Machine Learning, 28*(1), 41–75. doi:10.1023/A:1007379606734

Caruana, R., & de Sa, V. R. (2003). Benefiting from the variables that variable selection discards. *Journal of Machine Learning Research, 3*, 1245–1264. doi:10.1162/153244303322753652

Chan, V., Graves, D. J., & McKenzie, S. E. (1995). The biophysics of DNA hybridization with immobilized oligonucleotide probes. *Biophysical Journal, 69*(6), 2243–2255. doi:10.1016/S0006-3495(95)80095-0

Chang, Y. M., Burgoyne, L. A., & Both, K. (2003). Higher failures of amelogenin sex test in an Indian population group. *Journal of Forensic Sciences, 48*(6), 1309–1313.

Chattopadhyay, A. (2010). *Oral health epidemiology: Principles and practice*. Sudbury, MA: Jones & Bartlett publishers.

Chatziioannou, A., Moulos, P., & Kolisis, F. N. (2009). Gene ARMADA: An integrated multi-analysis platform for microarray data implemented in MATLAB. *BMC Bioinformatics, 10*, 354. doi:10.1186/1471-2105-10-354

Chen, J., & Rattray, M. (2006). Analysis of tag-position bias in MPSS technology. *BMC Genomics, 7*, 77. doi:10.1186/1471-2164-7-77

Chen, K., & Rajewsky, N. (2007). The evolution of gene regulation by transcription factors and microRNAs. *Nature Reviews. Genetics, 8*(2), 93–103. doi:10.1038/nrg1990

Chen, N.-Y., Lu, W.-C., Yang, J., & Li, G.-Z. (2004). *Support vector machines in chemistry*. Singapore: World Scientific Publishing Company. doi:10.1142/9789812794710

Cheng, S., Wu, Q., & Castleman, K. R. (2005). Non-ubiquitous digital watermarking for record indexing and integrity protection of medical images. *Proceedings of ICIP, 2*, 1062–1065.

Cheung, M., Mak, M., & Kung, S. (2005). A two-level fusion approach to multimodal biometric verification. *International Conference on Acoustics, Speech, and Signal Processing, 5*, 485–488. Philadelphia, PA, USA.

Cho, H., Stout, S. D., Madsen, R. W., & Streeter, M. A. (2002). Population specific histological age-estimating method: A model for known African-American and European-American skeletal remains. *Journal of Forensic Sciences, 47*(1), 12–18.

Chou, H. H., Hsia, A. P., Mooney, D. L., & Schnable, P. S. (2004). Picky: Oligo microarray design for large genomes. *Bioinformatics (Oxford, England), 20*(17), 2893–2902. doi:10.1093/bioinformatics/bth347

Chow, L. K., Gobin, Y. P., Cloughesy, T. F., Sayre, J. W., Villablanca, J. P., & Vinuela, F. (2000). Prognostic factors in recurrent glioblastoma multiforme and anaplastic astrocytoma, treated with selective intra-arterial chemotherapy. *AJNR. American Journal of Neuroradiology, 21*, 471–478.

Christensen, A. M. (2004). The impact of Daubert: Implications for testimony and research in forensic anthropology (and the use of frontal sinuses in personal identification). *Journal of Forensic Sciences, 49*(3), 427–430. doi:10.1520/JFS2003185

Churchill, G. A. (2002). Fundamentals of experimental design for cDNA microarrays. *Nature Genetics, 32*, 490–495. doi:10.1038/ng1031

Claes, P., Vandermeulen, D., De Greef, S., Willems, G., & Suetens, P. (2006). Craniofacial reconstruction using a combined statistical model of face shape and soft tissue depths: Methodology and validation. *Forensic Science International, 159*, 147–158. doi:10.1016/j.forsciint.2006.02.035

Clark, A. (1996). *Seeing beneath the soil: Preparing methods in archaeology* (2nd ed.). London: B.T. Batsford.

Clark, M. W. (1981). Quantitative shape analysis: A review. *Mathematical Geology, 13*(4), 303–320. doi:10.1007/BF01031516

Clark, H. C. (2008). *Practical forensic odontology.* Oxford: Wright.

Clement, J. G., & Ranson, D. L. (1998). *Craniofacial identification in forensic medicine.* London: Arnold.

Clement, J. G., & Marks, M. K. (2005). *Computer-graphic craniofacial reconstruction.* Boston: Academic Press.

Coatrieux, G., le Guillou, C., Cauvin, J.-M., & Roux, C. (2009). Reversible watermarking for knowledge digest embedding and reliability control in medical images. *IEEE Transactions on Information Technology in Biomedicine, 13*(2), 158–165. doi:10.1109/TITB.2008.2007199

Coatrieux, G., Lamard, M., Daccache, W., Puentes, J., & Roux, C. (2005). A low distortion and reversible watermark application to angiographic images of the retina. *Proceedings of the IEEE EMBC Conference, Shanghai, China, 2005*, (pp. 2224–2227).

Coatrieux, G., Lecornu, L., Roux, C., & Sankur, B. (2006). *A review of image watermarking applications in healthcare.* (pp. 4691–4694). 28th IEEE EMBS Annual International Conference, Aug 30-Sept. 3, 2006, New York.

Coatrieux, G., Maître, H., Sankur, B., Rolland, Y., & Collorec, R. (2000). Relevance of watermarking in medical imaging. (pp. 250–255). *Proceedings of the IEEE International Conference ITAB, USA.*

Cohen, M. M., Massaro, D. W., & Clark, R. (2002). Training a talking head. In *Proceedings of IEEE Fourth International Conference on MultiModal Interfaces,* (pp. 499–504).

Colman-Lerner, A., Gordon, A., Serra, E., Chin, T., Resnekov, O., & Endy, D. (2005). Regulated cell-to-cell variation in a cell-fate decision system. *Nature, 437*(7059), 699–706. doi:10.1038/nature03998

Combrinck, S., Duplooy, G. W., McCrindle, R. I., & Both, B. M. (2007). Morphology and histochemistry of the glandular trichomes of Lippia scaberrima (Verbenaceae). *Annals of Botany, 99*, 1111–1119. doi:10.1093/aob/mcm064

Conyers, L. B. (2004). *Ground-penetrating radar for archaeology.* Walnut Creek, CA: AltaMira Press.

Cootes, T. F., Taylor, C. J., Cooper, D., & Graham, J. (1995). Active shape models-their training and application. *Computer Vision and Image Understanding, 61*(1), 38–59. doi:10.1006/cviu.1995.1004

Corcuff, P., Gremillet, P., Jourlin, M., Duvault, Y., Leroy, F., & Leveque, J. L. (1993). 3D reconstruction of human hair by confocal microscopy. *Journal of the Society of Cosmetic Chemists, 44*, 1–12.

Costa, L. F., & Cesar, R. M. (2000). *Shape analysis and classification: Theory and practice.* Boca Raton, FL: CRC Press.

Cowell, R. G., Lauritzen, S. L., & Mortera, J. (2007). Identification and separation of DNA mixtures using peak area information. *Forensic Science International, 166*(1), 28–34. doi:10.1016/j.forsciint.2006.03.021

Crabtree, N., Wrigh,t J., Walgrove, A., et al. (2000). Vertebral morphometry: Repeat scan precision using the Lunar Expert-XL and the Hologic 4500A. A study for the WISDOM RCT of hormone replacement therapy. *Osteoporosis International, 11*, 537–543. doi:10.1007/s001980070098

Crans, G. G., Genant, H. K., & Krege, J. H. (2005). Measurement of vertebral heights. *Bone, 37*, 175–179. doi:10.1016/j.bone.2005.04.003

Cristianini, N., & Shawe-Taylor, J. (2000). *An introduction to support vector machines.* Cambridge, UK: Cambridge University Press.

Cros, P., Chollat, L., & Dumas, P. (1977). Dissymétrie des axes des condyles mandibulaires sur le plan horizontal. *Revue de Stomatologie et de Chirurgie Maxillo-Faciale, 78*, 429–432.

Crowder, C. M. (2009). Histological age estimation. In Blau, S., & Ubelaker, D. H. (Eds.), *Handbook of forensic anthropology and archeology* (pp. 222–235). Walnut Creek, CA: Left Coast Press, Inc.

Curran, J. M., Triggs, C. M., Buckleton, J., & Weir, B. S. (1999). Interpreting DNA mixtures in structured populations. *Journal of Forensic Sciences, 44*(5), 987–995.

Curran, J.M. & Buckleton, J. (2010). Inclusion probabilities and dropout. *Journal of Forensic Science.*

Dalma-Weiszhausz, D. D., Warrington, J., Tanimoto, E. Y., & Miyada, C. G. (2006). The Affymetrix GeneChip platform: An overview. *Methods in Enzymology, 410*, 3–28. doi:10.1016/S0076-6879(06)10001-4

Dalrymple, B. E., Duff, J. M., & Menzel, E. R. (1977). Inherent fingerprint luminescence-detection by laser. *Journal of Forensic Sciences, 22*, 106–1510.

Dawid, A. P., Mortera, J., & Pascali, V. L. (2001). Non-fatherhood or mutation? A probabilistic approach to parental exclusion in paternity testing. *Forensic Science International, 124*(1), 55–61. doi:10.1016/S0379-0738(01)00564-3

de Bruijne, M., & Nielsen, M. (2004). Image segmentation by shape particle filtering. In *Proceedings of the 17th International Conference on Pattern Recognition 2004,* (pp. 722–725).

De Greef, S., Claes, P., Vandermeulen, D., Mollemans, W., Suetens, P., & Willems, G. (2006). Large-scale in-vivo Caucasian facial soft tissue thickness database for craniofacial reconstruction. *Forensic Science International, 159S*, S126–S146. doi:10.1016/j.forsciint.2006.02.034

De Greef, S., & Willems, G. (2005). Three-dimensional craniofacial reconstruction in forensic identification: Latest progress and new tendencies in the 21st century. *Forensic Science International, 50*(1), 12–17.

Deborde, S., Perret, E., Gravotta, D., Deora, A., Salvarezza, S., & Sch, R. (2008). Clathrin is a key regulator of basolateral polarity. *Nature, 452*, 719–723. doi:10.1038/nature06828

del Angel, A., & Cisneros, H. B. (2004). Technical note: Modification of regression equations used to estimate stature in Mesoamerican skeletal remains. *American Journal of Physical Anthropology, 125*(3), 264–265. doi:10.1002/ajpa.10385

Delson, E., Harcourt-Smith, W. E. H., Frost, S. R., & Norris, C. A. (2007). Databases, data access, and data sharing in paleoanthropology: First steps. *Evolutionary Anthropology: Issues. News Review (Melbourne), 16*(5), 161–163.

Demirjian, A., Buschang, P. H., Tenguay, T., & Patterson, D. K. (1985). Interrelationships among measures of somatic, skeletal, dental, and sexual maturity. *American Journal of Orthodontics, 88*, 433–438. doi:10.1016/0002-9416(85)90070-3

Demirjian, A., & Goldstein, H. (1976). New systems for dental maturity based on seven and four teeth. *Annals of Human Biology, 3*, 411–421. doi:10.1080/03014467600001671

Demirjian, A., Goldstein, H., & Tanner, J. M. (1973). A new system of dental age assessment. *Human Biology, 45*, 211–227.

Demuth, H., & Beale, M. (2001). *Neural network toolbox user's guide for use with MATLAB* (4th ed.). The Mathworks Inc.

Dept. of Health. (2000). The ionising radiation (medical exposure) regulations 2000. Retrieved from www.opsi.gov.uk/si/si2000/20001059.htm

Di Maio, V. J. (1984). Basic principles in the investigation of homicides. *Pathology Annual, 19*(2), 149–164.

Diacinti, D., Acca, M., & Tomei, E. (1995). Metodica di radiologia digitale per la valutazione dell'osteoporosi vertebrale. *La Radiologia Medica, 91*, 1–5.

DICOM standard. (2010). *NEMA information.* Retrieved from http://medical.nema.org

Diehl, F., Grahlmann, S., Beier, M., & Hoheisel, J. D. (2001). Manufacturing DNA microarrays of high spot homogeneity and reduced background signal. *Nucleic Acids Research, 29*(7), E38. doi:10.1093/nar/29.7.e38

Diercks, A., Kostner, H., & Ozinsky, A. (2009). Resolving cell population heterogeneity: Real-time PCR for simultaneous multiplexed gene detection in multiple single-cell samples. *PLoS ONE, 4*(7), e6326. doi:10.1371/journal.pone.0006326

Dirnhofer, R., Jackowski, C., Vock, P., Potter, K., & Thali, M. J. (2006). Virtopsy: Minimally invasive, imaging-guided virtual autopsy. *Radiographics, 26*, 1305–1333. doi:10.1148/rg.265065001

DNA.gov. (2010). DNA *initiative: Advancing criminal justice through DNA technology*. Retrieved June 9, 2010, from www page: http://www.dna.gov/more/contactus/

Dobbin, K., Shih, J. H., & Simon, R. (2003a). Questions and answers on design of dual-label microarrays for identifying differentially expressed genes. *Journal of the National Cancer Institute, 95*(18), 1362–1369.

Dobbin, K., Shih, J. H., & Simon, R. (2003b). Statistical design of reverse dye microarrays. *Bioinformatics (Oxford, England), 19*(7), 803–810. doi:10.1093/bioinformatics/btg076

Dobbin, K., & Simon, R. (2002). Comparison of microarray designs for class comparison and class discovery. *Bioinformatics (Oxford, England), 18*(11), 1438–1445. doi:10.1093/bioinformatics/18.11.1438

Doench, J., & Sharp, P. (2004). Specificity of microRNA target selection in translational repression. *Genes & Development, 16*(1), 504–511. doi:10.1101/gad.1184404

Dolhenty, J. (2010). *Logic and critical thinking*. The Jonathan Dolhenty Archive.

Dolinak, D., Evan, M., & Lew, E. (2005). *Forensic pathology: Principles and practice*. Burlington, MA: Elsevier Academic Press.

Donchin, Y., Rivkind, A. I., Bar-Ziv, J., Hiss, J., Almog, J., & Drescher, M. (1994). Utility of postmortem computed tomography in trauma victims. *The Journal of Trauma, 37*, 552–556. doi:10.1097/00005373-199410000-00006

Dorak, M. T. (2007). Statistical analysis in HLA and disease association studies. Retrieved from www.dorak.info/hla/stat.html

Driessen, M. N. B. M., Willemse, M. T. M., & van Luijn, J. A. G. (1989). Grass pollen grain determination by light- and UV-microscopy. *Grana, 28*, 115–122. doi:10.1080/00173138909429962

Drmanac, S., Kita, D., Labat, I., Hauser, B., Schmidt, C., & Burczak, J. D. (1998). Accurate sequencing by hybridization for DNA diagnostics and individual ge-

nomics. *Nature Biotechnology, 16*(1), 54–58. doi:10.1038/nbt0198-54

Drygajlo, A., Meuwly, D., & Alexander, A. (2003). Statistical methods and Bayesian interpretation of evidence in forensic automatic speaker recognition. In [Geneva, Switzerland.]. *Proceedings of Eurospeech, 2003*, 689–692.

Dudar, J. C., Pfeiffer, S., & Saunders, S. R. (1993). Evaluation of morphological and histological adult skeletal age-at-death estimation techniques using ribs. *Journal of Forensic Sciences, 38*(3), 677–685.

Dudoit, S., Fridlyand, J., & Speed, T. P. (2002). Comparison of discrimination methods for the classification of tumors using gene expression data. *Journal of the American Statistical Association, 97*(457), 77–87. doi:10.1198/016214502753479248

Duggleby, R. G. (1994). Product inhibition of reversible enzyme-catalized reactions. *Biochimica et Biophysica Acta, 1209*, 238–240. doi:10.1016/0167-4838(94)90190-2

Eastell, R., Cedel, S. L., & Wahner, H. (1991). Classification of vertebral fractures. *Journal of Bone and Mineral Research, 6*, 207–215. doi:10.1002/jbmr.5650060302

Eder, A. F., McGrath, C. M., Dowdy, Y. G., Tomaszewski, J. E., Rosenberg, F. M., & Wilson, R. B. (1998). Ethylene glycol poisoning: Toxicokinetic and analytical factors affecting laboratory diagnosis. *Clinical Chemistry, 44*, 168–177.

Edgar, R., Domrachev, M., & Lash, A. E. (2002). Gene expression omnibus: NCBI gene expression and hybridization array data repository. *Nucleic Acids Research, 30*(1), 207–210. doi:10.1093/nar/30.1.207

Edmondston, S. J., Price, R. I., & Valente, B. (1999). Measurement of vertebral body height: Ex vivo comparison between morphometric X-ray absorptiometry, morphometric radiography and direct measurements. *Osteoporosis International, 10*, 7–13. doi:10.1007/s001980050187

Efron, B., Tibshirani, R., Storey, J. D., & Tusher, V. (2001). Empirical Bayes analysis of a microarray experiment. *Journal of the American Statistical Association, 96*, 1151–1160. doi:10.1198/016214501753382129

Egeland, T., Dalen, I., & Mostad, P. F. (2003). Estimating the number of contributors to a DNA profile. *International*

Journal of Legal Medicine, 117(5), 271–275. doi:10.1007/s00414-003-0382-7

Egli, N. M., Champod, C., & Margot, P. (2007). Evidence evaluation in fingerprint comparison and automated fingerprint identification systems-modelling within finger variability. *Forensic Science International, 167*, 189–195. doi:10.1016/j.forsciint.2006.06.054

Ekstrand, K. R., Christiansen, J., & Christiansen, M. E. C. (2003). Time and duration of eruption of first and second permanent molars: A longitudinal investigation. *Community Dentistry and Oral Epidemiology, 31*, 344–350. doi:10.1034/j.1600-0528.2003.00016.x

Elowitz, M. B., Levine, A. J., Siggia, E. D., & Swain, P. S. (2002). Stochastic gene expression in a single cell. *Science, 297*(5584), 1183–1186. doi:10.1126/science.1070919

Elton, S., & Cardini, A. (2008). Anthropology from the desk? The challenges of the emerging era of data sharing. *Journal of Anthropological Sciences, 86*, 209–212.

Erdtman, G., & Praglowski, J. R. (1959). Six notes on pollen morphology and pollen morphological techniques. *Botaniska Notiser, 112*, 175–184.

Ericksen, M. F. (1991). Histologic estimation of age at death using the anterior cortex of the femur. *American Journal of Physical Anthropology, 84*(2), 171–179.

Esquela-Kerscher, A., & Clack, F. (2006). Oncomirs: MicroRNAs with a role in cancer. *Nature Reviews. Cancer, 6*, 259–269. doi:10.1038/nrc1840

Evenhouse, R., Rasmussen, M., & Sadler, L. (1992). Computer-aided forensic facial reconstruction. *The Journal of Biocommunication, 19*(2), 22–28.

Evett, I. W., Buffery, C., Willott, G., & Stoney, D. (1991). A guide to interpreting single locus profiles of DNA mixtures in forensic cases. *Journal - Forensic Science Society, 31*(1), 41–47. doi:10.1016/S0015-7368(91)73116-2

Evett, I. W., Gill, P. D., & Lambert, J. A. (1998). Taking account of peak areas when interpreting mixed DNA profiles. *Journal of Forensic Sciences, 43*(1), 62–69.

Evison, M. P., & Vorder Bruegge, R. W. (2009). *Computer-aided forensic facial comparison.* Boca Raton, FL: CRC Press.

Evison, M. P. (1996). Computerized three dimensional facial reconstruction. Retrieved from www.shef.ac.uk/assem/1/evison.html

Excoffier, L., & Heckel, G. (2006). Computer programs for population genetics data analysis: A survival guide. *Nature Reviews. Genetics, 7*(10), 745–758. doi:10.1038/nrg1904

Fægri, K., & Iversen, J. (1989). *Textbook of pollen analysis* (4th ed.). Chichester, UK: J. Wiley & Sons.

Fahmy, G., Nassar, D., Said, E., Chen, H., Nomir, O., Zhou, J., et al. (2004a). Towards an automated dental identification system. *IEEE International Conference of Biometric Authenticity,* (pp. 789–796). Hong Kong.

Fahmy, G., Nassar, D., Said, E., Chen, H., Nomir, O., Zhou, J., et al. (2004b). A Web based tool for an Automated Dental Identification System (ADIS). *Proceedings of National Conference on Digital Government Research,* (pp. 1–2). Seattle, WA, USA.

Fall, C. P., Marland, E. S., Wagner, J. M., & Tyson, J. J. (2002). *Computational cell biology.* New York: Springer-Verlag.

Faller, M., Matsunaga, M., Yin, S., Loo, J., & Guo, F. (2007). Heme is involved in microRNA processing. *Nature Structural & Molecular Biology, 14*(1), 23–29. doi:10.1038/nsmb1182

Faustino, N. A., & Cooper, T. A. (2003). Pre-mRNA splicing and human disease. *Genes & Development, 17*(4), 419–437. doi:10.1101/gad.1048803

Ferrar, L., Jiang, G., & Eastell, R. (2003). Visual identification of vertebral fractures in osteoporosis using morphometric X-ray absorptiometry. *Journal of Bone and Mineral Research, 18*, 933–938. doi:10.1359/jbmr.2003.18.5.933

Fife, P. C., & McLeod, J. B. (1977). The approach of solutions of nonlinear diffusion equations to traveling front solutions. *Archive for Rational Mechanics and Analysis, 65*, 335–361. doi:10.1007/BF00250432

Finkbeiner, W. E., Ursell, P. C., & Davis, R. L. (2004). *Autopsy pathology: A manual and atlas.* Philadelphia: Churchill Livingstone.

Finkelstein, D., Ewing, R., Gollub, J., Sterky, F., Cherry, J. M., & Somerville, S. (2002). Microarray data quality analysis: Lessons from the AFGC project. Arabidopsis Functional Genomics Consortium. *Plant Molecular Biology, 48*(1-2), 119–131. doi:10.1023/A:1013765922672

Fire, A., Hu, S., Mongomery, M. K., Kostas, S. A., Driver, S. E., & Mello, C. C. (1998). Potent and specific genetic interference by double-stranded RNA in Caenorhabditis elegans. *Nature, 391*, 806–811. doi:10.1038/35888

Flynt, A. S., Li, N., Thatcher, E. J., Solica-Krezel, L., & Patton, J. G. (2007). Zebrafish miR-214 modulates hedgehog signaling to specify muscle cell fate. *Nature Genetics, 39*(2), 259–263. doi:10.1038/ng1953

Fogelman, I. (Ed.). (1998). *The evaluation of osteoporosis. Dual energy x-ray absorptiometry in clinical practice* (pp. 281–288). London: Martin Dunitz, Ltd.

Foreman, L. A., Champod, I. W., Evett, J. A., Lambert, S., & Pope, S. (2003). Interpreting DNA evidence: A review. *International Statistical Review, 71*(3), 473–495. doi:10.1111/j.1751-5823.2003.tb00207.x

Forensic Osteology. (2010). *Home page information.* Retrieved from http://www.forost.org

Foresee, F. D., & Hagan, M. T. (1997). Gauss-newton approximation to bayesian regularization. In *Proceedings of the 1997 International Joint Conference on Neural Networks,* (pp. 1930-1935).

Frangi, A., Rueckert, D., Schnabel, J., & Niessen, W. (2002). Automatic construction of multiple object three-dimensional statistical shape models: Application to cardiac modeling. *IEEE Transactions on Medical Imaging, 21*(9), 1151–1166. doi:10.1109/TMI.2002.804426

Fridrich, J., Goljan, J., & Du, R. (2001). Invertible authentication. *Proceedings of International Conference SPIE, Security and Watermarking of Multimedia Content, San Jose, CA, Jan. 2001,* (pp. 197-208).

Froberg, K., Dorion, R. P., & McMartin, K. E. (2006). The role of calcium oxalate crystal deposition in cerebral vessels during ethylene glycol poisoning. *Clinical Toxicology, 44*, 315–318. doi:10.1080/15563650600588460

Fujifilm, U. S. A. (2010). *Finepix camera specifications.* Retrieved from http://www.fujifilmusa.com/products/digital_cameras/is/finepix_ispro/index.html

Fukshansky, N., & Bar, W. (1998). Interpreting forensic DNA evidence on the basis of hypotheses testing. *International Journal of Legal Medicine, 111*(2), 62–66. doi:10.1007/s004140050116

Fukshansky, N., & Bar, W. (2000). Biostatistics for mixed stains: The case of tested relatives of a non-tested suspect. *International Journal of Legal Medicine, 114*(1-2), 78–82. doi:10.1007/s004140000155

Fukunaga, K. (1990). *Introduction to Statistical pattern recognition* (2nd ed.). Academic Press.

Fung, W. K., & Hu, Y. Q. (2000a). Interpreting forensic DNA mixtures: Allowing for uncertainty in population substructure and dependence. *Journal of the Royal Statistical Society. Series A (General), 163*, 241–254.

Fung, W. K., & Hu, Y. Q. (2000b). *Interpreting DNA mixtures based on the NRC-II recommendation 4.1.* Forensic Science Communications.

Fung, W. K., & Hu, Y. Q. (2001). The evaluation of mixed stains from different ethnic origins: General result and common cases. *International Journal of Legal Medicine, 115*(1), 48–53. doi:10.1007/s004140100205

Fung, W. K., & Hu, Y. Q. (2002a). Evaluating mixed stains with contributors of different ethnic groups under the NRC-II Recommendation 4.1. *Statistics in Medicine, 21*(23), 3583–3593. doi:10.1002/sim.1313

Fung, W. K., & Hu, Y. Q. (2002b). The statistical evaluation of DNA mixtures with contributors from different ethnic groups. *International Journal of Legal Medicine, 116*(2), 79–86. doi:10.1007/s004140100256

Fung, W. K., Chung, Y. K., & Wong, D. M. (2002). Power of exclusion revisited: Probability of excluding relatives of the true father from paternity. *International Journal of Legal Medicine, 116*(2), 64–67. doi:10.1007/s004140100210

Gallagher, J. C., Hedlund, L. R., & Stoner, S. (1988). Vertebral morphometry: Normative data. *Bone and Mineral, 4*, 189–196.

Gallo, L. M., Airoldi, G. B., Airoldi, R. L., & Palla, S. (1997). Description of mandibular finite helical axis pathways in asymptomatic subjects. *Journal of Dental Research, 76*, 704–713. doi:10.1177/00220345970760021201

Gallo, L. M., Fushima, K., & Palla, S. (2000). Mandibular helical axis pathways during mastication. *Journal of Dental Research, 79*, 1566–1572. doi:10.1177/00220345000790080701

Gardner, J. C., von Ingersleben, G., & Heyano, S. L. (2001). An interactive tutorial-based training technique for vertebral morphometry. *Osteoporosis International, 12*, 63–70. doi:10.1007/s001980170159

Garn, S., Lewis, A. B., & Bonne, B. (1962). Third molar formation and its development course. *The Angle Orthodontist, 32*, 270–279.

Garn, S., Lewis, A. B., & Kerewsky, R. S. (1965). Genetic, nutritional, and maturational correlates of dental development. *Journal of Dental Research, 44*(1), 228–242. doi:10.1177/00220345650440011901

Garn, S. M., Lewis, A. B., & Blizzard, R. M. (1965). Endocrine factors in tooth development. *Journal of Dental Research, 44*(1), 243–257. doi:10.1177/00220345650440012001

Gaytán, E., Mansilla-Lory, J., Leboreiro, I., & Pineda, S. C. (2009). Facial reconstruction of a pathological case. *Forensic Science, Medicine, and Pathology, 5*(2), 95–99. doi:10.1007/s12024-009-9088-6

Genant, H. K., Jergas, M., & Palermo, L. (1996). Comparison of semiquantitative visual and quantitative morphometric assessment of prevalent and incident vertebral fractures in osteoporosis. *Journal of Bone and Mineral Research, 11*, 984–996. doi:10.1002/jbmr.5650110716

Genant, H. K., Siris, E., & Crans, G. G. (2005). Reduction in vertebral fracture risk in teriaparatide-treated postmenopausal women as assessed by spinal deformity index. *Bone, 37*, 170–174. doi:10.1016/j.bone.2005.04.023

Genant, H. K., Wu, C. Y., & van Kuijk, C. (1993). Vertebral fracture assessment using a semiquantitative technique. *Journal of Bone and Mineral Research, 8*, 1137–1148. doi:10.1002/jbmr.5650080915

Ghosh, D. (2004). Mixture models for assessing differential expression in complex tissues using microarray data. *Bioinformatics (Oxford, England), 20*(11), 1663–1669. doi:10.1093/bioinformatics/bth139

Giakoumaki, A., Pavlopulos, S., & Koutouris, D. (2003). A medical image watermarking scheme based on wavelet transform. *Proceedings of the 25th IEEE EMBS Annual International Conference, 17-21 Sept. 2003, Vol. 1*, (pp. 856-859).

Gibson, G., & Muse, S. V. (2004). *A primer of genome science* (2nd ed.). Sunderland, MA: Sinauer Associates.

Gill, J. R. (2006). 9/11 and the New York City Office of Chief Medical Examiner. *Forensic Science, Medicine, and Pathology, 2*(1), 29–32. doi:10.1385/FSMP:2:1:29

Gillies, D. (1998). The Duhem thesis and the Quine thesis. In M. Curd & J.A. (Eds.), *Philosophy of science: The central issues*. (pp. 302-319). New York: Norton

Ginsberg, L. E., Fuller, G. N., Hashmi, M., Leeds, N. E., & Schomer, D. F. (1998). The significance of lack of MR contrast enhancement of surpratentorial brain tumors in adults: Histopathological evaluation of a series. *Surgical Neurology, 49*, 436–440. doi:10.1016/S0090-3019(97)00360-1

Goldberg, D. E. (1998). *Genetic algorithms in search, optimization, and machine learning*. Boston: Addison Wesley.

Goldbeter, A., Gonze, D., & Pourquie, O. (2007). Sharp developmental thresholds defined through bistability by antagonistic gradients of retinoic acid and FGF signaling. *Developmental Dynamics, 236*, 1495–1508. doi:10.1002/dvdy.21193

Golden, G. S. (1994). Use of alternate light source illumination in bite mark photography. *Journal of Forensic Sciences, 39*(3), 815–823.

Golden, G. S., & Wright, F. D. (2005). Photography: Noninvasive analysis. In Dorion, R. B. J. (Ed.), *Bitemark evidence* (pp. 136–139). New York: Marcel Dekker.

Golub, T. R., Slonim, D. K., Tamayo, P., Huard, C., Gaasenbeek, M., & Mesirov, J. P. (1999a). Molecular classification of cancer: Class discovery and class prediction by gene expression. *Bioinformatics &. Computational Biology, 286*(5439), 531–537.

Gonzalez, R., & Wood, R. (2003). *Digital image processing*. Addison Wesley.

Gordon, P. M., & Sensen, C. W. (2004). Osprey: A comprehensive tool employing novel methods for the design of oligonucleotides for DNA sequencing and microarrays. *Nucleic Acids Research, 32*(17), e133. doi:10.1093/nar/gnh127

Götherström, A., Collins, M.J., & Angerbjörn, A. & Liden, K. (2002). Bone preservation and DNA amplification. *Archaeometry, 44*(3), 395–404. doi:10.1111/1475-4754.00072

Graham, E. A. M. (2007). DNA reviews: Hair. *Journal of Forensic Science, Medicine, and Pathology, 3*(2), 1556–2891.

Graves, D. J. (1999). Powerful tools for genetic analysis come of age. *Trends in Biotechnology, 17*(3), 127–134. doi:10.1016/S0167-7799(98)01241-4

Green, P. (1999). Phrap. Retrieved from http://phrap.org

Grohne, U. (1957). Die Bedeutung des Phasenkontrastverfahrens fur die Pollenanalyse, dargelegt am Beispiel der Gramineenpollen vom Getreideyp. *Photogr. Forsch, 7*, 237–248.

Guglielmi, G., Diacinti, D., van Kuijk, C., Aparisi, F., Krestan, C., & Adams, J. E. (2008). Vertebral morphometry: Current methods and recent advances. *European Journal of Radiology, 18*, 1484–1496. doi:10.1007/s00330-008-0899-8

Guglielmi, G., Palmieri, F., & Placentino, M. G. (2008). Assessment of osteoporotic vertebral fractures using specialized workflow software for six point morphometry. *European Journal of Radiology, 70*, 142–148. doi:10.1016/j.ejrad.2007.12.001

Guglielmi, G., Stoppino, L. P., & Placentino, M. G. (2007). Reproducibility of a semi-automatic method for 6-point vertebral morphometry in a multi-centre trial. *European Journal of Radiology, 69*, 173–178. doi:10.1016/j.ejrad.2007.09.040

Gunn, A. (2009). *Essential forensic biology* (2nd ed., pp. 335–342). Ed Whiley Pty.

Gunst, R., Webster, J., & Mason, R. (1976). A comparison of least squares and latent root regression estimator. *Technometrics, 18*, 75–83. doi:10.2307/1267919

Guo, Z., Guilfoyle, R. A., Thiel, A. J., Wang, R., & Smith, L. M. (1994). Direct fluorescence analysis of genetic polymorphisms by hybridization with oligonucleotide

arrays on glass supports. *Nucleic Acids Research, 22*(24), 5456–5465. doi:10.1093/nar/22.24.5456

Gupta, N., Jadhav, K., & Mujib, B. R. (2009). Is recration of human identity possible using tooth prints? An experimental study to aid in identification. *Forensic Science International, 192*, 67–71. doi:10.1016/j.forsciint.2009.07.017

Gurden, S. P., Monteiro, V. F., Longo, E., & Ferreira, M. M. C. (2004). Quantitative analysis and classification of AFM images of human hair. *Journal of Microscopy, 215*(1), 13–23. doi:10.1111/j.0022-2720.2004.01350.x

Gusev, V. (2008). Computational methods for analysis of cellular functions and pathways collectively targeted by differentially expressed microRNA. *Methods (San Diego, Calif.), 44*, 61–72. doi:10.1016/j.ymeth.2007.10.005

Guyon, I., Gunn, S., Nikravesh, M., & Zadeh, L. (2006). *Feature extraction, foundations and applications. Physica-Verlag.* Springer.

Haavikko, K. (1970). The formation and the alveolar and clinical eruption of the permanent teeth. *Suom Hammaslaken Toimen, 66*, 103–170.

Hacia, J. G., Brody, L. C., & Collins, F. S. (1998). Applications of DNA chips for genomic analysis. *Molecular Psychiatry, 3*(6), 483–492. doi:10.1038/sj.mp.4000475

Hacia, J. G., & Collins, F. S. (1999). Mutational analysis using oligonucleotide microarrays. *Journal of Medical Genetics, 36*(10), 730–736.

Hadjur, C., Daty, G., Madry, G., & Corcuff, P. (2002). Cosmetic assessment of the human hair by confocal microscopy. *Scanning, 24*, 59–64. doi:10.1002/sca.4950240202

Hagelberg, E., Gray, I. C., & Jeffreys, A. J. (1991). Identification of the skeletal remains of a murder victim by DNA analysis. *Nature, 352*, 427–429. doi:10.1038/352427a0

Hanks, S. S., & Fairbrothers, D. E. (1970). Effect of preparation technique on pollen prepared for SEM observation. *Taxon, 19*, 879–886. doi:10.2307/1218302

Harbison, S. A., & Buckleton, J. S. (1998). Applications and extensions of subpopulation theory: A caseworkers guide. *Science & Justice, 38*(4), 249–254. doi:10.1016/S1355-0306(98)72119-7

Harke, H. T., Levy, A. D., Abbott, R. M., Mallak, C. T., Getz, M. J., & Champion, H. R. (2007). Autopsy radiography: Digital radiographs (DR) vs. multidetector computed tomography (MDCT) in high velocity gunshot wound victims. *The American Journal of Forensic Medicine and Pathology, 29,* 13–19.

Harris, E. F., Mincer, H. H., Anderson, K. M., & Senn, D. R. (2010). Age estimation from oral and dental structures. In Senn, D., & Stimson, P. (Eds.), *Forensic dentistry* (2nd ed., pp. 279–293). Boca Raton, FL: Taylor & Francis.

Harvey, S. B., Hutchinson, K. M., & Rennie, E. C. (1998). Comparison of the precision of two vertebral morphometry programs for the Lunar Expert-XL imaging densitometer. *The British Journal of Radiology, 71,* 388–398.

Hayakawa, M., Yamamoto, S., Motani, H., Yajima, D., Sato, Y., & Iwase, H. (2006). Does imaging technology overcome problems of conventional postmortem examination? A trial of computed tomography imaging for post mortem examination. *International Journal of Legal Medicine, 120*(1), 24–26. doi:10.1007/s00414-005-0038-x

He, S., Kirovski, D., & Wu, M. (2009). High-fidelity data embedding for image annotation. *IEEE Transactions on Image Processing, 18*(2), 429–435. doi:10.1109/TIP.2008.2008733

Hedlund, L. R., & Gallagher, J. C. (1988). Vertebral morphometry in diagnosis of spinal fractures. *Bone and Mineral, 5,* 59–67. doi:10.1016/0169-6009(88)90006-2

Helmer, R. P., Buzug, T. M., & Hering, P. (2003). Plastic facial reconstruction on the skull-a transition in Germany from a conventional technique to a new one. *Proceedings of the First International Conference on Reconstruction of Soft Facial Parts.* (pp. 75–90). Wiesbaden: Bundeskriminalamt.

Hierl, T., Wollny, G., Peter, F., Scholz, E., Schmidt, J.-G., & Berti, G. (2006). CAD-CAM implants in esthetic and reconstructive craniofacial surgery. *Journal of Computing and Information Technology, 14*(1), 65–70. doi:10.2498/cit.2006.01.07

Higuchi, R., von Beroldingen, C. H., Sensabaugh, G. F., & Erlich, H. A. (1988). DNA typing from single hairs. *Nature, 332,* 543–546. doi:10.1038/332543a0

Hirata, H., Bessho, Y., Kokubu, H., Mazamizu, Y., Yamada, S., & Lewis, J. (2004). Instability of Hes7 protein is critical for the somite segmentation clock. *Nature Genetics, 36,* 750–754. doi:10.1038/ng1372

Hirata, H., Yoshiura, S., Ohtsuka, T., Bessho, Y., Harada, T., & Yoshikawa, K. (2002). Oscillatory expression of the bHLH factor Hes1 regulated by a negative feedback loop. *Science, 298,* 840–843. doi:10.1126/science.1074560

Hishiki, T., Kawamoto, S., Morishita, S., & Okubo, K. (2000). BodyMap: A human and mouse gene expression database. *Nucleic Acids Research, 28*(1), 136–138. doi:10.1093/nar/28.1.136

Hockton, A. (2002). *The law of consent to medical treatment.* London: Sweet & Maxwell.

Holland, M. M., Cave, C. A., Holland, C. A., & Bille, T. W. (2003). Development of a quality, high throughput DNA analysis procedure for skeletal samples to assist with the identification of victims from the World Trade Center attacks. *Croatian Medical Journal, 44*(3), 264–272.

Holland, M. M., & Parsons, T. J. (1999). Mitochondrial DNA sequence analysis–validation and use for forensic casework. *Forensic Science Review, 11,* 21–50.

Holland, T. D., & Connell, S. V. (2009). The search for and detection of human remains. In Blau, S., & Ubelaker, D. H. (Eds.), *Handbook of anthropology and archaeology* (pp. 129–140). Walnut Creek, CA: Left Coast Press, Inc.

Homer, N., Szelinger, S., Redman, M., Duggan, D., Tembe, W., & Muehling, J. (2008). Resolving individuals contributing trace amounts of DNA to highly complex mixtures using high-density SNP genotyping microarrays. *PLOS Genetics, 4*(8), e1000167. doi:10.1371/journal.pgen.1000167

Honsinger, C. W., Jones, P., Rabbani, M., & Stoffel, J. C. (1999). *Lossless recovery of an original image containing embedded data.* US patent, docket no.:77102/E-D.

Hoppa, R. D., & Vaupel, J. W. (Eds.). (2002). *Paleodemography: Age distributions from skeletal samples.* Cambridge, UK: Cambridge University Press. doi:10.1017/CBO9780511542428

Horner, H. T., & Wagner, B. L. (1995). Calcium oxalate formation in higher plants. In Khan, S. (Ed.), *Calcium oxalate in biological systems* (pp. 53–72). CRC Book Press.

Horrocks, M., & Walsh, K. A. J. (2001). Forensic palynology: Assessing the value of the evidence. *Review of Palaeobotany and Palynology, 103*, 69–74. doi:10.1016/S0034-6667(98)00027-X

Houck, M. M., & Budowle, B. (2002). Comparison of microscopic and mitochondrial DNA hair comparisons. *Journal of Forensic Sciences, 47*(5), 1–4.

Howe, B., Gururajan, A., Sari-Sarraf, H., & Long, L. R. (2004). Hierarchical segmentation of cervical and lumbar vertebrae using a customized generalized Hough transform and extensions to active appearance models. In *Proceedings of IEEE 6th* (pp. 182–186). SSIAI.

Hu, Y. Q., & Fung, W. K. (2003). Interpreting DNA mixtures with the presence of relatives. *International Journal of Legal Medicine, 117*(1), 39–45.

Hubbell, E., Liu, W. M., & Mei, R. (2002). Robust estimators for expression analysis. *Bioinformatics (Oxford, England), 18*(12), 1585–1592. doi:10.1093/bioinformatics/18.12.1585

Hughes, T. R., Mao, M., Jones, A. R., Burchard, J., Marton, M. J., & Shannon, K. W. (2001). Expression profiling using microarrays fabricated by an ink-jet oligonucleotide synthesizer. *Nature Biotechnology, 19*(4), 342–347. doi:10.1038/86730

Hurley, D., Nixon, M., & Carter, J. (2000). *Automatic ear recognition by force field transformation* (pp. 789–796). London, UK: IEEE Colloquium on Visual Biometrics.

Hurley, D., Nixon, M., & Carter, J. (2002). Force field energy function for image feature extraction. *Image and Vision Computing*, 311–317. doi:10.1016/S0262-8856(02)00003-3

Hurxthal, L. M. (1968). Measurement of vertebral heights. *AJR. American Journal of Roentgenology, 103*, 635–644.

Hutton, T. J., Cunningham, S., & Hammond, P. (2000). An evaluation of active shape models for the automatic identification of cephalometric landmarks. *European Journal of Orthodontics, 22*(5), 499–508. doi:10.1093/ejo/22.5.499

Ibrahim, J. G., Chen, M.-H., & Gray, R. J. (2002). Bayesian models for gene expression with DNA microarray data. *Journal of the American Statistical Association, 97*, 88–99. doi:10.1198/016214502753479257

Ingervall, B., Carlsson, G. E., & Thilander, B. (1976). Postnatal development of the human temporomandibular joint. A microradiographic study. *Acta Odontologica Scandinavica, 34*, 133–139. doi:10.3109/00016357609002560

Irizarry, R. A., Bolstad, B. M., Collin, F., Cope, L. M., Hobbs, B., & Speed, T. P. (2003). Summaries of Affymetrix GeneChip probe level data. *Nucleic Acids Research, 31*(4), e15. doi:10.1093/nar/gng015

Irizarry, R. A., Hobbs, B., Collin, F., Beazer-Barclay, Y. D., Antonellis, K. J., & Scherf, U. (2003). Exploration, normalization, and summaries of high density oligonucleotide array probe level data. *Biostatistics (Oxford, England), 4*(2), 249–264. doi:10.1093/biostatistics/4.2.249

Irizarry, R. A., Wu, Z., & Jaffee, H. A. (2006). Comparison of Affymetrix GeneChip expression measures. *Bioinformatics (Oxford, England), 22*(7), 789–794. doi:10.1093/bioinformatics/btk046

Ith, M., Bigler, P., Scheurer, E., Kreis, R., Hoffman, L., & Dirnhofer, R. (2002). Observation and identification of metabolites emerging during postmortem decomposition of brain tissue by means of in situ 1H-magnetic resonance spectroscopy. *Magnetic Resonance in Medicine, 48*, 915–920. doi:10.1002/mrm.10294

Jackowski, C., Aghayev, E., Sonnenschein, M., Dirnhofer, R., & Thali, M. J. (2006). Maximum intensity projection of cranial computed tomography data for dental identification. *International Journal of Legal Medicine, 120*(3), 165–167. doi:10.1007/s00414-005-0050-1

Jackowski, C., Lussi, A., Classens, M., Kilchoer, T., Bolliger, S., & Aghayev, E. (2006). Extended CT scale overcomes restoration caused streak artifacts-3D color encoded automatic discrimination of dental restorations for identification. *Journal of Computer Assisted Tomography, 30*(3), 510–513. doi:10.1097/00004728-200605000-00027

Jackowski, C., Schweitzer, W., Thali, M., Yen, K., Aghayev, E., & Sonnenschein, M. (2005). Virtopsy: Postmortem imaging of the human heart in situ using

MSCT and MRI. *Forensic Science International, 149*(1), 11–23. doi:10.1016/j.forsciint.2004.05.019

Jackowski, C., Sonnenschein, M., Thali, M. J., Aghayev, E., Allmen, G., & Yen, K. (2005). Virtopsy: Postmortem minimally invasive angiography using cross section techniques—implementation and preliminary results. *Journal of Forensic Sciences, 50*, 1175–1186. doi:10.1520/JFS2005023

Jaffe, E. C., Roberts, G. J., Chantler, C., & Carter, J. E. (1990). Dental maturity in children with chronic renal failure assessed ITom dental panoramic tomographs. *Journal of the International Association of Dentistry for Children, 20*, 54–58.

Jain, A., & Zongker, D. (1997). Feature selection: Evaluation, application, and small sample performance. *IEEE Transactions on Pattern Analysis and Machine Intelligence, 19*, 153–158. doi:10.1109/34.574797

Jain, A. K., Bolle, R. M., & Pankanti, S. (1999). *Biometrics: Personal identification in networked society.* Boston: Kluwer Academic Publishers.

Jain, A. K., & Ross, A. (2002). Learning user-specific parameters in a multibiometric System. [Rochester, New York, USA.]. *Proceedings of the International Conference on Image Processing, 1*, 57–60. doi:10.1109/ICIP.2002.1037958

Jain, A. K., Ross, A., & Prabhakar, S. (2004). An introduction to biometric recognition. *IEEE Transactions on Circuits and Systems for Video Technology. Special Issue on Image and Video-Based Biometrics, 14*(1), 4–20.

Jain, R., Kasturi, R., & Schnck, B. G. (1995). *Machine vision.* McGraw-Hill Inc.

Jain, A. K., Duin, R. P. W., & Mao, J. (2000). Statistical pattern recognition: A review. *IEEE Transactions on Pattern Analysis and Machine Intelligence, 22*, 4–37. doi:10.1109/34.824819

Jauhiainen, T., Jarvinen, V. M., & Hekali, P. E. (2002). Evaluation of methods for MR imaging of human right ventricular heart volumes and mass. *Acta Radiologica, 43*(6), 587–592. doi:10.1034/j.1600-0455.2002.430609.x

Jergas, M., & San Valentin, R. (1995). Techniques for the assessment of vertebral dimensions in quantitative morphometry. In Genant, H. K., Jergas, M., & van Juijk, C.

(Eds.), *Vertebral fracture in osteoporosis* (pp. 163–188). San Francisco: University of California Osteoporosis Research Group.

Jiang, J., Lee, E., & Schmittgen, T. (2006). Increased expression of microRNA-155 in Epstein-Barr virus transformed lymphoblastiodcell lines. *Genes, Chromosomes & Cancer, 45*, 103–106. doi:10.1002/gcc.20264

Jobling, M. A., Hurles, M. E., & Tyler-Smith, C. (2004). *Human evolutionary genetics: Origins, people and disease.* Garland Science, Taylor & Francis Group.

Johnson, J. M., Castle, J., Garrett-Engele, P., Kan, Z., Loerch, P. M., & Armour, C. D. (2003). Genome-wide survey of human alternative pre-mRNA splicing with exon junction microarrays. *Science, 302*(5653), 2141–2144. doi:10.1126/science.1090100

Jolliffe, I. T. (1986). *Principal component analysis.* Berlin: Springer Verlag.

Jones, M.W. (2001). *Facial reconstruction using volumetric data.*

Jongeneel, C. V., Delorenzi, M., Iseli, C., Zhou, D., Haudenschild, C. D., & Khrebtukova, I. (2005). An atlas of human gene expression from massively parallel signature sequencing (MPSS). *Genome Research, 15*(7), 1007–1014. doi:10.1101/gr.4041005

Just, R. S., Irwin, J. A., O'Callaghan, J. E., Saunier, J. L., Coble, M. D., & Vallone, P. M. (2004). Toward increased utility of mtDNA in forensic identifications. *Forensic Science International, 146*(Suppl.), S147–S149. doi:10.1016/j.forsciint.2004.09.045

Kaestle, F. A., & Horsburgh, K. A. (2002). Ancient DNA in anthropology: Methods, applications, and ethics. *American Journal of Physical Anthropology, 119*(S35), 92–130. doi:10.1002/ajpa.10179

Kähler, K., Haber, J., & Seidel, H.-P. (2003). Reanimating the dead: Reconstruction of expressive faces from skull data. In *ACM Transactions on Graphics (SIGGRAPH 2003 Conference Proceedings), 22*(3), 554–561.

Kalender, W. A., & Eidloth, H. (1991). Determination of geometric parameters and osteoporosis indices for lumbar vertebrae from lateral QCT localizer radiographs. *Osteoporosis International, 1*, 197–200.

Kalidis, L., Felsenberg, D., & Kalender, W. A. (1992). Morphometric analysis of digitized radiographs: Description of automatic evaluation. In Ring, E. F. J. (Ed.), *Current research in osteoporosis and bone mineral measurement II* (pp. 14–16). London: British Institute of Radiology.

Kane, M. D., Jatkoe, T. A., Stumpf, C. R., Liu, J., Thomas, J. D., & Madore, S. J. (2000). Assessment of the sensitivity and specificity of oligonucleotide (50 mer) microarrays. *Nucleic Acids Research, 28*(22), 4552–4557. doi:10.1093/nar/28.22.4552

Kapushesky, M., Emam, I., Holloway, E., Kurnosov, P., Zorin, A., & Malone, J. (2010). Gene expression atlas at the European Bioinformatics Institute. *Nucleic Acids Research, 38*(Database issue), D690–D698. doi:10.1093/nar/gkp936

Karush, W. (1939). *Minima of functions of several variables with inequalities as side constraints*. Unpublished master's thesis, Department of Mathematics, University of Chicago.

Kashyap, V. K., Sahoo, S., Sitalaximi, T., & Trivedi, R. (2006). Deletions in the Y-derived amelogenin gene fragment in the Indian population. *BMC Medical Genetics, 7*, 37. doi:10.1186/1471-2350-7-37

Katsavrias, E. G. (2002). Changes in articular eminence inclination during the craniofacial growth period. *The Angle Orthodontist, 72*, 258–263.

Keener, J., & Sneyd, J. (1998). *Mathematical physiology*. New York: Springer.

Kerley, E. R., & Ubelaker, D. H. (1978). Revisions in the microscopic method of estimating age at death in human cortical bone. *American Journal of Physical Anthropology, 49*(4), 545–546. doi:10.1002/ajpa.1330490414

Kermi, A., Bloch, I. & Laskri, M.T. (2007). A non-linear registration method guided by b-splines free-form deformations for three-dimensional facial reconstruction. *International Review on Computers and Software, 20*.

Kerr, M. K., & Churchill, G. A. (2001). Experimental design for gene expression microarrays. *Biostatistics (Oxford, England), 2*(2), 183–201. doi:10.1093/biostatistics/2.2.183

Khanin, R., & Higham, D. J. (2007). *A minimal mathematical model of post-transcriptional gene regulation by microRNAs*. Report to Glasgow University.

Khanin, R., & Vinciotti, V. (2008). Computational modelling of post-transcriptional gene regulation by microRNAs. *Journal of Computational Biology, 15*(3), 305–316. doi:10.1089/cmb.2007.0184

Kidd, J. M., Cooper, G. M., Donahue, W. F., Hayden, H. S., Sampas, N., & Graves, T. (2008). Mapping and sequencing of structural variation from eight human genomes. *Nature, 453*(7191), 56–64. doi:10.1038/nature06862

Kleerekoper, M., & Nelson, D. A. (1992). Vertebral fracture or vertebral deformity? *Calcified Tissue International, 50*, 5–6. doi:10.1007/BF00297288

Kohavi, R., & George, J. H. (1997). Wrappers for feature subset selection. *Artificial Intelligence, 97*, 273–324. doi:10.1016/S0004-3702(97)00043-X

Konigsberg, L. W., Hens, S. M., Jantz, L. M., & Jungers, W. L. (1998). Stature estimation and calibration: Bayesian and maximum likelihood perspectives in physical anthropology. *Yearbook of Physical Anthropology, 41*, 65–92. doi:10.1002/(SICI)1096-8644(1998)107:27+<65::AID-AJPA4>3.0.CO;2-6

Konigsberg, L. W., Ross, A. H., & Jungers, W. L. (2006). Estimation and evidence in forensic anthropology: Determining stature. In Schmitt, A., Cunha, E., & Pinheiro, J. (Eds.), *Forensic anthropology and forensic medicine: Complimentary sciences from recovery to cause of death* (pp. 317–331). Totowa, NJ: Humana Press, Inc.

Kosa, F., & Castellana, C. (2005). New forensic anthropological approachment for the age determination of human fetal skeletons on the base of morphometry of vertebral column. *Forensic Science International, 147*, 69–74. doi:10.1016/j.forsciint.2004.09.096

Kostara, A., Roberts, G. J., & Gelbier, M. (2000). Dental maturity in children with Dystrophic Epidermolysis Bullosa. *Pediatric Dentistry, 22*, 385–388.

Krane, D. (2003). Random match probability. In *Proceedings of Forensic Bioinformatics 2nd Annual Conference on Statistics and DNA Profiling*. August 29-30, 2003. Retrieved on June 9, 2010, from http://www.bioforensics.com/conference/RMP/index.html

Kreitner, K. F., Schweden, F. J., Reipert, T., Nafe, B., & Thelen, M. (1998). Bone age determination based on the study of the medial extremity of the clavicle. *European Radiology, 8*, 1116–1122. doi:10.1007/s003300050518

Krek, A., Grun, D., Poy, M. N., Woff, R., Roseberg, L., & Epstein, E. J. (2005). Combinatorial microRNA target predictions. *Nature Genetics, 37*, 495–500. doi:10.1038/ng1536

Kronick, M. N. (2004). Creation of the whole human genome microarray. *Expert Review of Proteomics, 1*(1), 19–28. doi:10.1586/14789450.1.1.19

Kubinova, L., Janacek, J., Karen, P., Radochova, B., DiFato, F., & Krekule, I. (2004). Confocal stereology and image analysis: Methods for estimating geometrical characteristics of cells and tissues from three-dimensional confocal images. *Physiological Research, 53*(Suppl. 1), S47–S55.

Kudo, M., & Sklansky, J. (2000). Comparison of algorithms that select features for pattern classifiers. *Pattern Recognition, 33*(1), 25–41. doi:10.1016/S0031-3203(99)00041-2

Kuhn, H. W., & Tucker, A. W. (1951). Nonlinear programming. In *Proceeding of the 2nd Berkeley Symposium on Mathematical Statistics and Probabilistic,* (p. 481-492). Berkeley, CA: University of California Press.

Kulesh, D. A., Clive, D. R., Zarlenga, D. S., & Greene, J. J. (1987). Identification of interferon-modulated proliferation-related cDNA sequences. *Proceedings of the National Academy of Sciences of the United States of America, 84*(23), 8453–8457. doi:10.1073/pnas.84.23.8453

Kullman, L. (1995). Accuracy of two dental and one skeletal age estimation method in Swedish adolescents. *Forensic Science International, 75*, 225–226. doi:10.1016/0379-0738(95)01792-5

Kullmer, O. (2008). Benefits and risks in virtual anthropology. *Journal of Anthropological Sciences, 86*, 205–207.

Kuratate, T., Vatikiotis-Bateson, E., & Yehia, H. (2003). Cross-subject face animation driven by facial motion mapping. In Proceedings of *CE2003: Advanced Design, Production, and Managements systems,* (pp. 971–979).

Kvaal, S., Kolltveit, K. M., Thornsen, O., & Solheim, T. (1995). Age estimation of adults from dental radiographs. *Forensic Science International, 74*, 175–185. doi:10.1016/0379-0738(95)01760-G

Ladd, C., Lee, H. C., Yang, N., & Bieber, F. R. (2001). Interpretation of complex forensic DNA mixtures. *Croatian Medical Journal, 42*(3), 244–246.

Lagarde, J. M., Peyre, P., Redoules, D., Black, D., Briot, M., & Gall, Y. (1994). Confocal microscopy of hair. *Cell Biology and Toxicology, 10*, 301–304. doi:10.1007/BF00755774

Lahdesmaki, H., Shmulevich, L., Dunmire, V., Yli-Harja, O., & Zhang, W. (2005). In silico microdissection of microarray data from heterogeneous cell populations. *BMC Bioinformatics, 6*, 54. doi:10.1186/1471-2105-6-54

Lal, T. N., Chapelle, O., Weston, J., & Elisseeff, A. (2006). Embedded methods. In Guyon, I., Gunn, S., & Nikravesh, M. (Eds.), *Feature extraction, foundations and applications. Physica-Verlag.* Springer.

Lalueza-Fox, C., Sampietro, M. L., Gilbert, M. T., Castri, L., Facchini, F., & Pettener, D. (2004). Unravelling migrations in the steppe: Mitochondrial DNA sequences from ancient central Asians. *Proceedings. Biological Sciences, 271*(1542), 941–947. doi:10.1098/rspb.2004.2698

Lambrou, G. I., Chatziioannou, A., Sifakis, E. G., Prentza, A., Koutsouris, D., Koultouki, E., et al. (2009). *Setting a rational framework for experimental design and analysis of high-throughput DNA microarray experiments and data.* Paper presented at the 9th International Workshop on Mathematical Methods in Scattering Theory and Biomedical Engineering, Patras, Greece.

Lander, E. S. (2001). Initial sequencing and analysis of the human genome. *Nature, 409*(6822), 860–921. doi:10.1038/35057062

Lander, E. S. (2002). Initial sequencing and comparative analysis of the mouse genome. *Nature, 420*(6915), 520–562. doi:10.1038/nature01262

Landis, J. R., & Koch, G. G. (1977). The measurement of observer agreement for categorical data. *Biometrics, 33*, 159–174. doi:10.2307/2529310

Lash, A. E., Tolstoshev, C. M., Wagner, L., Schuler, G. D., Strausberg, R. L., & Riggins, G. J. (2000). SAGEmap: A public gene expression resource. *Genome Research, 10*(7), 1051–1060. doi:10.1101/gr.10.7.1051

Lauffenburger, D. A., Linderman, J., & Berkowitz, L. (1987). Analysis of mammalian cell growth factor receptor dynamics. *Annals of the New York Academy of Sciences, 506,* 147–162. doi:10.1111/j.1749-6632.1987.tb23816.x

Lee, H. C., & Gaensslen, R. E. (1991). *Advances in fingerprint technology.* Boca Raton, FL: CRC Press.

Lee, S., Yoo, C. D., & Kalker, T. (2007). Reversible image watermarking based on integer-to-integer wavelet transform information forensics and security. *IEEE Transactions Information Forensics and Security, 2*(3), 321–330. doi:10.1109/TIFS.2007.905146

Lee, Y., Terzopoulos, D., & Walters, K. (1995). *Realistic modeling for facial animation* (pp. 55–62).

Lee, E., Myungwon, B., Gusev, Y., Brackett, D. J., Nuovo, G. J., & Schmittgen, T. D. (2008). Systematic evolution of microRNA processing patterns in tissues, cell lines, and tumors. *RNA (New York, N.Y.), 14,* 35–42. doi:10.1261/rna.804508

Lee, M., & Vasioukhin, V. (2008). Cell polarity and cancer-cell and tissue polarity as a non-canonical tumor suppressor. *Journal of Cell Science, 121,* 1141–1150. doi:10.1242/jcs.016634

Lee, Y., Kim, M., Han, J., Yeom, K. H., Lee, S., & Baek, S. H. (2004). MicroRNA genes are transcribed by RNA polymerase II. *The EMBO Journal, 23*(20), 4051–4060. doi:10.1038/sj.emboj.7600385

Lersten, N. R., & Horner, H. T. (2000). Types of calcium oxalate crystals in macro patterns in leaves of Prunus (Rosaceae: Prunoideae). *Plant Systematics and Evolution, 224,* 83–96. doi:10.1007/BF00985267

Leth, P. M., & Gregersen, M. (2005). Ethylene glycol poisoning. *Forensic Science International, 155*(2-3), 179–184. doi:10.1016/j.forsciint.2004.11.012

Levesque, G. Y., Demirjian, A., & Tanguay, R. (1981). Sexual dimorphism in the development, emergence, and agenesis of the mandibular third molar. *Journal of Dental Research, 60,* 1735–1741. doi:10.1177/00220345810600100201

Levine, E., Ben Jacob, E., & Levine, H. (2007). Target-specific and global effectors in gene regulation by microRNA. *Biophysical Journal, 93*(11), L52–L54. doi:10.1529/biophysj.107.118448

Lewis, M. K., & Blake, G. M. (1995). Patient dose in morphometric X-ray absorptiometry. *Osteoporosis International, 5,* 281–282. doi:10.1007/BF01774019

Lewis, B., Burge, C., & Bartel, D. (2005). Conserved seed pairing, often flanked by adenosines, indicates that thousands of human genes are microRNA targets. *Cell, 120,* 15–20. doi:10.1016/j.cell.2004.12.035

Lewis, J. (2003). Autoinhibition with transcriptional delay: A simple mechanism for the zebrafish somitogenesis oscillator. *Current Biology, 19,* 1398–1408. doi:10.1016/S0960-9822(03)00534-7

Lewis, A. B., & Gam, S. M. (1960). The relationship between tooth formation and other maturational factors. *The Angle Orthodontist, 30,* 70–77.

Li, L., Li, C. T., Li, R. Y., Liu, Y., Lin, Y., & Que, T. Z. (2006). SNP genotyping by multiplex amplification and microarrays assay for forensic application. *Forensic Science International, 162*(1-3), 74–79. doi:10.1016/j.forsciint.2006.06.010

Li, Y., Carroll, D. S., Gardner, S. N., Walsh, M. C., Vitalis, E. A., & Damon, I. K. (2007). On the origin of smallpox: Correlating variola phylogenics with historical smallpox records. *Proceedings of the National Academy of Sciences of the United States of America, 104*(40), 15787–15792. doi:10.1073/pnas.0609268104

Li, G.-Z., Bu, H.-L., Yang, M. Q., Zeng, X.-Q., & Yang, J. Y. (2008). Selecting subsets of newly extracted features from PCA and PLS in microarray data analysis. *BMC Genomics, 9*(S2), S24. doi:10.1186/1471-2164-9-S2-S24

Li, G.-Z., & Liu, T.-Y. (2006). Improving generalization ability of neural networks ensemble with multi-task learning. *Journal of Computer Information Systems, 2*(4), 1235–1239.

Li, G.-Z., Meng, H.-H., Yang, M., & Yang, J. (2009). Combining support vector regression with feature selection for multivariate calibration. *Neural Computing & Applications, 18*(7), 813–820.

Li, G.-Z., Yang, J., Kong, A.-S., & Chen, N.-Y. (2004). Clustering algorithm based selective ensemble. *Journal of Fudan University, 2,* 689–691.

Li, G.-Z., Yang, J., Ye, C.-Z., & Geng, D. (2006). Degree prediction of malignancy in brain glioma using support vector machines. *Computers in Biology and Medicine, 36*(3), 313–325. doi:10.1016/j.compbiomed.2004.11.003

Li, G.-Z., & Yang, J. Y. (2008). Feature selection for ensemble learning and its applications. In *Machine Learning in Bioinformatics*. New York: John Wiley & Sons. doi:10.1002/9780470397428.ch6

Li, G.-Z., & Zeng, X.-Q. (2009). Feature selection for partial least square based dimension reduction. In A. Abraham, A.-E. Hassanien & V. Snasel (Eds.), *Foundations of computational intelligence.* (pp. 3-37). Springer Berlin / Heidelberg.

Li, G.-Z., Liu, T.-Y., & Cheng, V. S. (2006). Classification of brain glioma by using SVMs bagging with feature selection. In *BioDM 2006, Lecture Notes in Bioinformatics 3916* (p. 124-130). Springer.

Li, G.-Z., Yang, J., Liu, G.-P., & Xue, L. (2004). Feature selection for multi-class problems using support vector machines. In *PRICAI 2004, Lecture Notes in Artificial Intelligence 3157,* (p. 292-300). Springer.

Li, G.-Z., Yang, J., Lu, J., Lu, W.-C., & Chen, N.-Y. (2004). *On multivariate calibration problems.* In ISNN2004, (LNCS 3173). (p. 389-394). Springer.

Liang, M., Briggs, A. G., Rute, E., Greene, A. S., & Cowley, A. W. (2003). Quantitative assessment of the importance of dye switching and biological replication in cDNA microarray studies. *Physiological Genomics, 14*(3), 199–207.

Linch, C., Smith, S., & Prahlow, J. (1998). Evaluation of the human hair root for DNA typing subsequent to microscopic comparison. *Journal of Forensic Sciences, 43*(2), 305–314.

Linderman, J. J., & Lauffenburger, D. A. (1986). Analysis of intracellular receptor/ligand sorting. Calculation of mean surface and bulk diffusion times within a sphere. *Biophysical Journal, 50*(2), 295–305. doi:10.1016/S0006-3495(86)83463-4

Liu, W. M., Mei, R., Di, X., Ryder, T. B., Hubbell, E., & Dee, S. (2002). Analysis of high density expression microarrays with signed-rank call algorithms. *Bioinformatics (Oxford, England), 18*(12), 1593–1599. doi:10.1093/bioinformatics/18.12.1593

Liu, G.-P., Li, G.-Z., Wang, Y.-L., & Wang, Y. (2010). Syndrome model of inquiry diagnosis for coronary heart disease in Chinese medicine by using multi-label learning. *BMC Complementary and Alternative Medicine, 10,* 37. doi:10.1186/1472-6882-10-37

Liu, H., & Yu, L. (2005). Toward integrating feature selection algorithms for classification and clustering. *IEEE Transactions on Knowledge and Data Engineering, 17*(3), 1–12.

Liu, T.-Y., Li, G.-Z., & Wu, G.-F. (2006). Degree prediction of malignancy in brain glioma using selective neural networks ensemble. *Journal of Shanghai University, 10*(3), 244–246. doi:10.1007/s11741-006-0123-5

Liversidge, H. M. (2008). Timing of human mandibular third molar formation. *Annals of Human Biology, 35,* 294–321. doi:10.1080/03014460801971445

Liversidge, H. M., Chaillet, N., Mornstad, H., Nystrom, M., Rowlings, K., & Taylor, J. (2006). Timing of Demirjian's tooth formation stages. *Annals of Human Biology, 33,* 454–470. doi:10.1080/03014460600802387

Liversidge, H. M., Dean, M. C., & Molleson, T. (1993). Increasing human tooth length between birth and 5.4 years. *American Journal of Physical Anthropology, 90,* 307–313. doi:10.1002/ajpa.1330900305

Liversidge, H. M., Kosmidou, A., Hector, M. P., & Roberts, G. J. (2005). Epidermolysis bullo'sa and dental development age. *International Journal of Paediatric Dentistry, 15,* 335–341. doi:10.1111/j.1365-263X.2005.00649.x

Liversidge, H. M., Lyons, M., & Hector, M. P. (2003). The accuracy of three methods of age estimation using radiographic measurements of developing teeth. *Forensic Science International, 131,* 22–29. doi:10.1016/S0379-0738(02)00373-0

Ljung, P., Winskog, C., Persson, A., Lundstrom, C., & Ynnerman, A. (2006). Full-body virtual autopsies using a stateof- the-art volume rendering pipeline. *IEEE Transactions on Visualization and Computer Graphics, 12*(5), 869–876. doi:10.1109/TVCG.2006.146

Lockhart, D. J., Dong, H., Byrne, M. C., Follettie, M. T., Gallo, M. V., & Chee, M. S. (1996). Expression monitoring by hybridization to high-density oligonucleotide arrays.

Nature Biotechnology, 14(13), 1675–1680. doi:10.1038/nbt1296-1675

Logan, W., & Kronfeld, R. (1933). Development of the human jaws and surrounding structures from birth to the age of fifteen years. *The Journal of the American Dental Association, 20*(3), 379–427.

Lopez Gonzalez, M. A., & Sotelo, J. (2000). Brain tumors in Mexico: Characteristics and prognosis of glioblastoma. *Surgical Neurology, 53*, 157–162. doi:10.1016/S0090-3019(99)00177-9

Lowenstein, J. M. (1980). Species-specific proteins in fossils. *Naturwissenschaften, 67*(7), 343–346. doi:10.1007/BF01106588

Lowenstein, J. M., Reuther, J. D., Hood, D. G., Scheuenstuhl, G., Gerlach, S. C., & Ubelaker, D. H. (2006). Identification of animal species by protein radioimmunoassay of bone fragments and bloodstained stone tools. *Forensic Science International, 159*(2), 182–188. doi:10.1016/j.forsciint.2005.08.007

Lu, J., Lal, A., Merriman, B., Nelson, S., & Riggins, G. (2004). A comparison of gene expression profiles produced by SAGE, long SAGE, and oligonucleotide chips. *Genomics, 84*(4), 631–636. doi:10.1016/j.ygeno.2004.06.014

Lu, P., Nakorchevskiy, A., & Marcotte, E. M. (2003). Expression deconvolution: A reinterpretation of DNA microarray data reveals dynamic changes in cell populations. *Proceedings of the National Academy of Sciences of the United States of America, 100*(18), 10370–10375. doi:10.1073/pnas.1832361100

Luder, H.-U. (2002). Factors affecting degeneration in human temporomandibular joints as assessed histologically. *European Journal of Oral Sciences, 110*, 106–113. doi:10.1034/j.1600-0722.2002.11212.x

Lunt, R. C., & Law, D. B. (1974). A review of the chronology of calcification of deciduous teeth. *The Journal of the American Dental Association, 89*(3), 599–606.

Lynnerup, N., Clausen, M. L., Kristoffersen, A. M., & Steglich-Arnholm, H. (2009). Facial recognition and laser surface scan: A pilot study. *Forensic Science, Medicine, and Pathology, 5*(3), 167–173. doi:10.1007/s12024-009-9094-8

Maber, M., Liversidge, H. M., & Hector, M. P. (2006). Accuracy of age estimation of radiographic methods using developing teeth. *Forensic Science International, 159S*, S68–S73. doi:10.1016/j.forsciint.2006.02.019

Macgregor, S., Zhao, Z. Z., Henders, A., Nicholas, M. G., Montgomery, G. W., & Visscher, P. M. (2008). Highly cost-efficient genome-wide association studies using DNA pools and dense SNP arrays. *Nucleic Acids Research, 36*(6), e35. doi:10.1093/nar/gkm1060

Madden, S. L., Wang, C. J., & Landes, G. (2000). Serial analysis of gene expression: From gene discovery to target identification. *Drug Discovery Today, 5*(9), 415–425. doi:10.1016/S1359-6446(00)01544-0

Madea, B., Henssge, C., & Lockhoven, H. B. (1986). Priority of multiple gunshot injuries of the skull. *Zeitschrift fur Rechtsmedizin, 97*, 213–218.

Magid, D., Bryan, B. M., Drebin, R. A., Ney, D., & Fishman, E. K. (1989). Three-dimensional imaging of an Egyptian mummy. *Clinical Imaging, 13*, 239–240. doi:10.1016/0899-7071(89)90156-3

Mahoor, M., & Abdel-Mottaleb, M. (2005). Classification and numbering of teeth in Bitewing dental images. *Journal of Pattern Recognition, 38*, 577–586. doi:10.1016/j.patcog.2004.08.012

Mang, A., Müller, J., & Buzug, T. M. (2006). A multimodality computer-aided framework towards postmortem identification. *Journal of Computing and Information Technology, 14*(1), 7–19. doi:10.2498/cit.2006.01.02

Mang, A., Müller, J., & Buzug, M. T. (2005). Soft-tissue segmentation in forensic applications. In Buzug, T. M., Sigl, K.-M., Bongartz, J., & Prüfer, K. (Eds.), *Facial reconstruction* (pp. 62–67). München: Wolters/Kluwer.

Manhein, M. H., Listi, G. A., Barsley, R. E., Musselman, R., Barrow, N. E., & Ubelaker, D. H. (2000). In vivo facial tissue depth measurements for children and adults. *Journal of Forensic Sciences, 45*(1), 48–60.

Manjunath, K., Sriram, G., Saraswathi, T. R., & Sivapathasungharam, B. (2008). Enamel rod end patterns: a preliminary study using acetate peel technique adnd automated biometrics. *The Journal of Forensic Odonto-Stomatology, 1*(1), 33–36.

Marécaux, C., Sidjilani, B. M., Chabanas, M., Chouly, F., Payan, Y., & Boutault, F. (2003). A new 3D cephalometric analysis for planning in computer aided orthognatic surgery. *Computer Aided Surgery, 8*(4), 217.

Margolis, B., & Borg, J. P. (2005). Apicobasal polarity complexes. *Journal of Cell Science, 118*, 5157–5159. doi:10.1242/jcs.02597

Margulies, E. H., Kardia, S. L., & Innis, J. W. (2001). Identification and prevention of a GC content bias in SAGE libraries. *Nucleic Acids Research, 29*(12), E60–E0. doi:10.1093/nar/29.12.e60

Margulies, M., Egholm, M., Altman, W. E., Attiya, S., Bader, J. S., & Bemben, L. A. (2005). Genome sequencing in microfabricated high-density picolitre reactors. *Nature, 437*(7057), 376–380.

Matsumura, H., Reich, S., Ito, A., Saitoh, H., Kamoun, S., & Winter, P. (2003). Gene expression analysis of plant host-pathogen interactions by SuperSAGE. *Proceedings of the National Academy of Sciences of the United States of America, 100*(26), 15718–15723. doi:10.1073/pnas.2536670100

Maziere, P., & Enright, A. (2007). Prediction of mictoRNA targets. *Drug Discovery Today, 12*, 452–458. doi:10.1016/j.drudis.2007.04.002

Mc Closkey, E. V., Spector, T. D., & Eyres, K. S. (1993). The assessment of vertebral deformity: A method for use in population studies and clinical trials. *Osteoporosis International, 3*, 138–147. doi:10.1007/BF01623275

McAdams, H. H., & Arkin, A. (1997). Stochastic mechanisms in gene expression. *Proceedings of the National Academy of Sciences of the United States of America, 94*(3), 814–819. doi:10.1073/pnas.94.3.814

McMartin, K. E., & Wallace, K. B. (2005). Calcium oxalate monohydrate, a metabolite of ethylene glycol, is toxic for rat renal mitochondrial function. *Toxicological Sciences, 84*, 195–200. doi:10.1093/toxsci/kfi062

McQuain, M. K., Seale, K., Peek, J., Levy, S., & Haselton, F. R. (2003). Effects of relative humidity and buffer additives on the contact printing of microarrays by quill pins. *Analytical Biochemistry, 320*(2), 281–291. doi:10.1016/S0003-2697(03)00348-8

Meester, R., & Sjerps, M. (2003). The evidential value in the DNA database search controversy and the two-stain problem. *Biometrics, 59*(3), 727–732. doi:10.1111/1541-0420.00084

Menzel, E. R. (1999). Fingerprint detection with lasers, 2nd ed. [New York: Marcel Dekker.]. *Journal of Forensic Sciences, 42*, 303–306.

Mérida-Velasco, J. R., Rodriguez-Vazquez, J. F., Mérida-Velasco, J. A., Sanchez-Montesinos, I., Espin-Ferra, J., & Jimenez-Collado, J. (1999). Development of the human temporomandibular joint. *The Anatomical Record, 255*, 20–33. doi:10.1002/(SICI)1097-0185(19990501)255:1<20::AID-AR4>3.0.CO;2-N

Meyers, J. C., Okoye, M. I., Kiple, D., Kimmerle, E. H., & Reinhard, K. J. (1999). Three-dimensional (3-D) imaging in post-mortem examinations: Elucidation and identification of cranial and facial fractures in victims of homicide utilizing 3-D computerized imaging reconstruction techniques. *International Journal of Legal Medicine, 113*(1), 33–37. doi:10.1007/s004140050275

Meyers, B. C., Tej, S. S., Vu, T. H., Haudenschild, C. D., Agrawal, V., & Edberg, S. B. (2004a). The use of MPSS for whole-genome transcriptional analysis in Arabidopsis. *Genome Research, 14*(98), 1641–1653. doi:10.1101/gr.2275604

Meyers, B. C., Vu, T. H., Tej, S. S., Ghazal, H., Matvienko, M., & Agrawal, V. (2004b). Analysis of the transcriptional complexity of Arabidopsis thaliana by massively parallel signature sequencing. *Nature Biotechnology, 22*(8), 1006–1011. doi:10.1038/nbt992

Michael, A., & Brauner, P. (2004). Erroneous gender identification by the amelogenin sex test. *Journal of Forensic Sciences, 49*(2), 1–2. doi:10.1520/JFS2003223

Michael, S. D., & Chen, M. (1996). The 3-D reconstruction of facial features using volume distortion. *Proceedings of 14th Annual Conference of Eurographics*, (pp. 297-305).

Millikan, R. C. (2001). Re: Population stratification in epidemiologic studies of common genetic variants and cancer: Quantification of bias. *Journal of the National Cancer Institute, 93*, 156. doi:10.1093/jnci/93.2.156

Mincer, H. H., Hams, E. F., & Berryman, H. E. (1993). The ABFO study of third molar development. *Journal of Forensic Sciences, 38*, 379–390.

Minne, H. W., Leidig, C., & Wuster, C. H. R. (1988). A newly developed spine deformity index (SDI) to quantitative vertebral crush fractures in patients with osteoporosis. *Bone and Mineral*, *3*, 335–349.

Mirnics, K., Middleton, F. A., Marquez, A., Lewis, D. A., & Levitt, P. (2000). Molecular characterization of schizophrenia viewed by microarray analysis of gene expression in prefrontal cortex. *Neuron*, *28*(1), 53–67. doi:10.1016/S0896-6273(00)00085-4

Misner, L. M., Halvorson, A. C., Dreier, J. L., Ubelaker, D. H., & Foran, D. R. (2009). The correlation between skeletal weathering and DNA quality and quantity. *Journal of Forensic Sciences*, *54*(4), 822–828. doi:10.1111/j.1556-4029.2009.01043.x

Mitchell, P., Parkin, R., Kroh, E., Fritz, B., Wimen, S., & Pogosova-Agadjanyan, E. (2008). Circulating microRNAs as stable blood-based markers for cancer detection. [PNAS]. *Proceedings of the National Academy of Sciences of the United States of America*, *105*(30), 10513–10518. doi:10.1073/pnas.0804549105

Mitchell, J. C., Roberts, G., Donaldson, A. N., & Lucas, V. S. (2009). Dental Age Asessment (DAA): Reference data for British caucasians at the 16 year threshold. *Forensic Science International*, *189*, 19–23. doi:10.1016/j.forsciint.2009.04.002

Mitra, P., Murthy, C. A., & Pal, S. K. (2002). Unsupervised feature selection using feature similarity. *IEEE Transactions on Pattern Analysis and Machine Intelligence*, *24*(3), 301–312. doi:10.1109/34.990133

Modrek, B., & Lee, C. J. (2003). Alternative splicing in the human, mouse and rat genomes is associated with an increased frequency of exon creation and/or loss. *Nature Genetics*, *34*(2), 177–180. doi:10.1038/ng1159

Molina, D. K. (2010). Forensic medicine and human identification. In Senn, D., & Stimson, P. (Eds.), *Forensic dentistry* (2nd ed., pp. 61–78). Boca Raton, FL: Taylor & Francis.

Monjunath, K., Sriram, G., Sarawathi, T., Sivapathasundharam, B., & Porchelvam, S. (2009). Reliability of automated biometrics in the analysis of enamel rod end patterns. *Journal of Forensic Dental Sciences*, *1*(1), 32–36. doi:10.4103/0974-2948.50887

Monk, N. A. (2003). Oscillatory expression of Hes1, p53, and NF-kappaB driven by transcriptional time delays. *Current Biology*, *13*, 1409–1413. doi:10.1016/S0960-9822(03)00494-9

Moody, J., & Utans, J. (1992). Principled architecture selection for neural networks: Application to corporate bond rating prediction. In Moody, J. E., Hanson, S. J., & Lippmann, R. P. (Eds.), *Advances in neural information processing systems* (pp. 683–690). Morgan Kaufmann Publishers, Inc.

Moore, J. E. (1988). A key for the identification of animal hairs. *Proceedings of the Forensic Science Society*, (pp. 335-339).

Morimoto, K., Hashimoto, N., & Suetsugu, T. (1987). Prenatal developmental process of human temporomandibular joint. *The Journal of Prosthetic Dentistry*, *57*, 723–729. doi:10.1016/0022-3913(87)90372-6

Morrees, C. F. A., & Kent, R. L. (1978). A step function model using tooth counts to assess the developmental timing of dentititon. *Annals of Human Biology*, *5*, 55–68. doi:10.1080/03014467800002641

Morse, S. A., & Budowle, B. (2006). Microbial forensics: Application to bioterrorism preparedness and response. *Infectious Disease Clinics of North America*, *20*(2), 455–473. doi:10.1016/j.idc.2006.03.004

Mortera, J., Dawid, A. P., & Lauritzen, S. L. (2003). Probabilistic expert systems for DNA mixture profiling. *Theoretical Population Biology*, *63*(3), 191–205. doi:10.1016/S0040-5809(03)00006-6

Mulhern, D. M., & Ubelaker, D. H. (2001). Differences in osteon banding between human and nonhuman bone. *Journal of Forensic Sciences*, *46*(2), 220–222.

Mulhern, D. M., & Ubelaker, D. H. (2003). Histologic examination of bone development in juvenile chimpanzees. *American Journal of Physical Anthropology*, *122*(2), 127–133. doi:10.1002/ajpa.10294

Mulhern, D. M., & Ubelaker, D. H. (2009). Bone microstructure in juvenile chimpanzees. *American Journal of Physical Anthropology*, *140*(2), 368–375. doi:10.1002/ajpa.20959

Mulhern, D. M. (2009). Differentiating human from nonhuman skeletal remains. In Blau, S., & Ubelaker,

D. H. (Eds.), *Handbook of forensic anthropology and archaeology* (pp. 153–163). Walnut Creek, CA: Left Coast Press, Inc.

Naef, F., & Magnasco, M. O. (2003). Solving the riddle of the bright mismatches: Labeling and effective binding in oligonucleotide arrays. *Physical Review E: Statistical, Nonlinear, and Soft Matter Physics, 68*(1 Pt 1), 011906. doi:10.1103/PhysRevE.68.011906

Naef, F., Socci, N. D., & Magnasco, M. (2003). A study of accuracy and precision in oligonucleotide arrays: Extracting more signal at large concentrations. *Bioinformatics (Oxford, England), 19*(2), 178–184. doi:10.1093/bioinformatics/19.2.178

Naef, F., Hacker, C.R., Patil, N. & Magnasco, M. (2002). Characterization of the expression ratio noise structure in high-density oligonucleotide arrays. *Genome Biology, 3*(1), 01.

Najarian, K., Zaheri, M., Rad, A. A., Najarian, S., & Dargahi, J. (2004). A novel mixture model method for identification of differentially expressed genes from DNA microarray data. *BMC Bioinformatics, 5*, 201. doi:10.1186/1471-2105-5-201

Nakano, M., Nobuta, K., Vemaraju, K., Tej, S. S., Skogen, J. W., & Meyers, B. C. (2006). Plant MPSS databases: signature-based transcriptional resources for analyses of mRNA and small RNA. *Nucleic Acids Research, 34*(Database issue), D731–D735. doi:10.1093/nar/gkj077

Nakasone, H., & Beck, S. D. (2001). Forensic automatic speaker recognition. *2001: A Speaker Odyssey - The Speaker Recognition Workshop.* June 18-22, 2001, Crete, Greece.

Nandi, A., Vaz, C., Bhattacharya, A., & Ramaswamy, R. (2008). MiRNA-regulated dynamics in circadian oscillator models. *RNA (New York, N.Y.), 14*, 1480–1491.

Nassar, D., Said, E. H., Abaza, A., Chekuri, S., Zhou, J., Mahoor, M., et al. (2005). Automated Dental Identification System (ADIS). *Proceedings of National Conference on Digital Government Research,* (pp. 165–166). Atlanta, GA, USA.

National Academies Press. (2009). *Strengthening forensic science in the United States: A path forward.* Retrieved from http://www.nap.edu/catalogue.php?record_id=12589

Nelson, D., Peterson, E., & Tilley, B. (1990). Measurement of vertebral area on spine X-rays in osteoporosis: Reliability of digitizing techniques. *Journal of Bone and Mineral Research, 5*, 707–716. doi:10.1002/jbmr.5650050707

Nelson, L. A., & Michael, S. D. (1998). The application of volume deformation to three dimensional facial reconstruction: A comparison with previous techniques. *Forensic Science International, 94*, 167–181. doi:10.1016/S0379-0738(98)00066-8

Neri, M. (2010). Beyond and together with autopsy techniques: Confocal scanning laser microscopy in forensic medicine. In Pomara, C., Karch, S. B., & Fineschi, V. (Eds.), *Forensic autopsy: A handbook and altas* (pp. 113–120). CRC press. doi:10.1201/EBK1439800645-c5

Newman, J. R., Ghaemmaghami, S., Ihmels, J., Breslow, D. K., Noble, M., & DeRisi, J. L. (2006). Single-cell proteomic analysis of S. cerevisiae reveals the architecture of biological noise. *Nature, 441*(7095), 840–846. doi:10.1038/nature04785

Newton, M. A., Kendziorski, C. M., Richmond, C. S., Blattner, F. R., & Tsui, K. W. (2001). On differential variability of expression ratios: Improving statistical inference about gene expression changes from microarray data. *Journal of Computational Biology, 8*(1), 37–52. doi:10.1089/106652701300099074

NHGRI. (2008). National Human Genome Research Institute methods for discovering and scoring single nucleotide polymorphisms. Retrieved from www.genome.gov/10001029

Ni, Z., Shi, Y. Q., Ansari, N., Su, W., Sun, Q., & Lin, X. (2008). Robust lossless image data hiding designed for semi-fragile image authentication. *IEEE Transactions on Circuits and Systems for Video Technology, 18*(4), 497–508. doi:10.1109/TCSVT.2008.918761

Nicholson, P. H. F., Haddaway, M. J., & Davie, M. W. J. (1993). A computerized technique for vertebral morphometry. *Physiological Measurement, 14*, 195–204. doi:10.1088/0967-3334/14/2/010

Nickell, J., & Fischer, J. F. (1999). *Crime science: Methods of forensic detection.* Lexington, KY: University of Kentucky Press.

Nikolov, S., Vera, J., Herwig, R., Wolkenhauer, O. & Petrov, V. (2010). Dynamics of microRNA regulation of a cancer network, *Comptes rendus de l'Academie bulgare des Sciences, 63*(1), 61-70.

Nikolova, E., Herwig, R., & Petrov, V. (2009a). Quasi-stationary approximation of a dynamical model of microRNA target regulation. Part I. Establishment of time hierarchy in the model dynamics. *International Journal Bioautomation, 13*(4), 127–134.

Nikolova, E., Herwig, R., & Petrov, V. (2009b). Quasi-stationary approximation of a dynamical model of microRNA target regulation. Part II. Application of the QSSA theorem. *International Journal Bioautomation, 13*(4), 135–142.

Nissan, T., & Parker, R. (2008). Computational analysis of miRNA-mediated repression of translation: Implications for models of translation initiation inhibition. *RNA (New York, N.Y.), 14*, 1480–1491. doi:10.1261/rna.1072808

Njeh, C. F., Fuerst, T., & Hans, D. (1999). Radiation exposure in bone mineral density assessment. *Applied Radiation and Isotopes, 50*, 215–236. doi:10.1016/S0969-8043(98)00026-8

Nomir, O., & Abdel-Mottaleb, M. (2005). A system for human identification from X-ray dental radiographs. *Journal of Pattern Recognition, 38*(8), 1295–1305. doi:10.1016/j.patcog.2004.12.010

Nomir, O., & Abdel-Mottaleb, M. (2007a). Dental biometrics: Matching X-ray dental images using teeth shapes and appearances. *IEEE Transactions on Information Forensics and Security, 2*(2), 188–197. doi:10.1109/TIFS.2007.897245

Nomir, O., & Abdel-Mottaleb, M. (2008a). Hierarchical contour matching for dental X-ray radiographs. *Journal of Pattern Recognition, 41*(1), 130–138. doi:10.1016/j.patcog.2007.05.015

Nomir, O., & Abdel-Mottaleb, M. (2008b). Fusion of matching algorithms for human identification using dental X-ray radiographs. *IEEE Transactions on Information Forensics and Security, 3*(2), 223–233. doi:10.1109/TIFS.2008.919343

Nomir, O. (2006). *A framework for automating human identification using dental X-ray radiograph.* Unpublished doctoral dissertation, University of Miami, 2006.

Nomir, O., & Abdel-Mottaleb, M. (2006). Hierarchical dental X-ray radiographs matching. *International Conference on Image Processing ICIP*, (pp. 2677–2680). Atlanta, GA, USA.

Nomir, O., & Abdel-Mottaleb, M. (2007b). Combining matching algorithms for human identification using dental X-ray radiographs. *International Conference on Image Processing ICIP*, (pp. 409–412). San Antonio, Texas, USA.

Nomir, O., & Abdel-Mottaleb, M. (2007c). Human identification based on fusing matching algorithms using dental X-ray radiographs. *International Conference on Computer Theory and Applications*, (pp. 85–88). Alexandria, Egypt.

Nortje, C. J. (1983). The permanent mandibular third molar. It's value in age determination. *The Journal of Forensic Odonto-Stomatology, 1*, 27–31.

Notman, D. N., Tashjian, J., Aufderheide, A. C., Cass, O. W., Shane, O. C. III, & Berquist, T. H. (1986). Modern imaging and endoscopic biopsy techniques in Egyptian mummies. *AJR. American Journal of Roentgenology, 146*, 93–96.

O'Neill, T. W., Felsenberg, D., & Varlow, J. (1996). The prevalence of vertebral deformity in European men and women: The European vertebral osteoporosis study. *Journal of Bone and Mineral Research, 11*, 1010–1018. doi:10.1002/jbmr.5650110719

O'Rourke, D. H., Hayes, M. G., & Carlyle, S. W. (2000). Ancient DNA studies in physical anthropology. *Annual Review of Anthropology, 29*, 217–242. doi:10.1146/annurev.anthro.29.1.217

Öberg, T., Carlsson, G. E., & Fajers, C.-M. (1971). The temporomandibular joint. A morphologic study on a human autopsy material. *Acta Odontologica Scandinavica, 29*, 349–389. doi:10.3109/00016357109026526

Okamoto, T., Suzuki, T., & Yamamoto, N. (2000). Microarray fabrication with covalent attachment of DNA using bubble jet technology. *Nature Biotechnology, 18*(4), 438–441. doi:10.1038/74507

Okubo, K., Hori, N., Matoba, R., Niiyama, T., & Matsubara, K. (1991). A novel system for large-scale sequencing of cDNA by PCR amplification. *DNA Sequence, 2*(3), 137–144. doi:10.3109/10425179109039684

Oliver, W. R., Chancellor, A. S., Soitys, J., Symon, J., Cullip, T., & Rosenman, J. (1995). Three-dimensional reconstruction of a bullet path: Validation by computed radiography. *Journal of Forensic Sciences, 40*(2), 321–324.

Olze, A., Bilang, D., Schmidt, S., Wemecke, K. D., Geserick, G., & Schmeling, A. (2005). Validation of common classification systems for assessing mineralization of third molars. *Internal Journal of Legal Medicine, 119*, 22–26. doi:10.1007/s00414-004-0489-5

Olze, A., Schmeling, A., Taniguchi, M., Van Niekerk, P., Wemecke, K. D., & Geserick, G. (2004). Forensic age estimation in living subjects: The ethnic factor in wisdom teeth mineralization. *International Journal of Legal Medicine, 118*, 170–173. doi:10.1007/s00414-004-0434-7

Olze, A., van Nierkerk, P., Ishikawa, T., Zhu, B. L., Schulz, R., & Maeda, H. (2007). Comparative study on the effect of ethnicity on wisdom tooth eruption. *International Journal of Legal Medicine, 121*, 445–448. doi:10.1007/s00414-007-0171-9

Ousley, S. D., & Jantz, R. L. (1996). *FORDISC 2.0: Personal computer forensic discriminant functions.* Knoxville, TN: University of Tennessee Press.

Ozbudak, E. M., Thattai, M., Kurtser, I., Grossman, A. D., & van Oudenaarden, A. (2002). Regulation of noise in the expression of a single gene. *Nature Genetics, 31*(1), 69–73. doi:10.1038/ng869

Palla, S., Gallo, L. M., & Gossi, D. (2003). Dynamic stereometry of the temporomandibular joint. *Orthodontics & Craniofacial Research, 1*, 37–47. doi:10.1034/j.1600-0544.2003.233.x

Palmeirim, I., Henrique, D., Ish-Horowicz, D., & Pourquie, O. (1997). Avian hairy gene expression identifies a molecular clock linked to vertebrate segmentation and somitogenesis. *Cell, 91*, 639–648. doi:10.1016/S0092-8674(00)80451-1

Pan, W., Coatrieux, G., Montagner, J., Cuppens, N., Cuppens, F., & Roux, C. (2009). Comparison of some reversible watermarking methods in application to medical images. *Proceedings of the 31ˢᵗ IEEE EMBS Annual International Conference, September 2-6, 2009, Minneapolis, Minnesota, US,* (pp. 2172 – 2175).

Pandzic, I. S., & Forchheimer, R. (2002). *MPEG-4 facial animation. The standard, implementation, and applications.* Chichester, UK: John Wiley & Sons. doi:10.1002/0470854626

Parkinson, H., Kapushesky, M., Kolesnikov, N., Rustici, G., Shojatalab, M., & Abeygunawardena, N. (2009). ArrayExpress update-from an archive of functional genomics experiments to the atlas of gene expression. *Nucleic Acids Research, 37*(Database issue), D868–D872. doi:10.1093/nar/gkn889

Parmigiani, G., Garret, E. S., Andazhagan, R., & Gabrielson, E. (2002). A statistical framework for molecular-based classification in cancer. *Journal of the Royal Statistical Society. Series B. Methodological, 64*, 717–736. doi:10.1111/1467-9868.00358

Parsons, T. J., & Weedn, V. W. (1997). Preservation and recovery of DNA in postmortem specimens and trace samples. In Haglund, W. D., & Sorg, M. H. (Eds.), *Forensic taphonomy: The postmortem fate of human remains* (pp. 109–138). Boca Raton, FL: CRC Press.

Patriquin, L., Kassarjian, A., O'Brien, M., Andry, C., & Eustace, S. (2001). Postmortem whole-body magnetic resonance imaging as an adjunct to autopsy: Preliminary clinical experience. *Journal of Magnetic Resonance Imaging, 13*, 277–287. doi:10.1002/1522-2586(200102)13:2<277::AID-JMRI1040>3.0.CO;2-W

Payan, Y., Chabanas, M., Pelorson, X., Vilain, C., Levy, P., & Luboz, V. (2002). Biomechanical models to simulate consequences of maxillofacial surgery. *Comptes Rendus Biologies, 325*, 407–417. doi:10.1016/S1631-0691(02)01443-9

Paysan, P., Luthi, M., Albrecht, T., Lerch, A., Amberg, B., & Santini, F. (2009). Face reconstruction from skull shapes and physical attributes. In. *Proceedings of DAGM-Symposium, 2009*, 232–241.

Pearson, J. V., Huentelman, M. J., Halperin, R. F., Tembe, W. D., Melquist, S., & Homer, N. (2007). Identification of the genetic basis for complex disorders by use of pooling-based genomewide single-nucleotide-polymorphism association studies. *American Journal of Human Genetics, 80*(1), 126–139. doi:10.1086/510686

Peltre, G., Cerceau-Larrival, M.-T., Hideux, M., Abadie, M., & David, B. (1987). Scanning and transmission electron microscopy related to immunochemical analysis of grass pollen. *Grana, 26*, 158–170. doi:10.1080/00173138709429945

Petersen, C., Bordelean, M., Pelletier, J., & Sharp, P. (2006). Short RNAs repress translation after initiation in mammalian cells. *Molecular Cell, 21*, 533–542. doi:10.1016/j.molcel.2006.01.031

Petraco, N. (1987). A microscopical method to aid in the identification of animal hair. *Microscope (Carshalton Beeches (Surrey)), 35*, 83–92.

Petricoin, E. F., Ardekani, A. M., Hitt, B. A., Levine, P. J., Fusaro, V. A., & Steinberg, S. M. (2002). Use of proteomic patterns in serum to identify ovarian cancer. *Lancet, 359*(9306), 572–577. doi:10.1016/S0140-6736(02)07746-2

Petrie, A., & Sabin, C. (2009). *Medical statistics at a glance* (3rd ed.). Oxford: Wiley Blackwell.

Petrov, V., Nikolova, E., & Timmer, J. (2004). Dynamical analysis of cell function models. A review. *Journal of Theoretical Applied Mechanics, 34*(3), 55–78.

Petrov, V., Nikolova, E., & Wolkenhauer, O. (2007). Reduction of nonlinear dynamic system with an application to signal transduction pathways. *IET Systems Biology, 1*, 2–9. doi:10.1049/iet-syb:20050030

Petrov, V., & Timmer, J. (2009). One-dimensional model of somitic cells polarization in a bistability window of embryonic mesoderm. *Journal of Mechanics in Medicine and Biology, 9*, 359–272. doi:10.1142/S0219519409003061

Pighin, F., Szeliski, R., & Salesin, D. H. (1999). Resynthesizing facial animation through 3D model-based tracking. In. *Proceedings of International Conference on Computer Vision, 1*, 143–150. doi:10.1109/ICCV.1999.791210

Pinkel, D., Segraves, R., Sudar, D., Clark, S., Poole, I., & Kowbel, D. (1998). High resolution analysis of DNA copy number variation using comparative genomic hybridization to microarrays. *Nature Genetics, 20*(2), 207–211. doi:10.1038/2524

Piriyapongsa, J., & King Jordan, I. (2008). Dual coding of siRNAs and miRNAs by plant transposable elements. *RNA (New York, N.Y.), 14*, 814–821. doi:10.1261/rna.916708

Pirttiniemi, P., & Kantomaa, T. (1992). Relation of glenoid fossa morphology to mandibulofacial asymmetry, studied in dry human Lapp skulls. *Acta Odontologica Scandinavica, 50*, 235–243. doi:10.3109/00016359209012768

Piva, A., Barni, M., Bartolini, F., & De Rosa, A. (2005). Data hiding technologies for digital radiography. *IEEE Proceedings of Visual Image Signal Processing, 152*(5), 604–610. doi:10.1049/ip-vis:20041240

Planz, J. V. (2008). *Validation theory and its effect on the interpretation of DNA mixtures.* 19th International Symposium on Human Identification, October 15, 2008. Hollywood, CA.

Plasterk, R. (2002). RNA silencing: The genome's immune system. *Science, 296*(5571), 1263–1265. doi:10.1126/science.1072148

Pomara, C., Fiore, C., D'Errico, S., Riezzo, I., & Fineschi, V. (2008). Calcium oxalate crystals in acute ethylene glycol poisoning: A confocal laser scanning microscope study in a fatal case. *Clinical Toxicology, 46*(4), 322–324. doi:10.1080/15563650701419011

Pomara, C., & Fineschi, V. (2007). *Manuale atlante di tecniche autoptiche.* Padova: Piccin.

Pomara, C., Fineschi, V., Scalzo, G., & Guglielmi, G. (2009). Virtopsy versus digital autopsy: Virtuous autopsy. *La Radiologia Medica, 114*(8), 1367–1382. doi:10.1007/s11547-009-0435-1

Pomara, C., Karch, S. B., & Mallegni, F. (2008). A medieval murder. *The American Journal of Forensic Medicine and Pathology, 29*, 72–74. doi:10.1097/PAF.0b013e31816520bf

Poole, C. (2001). Low p-values or narrow confidence intervals: Which are more durable? *Epidemiology (Cambridge, Mass.), 12*, 291–294. doi:10.1097/00001648-200105000-00005

Poulsen, K., & Simonsen, J. (2007). Computed tomography as routine connection with medico-legal autopsies. *Forensic Science International, 171*, 190–197. doi:10.1016/j.forsciint.2006.05.041

Praglowski, J., & Punt, W. (1973). An elucidation of the microreticulate structure of the exine. *Grana, 13*, 45–50. doi:10.1080/00173137309428842

Primorac, D., Andelinovic, S., Definis-Gojanovic, M., Drmic, I., Rezic, B., & Baden, M. M. (1996). Identification of war victims from mass graves in Croatia, Bosnia, and Herzegovina by the use of standard forensic methods and DNA typing. *Journal of Forensic Sciences*, *41*(5), 891–894.

Provost, F. J., & Fawcett, T. (2001). Robust classification for imprecise environments. *Machine Learning*, *42*(3), 203–231. doi:10.1023/A:1007601015854

Pudil, P., Novovicova, J., & Kittler, J. (1994). Floating search methods in feature selection. *Pattern Recognition Letters*, *15*, 1119–1125. doi:10.1016/0167-8655(94)90127-9

Quackenbush, J., Liang, F., Holt, I., Pertea, G., & Upton, J. (2000). The TIGR Gene Indices: reconstruction and representation of expressed gene sequences. *Nucleic Acids Research*, *28*(1), 141–145. doi:10.1093/nar/28.1.141

Quackenbush, J. (2001). Computational analysis of microarray data. *Nature Reviews. Genetics*, *2*(6), 418–427. doi:10.1038/35076576

Quatrehomme, G., Lacoste, A., Bailet, P., Grevin, G., & Ollier, A. (1997). Contribution of microscopic plant anatomy to postmortem bone dating. *Journal of Forensic Sciences*, *42*(1), 140–143.

Quatrehomme, G., Cotin, S., Subsol, G., Delingette, H., Garidel, Y., & Ollier, A. (1997). A fully three-dimensional method for facial reconstruction based on deformable models. *Journal of Forensic Sciences*, *42*(3), 649–652.

Rajewsky, N. (2006). MicroRNA target predictions in animals. *Nature Genetics*, *38*, S8–S13. doi:10.1038/ng1798

Ramsey, S., Ozinsky, A., Clark, A., Smith, K. D., de Atauri, P., & Thorsson, V. (2006). Transcriptional noise and cellular heterogeneity in mammalian macrophages. *Philosophical Transactions of the Royal Society of London. Series B, Biological Sciences*, *361*(1467), 495–506. doi:10.1098/rstb.2005.1808

Randall, B. B., Fierro, M. F., & Froede, R. C. (1998). Practice guideline for forensic pathology. *Archives of Pathology & Laboratory Medicine*, *122*, 1056–1064.

Rea, J. A., Chen, M. B., & Li, J. (2000). Morphometry X-ray absorptiometry and morphometric radiography of the spine: A comparison of prevalent vertebral deformity identification. *Journal of Bone and Mineral Research*, *15*, 564–574. doi:10.1359/jbmr.2000.15.3.564

Rea, J. A., Li, J., & Blake, G. M. (2000). Visual assessment of vertebral deformity by X-ray absorptiometry: A highly predictive method to exclude vertebral deformity. *Osteoporosis International*, *11*, 660–668. doi:10.1007/s001980070063

Reeder, D. J. (1999). Impact of DNA typing on standards and practice in the forensic community. *Archives of Pathology & Laboratory Medicine*, *123*(11), 1063–1065.

Relogio, A., Schwager, C., Richter, A., Ansorge, W., & Valcarcel, J. (2002). Optimization of oligonucleotide-based DNA microarrays. *Nucleic Acids Research*, *30*(11), e51. doi:10.1093/nar/30.11.e51

Ren, B., Robert, F., Wyrick, J. J., Aparicio, O., Jennings, E. G., & Simon, I. (2000). Genome-wide location and function of DNA binding proteins. *Science*, *290*(5500), 2306–2309. doi:10.1126/science.290.5500.2306

Reuther, J. D., Lowenstein, J. M., Gerlach, S. C., Hood, D., Scheuenstuhl, G., & Ubelaker, D. H. (2006). The use of an improved pRIA technique in the identification of protein residues. *Journal of Archaeological Science*, *33*(4), 531–537. doi:10.1016/j.jas.2005.09.008

Rhine, J. S., & Campell, H. R. (1980). Thickness of facial tissue in American blacks. *Journal of Forensic Sciences*, *25*(4), 847–858.

Rhine, J. S., & Moore, C. E. (1984). *Facial reproduction: Tables of facial tissue thickness of American caucasoids in forensic anthropology. Technical series 1*. Albuquerque: University of New Mexico.

Rimour, S., Hill, D., Militon, C., & Peyret, P. (2005). GoArrays: Highly dynamic and efficient microarray probe design. *Bioinformatics (Oxford, England)*, *21*(7), 1094–1110. doi:10.1093/bioinformatics/bti112

Ritchie, M. E., Silver, J., Oshlack, A., Holmes, M., Diyagama, D., & Holloway, A. (2007). A comparison of background correction methods for two-colour microarrays. *Bioinformatics (Oxford, England)*, *23*(20), 2700–2707. doi:10.1093/bioinformatics/btm412

Robbins, C. R. (1988). *Chemical and physical behavior of human hair* (2nd ed., pp. 1–36). New York: Springer-Verlag.

Roberts, M., Cootes, T. F., & Adams, J. E. (2006). Vertebral morphometry: Semiautomatic determination of detailed shape from dual-energy X-ray absorptiometry images using active appearance models. *Investigative Radiology, 41*(12), 849–859. doi:10.1097/01.rli.0000244343.27431.26

Roberts, G. L., & Lucas, V. S. (1994). Growth of the nasal septum of in the Snell strain of hypopituitary dwarf mouse. *European Journal of Orthodontics, 16*, 138–148.

Roberts, G. L., Parekh, S., Petrie, A., & Lucas, V. S. (2008). Dental age assessment (DAA): A simple method for children and emerging adults. *British Dental Journal, 204*, E7–E9. doi:10.1038/bdj.2008.21

Robertson, J. (1999). Forensic and microscopic examination of human hair. In Robertson, J. (Ed.), *Forensic examination of hair* (pp. 79–154). London: Taylor & Francis.

Romanovskii, U. M., Stepanova, N. V., & Chernavskii, D. S. (1975). *Matematicheskoe modelirovanie v biofizike.* Nauka, Moskva.

Ros, P. R., Li, K. C., Vo, P., Baer, H., & Staab, E. V. (1990). Preautopsy magnetic resonance imaging: Initial experience. *Magnetic Resonance Imaging, 8*, 303–308. doi:10.1016/0730-725X(90)90103-9

Rosas, A., & Bastir, M. (2002). Thin-plate spine analysis of allometry and sexual dimorphism in the human craniofacial complex. *American Journal of Physical Anthropology, 117*(3), 236–245. doi:10.1002/ajpa.10023

Ross, A. H., McKeown, A. H., & Konigsburg, L. W. (1999). Allocation of crania to groups via the New Morphometry. *Journal of Forensic Sciences, 44*(3), 584–587.

Ross, A. H., & Ubelaker, D. H. (2009). Effect of intentional cranial modification of craniofacial landmarks: A three-dimensional perspective. *The Journal of Craniofacial Surgery, 20*(6), 2185–2187. doi:10.1097/SCS.0b013e3181bf038c

Ross, S., Spendlove, D., Bolliger, S., Christe, A., Oesterhelweg, L., & Grabherr, S. (2008). Postmortem whole-body CT angiography: Evaluation of two contrast media solutions. *AJR. American Journal of Roentgenology, 190*, 1380–1389. doi:10.2214/AJR.07.3082

Ross, A., & Jain, A. K. (2003). Information fusion in biometrics. *Pattern Recognition Letters, 24*, 2115–2125. doi:10.1016/S0167-8655(03)00079-5

Ross, A., Nandakumar, K., & Jain, A. K. (2006). *Handbook of biometrics.* Springer-Verlag.

Ross, A. H., & Kimmerle, E. H. (2009). Contribution of quantitative methods in forensic anthropology: A new era. In Blau, S., & Ubelaker, D. H. (Eds.), *Handbook of forensic anthropology and archaeology* (pp. 479–489). Walnut Creek, CA: Left Coast Press, Inc.

Rowley, J. R., Skvarla, J. J., & Vezey, E. L. (1988). Evaluating the relative contributions of SEM, TEM and LM to the description of pollen grains. *Journal of Palynology, 23-24*, 27–28.

Ryszard, T., & Marek, R. O. (2004). *Medical imaging understanding technology.* Springer Verlag.

Saferstein, R. (2004). *Criminalistics: An introduction to forensic science* (8th ed.). Upper Saddle River, NJ: Pearson Education Inc.

Saha, S., Sparks, A. B., Rago, C., Akmaev, V., Wang, C. J., & Vogelstein, B. (2002). Using the transcriptome to annotate the genome. *Nature Biotechnology, 20*(5), 508–512. doi:10.1038/nbt0502-508

Sakurada, K., Ikegaya, H., Fukushima, H., Akutsu, T., Watanabe, K., & Yoshino, M. (2009). Evaluation of mRNA-based approach for identification of saliva and semen. *Legal Medicine, 11*(3), 125–128. doi:10.1016/j.legalmed.2008.10.002

Salama, N. R., Gonzalez-Valencia, G., Deatherage, B., Aviles-Jimenez, F., Atherton, J. C., & Graham, D. Y. (2007). Genetic analysis of Helicobacter pylori strain populations colonizing the stomach at different times post-infection. *Journal of Bacteriology, 189*(10), 3834–3845. doi:10.1128/JB.01696-06

Salih, A., Jones, A. S., Bass, D., & Cox, G. (1997). Confocal imaging of exine as a tool for grass pollen analysis. *Grana, 36*, 215–224. doi:10.1080/00173139709362610

Saunders, E. (1837). *The teeth a test of age, considered with reference to the factory children: Addressed to both Houses of Parliament, Westminster, London UK.* London: H. Renshaw.

Schena, M., Shalon, D., Davis, R. W., & Brown, P. O. (1995). Quantitative monitoring of gene expression patterns with a complementary DNA microarray. *Science, 270*(5235), 467–470. doi:10.1126/science.270.5235.467

Schmeling, A., Olze, A., Reisinger, W., Rosing, F. W., Muhler, M., & Wemecke, K. D. (2003). Forensic age diagnostics of living individuals in criminal proceedings. *Homo, 54*, 162–169. doi:10.1078/0018-442X-00066

Schmitt, A. O., Specht, T., Beckmann, G., Dahl, E., Pilarsky, C. P., & Hinzmann, B. (1999). Exhaustive mining of EST libraries for genes differentially expressed in normal and tumour tissues. *Nucleic Acids Research, 27*(21), 4251–4260. doi:10.1093/nar/27.21.4251

Schmittgen, T., Jiang, J., Lin, Q., & Yang, L. (2004). A high-throughput method to monitor the expression of microRNA precursors. *Nucleic Acids Research, 32*, E43. doi:10.1093/nar/gnh040

Schneider, K. R., & Wilhelm, T. (2000). Model reduction by extended quasi-steady-state approximation. *Journal of Mathematical Biology, 40*, 443–450. doi:10.1007/s002850000026

Schou, C. D., Frost, J., & Maconachy, W. V. (2004). Information assurance in biomedical informatics systems. *IEEE Engineering in Medicine and Biology Magazine, 23*(1), 110–118. doi:10.1109/MEMB.2004.1297181

Schour, I., & Massler, M. (1940a). Studies in tooth development: The growth pattern of human teeth, part 1. *The Journal of the American Dental Association, 27*(11), 1778–1793.

Schramm, A., Schön, R., Rüker, M., Barth, E.-L., Zizelmann, C., & Gellrich, N.-C. (2006). Computer assisted oral and maxillofacial reconstruction. *Journal of Computing and Information Technology, 14*(1), 71–77. doi:10.2498/cit.2006.01.08

Schutzer, S. E., Budowle, B., & Atlas, R. M. (2005). Biocrimes, microbial forensics, and the physician. *PLoS Medicine, 2*(12), e337. doi:10.1371/journal.pmed.0020337

Seah, L. K., Dinish, U. S., Phang, W. F., Chao, Z. X., & Murukeshan, V. M. (2005). Fluorescence optimisation and lifetime studies of fingerprints treated with magnetic powders. *Forensic Science International, 152*, 249–257. doi:10.1016/j.forsciint.2004.09.121

Sellin, S., & Mannervik, B. (1983). Reversal of the reaction catalyzed by glyoxalase I: Calculation of the equilibrium constant for the enzymatic reaction. *The Journal of Biological Chemistry, 258*, 8872–8875.

Seta, S., Sato, H., & Miyake, B. (1988). Forensic hair investigation. In Maehly, A., & Williams, R. L. (Eds.), *Forensic science progress*. Berlin, Heidelberg: Springer-Verlag.

Sethian, J. (1999). *Level sets methods and fast marching methods*. Cambridge University Press.

Shahrom, A. W., Vanezis, P., Chapman, R. C., Gonzales, A., Blenkinsop, C., & Rossi, M. L. (1996). Techniques in facial identification: Computer-aided facial reconstruction using a laser scanner and video superimposition. *International Journal of Legal Medicine, 108*, 194–200. doi:10.1007/BF01369791

Shannon, K. W., Wolber, P. K., Delenstarr, G. C., Webb, P. G., & Kincaid, R. H. (2001). *Method for evaluating oligonucleotide probe sequences*. Palo Alto, CA: Agilent Technologies Inc.

Sheng-Bo, Y., U-Young, L., Dai-Soon, K., Yong-Woo, A., Chang-Zhu, J., Jie, Z., et al. (2008). Determination of sex for the 12th thoracic vertebra by morphometry of three-dimensional reconstructed vertebral models. *Journal of Forensic Sciences, 53*(3), 620–625. doi:10.1111/j.1556-4029.2008.00701.x

Sheppard, S. M. (1982). Asymptomatic morphologic variations in the mandibular condyle-ramus region. *The Journal of Prosthetic Dentistry, 47*, 539–544. doi:10.1016/0022-3913(82)90306-7

Sidler, M., Jackowski, C., Dirnhofer, R., Vock, P., & Thali, M. J. (2007). Use of multislice computed tomography in disaster victim identification: Advantages and limitations. *Forensic Science International, 169*, 118–128. doi:10.1016/j.forsciint.2006.08.004

Simon, R., Mirlacher, M., & Sauter, G. (2004). Tissue microarrays. *Methods in Molecular Medicine, 97*, 377–389.

Smith, W. C., Kinney, R. W., & De Partee, D. G. (1993). Latent fingerprints—a forensic approach. *Journal of Forensic Identification, 43*(6), 563–570.

Smith, B. C., & Sweet, D. (2010). DNA and DNA evidence. In Senn, D., & Stimson, P. (Eds.), *Forensic dentistry* (2nd ed., pp. 103–136). Boca Raton, FL: Taylor & Francis.

Smyth, P. P., Taylor, C. J., & Adams, J. E. (1999). Vertebral shape: Automatic measurement with active shape models. *Radiology, 211,* 571–578.

Smyth, G. K., & Speed, T. P. (2003). Normalization of cDNA microarray data. *Methods (San Diego, Calif.), 31,* 265–273. doi:10.1016/S1046-2023(03)00155-5

Snelick, R., Uludag, U., Mink, A., Indovina, M., & Jain, A. K. (2005). Large-scale evaluation of multimodal biometric authentication using state-of-the-art systems. *IEEE Transactions on Pattern Analysis and Machine Intelligence, 27*(3). doi:10.1109/TPAMI.2005.57

Soares, M. B., Bonaldo, M. F., Jelene, P., Su, L., Lawton, L., & Efstratiadis, A. (1994). Construction and characterization of a normalized cDNA library. *Proceedings of the National Academy of Sciences of the United States of America, 91*(20), 9228–9232. doi:10.1073/pnas.91.20.9228

Sodhi, G. S., & Kaur, J. (2001). Powder method for detecting latent fingerprints: A review. *Forensic Science International, 120,* 172–176. doi:10.1016/S0379-0738(00)00465-5

Solberg, W. K., Hansson, T. L., & Nordtrom, B. (1985). The temporomandibular joint in young adults at autopsy: A morphologic classification and evaluation. *Journal of Oral Rehabilitation, 12,* 303–321. doi:10.1111/j.1365-2842.1985.tb01285.x

Southern, E. M. (1975). Detection of specific sequences among DNA fragments separated by gel electrophoresis. *Journal of Molecular Biology, 98*(3), 503–517. doi:10.1016/S0022-2836(75)80083-0

Speed, T. (2003). *Interdisciplinary statistics: Statistical analysis of gene expression microarray data.* Chapman & Hall/CRC.

Staal, F. J., van der Burg, M., Wessels, L. F., Barendregt, B. H., Baert, M. R., & van den Burg, C. M. (2003). DNA microarrays for comparison of gene expression profiles between diagnosis and relapse in precursor-B acute lymphoblastic leukemia: Choice of technique and purification influence the identification of potential diagnostic markers. *Leukemia, 17*(7), 1324–1332. doi:10.1038/sj.leu.2402974

Stark, A., Brennecke, J., Bushati, N., Russel, R. B., & Cohen, S. M. (2005). Animal microRNAs confer robustness to gene expression and have a significant impact on 3'UTR evolution. *Cell, 123,* 1133–1146. doi:10.1016/j.cell.2005.11.023

Statacorp, L. P. (2007). *Stata reference manual* (10th ed.).

Stearns, S. C., & Magwene, P. (2003). American Society of Naturalists. The naturalist in a world of genomics. *American Naturalist, 161*(2), 171–180. doi:10.1086/367983

Steiger, P., Cummings, S. R., Genant, H. K., & Weiss, H. (1994). Morphometric X-ray absorptiometry of the spine: Correlation in vivo with morphometric radiography. *Osteoporosis International, 4,* 238–244. doi:10.1007/BF01623347

Steiger, P. & Wahner, H. (1994). Instruments using fan-beam geometry.

Steinlechner, M., Berger, B., Niederstätter, H., & Parson, W. (2002). Rare failures in the amelogenin sex test. *International Journal of Legal Medicine, 116*(2), 117–120. doi:10.1007/s00414-001-0264-9

Stephan, C. N. (2009). Craniofacial identification: Techniques of facial approximation and craniofacial superimposition. In Blau, S., & Ubelaker, D. H. (Eds.), *Handbook of forensic anthropology and archaeology* (pp. 304–321). Walnut Creek, CA: Left Coast Press, Inc.

Sterne, J. A. C. (2009). *Meta-analysis in stata.* College Station, TX: Stata Corp LP.

Sterne, C.M.M. (2008). *Age assessment in young people: Witness statement to the courts.*

Stockmarr, A. (1999). Likelihood ratios for evaluating DNA evidence when the suspect is found through a database search. *Biometrics, 55,* 671–677. doi:10.1111/j.0006-341X.1999.00671.x

Stollberg, J., Urschitz, J., Urban, Z., & Boyd, C. D. (2000). A quantitative evaluation of SAGE. *Genome Research, 10*(8), 1241–1248. doi:10.1101/gr.10.8.1241

Stolovitzky, G. A., Kundaje, A., Held, G. A., Duggar, K. H., Haudenschild, C. D., & Zhou, D. (2005). Statistical analysis of MPSS measurements: Application to the study of LPS-activated macrophage gene expression. *Proceedings of the National Academy of Sciences of the United States of America, 102*(5), 1402–1407. doi:10.1073/pnas.0406555102

Storvik, G., & Egeland, T. (2007). The DNA database search controversy revisited: Bridging the Bayesian-frequentist gap. *Biometrics, 63*(3), 922–925. doi:10.1111/j.1541-0420.2007.00751.x

Stout, S. D., Dietze, W. H., Işcan, M. Y., & Loth, S. R. (1994). Estimation of age at death using cortical histomorphometry of the sternal end of the fourth rib. *Journal of Forensic Sciences, 39*(3), 778–784.

Stratomeier, H., Spee, J., Wittwer-Backofen, U. & Bakker, R. (2005). *Methods of forensic facial reconstruction.*

Surazhsky, V., Surazhsky, T., & Kirsanov, D. (2005). Fast, exact, and approximate geodesics on meshes. In *Proceedings of ACM SIGGRAPH 2005, 24*(3).

Suzuki, A., & Ohno, S. (2006). The PAR-aPKS system: Lessons in polarity. *Journal of Cell Science, 119*, 979–987. doi:10.1242/jcs.02898

Sweetman, D., Rathjen, T., Jefferson, M., Wheeler, G., Smith, T. G., & Wheeler, G. N. (2006). FGF-4 signaling is involved in mir-206 expression in developing somites of chicken embryos. *Developmental Dynamics, 235*, 2185–2191. doi:10.1002/dvdy.20881

Szeliski, R., & Lavallee, S. (1996). Matching 3-D anatomical surfaces with non-rigid deformation using octree splines. *International Journal of Computer Vision, 18*(2), 171–186. doi:10.1007/BF00055001

Tabor, M. P., & Schrader, B. A. (2010). Forensic dental identification. In Senn, D., & Stimson, P. (Eds.), *Forensic dentistry* (2nd ed., p. 167). Boca Raton, FL: Taylor & Francis.

Takahashi, S., Kanetake, J., Kanawaku, Y., & Funayama, M. (2008). Brain death with calcium oxalate deposition in the kidney: Clue to the diagnosis of ethylene glycol poisoning. *Legal Medicine, 10*(1), 43–45. doi:10.1016/j.legalmed.2007.05.010

Tanner, J. M., Healy, M. J. R., Goldstein, H., & Cameron, N. (2001). *Assessment of skeletal maturity* (3rd ed.). London: W.B. Saunders.

Taroni, F., Bozza, S., & Aitken, C. (2005). Decision analysis in forensic science. *Journal of Forensic Sciences, 50*(4), 894–905. doi:10.1520/JFS2004443

Taupin, J. M. (2004). Forensic hair morphology comparison-a dying art or junk science? *Science & Justice, 44*(2), 95–100. doi:10.1016/S1355-0306(04)71695-0

Taylor, B., & Skene, K. R. (2003). Forensic palynology: Spatial and temporal considerations of spora deposition in forensic investigations. *The Australian Journal of Forensic Sciences, 35*(2), 193–204. doi:10.1080/00450610309410582

Thali, M. J., Braun, M., Markwalder, T. H., Brueschweiler, W., Zollinger, U., & Malik, N. J. (2003). Bite mark documentation and analysis: The forensic 3D/CAD supported photogrammetry approach. *Forensic Science International, 135*, 115–121. doi:10.1016/S0379-0738(03)00205-6

Thali, M. J., Braun, M., Wirth, J., Vock, P., & Dirnhofer, R. (2003). 3D surface and body documentation in forensic medicine: 3-D/CAD photogrammetry merged with 3D radiological scanning. *Journal of Forensic Sciences, 48*, 1356–1365.

Thali, M. J., Dirnhofer, R., Becker, R., Oliver, W., & Potter, K. (2004). Is virtual histology the next step after the virtual autopsy? Magnetic resonance microscopy in forensic medicine. *Magnetic Resonance Imaging, 22*, 1131–1138. doi:10.1016/j.mri.2004.08.019

Thali, M. J., Jackowski, C., Oesterhelweg, L., Ross, S. G., & Dirnhofer, R. (2007). Virtopsy: The Swiss virtual autopsy approach. *Legal Medicine, 9*, 100–104. doi:10.1016/j.legalmed.2006.11.011

Thali, M. J., Markwalder, T., Jackowski, C., Sonnenschein, M., & Dirnhofer, R. (2006). Dental CT imaging as a screening tool for dental profiling: Advantages and limitations. *Journal of Forensic Sciences, 51*, 113–119. doi:10.1111/j.1556-4029.2005.00019.x

Thali, M. J., Schweitzer, W., Yen, K., Vock, P., Ozdoba, C., & Spielvogel, E. (2003). New horizons in forensic radiology: The 60-second digital autopsy–full-body examination of a gunshot victim by multislice computed tomography. *The American Journal of Forensic Medicine and Pathology, 24*, 22–27. doi:10.1097/00000433-200303000-00004

Thali, M. J., Taubenreuther, U., Karolczak, M., Braun, M., Brueschweiler, W., & Kalender, W. A. (2003). Forensic microradiology: Micro-computed tomography (micro-

CT) and analysis of patterned injuries inside of bone. *Journal of Forensic Sciences, 48*, 1336–1342.

Thali, M. J., Yen, K., Plattner, T., Schweitzer, W., Vock, P., & Ozdoba, C. (2002). Charred body: Virtual autopsy with multi-slice computed tomography and magnetic resonance imaging. *Journal of Forensic Sciences, 47*, 1326–1331.

Thali, M. J., Yen, K., Schweitzer, W., Vock, P., Boesch, C., & Ozdoba, C. (2003). Virtopsy, a new imaging horizon in forensic pathology: Virtual autopsy by postmortem multislice computed tomography (MSCT) and magnetic resonance imaging MRI)—a feasibility study. *Journal of Forensic Sciences, 48*, 386–403.

Thali, M. J., Yen, K., Schweitzer, W., Vock, P., Ozdoba, C., & Dirnhofer, R. (2003). Into the decomposed body-forensic digital autopsy using multislice-computed tomography. *Forensic Science International, 134*, 109–114. doi:10.1016/S0379-0738(03)00137-3

Thali, M. J., Yen, K., Vock, P., Ozdoba, C., Kneubue, W. B. P., & Sonneschein, M. (2003). Image guided virtual autopsy findings of gunshot victims performed with multislice computed tomography (MSCT) and magnetic resonance imaging (MRI) and subsequent correlation between radiology and autopsy findings. *Forensic Science International, 138*, 8–16. doi:10.1016/S0379-0738(03)00225-1

Thali, M. J., & Vock, P. (2003). Role of and techniques in forensic imaging. In James, J. P., Busuttil, A., & Smock, W. (Eds.), *Forensic medicine: Clinical and pathological aspects* (pp. 731–745). San Francisco: GMM.

Thangaraj, K., Reddy, A. G., & Singh, L. (2002). Is the amelogenin gene reliable for gender identification in forensic casework and prenatal diagnosis? *International Journal of Legal Medicine, 116*(2), 121–123. doi:10.1007/s00414-001-0262-y

The ENCODE Project Consortium et al. (2007). Identification and analysis of functional elements in 1% of the human genome by the ENCODE pilot project. *Nature, 447*(7146), 799–816. doi:10.1038/nature05874

The Royal Statistical Society. (2005). *A career as a forensic statistician.* Retrieved June 9, 2010, from http://www.rss.org.uk/pdf/Careers_forensic4.pdf

Thomson, J., Newman, M., Parker, J., Morin-Kensicki, E. M., Wright, T., & Hammond, S. M. (2006). Extensive post-transcriptional regulation of microRNAs and its implications for cancer. *Genes & Development, 20*, 2202–2207. doi:10.1101/gad.1444406

Tian, J. (2003). Reversible data embedding using a difference expansion. *IEEE Transactions on Circuits and Systems for Video Technology, 13*(8), 890–896. doi:10.1109/TCSVT.2003.815962

Tichonov, A.N. (1952) Systemy differentsialnyh uravneniy, soderjashchie malye parametry pri proizvodnyh. *Matematicheskiy sbornik, 31*(3), 575-586.

Tilotta, F., Richard, F., Glaunès, J., Bérar, M., Gey, S., & Verdeille, S. (2009). Construction and analysis of a head CT-scan database for craniofacial reconstruction. *Forensic Science International, 191*(1), 112–118. doi:10.1016/j.forsciint.2009.06.017

Tilotta, F., et al. (2007). Statistical facial reconstruction by tree functional regression on surfaces. *Proceedings of the Third Mediterranean Academy of Forensic Sciences Congress, Porto, Portugal.*

Townsend, J. P. (2003). Multifactorial experimental design and the transitivity of ratios with spotted DNA microarrays. *BMC Genomics, 4*(1), 41. doi:10.1186/1471-2164-4-41

Tseng, G. C., Oh, M. K., Rohlin, L., Liao, J. C., & Wong, W. H. (2001). Issues in cDNA microarray analysis: Quality filtering, channel normalization, models of variations and assessment of gene effects. *Nucleic Acids Research, 29*(12), 2549–2557. doi:10.1093/nar/29.12.2549

Tsoumakas, G., Katakis, I., & Vlahavas, I. (2009). Data mining and knowledge discovery handbook. In Maimon, O., & Rokach, L. (Eds.), *Mining multi-label data* (2nd ed.). Springer.

Tsuchiya, S., Oku, M., Imanaka, Y., Kunimoto, R., Okuno, Y., & Terasawa, K. (2009). MicroRNA-338-3p and microRNA-451 contribute to the formation of basolateral polarity in epithelial cells. *Nucleic Acids Research, 37*(11), 3821–3827. doi:10.1093/nar/gkp255

Tu, P., Book, R., Liu, X., Krahnstoever, N., Adrian, C., & Williams, P. (2007). Automatic face recognition from skeletal remains. In *IEEE Computer Society Conference on Computer Vision and Pattern Recognition (CVPR 2007)*, Minneapolis.

Turillazzi, E., Karch, S. B., Neri, M., Pomara, C., Riezzo, I., & Fineschi, V. (2008). Confocal laser scanning microscopy: Using new technology to answer old questions in forensic investigations. *International Journal of Legal Medicine, 122,* 173–177. doi:10.1007/s00414-007-0208-0

Tzafriri, A. R., & Edelman, E. R. (2004). The total quasi-state-approximation is valid for reversible enzyme kinetics. *Journal of Theoretical Biology, 226,* 303–313. doi:10.1016/j.jtbi.2003.09.006

Ubelaker, D. H. (1999). *Human skeletal remains: Excavation, analysis, interpretation* (3rd ed.). Washington, DC: Taraxacum.

Ubelaker, D. H. (2001). Artificial radiocarbon as an indicator of recent origin of organic remains in forensic cases. *Journal of Forensic Sciences, 46*(6), 1285–1287.

Ubelaker, D. H., Buchholz, B. A., & Stewart, J. E. B. (2006). Analysis of artificial radiocarbon in different skeletal and dental tissue types to evaluate date of death. *Journal of Forensic Sciences, 51*(3), 484–488. doi:10.1111/j.1556-4029.2006.00125.x

Ubelaker, D. H., Lowenstein, J. M., & Hood, D. G. (2004). Species identification of small skeletal fragments using protein radioimmunoassay (pRIA). *Proceedings of the American Academy of Forensic Sciences, 10,* 327–328.

Ubelaker, D. H., Ward, D. C., Braz, V. S., & Stewart, J. (2002). The use of SEM/EDS analysis to distinguish dental and osseus tissue from other materials. *Journal of Forensic Sciences, 47*(5), 940–943.

Ubelaker, D. H. (1998). The evolving role of the microscope in forensic anthropology. In Reichs, K. J. (Ed.), *Forensic osteology: Advances in the identification of human remains* (2nd ed., pp. 514–532). Springfield, IL: Charles C. Thomas.

Ubelaker, D. H. (2009). Approaches to facial reproduction and photographic superimposition. In Steadman, D. W. (Ed.), *Hard rvidence: Case studies in forensic anthropology* (2nd ed., pp. 248–257). Upper Saddle River, NJ: Prentice Hall.

Ubelaker, D. H., Jumbelic, M., Wilson, M., & Levinsohn, E. M. (2009). Multidisciplinary approach to human identification in homicide investigation: A case study from New York. In Steadman, D. W. (Ed.), *Hard evidence: Case studies in forensic anthropology* (2nd ed., pp. 29–33). Upper Saddle River, NJ: Prentice Hall.

Ubelaker, D. H., & Smialek, J. E. (2009). The interface of forensic anthropology and forensic pathology in trauma interpretation. In Steadman, D. W. (Ed.), *Hard evidence: Case studies in forensic anthropology* (2nd ed., pp. 221–224). Upper Saddle River, NJ: Prentice Hall.

Ubelaker, D. H. (2007a). Cranial photographic superimposition. In C.H. Wecht (Ed), *Forensic sciences, volume 2.* (pp. 27C-1-27C-41). New York: Matthew Bender and Company.

Ubelaker, D. H. (2007b). Facial reproduction. In C.H. Wecht (Ed.), *Forensic sciences, volume 3.* (pp. 28E-1-28E-70). New York: Matthew Bender and Company.

Ubelaker, D.H. & B.A. Buchholz. (2006). Complexities in the use of bomb-curve radiocarbon to determine time since death of human skeletal remains. *Forensic Science Communications, 8,* online journal.

Uhle, A. J. (2010). Fingerprints and human identification. In Senn, D., & Stimson, P. (Eds.), *Forensic dentistry* (2nd ed., pp. 79–102). Boca Raton, FL: Taylor & Francis.

Utech, M., Ivanov, A. I., Samarin, S. N., Bruewer, M., Turner, J. R., & Mrsny, R. J. (2005). Mechanism of IFN-gamma-induced endocytosis of tight junction proteins: Myosin II-dependent vacuolarization of the apical plasma membrane. *Molecular Biology of the Cell, 16,* 5040–5052. doi:10.1091/mbc.E05-03-0193

Vallejo-Bollanos, E., & Espana-Lopez, A. J. (1997). The relationship between dental age, bone age and chronological age in 54 children with short familial stature. *International Journal of Paediatric Dentistry, 7,* 15–17. doi:10.1111/j.1365-263X.1997.tb00267.x

Van Gelder, R. N., von Zastrow, M. E., Yool, A., Dement, W. C., Barchas, J. D., & Eberwine, J. H. (1990). Amplified RNA synthesized from limited quantities of heterogeneous cDNA. *Proceedings of the National Academy of Sciences of the United States of America, 87*(5), 1663–1667. doi:10.1073/pnas.87.5.1663

van Hal, N. L., Vorst, O., van Houwelingen, A. M., Kok, E. J., Peijnenburg, A., & Aharoni, A. (2000). The application of DNA microarrays in gene expression analysis. *Journal of Biotechnology, 78*(3), 271–280. doi:10.1016/S0168-1656(00)00204-2

Van Neste, D., & Houbion, Y. (1989). Office diagnosis of pathological changes in hair cuticular cell pattern. In Van Neste, D., Lachapelle, J. M., & Antoine, J. L. (Eds.), *Trends in human hair growth and alopecia research* (pp. 173–179). Dordrecht: Kluwer.

Van't Veer, L. V., Dai, H., Vijver, M. V., He, Y., Hart, A., & Mao, M. (2002). Gene expression profiling predicts clinical outcome of breast cancer. *Nature, 415*(6871), 530–536. doi:10.1038/415530a

Vandermeulen, D., Claes, P., Loeckx, D., De Greef, S., Willems, G., & Suetens, P. (2006). Computerized cranio-facial reconstruction using CT-derived implicit surface representations. *Forensic Science International, 159S*, S164–S174. doi:10.1016/j.forsciint.2006.02.036

Vanezis, P., Vanezis, M., McCombe, G., & Niblett, T. (2000). Facial reconstruction using 3-D computer graphics. *Forensic Science International, 108*(2), 81–95. doi:10.1016/S0379-0738(99)00026-2

Vapnik, V. (1995). *The nature of statistical learning theory.* New York: Springer.

Vaughn, C. J. (1986). Ground-penetrating radar survey used in archaeological investigations. *Geophysics, 51*(3), 595–604. doi:10.1190/1.1442114

Veeramachaneni, K., Osadciw, L., & Varshney, P. K. (2005). An adaptive multimodal biometric management algorithm. *IEEE Transactions on Systems, Man, and Cybernetics, 35*(3).

Velculescu, V. E., Zhang, L., Vogelstein, B., & Kinzler, K. W. (1995). Serial analysis of gene expression. *Science, 270*(5235), 484–487. doi:10.1126/science.270.5235.484

Venables, J. P. (2006). Unbalanced alternative splicing and its significance in cancer. *BioEssays, 28*(4), 378–386. doi:10.1002/bies.20390

Venet, D., Pecasse, F., Maenhaut, C., & Bersini, H. (2001). Separation of samples into their constituents using gene expression data. *Bioinformatics (Oxford, England), 17*(1), S279–S287.

Venter, J. C. (2001). The sequence of the human genome. *Science, 291*(5507), 1304–1351. doi:10.1126/science.1058040

Vigneau, E., & Qannari, M. (2002). A new algorithm for latent root regression analysis. *Computational Statistics & Data Analysis, 41*, 231–242. doi:10.1016/S0167-9473(02)00071-3

Vilar, J. M., Guet, C. C., & Leibler, S. (2003). Modeling network dynamics: The lac operon, a case study. *The Journal of Cell Biology, 161*(3), 471–476. doi:10.1083/jcb.200301125

Vinciotti, V., Khanin, R., D'Alimonte, D., Liu, X., Cattini, N., & Hotchkiss, G. (2005). An experimental evaluation of a loop versus a reference design for two-channel microarrays. *Bioinformatics (Oxford, England), 21*(4), 492–501. doi:10.1093/bioinformatics/bti022

Wacholder, S. (2000). Population stratification in Epidemiologic studies of common genetic variants and cancer: Quantification of bias. *Journal of the National Cancer Institute, 92*, 1151–1158. doi:10.1093/jnci/92.14.1151

Wakatani, A. (2002). Digital watermarking for ROI medical images by using compressed signature image. *Proceedings of the the Annual Hawaii International Conference on System Sciences (HICSS) 2002, Jan. 7-10*, (pp. 2043-2048).

Wakiyama, M., Takimoto, K., Ohara, O., & Yokoyama, K. (2007). Let-7 microRNA-mediated mRNA deadenylation and translational repression in a mammalian cell-free system. *Genes & Development, 21*, 857–1862. doi:10.1101/gad.1566707

Wallace, S. K., Cohen, W. A., Stern, E. J., & Reay, D. T. (1994). Judicial hanging: Postmortem radiographic CT, and MR imaging features with autopsy confirmation. *Radiology, 193*(1), 263–267.

Wang, D., Gou, S. Y., & Axelrod, D. (1992). Reaction rate enhancement by surface diffusion of adsorbates. *Biophysical Chemistry, 43*(2), 117–137. doi:10.1016/0301-4622(92)80027-3

Wang, T., Xue, N., & Birdwell, J. D. (2006). Least-square deconvolution: A framework for interpreting short tandem repeat mixtures. *Journal of Forensic Sciences, 51*(6), 1284–1297. doi:10.1111/j.1556-4029.2006.00268.x

Wang, C., Zhang, J., Liu, A., Sun, B., & Zhao, Y. (2000). Surgical treatment of primary midbrain gliomas. *Surgical Neurology, 53*, 41–51. doi:10.1016/S0090-3019(99)00165-2

Wang, Y., Peterson, B., & Staib, L. (2000). Shape-based 3D surface correspondence using geodesics and local geometry. *IEEE Conference on Computer Vision and Pattern Recognition, 2*, 644-651.

Watanabe, Y., Tonita, M., & Kanai, A. (2007). Computational methods for microRNA target prediction. *Methods in Enzymology, 427*, 65–86. doi:10.1016/S0076-6879(07)27004-1

Waterhouse, P., Wang, M., & Lough, T. (2001). Gene silencing as an adaptive defence against viruses. *Nature, 411*, 834–842. doi:10.1038/35081168

Watson, J. T., Jones, R. C., Siston, A. M., Diaz, P. S., Gerber, S. I., & Crowe, J. B. (2005). Outbreak of food-borne illness associated with plant material containing raphides. *Clinical Toxicology, 43*(1), 17–21.

Watson, L., & Bell, E. M. (1975). A surface-structural survey of some taxonomically diverse grass pollens. *Australian Journal of Botany, 23*, 981–990. doi:10.1071/BT9750981

Watson, C. L., & Lockwood, D. N. (2009). Single nucleotide polymorphism analysis of European archaeological M. leprae DNA. *PLoS ONE, 4*(10), e7547. doi:10.1371/journal.pone.0007547

Weber, A. P., Weber, K. L., Carr, K., Wilkerson, C., & Ohlrogge, J. B. (2007). Sampling the Arabidopsis transcriptome with massively parallel pyrosequencing. *Plant Physiology, 144*(1), 32–42. doi:10.1104/pp.107.096677

Wedel, A., Carlsson, G. E., & Sagne, S. (1978). Temporomandibular joint morphology in a medieval skull material. *Swedish Dental Journal, 2*, 177–187.

Weems, R. A. (2010). Forensic dental radiography. In Senn, D., & Stimson, P. (Eds.), *Forensic dentistry* (2nd ed., pp. 190–191). Boca Raton, FL: Taylor & Francis.

Weir, B. S. (1995). DNA statistics in the Simpson matter. *Nature Genetics, 11*(4), 365–368. doi:10.1038/ng1295-365

Weir, B. S., Triggs, C. M., Starling, L., Stowell, L. I., Walsh, K. A., & Buckleton, J. (1997). Interpreting DNA mixtures. *Journal of Forensic Sciences, 42*(2), 213–222.

Wells, C. G., & Hintze, J. M. (2007). Dealing with assumptions underlying statistical tests. *Psychology in the Schools, 44*, 495–502. doi:10.1002/pits.20241

Wessel, S., Pagel, M., Ritter, H., & Hohenberg, R. (2003). Topographic measurements of real structures in reflection confocal laser scanning microscope (CLSM). *Microscopy and Microanalysis, 3*, 162.

Wheeler, G., Ntounia-Fousara, S., Granda, B., Rathjen, T., & Dalmay, T. (2006). Identification of new central nervous system specific mouse microRNAs. *FEBS Letters, 580*, 2195–2200. doi:10.1016/j.febslet.2006.03.019

Whittaker, D. K., Davies, G., & Brown, M. (1985). Tooth loss, attrition and temporomandibular joint changes in a Romano-British population. *Journal of Oral Rehabilitation, 12*, 407–419. doi:10.1111/j.1365-2842.1985.tb01546.x

Wienholds, E., Kloosterman, W., Miska, E., Alvarez-Saavedra, E., Berezikov, E., & de Bruijn, E. (2005). MicroRNA expression in zebrafish embrionic development. *Science, 309*, 310–311. doi:10.1126/science.1114519

Wilkinson, C. (2004). *Forensic facial reconstruction.* Cambridge, UK: Cambridge University Press.

Wilkinson, C. (2005). Computerized forensic facial reconstruction: A review of current systems. *Forensic Science, Medicine, and Pathology, 1*(3), 173–177. doi:10.1385/FSMP:1:3:173

Willerhausen, B., Loffler, N., & Schulze, R. (2001). Analysis of 1202 orthopantomograms to evaluate the potential of forensic age determination based on third molar developmental stages. *European Journal of Medical Research, 6*, 377–384.

Williams, R. M., Zipfel, W. R., & Webb, W. W. (2001). Multiphoton microscopy in biological research. *Current Opinion in Chemical Biology, 5*(5), 603–608. doi:10.1016/S1367-5931(00)00241-6

Witze, E. S., Litman, E. S., Argast, G. M., Moon, R. T., & Ahn, N. G. (2008). Wnt5a control of cell polarity and directional movement by polarized redistribution of adhesion receptors. *Science, 320*, 365–369. doi:10.1126/science.1151250

Wodarz, A. (2005). Molecular control of cell polarity and asymmetric cell division in Drosophila neuroblasts. *Cur-*

rent Opinion in Cell Biology, *17*, 475–481. doi:10.1016/j.ceb.2005.08.005

Wodehouse, R. P. (1935). *Pollen grains. Their structure, identification and significance in science and medicine*. New York, London: McGraw-Hill.

Wolber, P. K., Collins, P. J., Lucas, A. B., De Witte, A., & Shannon, K. W. (2006). The agilent in situ-synthesized microarray platform. *Methods in Enzymology*, *410*, 28–57. doi:10.1016/S0076-6879(06)10002-6

Wolff, C., Roy, S., & Ingham, P. W. (2003). Multiple muscle cell identities induced by distinct levels and timing of hedgehog activity in the zebrafish embryo. *Current Biology*, *13*(14), 1169–1181. doi:10.1016/S0960-9822(03)00461-5

Woo, Y., Krueger, W., Kaur, A., & Churchill, G. (2005). Experimental design for three-color and four-color gene expression microarrays. *Bioinformatics (Oxford, England)*, *21*(1), i459–i467. doi:10.1093/bioinformatics/bti1031

Wright, F. D., & Dailey, J. C. (2001). Human bite marks in forensic dentistry. *Dental Clinics of North America*, *45*(2), 365–397.

Wright, F. D., & Golden, G. S. (2010). Forensic dental photography. In Senn, D., & Stimson, P. (Eds.), *Forensic dentistry* (2nd ed., p. 219). Boca Raton, FL: Taylor & Francis.

Wu, Z., Irizarry, R. A., Gentleman, R., Martinez-Murillo, F., & Spencer, F. (2004). A model based background adjustment for oligonucleotide expression arrays. *Journal of the American Statistical Association*, *99*(468), 909–917. doi:10.1198/016214504000000683

Xi, Y., Nakajima, G., Gavin, E., Morris, K. K., Hayashi, K., & Ju, J. (2007). Systematic analysis of microRNA expression of RNA extracted from fresh frozen and formalin-fixed paraffin-embedded samples. *RNA (New York, N.Y.)*, *13*, 1668–1674. doi:10.1261/rna.642907

Xie, Zh., Yang, H., Liu, W., & Hwang, M. (2007). The role of microRNA in the delayed negative feedback regulation of gene expression. [BBRC]. *Biochemical and Biophysical Research Communications*, *358*, 722–726. doi:10.1016/j.bbrc.2007.04.207

Xu, J., & Wong, Ch. (2008). A computational screen for mouse signalling pathways targeted by microRNA clusters. *RNA (New York, N.Y.)*, *14*, 1276–1283. doi:10.1261/rna.997708

Xuan, G. R., Yao, Q. M., Yang, C., & Gao, J. (2006). *Lossless data hiding using histogram shifting method based on integer wavelets*. (LNCS-4283). (pp. 323-332).

Yamany, S., & Farag, A. (2003). Adaptive object identification and recognition using neural networks and surface signatures. *IEEE Conference on Advanced Video and Signal Based Surveillance*, (pp. 137–142). Miami, FL, USA.

Yang, I. V., Chen, E., Hasseman, J. P., Liang, W., Frank, B. C., & Wang, S. (2002). Within the fold: Assessing differential expression measures and reproducibility in microarray assays. *Genome Biology*, *3*(11), 62.

Yang, Y. H., & Speed, T. (2002). Design issues for cDNA microarray experiments. *Nature Reviews. Genetics*, *3*(8), 579–588.

Yang, J., & Honavar, V. (1998). Feature subset selection using a genetic algorithm. *IEEE Intelligent Systems*, *13*, 44–49. Retrieved from citeseer.ist.psu.edu/yang98feature.html. doi:10.1109/5254.671091

Yang, J. Y., Li, G.-Z., Meng, H.-H., & Yang, M. Q. (2008). Improving prediction accuracy of tumor classification by reusing the discarded genes during gene selection. *BMC Genomics*, *9*(1), S3. doi:10.1186/1471-2164-9-S1-S3

Yang, J. Y., Li, G.-Z., Liu, L.-X., & Yang, M. Q. (2007). Classification of brain glioma by using neural networks ensemble with multi-task learning. In *Proceedings of the 2007 International Conference on Bioinformatics and Computational Biology (BIOCOMP '07)*, (p. 515-522). Las Vegas: CSREA Press.

Ye, C.-Z., Yang, J., Geng, D.-Y., Zhou, Y., & Chen, N.-Y. (2002). Fuzzy rules to predict degree of malignancy in brain glioma. *Medical & Biological Engineering & Computing*, *40*, 145–152. doi:10.1007/BF02348118

Yen, K., Lovblad, K. O., Scheurer, E., Ozdoba, C., Thali, M. J., & Aghayev, E. (2007). Post-mortem forensic neuroimaging: Correlation of MSCT and MRI findings with autopsy results. *Forensic Science International*, *173*, 21–35. doi:10.1016/j.forsciint.2007.01.027

Yen, K., Thali, M. J., Aghayev, E., Jackowski, C., Schweitzer, W., & Boesch, C. (2005). Strangulation signs: Initial correlation of MRI, MSCT, and forensic neck findings. *Journal of Magnetic Resonance Imaging, 22*, 501–510. doi:10.1002/jmri.20396

Yen, K., Vock, P., Tiefenthaler, B., Ranner, G., Scheurer, E., & Thali, M. J. (2004). Virtopsy: Forensic traumatology of the subcutaneous fatty tissue. Multislice computed tomography (MSCT) and magnetic resonance imaging (MRI) as diagnostic tools. *Journal of Forensic Sciences, 49*(4), 799–806. doi:10.1520/JFS2003299

Yoon, C. K. (1993). Botanical witness for the prosecution. *Science, 260*, 894–895. doi:10.1126/science.8493521

Yu, L., & Liu, H. (2004). Efficient feature selection via analysis of relevance and redundancy. *Journal of Machine Learning Research, 5*, 1205–1224.

Zachow, S., Hege, H.-C., & Deuflhard, P. (2006). Computer assisted planning in cranio-maxillofacial surgery. *Journal of Computing and Information Technology, 14*(1), 53–64. doi:10.2498/cit.2006.01.06

Zain, J. M., Fauzi, A. R. M., & Aziz, A. A. (2006). Clinical evaluation of watermarked medical images. *Proceedings of the 28th IEEE EMBS Annual International Conference, New York City, USA, Aug 30-Sept 3, 2006,* (pp. 5459-5462).

Zamora, G., Sari-Sarraf, H., & Long, L. R. (2003). Hierarchical segmentation of vertebrae from X-ray images. In. *Proceedings of SPIE Medical Imaging, 5032*, 631–642.

Zehner, R., Amendt, J., & Boehme, P. (2009). Gene expression analysis as a tool for age estimation of blowfly pupae. *Forensic Science International. Genetics Supplement Series, 2*(1), 292–293. doi:10.1016/j.fsigss.2009.08.008

Zeng, X.-Q., Li, G.-Z., Wu, G.-F., Yang, J., & Yang, M. (2009b). Orthogonal projection weights in dimension reduction based on partial least squares. *International Journal of Computational Intelligence of Bioinformatics &. Systematic Biology, 1*(1), 100–115.

Zeng, X.-Q., Li, G.-Z., Wu, G.-F., Yang, J. Y., & Yang, M. Q. (2009a). Irrelevant gene elimination for partial least squares based dimension reduction by using feature probes. *International Journal of Data Mining &. Bioinformatics (Oxford, England), 3*(1), 85–103.

Zeng, X.-Q., Li, G.-Z., Yang, J. Y., Yang, M. Q., & Wu, G.-F. (2008). Dimension reduction with redundant genes elimination for tumor classification. *BMC Bioinformatics, 9*(6), S8. doi:10.1186/1471-2105-9-S6-S8

Zhang, L., Foxman, B., Drake, D. R., Srinivasan, U., Henderson, J., & Olson, B. (2009). Comparative whole-genome analysis of Streptococcus mutans isolates within and among individuals of different caries status. *Oral Microbiology and Immunology, 24*(3), 197–203. doi:10.1111/j.1399-302X.2008.00495.x

Zhang, Y., Hammer, D. A., & Graves, D. J. (2005). Competitive hybridization kinetics reveals unexpected behavior patterns. *Biophysical Journal, 89*(5), 2950–2959. doi:10.1529/biophysj.104.058552

Zhang, M.-L., & Zhou, Z.-H. (2007). Ml-knn: A lazy learning approach to multi-label learning. *Pattern Recognition, 40*(7), 2038–2048. doi:10.1016/j.patcog.2006.12.019

Zhou, Z.-H., Wu, J.-X., & Tang, W. (2002). Ensembling neural networks: Many could be better than all. *Artificial Intelligence, 137*(1-2), 239–263. doi:10.1016/S0004-3702(02)00190-X

Zhuo, L., Hu, L. S., Zhou, L., Zheng, N., Liang, M., & Yang, F. (2009). Application of confocal laser scanning microscope in forensic pathology. *Fa Yi Xue Za Zhi, 25*(6), 455–458.

zur Nedden, D., Knapp, R., Wicke, K., Judmaier, W., Murphy, W. A., & Seidler, H. (1994). Skull of a 5,300-yearold mummy: Reproduction and investigation with CT-guided stereolithography. *Radiology, 193*, 269–272.

About the Contributors

Andriani Daskalaki is a dentist and bioinformatician. She presently works in the field of molecular medicine and bioinformatics at the Max Planck Institute for Molecular Genetics in Berlin. She completed her PhD in 2002 on working in the applications of photodynamic therapy in the area of oral medicine from the Free University of Berlin. She received a two-year DAAD scholarship for her research in the field of PDT. Dr. Daskalaki received a MS in Medical Informatics from TFH Berlin with her work in "Development of a Documentation Software for Robot-Assisted Intraoral Operations" and a MS degree in bioinformatics with her work in "Variance Analysis of Multifactor Models in Gene Expression Experiments with Application to the Identification of Genetic Markers for Hypertension." She received a poster prize for her participation in the International Photodynamic Association Meeting in Nantes. She is the editor of the "Handbook of Research on Systems Biology Applications in Medicine" and has presented many oral presentations at national and international meetings. She is a founding member and committee member of the Greek Dental Laser Association. Her research interest areas include systems biology, PDT, and laser applications in dentistry.

* * *

Mohamed Abdel-Mottaleb received the PhD degree in computer science from the University of Maryland, College Park, in 1993. Currently, he is a Professor and Chairman of the Department of Electrical and Computer Engineering, University of Miami, where his research focuses on 3-D face recognition, dental biometrics, visual tracking, and human activity recognition. Prior to joining the University of Miami, from 1993 to 2000, he was with Philips Research, Briarcliff Manor, NY. While there, he was a Principal Member of the Research Staff and a Project Leader, where he led several projects in image processing, and content-based multimedia retrieval. He holds 20 U.S. patents and has published many journal and conference papers in the areas of image processing, computer vision, and content-based retrieval. He is an associate editor for the *Pattern Recognition* journal.

Maria Adamaki is a Molecular Biologist currently occupied at the oncology lab of Aghia Sofia Children's Hospital. She possesses a BSc (Hons) in Molecular Biology, an MSc in Molecular Medicine, and has scientific research experience in inherited blood disorders and in children's leukemias. Her current work is focused on investigating the expression and analysis of certain genes in childhood leukemias.

Stilianos Arhondakis received his BSc degree (2001) in Biology (University of Bari, Italy), with thesis in Molecular Biology–Bioinformatics entitled "Study of mammalian interspecies variability in mitochondria genes and genomes." In 2002, he joined the Laboratory of Molecular Evolution (Stazione Zoologica A. Dohrn, Naples, Italy) directed by Prof. Giorgio Bernardi. In 2008, he received his PhD in Human Genetics (University of Paris VII, Paris, France), with the honors and felicitation of the jury entitled "Correlation entrè expression des genes et isochores". Currently, he holds a Post-Doc fellowship at the Bioinformatics and Medical Informatics Team in the Biomedical Research Foundation of the Academy of Athens (BRFAA), working on structural genomics and evolution.

Maxime Berar is an assistant professor at University of Rouen, France. After an engineering degree in electronics and a Master Degree in cognitive sciences, he received his PhD in Signal and Images Processing from the Institut National Polytechnique de Grenoble. He then spent two years in MAP5 laboratory in University Paris Descatres for a post-doctoral training. Since 2009, he has been affiliated with LITIS laboratory (Laboratoire d'Informatique, de Traitement de l'Information et des Systèmes) in Rouen. His scientific interests include modelling of the variability observed in anatomical structures and cover all the steps of the data treatment. In this context, facial reconstruction is a challenging application.

Marek Bucki received his PhD from the Joseph Fourier University (Grenoble, France) and the Universidad de Chile (Santiago, Chile) in 2008. He is currently a post-doctoral fellow in the Computer Assisted Medical Interventions team at the TIMC-IMAG laboratory (La Tronche, France), where he collaborates with the department of neurosurgery of the Michallon Hospital, working on brain-shift compensation strategies based on Finite Element modeling of the patient's brain soft tissues coupled with intraoperative Doppler ultrasound tracking of the vascular tree. His activities also include the development of MMRep, a fast and automatic FE mesh registration procedure for subject-specific biomedical modeling.

Amit Chattopadhyay recently joined the National Institute of Dental and Craniofacial Research, Office of Science Policy and Analysis at the National Institutes of Health in Bethesda, Maryland. His varied duties will include serving as oral epidemiologist, faculty to the dental public health residency program, and representative to the national Healthy People initiative. Dr. Chattopadhyay earned a dental degree with honors (Calcutta University, India); master's degrees in: Oral Pathology (Gujarat University, India) and Public Health – Epidemiology (Oklahoma University); and a residency training certificate in Dental Public Health (SUNY, Albany & New York State Department of Health). He is board certified by the American National Board of Public Health Examiners and by the American Board of Dental Public Health; and is a Fellow of the Faculty of Public Health of the Royal College of Physicians (London, UK). Dr. Chattopadhyay also earned a PhD in Epidemiology from the University of North Carolina at Chapel Hill with National Research Service Award funding, serving as an adjunct Assistant Professor in the Department of Dental Ecology in the School of Dentistry. He has also earned a diploma in journalism and a doctorate certificate in Family Medicine from India, and graduate certificates in international development and in public health outcomes from the University of North Carolina at Chapel Hill and a diploma in Global ethics from the University of Joensuu, Finland. At various times, he has taught Epidemiology, Oral Epidemiology, Public Health Biology, Research Methods and Dental Public Health at Universities of Kentucky, North Carolina, and Temple University. He is the author of chapters in several text books and was Guest Editor of the first-ever issue on Dental Public Health published in

Dental Clinics of North America. He has been an invited speaker in several meetings and conferences around the world. He serves on the Ethics Committee of the American Association for Dental Research, the Editorial Committee of the Journal of Dental Research and several other international dental and medical journals.

Jan Pieter Clarys started as a researcher for the Belgian National Fund for Scientific Research at the University of Ghent and Brussels in 1969. He became associate Professor in 1977 and full Professor in Anatomy and Electromyography in 1988. He teaches Topographical, Functional, and Clinical Anatomy to Medical and Physical Education, Physiotherapy, Pharmacy, Manual Therapy, and Clinical Engineering students. He is Past-President of the World Commission of Sports Biomechanics (WCSB) (ICSSPE-UNESCO) and Past-President of ISEK (International Society of Electrophysiology and Kinesiology). He presented 140 keynote or invited lectures on International Congresses of Sport Sciences, Sport Medicine, Biomechanics, Ergonomics and Body Composition and presented another 150 papers on conferences with a scientific committee. Prof. Clarys wrote 9 books and published over 250 articles. He is editorial board member of the Journal of Electromyography and Kinesiology, The Journal of Sports Medicine and Physical Fitness and International Journal of Training and Coaching. He was awarded the Dutch Prize of Sport Medicine in 1978 (Amsterdam) and the Philip Noel Baker Research award - ICSSPE - UNESCO in 1995 (Ottawa). He is doctor Honoris Causa of the John Moores University of Liverpool since July 1996 and honorary citizen of Montpellier (France) and Florence (Italy).

Thomas J. David has been active in Forensic Odontology for the last 27years. He is a member of the ASFO, a Fellow of the AAFS and a Diplomate of the ABFO. During that time he has served as Chair of the Odontology Section of the AAFS and is currently the Secretary of the ABFO. He serves as a Consultant to the Georgia Bureau of Investigation, Division of Forensic Sciences. In addition, he is a Forensic Odontologist with DMORT (Disaster Mortuary Operational Response Team) and has been deployed to the World Trade Center after 9/11 as well as Mississippi and Louisiana after hurricane Katrina. He is also on the Editorial Board of the Journal of Forensic Sciences. He is Fellow of the American College of Dentists (FACD), International College of Dentists (FICD) and the Pierre Fauchard Academy (F-PFA).

Michel Desvignes received the MS degree from the ENSICAEN, Caen, France and the PhD degree in computer science from the University of Caen. After being an assistant professor, he received the Habilitation a Diriger des Recherches in 2002, and he became a professor in computer science at INPG (Grenoble). His research interests include statistical models, shape representation, image distortions, segmentation and image analysis, video processing and interpretation and pattern recognition.

Stefano D'Errico's research in the field of clinical risk management. After a first degree in Medicine from the University of Florence (Italy) in 2000, he attended specialization in Legal Medicine at University of Foggia in 2006. In 2007, he conducted doctoral research in forensic pathology, graduating in 2010. He is active in the field of forensic pathology, and engaged in the University staff for post mortem scenes and hystopathological reports. He has also been an expert witness for the Court of Italy in cases of medical malpractice and gunshot wounds, as well as co-author of chapters in manuscripts in the field of crime scene investigation and forensic radiology.

Vittorio Fineschi is Full Professor of Legal Medicine at the University of Foggia, School of Medicine, in Italy. He grew up in Italy and received his basic medical degree from the University of Perugia, Italy, where he graduated in 1984. He received his Post-Graduate Corse in Forensic Medicine from the University of Siena, Italy, in 1987 and the Clinical Doctorate in Legal Medicine from the Universities of Siena and Perugia in 1990 and conducted his post-doctoral training in Forensic Pathology at the University of Siena ("Le Scotte" Research Institutes in Siena). In 1988, 1989, and 1993 Prof. Vittorio Fineschi received the National Awards for the Best Scientific Paper of the Year from the Italian Society of Legal Medicine. His main research interests are generally in medical ethics and forensic pathology. He is author and co-author of an extensive number of papers published in major scientific journals. His primary research achievements are related to his studies on traumatic agents and their effects related to sudden cardiac death.

Joan Alexis Glaunès, born 1976, is an assistant professor (Maître de Conférences) in mathematics at Paris Descartes University. He completed the Ecole Nationale Supérieure of Cachan in 2001, and received a PhD from Paris Nord University, under the joint supervision of Pr. Alain Trouvé (ENS Cachan) and Pr. Laurent Younes (Johns Hopkins University). During years 2005-2006, J. Glaunès was a post-doc fellow at Johns Hopkins University and Brown University, USA. From the beginning of his Ph.D, he has worked on improvements and extensions of diffeomorphic models for the analysis of deformations of geometric data such as clouds of points, curves and surfaces.

Gregory S. Golden received his dental degree from the University of Southern California in 1975 and practices general dentistry four days a week in Rancho Cucamonga, California. Upon developing an interest in Forensic Dentistry in 1980, he became a Diplomate of the American Board of Forensic Odontology in 1982 and continues to support the ABFO, serving on the Board of Directors and member of numerous committees. He is currently the Treasurer of the ABFO. In 1992, he became the Chief Forensic Odontologist for San Bernardino County and has contracts with Riverside and Los Angeles Counties as a consultant. As a past Chairman of the Odontology Section in the American Academy of Forensic Sciences and former Trustee to the Forensic Sciences Foundation, he has presented numerous papers, is a contributing author to several textbooks, and has published several articles applicable to his field, including research in Fluorescent, Infra-Red, and Ultra-Violet Photography. He is a guest editorial reviewer for the Journal of Forensic Sciences and is currently an instructor at Loma Linda University School of Dentistry and at the University of Texas, San Antonio Health Sciences Center. He has also taught advanced photographic techniques at the biannual International Forensic Photography Workshops and Odontology Practicum Seminars held in Miami, Florida. Dr. Golden has qualified as an expert witness numerous times in Superior Courts of eight California counties, as well as in the states of Ohio, Louisiana, Nevada, and Florida. Other accomplishments include his assistance in identification of victims of the World Trade Center disaster, receiving the Meritorious Service Medal from the San Bernardino County Sheriff, and multiple commendations from the California Attorney General for his help in implementing the Missing Unidentified Persons System at the California Department of Justice. He is a Director of the California Dental Association's Committee on Mass Disasters and a Southern Regional Director for the California Dental Identification Team.

Julia A. Grossman received her MS in Forensic DNA/Serology from the University of Florida in 2008. Since that time, she has been working at the Smithsonian Institution's National Museum of

Natural History in the Department of Anthropology as a lab assistant/researcher under the direction of Dr. Douglas H. Ubelaker. Her interest in Forensic Anthropology is in the evaluation of traumatic events to bones, including the identification of remains from healed injuries and the remodeling of bone after injuries. She has also cultivated an interest in the creation of an online database for the various osteological research collections throughout the United States. Julia is currently preparing to apply for doctoral programs in Forensic Anthropology.

Giuseppe Guglielmi is Professor of Radiology at the University of Foggia and the Scientific Institute Hospital in San Giovanni Rotondo in Italy, and a specialist in musculoskeletal radiology, particularly metabolic bone disease. He is a research associate within the Osteoporosis and Arthritis Research Group in the Department of Radiology at the University of California, San Francisco. Giuseppe Guglielmi, Radiological Society North America Editorial Fellow in 2003, has been named deputy editor of La Radiologia Medica, the official journal of the Italian Society of Medical Radiology. He was also recently named a subspecialty editor in musculoskeletal radiology for EURORAD, a teaching database facilitating searches of Web-based radiologic documents. He is the reference radiologist of the European Society of Musculoskeletal Radiology (ESSR) and of the Italian Society of Medical Radiology (SIRM) of the International Osteoporosis Foundation (IOF) Invest in Your Bones Meetings – Italian Campaign for many years, and he has collaborated in the Vertebral Fracture Initiative of the IOF and has translated into Italian the Vertebral Fracture Initiative CD-ROM. Giuseppe Guglielmi is a consultant of the Italian Ministry of Health and has authored more than 100 scientific articles, 115 scientific abstracts, and 21 book chapters. He has co-authored 6 books and has contributed to a teaching video and CD-ROM on bone densitometry and osteoporosis. He serves on the Editorial boards of Skeletal Radiology, European Radiology and Singapore Medical Journal and holds memberships in the Radiological Society of North America; the European Skeletal Society of Radiology, where he is one of the founding members of the osteoporosis subcommittee; the Italian Society of Medical Radiology; the International Skeletal Society; the American Society for Bone and Mineral Research and the International Osteoporosis Foundation.

Ralf Herwig studied Physics and Mathematics at the Technical and the Free University Berlin and finished his PhD in 2001 on clustering methods for gene expression data. He was awarded the Heinz-Billing-Price Award for Scientific Computation of the Max-Planck Society in 1999 and was an Honor Student of the American Academy of Achievement in 2000. Since 2001, he has been group leader at the Max-Planck-Institute for Molecular Genetics. His research focuses on multivariate statistical methods, data integration systems and computational modelling. Ralf Herwig has contributed to fifty scientific publications and was co-author of the first textbook on systems biology in 2005

Sophia Kossida received her BSc degree (1995) in Biology from the University of Crete, Greece. She was awarded her DPhil in Bioinformatics, from Oxford University, UK (1998). She worked at Harvard University, USA, within the FlyBase group. She was employed as Senior Scientist within Lion Bioscience Research Inc. in MA, USA, where she worked on the human genome mining project. She was appointed Director of Bioinformatics of Endocube in Toulouse, France. She joined Novartis in Switzerland as Lab Head within the Functional Genomics Group. She joined the Biomedical Research Foundation of the Academy of Athens (2004) as tenure track Bioinformatician.

Eleftheria Koultouki, was born in Greece. She studied Medicine in the Aristotle University of Thessaloniki, Greece, and specialized in Pediatrics in Hospitals in the United Kingdom and in Greece; qualified in 2003. Since then she has worked in the Hematology / Oncology Unit of the 1st Department of Pediatrics of the University of Athens. Currently working on her PhD thesis, she is involved in cell biology studies, flow cytometry, and microarray techniques.

George I. Lambrou is a biologist, born in Greece. He received his biology training at the Philipps-Universität, Marburg Germany (Diplom). He has specialized in developmental biology and neurochemistry. His main research interests include tumor cell proliferation dynamics, in particular nonlinear and chaotic models, as well as pharmacogenomics with emphasis on the glucocorticoid receptor NF?B signal transduction pathway and resistance to glucocorticoid-induced apoptosis. He is also occupied with modeling methodologies and computational biology approaches, along with high-throughput methodologies, such as microarrays.

Guo-Zheng Li is a Professor in the Department of Control Science & Engineering at Tongji University, China, Committee Member of CAAI Machine Learning Society and CCF Artificial Intelligence & Pattern Recognition Society, Fellow of The International Society of Intelligent Biological Medicine (ISIBM). He obtained his Ph.D. degree from Shanghai Jiao Tong University in 2004. Dr. Li is interested in machine learning and medical informatics. He is Principle Investigator of projects under grants of Natural Science Foundation of China. Li has published 50+ refereed papers in several professional journals and conferences and three chapters. He is Associate Editor and/or Editor on board of 8 international journals like IJDMB, and Program co-Chair of IJCBS 2009, ITCM 2010. He has obtained Best paper awards at PRICAI 2006, ICAI 2007 and BIBE 2007, Academic Service Award by ISIBM at IJCBS 2009. His homepage: http://levis.tongji.edu.cn.

Maria Moschovi is an Assistant Professor of Pediatric Hematology and Oncology at the Medical School of the Kapodestrian University of Athens and the Director of the Hematology / Oncology Unit of Aghia Sofia Children's Hospital. She has extensive knowledge and experience in the field of medical oncology and is currently responsible for the running of various laboratory-based scientific research projects. Her main scientific interests lie in the investigation of metabolic and genetic changes that contribute to the development of childhood cancers, aiming for a more targeted therapeutic outcome in the clinical practice.

Elena Nikolova's research and educational interests are in the fields of systems biology, non-linear dynamics, mathematical modeling and simulations of immune and intracellular processes, based on enzyme kinetics. She graduated with a M.Sc. degree at Faculty of Physics, Sofia University "St. Kliment Ohridski" (Bulgaria) in 2002 and defended a Ph.D. thesis in the Institute of Mechanics at Bulgarian Academy of Sciences (BAS) in 2007. Since 2008 Elena Nikolova has occupied a permanent position in the same institute as a research fellow.

Svetoslav Nikolov received a M.Sc. in Mechanical Engineering from the Technical University Sofia (Bulgaria) in 1994, and a PhD in Biomechanics from the Institute of Mechanics and Biomechanics (IMech), Bulgarian Academy of Sciences in 1999. During 1999, he was a researcher at IMech. Since 2003, he has been a tenured associate professor position at the Sofia University, Biological Department, and since 2005 the same position at the IMech. His research interests are in application of methods of nonlinear dynamics and systems theory to systems biology.

Omaima Nomir received her PhD degree in electrical and computer engineering from University of Miami, Coral Gables, FL, US in 2006. Currently, she is an assistant professor in the department of Computer Science, School of Computer and Information Sciences, University of Manosura, Egypt. Prior joining the school, she was a systems analyst. Her duties included analyzing and designing systems for banking, and some government agencies, and systems supported by U.S. Agency for International Development (USAID). Her PhD research was on automating human identification using dental X-ray radiographs. Her research interests include human identification, pattern recognition, medical image processing, and neural networks. She has published 17 research papers in fields related to forensic identification, medical image processing and pattern recognition.

Yohan Payan received the PhD degree in computer science and signal processing, from the Institut National Polytechnique of Grenoble, Grenoble, France, in 1996. Currently, he is Director of Research at the French National Research Institute (CNRS), La Tronche, France, in the TIMC-IMAG Laboratory (http://www-timc.imag.fr/), with interests including biomechanics, computer-assisted surgery, signal processing, technologies for handicaps, and neurosciences.

Aviva Petrie obtained her degrees in Statistics from University College London (UCL) and Medical Statistics from the London School of Hygiene and Tropical Medicine (LSHTM). She is a Chartered Statistician, a Chartered Scientist and a Fellow of the Higher Education Academy. She is currently a part-time Senior Lecturer and Head of the Biostatistics Unit at the UCL Eastman Dental Institute where she has been since 1991. She also holds an honorary appointment in the Medical Statistics Department of the LSHTM and acts as a statistical consultant. Previous academic appointments have included roles in London as a lecturer/senior lecturer at the Royal Postgraduate Medical School, the Royal Free Hospital Medical School and the Royal Veterinary College, and in California as a visiting Professor in the Statistics Department at Stanford University. She has published eight books on statistics in the fields of Dentistry, Medicine and Veterinary Science.

Valko Petrov is a theoretical physicist by education, but for 20 years his interests are in the scope of mathematical biophysics. He is a doctor and a senior researcher on biomechanics and head of section "Biodynamics and Biorheology" at Bulgarian Academy of Sciences. He deals with modeling biophysical processes at macroscopic, cellular and molecular levels by using the methods of qualitative theory of dynamical systems. As an associate professor on biomechanics in the Faculty of Physics, Sofia University "St. Kliment Ohridski," he published a textbook entitled "Lectures on biodynamics and biorheology" as well as many scientific articles in various journals on the related subject.

Cristoforo Pomara's research is in the field of forensic pathology and autopsy techniques. After a first degree in Medicine from the University of Palermo (Italy) in 1998, he attended specialization in Legal Medicine at University of Foggia in 2002. In 2002, he conducted doctoral research in forensic pathology, graduating in 2005, and in 2007, he became research professor of Legal Medicine at the Department of Forensic Pathology of the University of Foggia (Italy). Active in the field of forensic pathology, he is engaged in the University staff for post-mortem scenes and hystopathological reports. He has also been an expert witness for the Court of Italy in cases of gunshot wounds and medical malpractice, and an author of manuscripts in the field of forensic medicine and autopsy practice.

Steven Provyn obtained his degree of Doctor in Physiotherapy and Rehabilitation Sciences at the Vrije Universiteit Brussel in 2010. (Thesis title: Quality control and critical appraisal of the reliability of selected body composition data acquisition techniques and systems). In 2000 he started as a voluntary scientific collaborator for two years, followed by an assistantship in 2004 at the Experimental Anatomy department. His teaching and research interest in the anatomy of the human body initiated research in body composition and has led to five publications in peer reviewed journals as a first author and several as co-author. Since December 2009, he has worked at the Haute École Paul Henri Spaak as a researcher for the Anatomy, Morphology and Biomechanics department. Besides his academic work, he is still active in a multidisciplinary private practice.

Mehul S. Raval (Member, IEEE) received the Bachelor of Engineering degree in 1996, Master of Engineering in 2002 and PhD degree from University of Pune, India, in 2008. All the degrees were obtained in Electronics and Telecommunication Engineering. He joined Sarvajanik College of Engineering and Technology, Surat, India as Lecturer in 1997. Currently, he is serving as Assistant Professor at Dhirubhai Ambani Institute of Information and Communication Technology, Gandhinagar. His research interests lie in the area of digital data hiding, steganography, and security aspects of digital data hiding. He is reviewer for many international and national journals and conferences. He has research publications in peer reviewed journals and conferences.

Graham Roberts, MDS(Lond), PhD, MPhil, BDS, FDSRCS(Eng), ILTIM, DipFHID (Apothecaries), qualified as a Dental Surgeon in 1971. Since that time he has had a long career as a Specialist and Consultant in Paediatric Dentistry in the UK National Health Service. He became a Professor of Paediatric Dentistry in 1996 at the Institute of Child Health and the Eastman Dental Institute London. He holds Honorary Professor appointments at University College London. His major research interest has been bacteraemia following dental procedures. Since 2003 he has had a rapidly developing involvement in estimating the age of children and adolescents for whom birth records do not exist. This has led to the establishment of an International Database of over 5,000 cases.

Yves Rozenholc is Assistant Professor in the Applied Mathematical department of University Paris Descartes. His research focuses on Mathematical Statistics: model selection, test, classification, et cetera, with a special interest on finding proper algorithms for complex statistical problems. He has been team leader for the facial reconstruction group at the University Paris Descartes for the last 5 years.

Anya Salih is a biologist who uses confocal imaging to investigate structural, physiological, biochemical and biological characteristics of a wide range of samples. She obtained her PhD at the University of Sydney in 2001, during which, she conducted research into the stress responses of reef corals to climate change and the role of GFP-type fluorescent proteins in reducing stressful effects. Anya continues to research the diversity, characteristics, and biology of fluorescent proteins of reef organisms. She also works on developing these proteins into molecular fluorescent labels for confocal imaging for cell biology and biomedicine. Since 2007, she has been a research scientist at the Confocal Bio-Imaging Facility at

University of Western Sydney, Australia, where she applies bio-imaging skills to solve research questions in biological, biomedical, and forensic disciplines.

David R. Senn, D.D.S., is a Clinical Assistant Professor at the University of Texas Health Science Center-San Antonio (UTHSCSA), Director of the Center for Education and Research in Forensics (C.E.R.F), Director of Southwest Symposium on Forensic Dentistry, and Director of the postdoctoral Fellowship in Forensic Odontology. He is the Chief Forensic Odontology consultant to the Bexar County Medical Examiner, and is a member DMORT region VI. He is a Diplomate of the American Board of Forensic Odontology, a Fellow in the American Academy of Forensic Sciences, and a member of the American Society of Forensic Odontology. He is a Fellow of the American College of Dentists and the International College of Dentists , a member of the American Dental Association, Texas Dental Association, and the San Antonio District Dental Society. Dr. Senn practiced general dentistry for 23 years and has practiced and taught forensic odontology since 1992.

Aldo Scafoglieri is a PhD student in Physiotherapy and Revalidation Sciences at the Experimental Anatomy department of the Vrije Universiteit Brussel (VUB). He is an assistant of Prof. Jan Pieter Clarys since 2007. His PhD work is on the validation, quality control improvement, and implementation of body composition technologies and techniques for long-term public health use. He graduated from the VUB with an honours degree in Manual Therapy in 2003. He subsequently worked as a physiotherapist at the Ghent University Hospital and as a private practitioner.

Françoise Tilotta is Doctor in Dental Surgery of the University Paris Descartes – France (1998). She received a PhD in facial reconstruction from the University Paris 11 – France (2008). She works at the Anatomo-Pathology and Forensic Medicine Department of the Raymond Poincaré Hospital, Garches in human dental identification. For the last several years, her focus has been to attempt to increase the accuracy of facial reconstruction methods by analyzing the relationships between the soft and hard tissues of the face with a local and individual approach using dense meshes associated to a large collection of landmarks directly extracted from CT-scans.

Jonathan Tresignie graduated from the Vrije Universiteit Brussel (VUB) with an honours degree in Rehabilitation Sciences and Physiotherapy in July 2009. Subsequently he started his PhD in Revalidation Sciences and Physiotherapy at the Experimental Anatomy department of the VUB. He is a PhD student and an assistant of Prof. Jan Pieter Clarys since October 2009. His PhD work is on the validation, quality control improvement, and implementation of body composition technologies and techniques to provide aggregated data for long-term public health use.

Georgia Tsiliki received her BSc degree (2000) in Statistics and Actuarial Science from the University of Piraeus, Greece. She was awarded a Masters of Science in Statistics from University College London, UK (2003). She received her PhD in Statistical Genetics from the Department of Mathematics, Imperial College of Science, Technology and Medicine, UK (2007). She was employed as a Post-Doc fellow at the Institute of Molecular Biology and Biotechnology - FORTH, working on breast cancer microarray data analysis. She joined the Bioinformatics and Medical Informatics Team, in the Biomedical Research Foundation of the Academy of Athens (2010) as a research fellow.

Peter Van Roy, has a PhD in motor rehabilitation and physiotherapy (1988), is full professor of anatomy and applied biomechanics, has been a lecturer and/or director at Institutes for Higher Education in Physiotherapy in Brussels, Utrecht (the Netherlands) and Landquart (Switzerland) from 1972-1991. He was awarded the Sport Science Award of the I.O.C.-President for the paper "Three-dimensional kinematic study of the screw-home movement of the knee joint using magnetic resonance imaging" in 1989. His research lines include anatomical variants of the musculoskeletal system, 3D joint kinematics, and correlative anatomy with medical imaging. He has been vice-dean (2004-2008) and currently he is dean (2008-) of the faculty of physical education and physiotherapy of the Vrije Universiteit Brussel (VUB). He is the co-ordinator of the master in manual therapy of the VUB since 1991 and chairman of the scientific commission of the National council of Physiotherapy (Belgium) since 2007. He is also panel member of the Netherlands Quality Agency and Bologna expert (Flanders).

Douglas Ubelaker received his PhD from the University of Kansas in 1973. Currently, he is a senior scientist and curator of physical anthropology at the Smithsonian Institution's National Museum of Natural History in Washington D.C. He has served as a consultant in forensic anthropology since 1977 and currently is President-Elect of the American Academy of Forensic Sciences. He has published extensively on methods to extract information from human skeletal material and the applications to forensic cases as well remains from archaeological contexts.

Franklin D. Wright, DMD, D-ABFO is the forensic dental consultant for the Hamilton County, Cincinnati, Ohio Coroner's Office. He graduated from the University of Kentucky College of Dentistry in 1984 and was certified as a diplomate of the American Board of Forensic Odontology (ABFO) in 1989. Dr. Wright is the President-elect of the ABFO, Chairman of the Ohio Dental Association Forensic Dental Team. He has presented courses and workshops on forensic dentistry throughout the United States as well as Central and South America. His research interest is non-visible light photography of patterned injuries and bitemarks in skin.

Index

Symbols

2D images 71
3D computerised forensic facial reconstruction 83
3D digital data 14, 22
3D geometric morphometrics 6
3D imagery 6
3D imaging techniques 28
3D models 71
4D microscopy 14

A

Active Shape Model (ASM) 53, 54
adaptive thresholding 283, 284, 285, 288
Adobe Photoshop 222
Age Assessment 226, 227, 228, 232, 235, 255, 256, 259, 261
Allele (AF) 340
alternate light imaging (ALI) 220, 221, 225
American Board of Forensic Odontology (ABFO) 223
American College of Radiology (ACR) 30
AM teeth 288, 292, 293, 294, 298, 300
animal activity 2
antemortem (AM) 280, 281, 282, 287, 288, 290, 291, 292, 293, 294, 295, 296, 298, 299, 300, 301, 302, 310, 311, 313, 314
anthropologists 1, 3
anthropology 1, 3, 4, 6, 7, 8, 9, 10, 11, 12, 72, 85, 219
approach for the qualitative (ABQ) 58
articular eminences 315, 317, 319, 320
artificial neural networks (ANN) 194, 196, 205, 206

asymmetrical 248
asymmetric development 248
audio clips 33
Automated Dental Identification System (ADIS) 282, 312
automatic system 281, 311
autopsy 317, 325

B

background correction (BC) 115, 149, 152
backward floating search (BFS) 197, 198, 199, 200, 201
Bayesian framework 302, 305, 307, 308, 311
Bayesian interpretation (BI) 332
behavioral biometrics 314
biological observations 100
biological processes 94, 100
biological systems 118
biology 13, 25
Biometrics 281, 312, 313
bistable equations 164, 170
Bland and Altman diagram 238
brain glioma 193, 194, 195, 196, 198, 199, 200, 201, 202, 203, 210, 213, 214, 215

C

Caenorhabditis elegans 157, 171, 189
causal associations 327
cell polarity 163, 171, 191, 192
cervical vertebra 59
chemistry 13
clinical goniometer 315, 319
clinical photographs 239
clustering algorithm based selective ensemble method (CLUSEN) 195, 196, 202, 203

Combined DNA Index System (CODIS) 334, 337, 338
comparative genomic hybridization (aCGH) 96
Comparative Genomic Hybridization (CGH) 110, 112, 118, 149, 150
complex structures 193, 212
computerized tomography 6, 7, 30, 45, 49, 50, 51, 59, 62, 64, 65, 69, 72, 86, 87
computer sciences 13
cone beam tomography (CBT) 254
confocal imaging 13, 14, 16, 17, 18, 22, 23, 24, 28
confocal microscopes 14, 15, 17, 18, 28
confocal microscopy 13, 15, 20, 21, 22, 23, 24, 25, 26, 28
construction activity 2
cooperative working 29
craniofacial reconstruction 69, 77, 84, 86
criminal cases 326
Criminal Justice Information Service (CJIS) 287, 313
cryptographic security mechanisms 32
cryptographic tools 32
cryptography 33
CT (computerised tomography) scanner 6, 72

D

data mining 330
date of radiograph (dor) 232, 235
deciphering evidence 326
decision boundary 331
dendrogram 123
dental age 226, 227, 228, 238, 244, 246, 247, 248, 253, 255, 256, 257, 259
dental age assessment (DAA) 226, 227, 228, 232, 233, 237, 239, 244, 245, 248, 251, 252, 253, 254, 255, 256, 257, 258, 259, 261
dental aging 219
dental characteristics 280, 281
dental features 281, 314
dental identification 217
dental image 280, 282
dental panoramic tomographs (DPT) 227, 229, 232, 233, 237, 244, 247, 254, 255
dental wax 223

dental X-ray images 280
dental X-ray teeth matching 288, 293, 294, 295, 299, 300
deoxyribonucleic acid (DNA) 3, 4, 5, 8, 9, 10, 12, 109, 110, 111, 112, 113, 124, 125, 126, 128, 129, 130, 135, 136, 137, 139, 140, 142, 143, 144, 145, 146, 147, 148, 149, 150, 152, 172, 192, 196, 211, 218, 222, 224
detection call (DC) 97, 115
developing tooth stage 246
differential interference contrast (DIC) 15
digital caliper 315, 318
digital cameras 220
Digital Differential Display (DDD) 91, 106
digital image-subtraction 218
Digital Imaging and Communications in Medicine (DICOM) 30, 31, 45, 47
digital imaging programs 222
digital photography 3, 217, 222, 223
digital processing 51
digital radiography 218, 221
digital revolution 217
digital signature (DS) 32
digital technologies 29
dimethyl sulfoxide (DMSO) 113, 114
disaster victim identification (DVI) 218, 219
Discrete Fourier transformation (DFT) 296
discrimination 326, 330, 331, 338, 344
distance transformation (DT) 292, 293, 294
DNA database 338, 341, 342, 343
DNA evidence 328, 333, 337, 338, 343
DNA forensics 333
DNA profile matching 326
DNA profiles 326, 334, 336, 337, 338, 339, 340, 341
DNA profiling 328, 334
dual X-ray absorptiometry (DXA) 48, 52, 53, 54, 55, 56, 57, 58, 66
Duhem-Quine thesis 327, 343

E

electronic databases 29
electronic patient records (EPR) 30, 33, 47
embryonic mesoderm 161, 163, 190
enchondral ossification 325

engineering 13

enhanced version of genetic algorithm based multi-task learning (e-GA-MTL) 196, 204, 205, 206, 207, 208

ensemble learning 193, 194, 196, 211, 214

ethylene glycol (EG) 18

European Vertebral Osteoporosis Study (EVOS) 53

evidence 326, 327, 328, 329, 331, 332, 333, 334, 337, 338, 339, 340, 341, 342, 343

expressed sequence tags (EST) 90, 91, 94, 98, 99, 100, 101, 105

extraction algorithms 32, 33

extreme values 326

F

face recognition 330

facial reconstruction 68, 69, 70, 71, 72, 76, 77, 79, 80, 81, 83, 84, 85, 86

fallacy 327, 328

feature extraction 281, 286, 292, 293, 296, 312, 314

feature matching 281

Federal Bureau of Investigation (FBI) 332, 334

fetal development 325

Fibroplast Growth Factor (FGF) 161, 162, 166, 187, 189, 191

fingerprint analysis 17, 21, 22

flipped-color sandwich 116

fluorescence correlation spectroscopic (FCS) 17

fluorescence lifetime imaging (FLIM) 17

force field 280, 282, 295, 296, 297, 298, 299, 300, 302, 312, 313, 314

forensic anthropology 1, 3, 4, 6, 7, 8, 9, 10, 11, 12

forensic automatic speaker recognition (FASR) 331, 332

forensic dentistry 217, 225, 280

forensic dentists 217, 218, 222, 223

forensic medicine 69

forensic odontology 217, 218, 222, 281

forensic pathologists 14, 17

forensics 108, 110, 111, 112, 114, 128, 129, 137, 143, 146, 148, 281, 314

forensic statistical methods 326

Fourier descriptors (FDs) 280, 282, 295, 296, 297, 299, 300, 301, 302, 311, 314

Frankfort horizontal 325

fusion 280, 282, 302, 303, 305, 306, 308, 309, 310, 311, 312, 314

fusion level 280

fuzzy rule extraction algorithm based on fuzzy min-max neural networks (FMMNN-FRE) 196, 198, 199, 200, 201, 203

G

Gaussian mixture model (GMM) 332

Gauss-Markov theorem 135

Gene Expression Database (GXD) 100

gene frequency (GF) 340

genetic algorithm based multi-task learning (GA-MTL) 196, 204, 205, 206, 207, 208

genetic algorithms (GA) 195, 196, 202, 204, 206, 207, 208, 214

genomic information 89

glenoid fossae 315, 316, 317, 318, 319, 320, 321, 323, 324, 325,

grid systems 2

ground penetrating radar (GPR) 1, 2

H

haplotype frequency (HF) 340

Hardy-Weinberg Equilibrium (HWE) 335, 336

Hedgehog (Hh) 162

heteroscedasticity 135

Hierarchical Chamfer 280, 282, 292, 311

hierarchical clustering 123, 150

hierarchical edge 282

homoscedasticity 135

human genome 89, 100, 103, 105, 106

human identification 281, 312, 313, 314

human visual systems (HVS) 36

hybridization-based techniques 90, 94, 98, 100

hypothesis testing 330

I

Identifiable Human Groups (IHG) 256

image rectification 218

information and communication technologies (ICT) 29

information fusion 314
infra-red (IR) 220, 221
instant vertebral assessment (IVA) 58, 59
integration 314
intelligent techniques 193
International Dental Federation (FDI) 228, 229, 260
International Human Genome Sequence Consortium (IHGSC) 89
intracellular systems 164
intra-oral periapical (IOP) 232, 254
iterative threshold 284
iterative thresholding 283, 284, 285

J

joint statistical shape model (JSSM) 79, 80, 81, 82
just noticeable difference (JND) 36

K

Karush-Kuhn-Tucker (KKT) 197

L

latent root regression (LRR) 76, 79, 80, 81, 82
lateral cephalogram 87
learning algorithms 197, 208, 209
leave-one-out cross-validation tests 83
left-right asymmetries 315, 316, 321, 322, 323, 324
Lethal giant larvae (Lgl) 171
Lower Standard Occlusals (LSOs) 232

M

machine-aided techniques 69
machine learning 193, 194, 195, 196, 202, 211, 212, 213, 215
machine learning researchers 193, 194
machine learning techniques 193, 194, 196, 212
magnetic nuclear resonance (MNR) 50, 52
magnetic resonance imaging (MRI) 6, 12, 48, 59, 62, 65, 69, 196, 210
magnetometer 2
magnetometry 2
mammalian skeletal systems 325

mandibular condyles 315, 316, 317, 318, 319, 320, 321, 322, 323, 324
marker frequencies (MF) 340
Massively Parallel Signature Sequencing (MPSS) 92, 93, 99, 101, 103, 104, 105
matching techniques 280, 282, 288, 299, 301, 302, 304, 306
mathematics 13
medical domain 29, 30, 31, 33, 44, 45
Melanoma Cell Adhesion Molecule (MCAM) 172
meta-analysis 237, 244, 246, 248, 259
metal detectors 2
microarray experiments 108, 110, 117, 118, 120, 121, 124, 142, 145, 146, 149
microarray method 108, 127
Micro Array Suite (MAS) 97
microarray technologies 108, 109, 111, 113, 117, 123, 128, 132, 138, 142, 150
mismatch (MM) 115, 124, 126, 152
missing and unidentified persons (MUP) 282
molecular biology 157
molecular mechanisms 161, 163, 187
morphology 316, 317, 323, 324, 325
morphometric methodologies 48
morphometric X-ray absorptiometry (MXA) 52, 55, 56, 57, 58, 66
morphometry 48, 52, 53, 54, 55, 56, 58, 59, 60, 61, 62, 63, 64, 66, 67
multi-label learning 193, 194, 196, 208, 209, 211, 214, 215
multimedia data 330
multiple fatality incident (MFI) 218
multi slice computed tomography (MSCT) 48, 49, 50, 60, 62, 65
multi-task learning (MTL) 193, 194, 195, 196, 203, 204, 205, 206, 207, 208, 211, 213, 214

N

National Electrical Manufacturers Association (NEMA) 30, 45
National Patient Dose Database (NPDD) 255
National Research Council (NRC) 338, 341
Next Generation Sequencing (NGS) 93, 94
Next Generation Sequencing (NGS) techniques 93

Normal distribution function (NORMDIST) 236, 250
nuclear magnetic resonance (NMR) 30
null hypothesis 328, 330
Numeric Aperture (N.A.) 14

O

odontologists 222, 223
odontology 217, 218, 219, 222
optical physics 13
orthodontics 87

P

partial least square (PLS) 77
peak signal to noise ratio (PSNR) 36, 44
perfect match (PM) 115, 124, 126, 152
photographic superimposition 4, 7, 11
photomultiplier tubes (PMT) 15, 16
physical anthropology 1, 9, 10, 72
pipeline excavation 2
PM identification 281, 314
PM teeth 280, 282, 290, 294, 296, 299, 314
Point Distribution Model (PDM) 55
point-to-point analysis 218
polymerase chain reaction (PCR) 113, 114, 118, 128, 140, 141, 144, 152
positron emission tomography (PET) 30, 31, 35, 45
posteroanterior (PA) 55
postmortem (PM) 280, 281, 282, 287, 288, 289, 290, 291, 292, 293, 294, 295, 296, 298, 299, 300, 301, 302, 310, 311, 313, 314
PreSomitic Mesoderm (PSM) 159, 160, 161, 165, 187
principal component analysis (PCA) 110
principal components regression (PCR) 75, 77, 78, 79, 80, 81, 82
probabilistic expert systems (PES) 135, 136, 137
probabilities 326, 328, 338, 339, 340, 342
Probe Logarithmic Intensity Error (PLIER) 98
protein radioimmunoassay (pRIA) 3, 4, 10, 12
public domain computer networks 29

Q

qualitative synthesis 157
quantitative 48, 52, 53, 55, 57, 58, 61, 62, 63, 66
quantitative morphometry (QM) 58
Quasi-Steady-State-Approximation (QSSA) 167, 168, 177, 178, 179, 182, 184, 185, 186, 190

R

racial groups 252
radiographic images 218, 219, 227, 244
radiographs 232, 237, 239, 240, 243, 244, 251, 280, 281, 287, 311, 312, 313
radiography 4, 49, 52, 56, 58, 60, 61, 63, 64, 218, 221, 224, 225
receiver operating characteristic (ROC) 307, 308, 309, 310
Receptor Tyrosine Kinase (RTK) 162
recognition techniques 330
red, green and blue (RGB) 16, 28
Reference Data Sets 256
reflectance confocal imaging (RCI) 16, 28
reflective ultraviolet (UVA) 220, 221
region of interest (ROI) 34, 36, 45, 46
region of no interest (RNI) 34, 35, 36, 45
regions of interests (ROI) 16
regression analysis 256
retinoic acid (RA) 161, 187
ribo nucleic acid interference (RNAi) 157, 187
Riken Expression Array Database (READ) 100
RNA Induced Silencing Complex (RISC) 160
robotic surgery 29
robust multi-array average (RMA) 97, 98
Robust Multichip Analysis (RMA) 116, 121
root canal 227, 228, 251

S

sagittal plane 317, 319, 323
scientific reliability 326
score level 280
score summation 302, 307
Scribble (Scrib) 171
self organizing maps (SOM) 123, 152, 153
semi-automatic system 281, 311

semiquantitative (SQ) 52, 57, 58, 66
sensor chips 221
sequential backward search (SBS) 198
sequential forward search (SFS) 198
Serial Analysis of Gene Expression (SAGE) 92, 93, 99, 103, 105
short vertebral height (SVH) 58
single nucleotide polymorphism (SNP) 94, 110, 111, 112, 114, 118, 128, 137, 138, 139, 142, 143, 145, 146, 152, 153
Single Tandem Repeats (STR) 336, 337
soil disturbance 2
spinal deformity index (SDI) 52, 63
squamotympanical fissure 318, 319
statistical analysis 326
statistical conclusions 328
statistical evidence 326, 328
statistical methods 72, 83, 326, 327, 329, 334, 336, 340
support vector machines (SVM) 123, 124, 153, 193, 194, 195, 196, 197, 198, 199, 200, 201, 202, 203, 211, 212, 213, 214
support vectors (sv) 197
symmetrical development 248
symmetry 244, 248
systematic difference 238, 246

T

technological developments 1
teeth matching 288, 292, 293, 294, 295, 299, 300, 301, 311
teeth numbering 289, 292
tele-diagnosis 29, 36
tele-medicine 29
tele-surgery 29
temporomandibular articular surfaces 315, 316, 317, 320, 321, 324
temporomandibular joint dysfunction 316
temporomandibular joint (TMJ) 315, 316, 317, 320, 321, 322, 323, 324, 325,

temporomandibular joint (TMJ) surfaces 315, 317, 321, 322
thermo vision images 30
three dimensional (3-D) 332
thresholding 283, 284, 285, 288
tooth development stage (TDS) 228, 229, 233, 234, 235, 236, 237, 238, 240, 243, 244, 246, 247, 248, 250, 259, 264, 265, 266, 267, 268, 270, 271, 272, 273, 274, 275, 276, 277, 278, 279
Tooth Morphology Type (TMT) 227, 229, 232, 235, 239, 244, 251, 254, 259
tooth stage 246
transcriptome 89, 90, 93, 94, 98, 100, 101, 105, 106, 107

U

ultra sonography (USG) 30, 35, 45
ultraviolet (UV) 220, 221
Upper Standard Occlusals (USOs) 232
US Food and Drug Administration (FDA) 54

V

vertebral fracture assessment (VFA) 57, 58
virtual skulls 69

W

watermarking 29, 32, 33, 34, 35, 36, 37, 41, 44, 45, 46, 47
watermarks 33, 34, 35, 36, 37, 38, 39, 40, 41, 44, 45
web searching 330
wide-field microscopy 13, 22, 28
Wnt/Wingless (Wg) 162

X

X-ray images 280, 283, 288, 290
X-ray spectroscopy 3